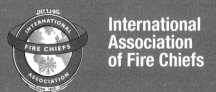
International Association of Fire Chiefs

Vehicle Rescue and Extrication

Principles and Practice

REVISED SECOND EDITION

David Sweet

JONES & BARTLETT LEARNING

World Headquarters
Jones & Bartlett Learning
25 Mall Road, 6th Floor
Burlington, MA 01803
978-443-5000
info@jblearning.com
www.jblearning.com
www.psglearning.com

National Fire Protection Association
1 Batterymarch Park
Quincy, MA 02169-7471
www.NFPA.org

International Association of Fire Chiefs
4025 Fair Ridge Drive
Fairfax, VA 22033
www.IAFC.org

Jones & Bartlett Learning books and products are available through most bookstores and online booksellers. To contact the Jones & Bartlett Learning Public Safety Group directly, call 800-832-0034, fax 978-443-8000, or visit our website, www.psglearning.com.

Substantial discounts on bulk quantities of Jones & Bartlett Learning publications are available to corporations, professional associations, and other qualified organizations. For details and specific discount information, contact the special sales department at Jones & Bartlett Learning via the above contact information or send an email to specialsales@jblearning.com.

Copyright © 2022 by Jones & Bartlett Learning, LLC, an Ascend Learning Company

All rights reserved. No part of the material protected by this copyright may be reproduced or utilized in any form, electronic or mechanical, including photocopying, recording, or by any information storage and retrieval system, without written permission from the copyright owner.

The content, statements, views, and opinions herein are the sole expression of the respective authors and not that of Jones & Bartlett Learning, LLC. Reference herein to any specific commercial product, process, or service by trade name, trademark, manufacturer, or otherwise does not constitute or imply its endorsement or recommendation by Jones & Bartlett Learning, LLC and such reference shall not be used for advertising or product endorsement purposes. All trademarks displayed are the trademarks of the parties noted herein. *Vehicle Rescue and Extrication: Principles and Practice, Revised Second Edition* is an independent publication and has not been authorized, sponsored, or otherwise approved by the owners of the trademarks or service marks referenced in this product.

There may be images in this book that feature models; these models do not necessarily endorse, represent, or participate in the activities represented in the images. Any screenshots in this product are for educational and instructive purposes only. Any individuals and scenarios featured in the case studies throughout this product may be real or fictitious but are used for instructional purposes only.

The NFPA & IAFC and the publisher have made every effort to ensure that contributors to *Vehicle Rescue and Extrication: Principles and Practice, Revised Second Edition* materials are knowledgeable authorities in their fields. Readers are nevertheless advised that the statements and opinions are provided as guidelines and should not be construed as official NFPA & IAFC policy. The recommendations in this publication or the accompanying resources do not indicate an exclusive course of action. Variations, taking into account the individual circumstances and local protocols, may be appropriate. The NFPA & IAFC and the publisher disclaim any liability or responsibility for the consequences of any action taken in reliance on these statements or opinions.

23233-2

Production Credits
VP, Product Development: Christine Emerton
Director of Product Management: Bill Larkin
Content Strategist: Jennifer Deforge-Kling
Project Manager: Kristen Rogers
Senior Digital Project Specialist: Angela Dooley
Director of Marketing Operations: Brian Rooney
VP, Sales, Public Safety Group: Matthew Maniscalco
Content Services Manager: Colleen Lamy
VP, Manufacturing and Inventory Control: Therese Connell
Project Management: S4Carlisle Publishing Services

Composition: S4Carlisle Publishing Services
Cover Design: Scott Moden
Text Design: Scott Moden
Media Development Editor: Faith Brosnan
Rights & Permissions Manager: John Rusk
Rights Specialist: Liz Kincaid
Cover Image (Title Page, Front Matter, Appendix, Glossary, Index Opener): Courtesy of David Sweet
Printing and Binding: LSC Communications

Library of Congress Cataloging-in-Publication Data
Names: Sweet, David, author. | National Fire Protection Association, author. | International Association of Fire Chiefs, author.
Title: Vehicle rescue and extrication : principles and practice / David Sweet, National Fire Protection Association, International Association of Fire Chiefs.
Description: Second edition revised. | Burlington, MA : Jones & Bartlett Learning, 2021. | Includes bibliographical references and index. | Summary: "This training solution is designed to prepare firefighters to extricate victims from common passenger vehicle collisions"-- Provided by publisher.
Identifiers: LCCN 2021010198 | ISBN 9781284245622 (paperback)
Subjects: LCSH: Traffic accidents. | Crash injuries. | Rescue work. | Transport of sick and wounded.
Classification: LCC RC88.9.T7 S94 2021 | DDC 617.1/028--dc23
LC record available at https://lccn.loc.gov/2021010198

6048

Printed in the United States of America
25 24 23 22   10 9 8 7 6 5 4 3 2

Dedication

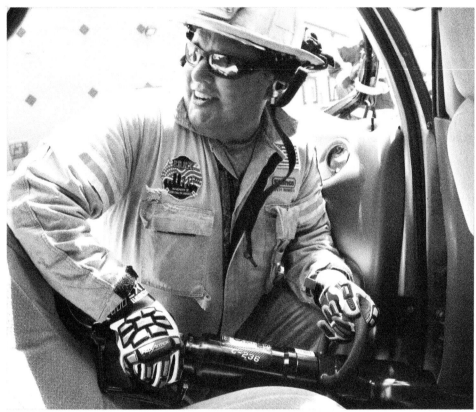

Courtesy of David Sweet.

To my friend and brother
Battalion Chief Juan Linares,

Your passion, excitement, and dedication to the
job are unsurpassed; your spirit lives forever.

"There is no greater love than one that
lays down his life for another."

Brief Contents

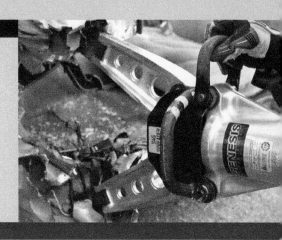

SECTION 1
Awareness Level

CHAPTER 1 Introduction to Vehicle Rescue and Extrication — 2

CHAPTER 2 Vehicle Rescue Incident Awareness — 19

CHAPTER 3 Tools and Equipment — 49

SECTION 2
Operations and Technician Levels

CHAPTER 4 Site Operations — 100

CHAPTER 5 Mechanical Energy and Vehicle Anatomy — 120

CHAPTER 6 Supplemental Restraint Systems — 149

CHAPTER 7 Advanced Vehicle Technology: Alternative-Fuel Vehicles — 168

CHAPTER 8 Vehicle Stabilization — 199

CHAPTER 9 Victim Access and Management — 221

CHAPTER 10 Alternative Extrication Techniques — 282

CHAPTER 11 Terminating the Incident — 317

SECTION 3
Heavy Vehicle Incidents

CHAPTER 12 Commercial Vehicles — 330

CHAPTER 13 School Buses — 353

Appendix: NFPA 1006 Correlation Guide — 399

GLOSSARY — 403

INDEX — 414

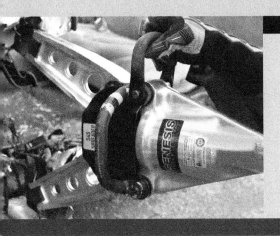

Contents

Skill Drills	x
Foreword: Honoring History	xiii
Acknowledgments	xv

SECTION 1
Awareness Level

CHAPTER 1
Introduction to Vehicle Rescue and Extrication — 2

Introduction	3
Standards and Qualifications	4
NFPA 1006, *Standard for Technical Rescue Personnel Professional Qualifications*	5
NFPA 1670, *Standard on Operations and Training for Technical Search and Rescue Incidents*	7
Compliance with NFPA 1006 and NFPA 1670	10
Vehicle Rescue and Extrication Resources	12
Specialists	12
Online Resources	12
Emergency Field Guide	12
Challenge Events	13
Scenario-Based Training	14
Continuous Improvement	16

CHAPTER 2
Vehicle Rescue Incident Awareness — 19

Introduction	20
Determining Level of Service	21
Risk Assessment	21
Hazard Analysis	21
Organizational Analysis	22
Risk–Benefit Analysis	23
Level of Response Analysis	24
Standard Operating Procedures	24
Incident Response Planning	25
Problem Identification	25
Resource Identification and Allocation	25
Operational Procedures	26
Incident Command System	26
Jurisdictional Authority	26
Unity of Command	27
Span of Control	27
Modular Organization	27
Common Terminology	27
Integrated Communications	27
Consolidated IAPs	27
Designated Incident Facilities	27
Resource Management	28
Victim Reconnaissance	28
ICS Organization	28
Incident Commander	28
Command Staff	29
ICS Sections	30
Additional ICS Terminology	32
Tracking Systems	32
Personnel Accountability	32
Equipment Inventory and Tracking Systems	34
Long-Term Operations	34
Safety	35
Time Management	35

Responding to the Scene	36	Cutting Torches	79
Personal Protective Equipment	36	Hydraulic Rescue Tools	80
Dispatch Information	36	Hydraulic Spreader	82
Preincident Assignments	37	Hydraulic Cutter	83
Traffic	38	Hydraulic Ram	84
Crowd Control	40	Hydraulic Combination Tool	84
Personnel Resources	40	Battery-Powered Hydraulic Rescue Tools	84
Scene Size-Up	42	Stabilization Tools	85
Scene Size-Up Report	44	Cribbing	86
Inner and Outer Surveys	44	Struts	87
Scene Safety Zones	44	Jacks	88
		Ratchet Strap	89
		Organization of Equipment	90

CHAPTER 3
Tools and Equipment 49

		Special Equipment	90
		Foam	90
Introduction	50	Signaling Devices	91
Personal Protective Equipment (PPE)	50	Power Detection	92
Head Protection	50	Victim Packaging and Removal Equipment	93
Body Protection	51	Immobilization Devices	93
Eye and Face Protection	52	Stretchers and Litters	93
Hand Protection	53	Research Tools	93
Foot Protection	54		
Hearing Protection	54		

SECTION 2
Operations and Technician Levels

Respiratory Protection	56		
Maintenance of PPE	57		
Hand Tools	57		

CHAPTER 4
Site Operations 100

Striking Tools	58		
Leverage Tools	60	Introduction	101
Cutting Tools	62	Safety	101
Lifting/Pushing/Pulling Tools	63	Personnel Rehabilitation	102
Pneumatic Tools	66	Equipment Resources	102
Pneumatic Cutting Tools	67	Communication and Documentation	103
Pneumatic Rotating Tools	70	Scene Size-Up	103
Pneumatic Lifting Tools	70	Scene Size-Up Report	105
Electric Tools	74	Inner and Outer Surveys	105
Electric Cutting Tools	75	Incident Action Plan	108
Electric Lifting and Pulling Tools	77	Establishing Scene Safety Zones	109
Electric Lighting	78	Specific Hazards	111
Fuel-Powered Cutting Tools	79	Fire Hazards	111
Chain Saws	79	Electrical Hazards	112
Rotary Saws	79		

Fuel Sources	113
Fuel Runoff	113
Ignition Sources	113
Hazardous Materials	114
Other Hazards	114
Air Medical Operations	115
Establishing a Landing Zone	115
Landing Zone Safety	116

CHAPTER 5
Mechanical Energy and Vehicle Anatomy — 120

Introduction	121
Energy	121
Sequence of Events in a Motor Vehicle Collision	122
Event 1: Vehicle Impact with Object	123
Event 2: Occupant Impact with Vehicle	123
Event 3: Occupant Organs Impact Solid Structures of the Body	124
Vehicular Collision Classifications	124
Front Impact Collisions	124
Rear-End Collisions	125
Lateral (Side-Impact) Collisions	125
Rollovers	125
Rotational Collisions	126
Vehicle Anatomy and Composition	126
Electricity	126
Metal, Carbon, and Composites	127
Frame Systems	130
Body-over-Frame Construction	130
Unibody Construction	130
Space Frame Construction	131
Structural Components	132
Rocker Panel	133
Doors	133
Roof Posts	136
Federal Safety Standards and Regulations	140
Vehicle Glass and Glazing	140
Laminated Safety Glass	140
Gorilla® Glass	141
Tempered Safety Glass	141

Polycarbonate	141
Ballistic Glass	142
Vehicle Classifications	142
Vehicle Identification Numbers	142
Vehicle Propulsion Systems	144
Conventional Vehicles	144
Hybrid Electric Vehicles	144
Hydrogen Fuel Cell Vehicles	144
Electric-Powered Vehicles	144

CHAPTER 6
Supplemental Restraint Systems — 149

Introduction	150
Air Bags	150
Air Bag Deployment Process	152
Air Bag Components	152
Rollover Protection System	158
Seat Belt Systems	158
Seat Belt Types	159
Pretensioning Systems	159
Emergency Procedures	161
Disconnecting Power	161
Recognizing and Identifying Air Bags	162
Distancing	163
Extrication Precautions	163

CHAPTER 7
Advanced Vehicle Technology: Alternative-Fuel Vehicles — 168

Introduction	169
Safety	170
Alternative Fuels	172
Ethanol and Methanol	172
Natural Gas	173
Liquefied Petroleum Gas	177
Biodiesel	179
Hydrogen	180
Hydrogen Storage Tanks	181
Hydrogen Fuel-Cell Vehicles	183

Hybrid Electric Vehicles (HEVs) 188
All-Electric Vehicles 193
Ongoing Education 194

CHAPTER 8
Vehicle Stabilization 199

Introduction 200
Cribbing 201
   Wood Characteristics 202
   Wood Box Cribbing 202
Vehicle Positioning 203
   The Vehicle in Its Normal Position 203
   The Vehicle Resting on Its Side 208
   The Vehicle Upside Down or Resting on Its Roof 212
   Vehicle on Vehicle or Multiple Concurrent Hazards 214
Monitoring Stabilization 216
Hidden Dangers and Energy Sources 216

CHAPTER 9
Victim Access and Management 221

Introduction 222
Access Points 222
   Access Through Doors 224
   Access Through Windows 224
   The Backboard Slide Technique 226
   Tempered Safety Glass 227
   Laminated Safety Glass 230
   Polycarbonate Windows and Ballistic-Rated Glass 235
   Removing the Windshield from a Partially Ejected Victim 235
Using Hydraulic Rescue Tools to Gain Door and Roof Access 235
   Door Access from the Latch Side: The Vertical Spread 237
   Door Access from the Hinge Side: Front Wheel Well Crush 239
   The Complete Side Removal Technique: The Side-Out 245
Removing the Vehicle from the Victim 249

Roof Removal 249
Relocating the Dash Section and/or Steering Wheel Assembly 255
   The Dash Roll Technique 255
   The Dash Lift Technique 260
   Steering Wheel Assembly Relocation 266
Providing Initial Medical Care 271
   Exsanguinating Hemorrhage 272
   Airway 272
   Breathing 273
   Circulation 274
   Disability 274
   Expose 274
   Compartment Syndrome 275
   Triage 275
Victim Packaging and Removal 276
   Transport 277

CHAPTER 10
Alternative Extrication Techniques 282

Introduction 283
Tunneling 283
Jacking the Trunk 284
Seat Removal 287
   Front Seat-Back Removal 287
   Front Seat-Back Relocation 290
Impingement and Penetrating Objects 291
   Impingement 293
   Roof Lift 295
   Penetrating Objects 298
Roof Removal 300
   Roof Removal Using the Air Chisel 301
   Roof Removal Using the Reciprocating Saw 301
   Rapid Roof Removal: Vehicle on Its Side 304
Door Removal on the Hinge Side 308
Side Removal: Vehicle Upside Down or Resting on Its Roof 310
Pedal Displacement and Removal 310
Removal of a Victim Under a Vehicle Using an FRJ 313

CHAPTER 11
Terminating the Incident — 317

Introduction	318
Securing the Scene	318
Securing Equipment	319
Securing Personnel	321
Stress	321
Critical Incident Stress	321
Critical Incident Stress Management	323
Peer Support Groups	323
Postincident Analysis	324
Documentation and Record Management	324

SECTION 3
Heavy Vehicle Incidents

CHAPTER 12
Commercial Vehicles — 330

Introduction	331
Commercial Trucks	331
Commercial Truck Classifications	332
Commercial Truck Anatomy	333
Hazardous Materials	343
Site Operations: Commercial Motor Vehicle	347
Victim Access: Commercial Motor Vehicle	348

CHAPTER 13
School Buses — 353

Introduction	354
School Buses	355
School Bus Anatomy	357
Site Operations: School Buses	360
Victim Access: School Buses	367
Lifting a School Bus Off of an Underride	390
Alternative-Fuel Buses	393
Appendix: NFPA 1006 Correlation Guide	**399**
Glossary	403
Index	414

Skill Drills

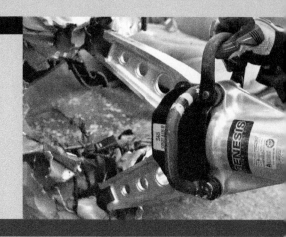

CHAPTER 2

SKILL DRILL 2-1 — 43
Conducting a Size-Up of a Motor Vehicle Collision NFPA 1006 8.1.1, 8.1.3

CHAPTER 4

SKILL DRILL 4-1 — 112
Extinguishing a Vehicle Fire NFPA 1006 8.2.2

CHAPTER 6

SKILL DRILL 6-1 — 161
Disconnect a Vehicle Battery to De-energize and Disable an Air Bag or a Rollover Protection System NFPA 1006 8.2.4

CHAPTER 7

SKILL DRILL 7-1 — 171
Applying Standard Safety Procedures to a Vehicle NFPA 1006 8.2.1, 8.2.2, 8.2.3, and 8.2.4

CHAPTER 8

SKILL DRILL 8-1 — 208
Stabilizing a Common Passenger Vehicle in Its Upright Normal Position NFPA 1006 8.2.3

SKILL DRILL 8-2 — 211
Stabilizing a Vehicle Resting on Its Side NFPA 1006 8.2.3

SKILL DRILL 8-3 — 213
Stabilizing a Vehicle Resting on Its Roof NFPA 1006 8.2.3

SKILL DRILL 8-4 — 215
Stabilizing/Marrying a Vehicle on Top of Another Vehicle NFPA 1006 8.2.3

SKILL DRILL 8-5 — 218
Mitigating Vehicle Electrical Hazards at an MVA NFPA 1006 8.2.3 and 8.2.4

CHAPTER 9

SKILL DRILL 9-1 — 226
The Assisted Backboard Slide Technique NFPA 1006 8.2.6, 8.2.7, 8.3.6, 8.3.9

SKILL DRILL 9-2 — 229
Breaking Tempered Glass Using a Spring-Loaded Center Punch NFPA 1006 8.2.6, 8.2.7, 8.3.6, 8.3.9

SKILL DRILL 9-3 — 230
Fracturing Tempered Safety Glass Using a Glass Handsaw NFPA 1006 8.2.6, 8.2.7, 8.3.6, 8.3.9

SKILL DRILL 9-4 — 232
Removing the Windshield Using a Glass Handsaw NFPA 1006 8.2.6, 8.2.7, 8.3.6, 8.3.9

SKILL DRILL 9-5 — 234
Removing the Windshield Using a Reciprocating Saw NFPA 1006 8.2.6, 8.2.7, 8.3.6, 8.3.9

SKILL DRILL 9-6 — 236
Removing the Windshield from a Partially Ejected Victim NFPA 1006 8.2.6, 8.2.7, 8.3.6, 8.3.9

SKILL DRILL 9-7 — 240
Releasing a Door from Its Frame or Performing the Vertical Spread (Hydraulic) NFPA 1006 8.2.6, 8.2.7, 8.3.6, 8.3.9

SKILL DRILL 9-8 242
Releasing a Door from Its Frame or Performing the Vertical Spread (Non-Hydraulic) NFPA 1006 8.2.6, 8.2.7, 8.3.6, 8.3.9

SKILL DRILL 9-9 244
The Wheel Well Crush Technique NFPA 1006 8.2.6, 8.2.7, 8.3.6, 8.3.9

SKILL DRILL 9-10 246
The Complete Side Removal/Side-Out Technique (Hydraulic) NFPA 1006 8.2.6, 8.2.7, 8.3.6, 8.3.9

SKILL DRILL 9-11 250
The Complete Side Removal/Side-Out Technique (Non-Hydraulic) NFPA 1006 8.2.6, 8.2.7, 8.3.6, 8.3.9

SKILL DRILL 9-12 253
Removing the Roof of an Upright Vehicle NFPA 1006 8.2.6, 8.2.7, 8.3.6, 8.3.9

SKILL DRILL 9-13 257
The Dash Roll Technique (Hydraulic) NFPA 1006 8.2.6, 8.2.7, 8.3.6, 8.3.9

SKILL DRILL 9-14 258
The Dash Roll Technique (Non-Hydraulic) NFPA 1006 8.2.6, 8.2.7, 8.3.6, 8.3.9

SKILL DRILL 9-15 261
The Dash Lift Technique (Hydraulic) NFPA 1006 8.2.6, 8.2.7, 8.3.6, 8.3.9

SKILL DRILL 9-16 264
The Dash Lift Technique (Non-Hydraulic) NFPA 1006 8.2.6, 8.2.7, 8.3.6, 8.3.9

SKILL DRILL 9-17 267
Relocating the Steering Wheel Assembly Utilizing a 2/4-Ton–Rated Come Along NFPA 1006 8.2.6, 8.2.7, 8.3.6, 8.3.9

SKILL DRILL 9-18 269
Relocating the Steering Wheel Assembly Utilizing a First Responder Jack NFPA 1006 8.2.6, 8.2.7, 8.3.6, 8.3.9

SKILL DRILL 9-19 277
Extricating a Victim from a Passenger Car NFPA 1006 8.2.8, 8.3.9

CHAPTER 10

SKILL DRILL 10-1 284
Tunneling Through the Trunk NFPA 1006 8.2.4, 8.2.6, 8.2.7, and 8.3.9

SKILL DRILL 10-2 288
Jacking the Trunk NFPA 1006 8.2.6, 8.2.7, and 8.3.9

SKILL DRILL 10-3 289
Front Seat-Back Removal NFPA 1006 8.2.4, 8.2.6, 8.2.7, and 8.3.9

SKILL DRILL 10-4 290
Front Seat-Back Relocation NFPA 1006 8.2.6, 8.2.7, and 8.3.9

SKILL DRILL 10-5 291
Relocate the B-Post or Door Frame with a Hydraulic Ram NFPA 1006 8.2.6, 8.2.7, and 8.3.9

SKILL DRILL 10-6 293
Relocate the B-Post or Door Frame with a First Responder Jack NFPA 1006 8.2.6, 8.2.7, and 8.3.9

SKILL DRILL 10-7 297
Performing a Cross-Ramming Operation Using a Hydraulic Ram NFPA 1006 8.2.4, 8.2.6, 8.2.7, and 8.3.9

SKILL DRILL 10-8 299
Stabilizing an Impaled Object NFPA 1006 8.2.4, 8.2.6, 8.2.7, and 8.3.9

SKILL DRILL 10-9 302
Removing a Roof Using an Air Chisel NFPA 1006 8.2.4, 8.2.6, 8.2.7, and 8.3.9

SKILL DRILL 10-10 304
Removing a Roof Using a Reciprocating Saw NFPA 1006 8.2.4, 8.2.6, 8.2.7, and 8.3.9

SKILL DRILL 10-11 306
Removing a Roof from a Vehicle Resting on Its Side NFPA 1006 8.2.4, 8.2.6, 8.2.7, and 8.3.9

SKILL DRILL 10-12 308
Removing a Door on the Hinge Side Using an Air Chisel NFPA 1006 8.2.4, 8.2.6, 8.2.7, and 8.3.9

SKILL DRILL 10-13	311
Performing a Side Removal on a Vehicle Upside Down or Resting on Its Roof NFPA 1006 8.2.6, 8.2.7, and 8.3.9	
SKILL DRILL 10-14	313
Relocating a Pedal NFPA 1006 8.2.6, 8.2.7, and 8.3.9	
SKILL DRILL 10-15	314
Removal of a Victim Under a Vehicle Using an FRJ NFPA 1006 8.2.3, 8.2.6, 8.2.7, and 8.3.9	

CHAPTER 11

SKILL DRILL 11-1	325
Terminating a Vehicle Rescue and Extrication Incident NFPA 1006 8.2.9	

CHAPTER 13

SKILL DRILL 13-1	263
Stabilizing a School Bus in Its Normal Position	
SKILL DRILL 13-2	365
Stabilizing a School Bus Resting on Its Side	
SKILL DRILL 13-3	366
Stabilizing a School Bus Resting on Its Roof	
SKILL DRILL 13-4	368
Stabilizing/Marrying a School Bus on Top of Another Vehicle	
SKILL DRILL 13-5	370
Gaining Access into a School Bus by Removing the Front Windshield	
SKILL DRILL 13-6	372
Removing a Bench Seat from a School Bus	
SKILL DRILL 13-7	374
Removing a Section of the Sidewall of a School Bus	
SKILL DRILL 13-8	376
Gaining Access Through the Roof of a School Bus on Its Side	
SKILL DRILL 13-9	378
Gaining Access Through the Rear Door of a School Bus in Its Normal Position	
SKILL DRILL 13-10	380
Gaining Access Through the Rear Door of a School Bus Resting on Its Side	
SKILL DRILL 13-11	383
Gaining Access Through the Front Door of a School Bus in Its Normal Position	
SKILL DRILL 13-12	385
Removing a Victim from Under a School Bus Resting on Its Side Utilizing FRJs	
SKILL DRILL 13-13	388
Removing a Victim from Under a School Bus Resting on Its Side Utilizing Air-Lift Bags	
SKILL DRILL 13-14	391
Lifting a School Bus Off of an Underride	
SKILL DRILL 13-15	395
Disabling the Hybrid System on a Type C or D School Bus	

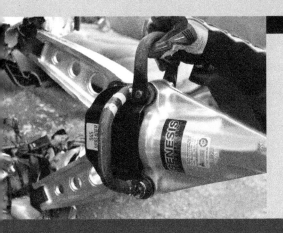

Foreword: Honoring History

In 1869, the first vehicle-related fatality in history ever to be recorded occurred in Birr, Ireland, when a 42-year-old female was thrown from an experimental steam engine vehicle. The first vehicle accident to be recorded in the United States occurred in 1891 in Ohio City, Ohio, when another experimental gas-powered vehicle veered off the road and crashed into a hitching post, causing minor injuries. These are the first ever recorded vehicle accidents with little to no mention of any rescue efforts. However, some form of first-aid or life-saving measures from vehicle accidents, whether occurring from horse and carriage or motorized vehicles accidents, has been rendered for centuries.

As motorized vehicles became more prevalent and the major form of transportation in the world, vehicle rescue evolved into a specialized and technical field that technical rescuers practice today.

Vehicle rescue and extrication could not have evolved into the vital skill it now is without the pioneers of extrication who helped propel it into a modern world with advanced hydraulic tools and equipment and the ever-changing automotive world. While no specific date or location can be pinpointed as the official beginnings of vehicle extrication, many important pioneers have contributed greatly to make the vehicle extrication field the necessary and critical part of society and victim rescue that it is today.

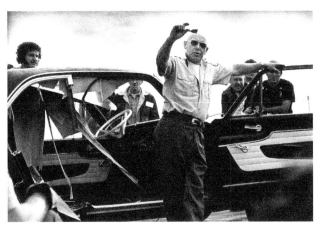
© Steve Larson/The Denver Post/Getty Images.

George Hurst of Hurst High Performance Products invented the first hydraulic tool in 1961, after he witnessed rescue crews take more than an hour to extricate a driver from a crashed race car. Hurst's hydraulic tool weighed 350 pounds and was carried in the back of a pickup truck. In 1971, Hurst engineering technician Mike Brick developed the first portable hydraulic rescue tool weighing 60 pounds. Mike Brick coined the term "Jaws of Life" after testing the new tool on several training evolutions. George Hurst registered this name as a trademark of Hurst Rescue tools. The Jaws of Life term is often generically used to describe the multitude of hydraulic rescue tools on the market today.

OB Streeper, the chief of the MacLean County Rescue Squad in Illinois and founder of the Emergency Squad Training Institute, also greatly influenced the field of vehicle rescue and extrication. OB toured the country from the 1960s to the 1990s teaching over 30,000 automobile extrication courses. He mastered hand and mechanical powered tools such as porta powers, come alongs, and chains, long before hydraulic power rescue tools became prevalent.

Yet another pioneer was Harvey Grant, a firefighter and chief who taught rescuers for over 40 years. He wrote his first automobile extrication book in 1975, and his teachings and knowledge form the foundation of most training programs taught today.

The discipline of vehicle rescue and extrication has benefited greatly from the veteran rescuers who established the foundation for this field, passing their knowledge and experience onto new rescuers who contribute passion, enthusiasm, and dedication to the critical role of technical rescuer. Dr. Martin Luther King, Jr. stated it best—"We are not makers of history. We are made by history."

Chief Rodney Turpel
North Lauderdale Fire and Rescue

References

1. Hurst Power Rescue Tool (Jaws of Life) Smithsonian Institution, National Museum of American History.
2. Getty Images Denver Post, September 1976.
3. The Pillars of Vehicle Rescue, Fire Engineering, June 5, 2018.

From the Author

Thanks to the guidance and prodding of my parents, Ray and Karen, and one of my oldest friends, Michael Clougherty, I started my career in the fire rescue service in 1984. From the moment I laid my hands on a hydraulic tool, I was hooked, but it wasn't until 1987 that this would turn into a never-ending quest to learn, perfect, and share my skills in vehicle extrication. That year, I was in a bad car accident in which a drunk driver collided with my vehicle head-on, causing my vehicle to roll over several times, trapping me inside. It took fire rescue crews from Broward County only a few minutes to get me out, but I remember being strapped to a backboard and slowly pulled out through the back of my SUV. I could have easily been killed that evening, but I believe that God had another plan. Ever since that night, I have had a desire to learn everything I can about vehicle extrication and eventually share what I have learned.

Over the years, I have been blessed to work with many great individuals and fire rescue departments across the country. I've had incredible opportunities to write articles for trade magazines and teach at Firehouse Expo in Las Vegas. I have been involved in organizing numerous vehicle extrication competitions, including co-chairing and organizing the 2005 International Extrication Competition as well as being a competition assessor at the Nationals. I have also had the incredible experience of working with Jones & Bartlett Learning in writing my first book in 2011 and now completing this second revised edition. I truly believe that there is always something new to learn and share, with the goal of serving and helping others. My hope and purpose for this book are to help emergency response personnel save the lives of those we serve.

There are so many friends and colleagues who have helped me with this book as well as those who helped with the first edition. First and always, I give thanks to my Lord and Savior; You are the rock on which I stand. To my wife and best friend, Devon, thank you, for this would not have been possible without your constant encouragement, love, and support. To my parents, Ray and Karen, thank you for the love, lessons, and foundation you set in me. To my children, Austin, Cameron, and my little angel Grace, you guys bring me joy that words cannot describe.

I would also like to thank the city of North Lauderdale Commission and Administrative staff, Fire Chief Rodney Turpel, The North Lauderdale Fire Rescue Department, Brett Holcombe and the Westway Towing family, Captain Eddie Monahan, Firefighter Sam Franco, Firefighter Houston Holcombe, Attorney Neil Taylor, the Linares family, Captain Jayson Lynn, Firefighter Rick Fernandez, Firefighter Ivan Chong, Firefighter Carlos "Iggy" Eguiluz, Fire Chief Neil DeJesus, District Chief Dan Zinge, Battalion Chief Nelson Canizares, Battalion Chief Steve Stillwell, Division Chief Mike Nugent, Chaplain Paul Schweinler, Firefighter Jeff Pugh, Firefighter Chris Burdyshaw, Assistant Chief Michael Clougherty, Fire Chief Josh Boone, Spruce Pine Fire Rescue Department, Fire Chief Julie Downey, Battalion Chief Vincent Martinez, Davie Fire Rescue, Nebraska City Fire Rescue, Deputy Chief Gregg Pagliarulo, Mike and Ralph at M and L Salvage, Hal Eastman and Kevin Bellucy at Genesis Rescue Systems, Mike Smith at BoronExtrication.com, Lydia Agurkis and Tim O'Connell at Rescue 42, Steve Dowden at Hi-Lift Jack Company/First Responder Jack, Michael Ens at HexArmor, Bill Benedict at Ajax Tools, Andrew Orchard at Packexe, Chris Pasto at Res-Q-Jack, Tammi Northrop at JYD Industries, Jeffrey Benker at BullDog Hose Company, and Jenny McPherson at TECGEN. And finally, to Director of Product Management Bill Larkin, Cindy Mosher, and the staff at Jones & Bartlett Learning—thank you, what an incredible team to work with.

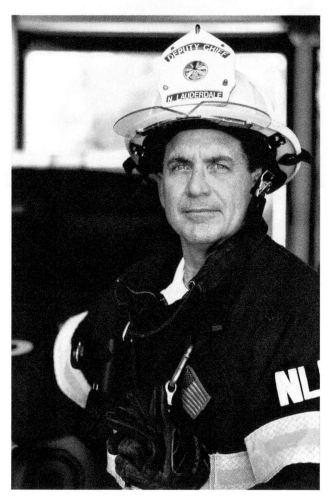

Deputy Fire Chief David Sweet of the North Lauderdale Fire Rescue Department.
Courtesy of David Sweet.

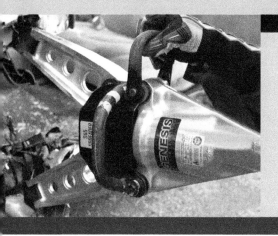

Acknowledgments

Author

David A. Sweet
Deputy Fire Chief
North Lauderdale Fire Rescue Department
North Lauderdale, Florida

Reviewers and Contributors

James Allen
Fire Training Officer, Technical Rescue & HazMat Coordinator
The Ohio Fire Academy
Reynoldsburg, Ohio

Hudson Babler
Dallas Fire Rescue
Dallas, Texas

Amy Brooks
Captain, Paramedic, Fire Science Director
Central Arizona College
Coolidge, Arizona

Jim Campbell
Battalion Chief
Pike Township Fire Department
Indianapolis, Indiana

Mark Cleveland
Fire Chief
Egelston Township Fire Department
Muskegon, Michigan

Mike Daley
Fire Service Performance Concepts, LLC
Monroe Township Fire Department
Monroe, New Jersey

Scott Floyd
Indianapolis Fire Department
Indianapolis, Indiana

Brian Grindstaff
Battalion Chief, Training Officer
Skyland Fire and Rescue
Skyland, North Carolina

Shawn Haynes
Fire Rescue Training Specialist, Captain
North Carolina Office of State Fire Marshal/Henderson County Rescue Squad
Raleigh, North Carolina

Harris Henbest
Broward Sheriff's Fire Rescue & Emergency Services Department
Fort Lauderdale, Florida

Brett Holcombe
Owner
Westway Towing
Fort Lauderdale, Florida

Houston Holcombe
North Lauderdale, Florida

Matthew Hull
Captain
Athens Fire Department
Athens, Ohio

Mark E. Karp
Fire Instructor, AEMT
Nicolet Area Technical College
Rhinelander, Wisconsin

Shawn S. Kelley
International Association of Fire Chiefs
Fairfax, Virginia

Jared Kimball, NRP
Tulane Trauma Education
New Orleans, Louisiana

Steve Knight
Coordinator, Professor
Lambton College Fire & Public Safety Centre of Excellence
Sarnia, Ontario, Canada

Jayson Lynn
Captain
North American Vehicle Rescue Association
Hillsborough County Fire Rescue
Tampa, Florida

Daniel Manning, PhD
Assistant Fire Chief of Special Operations, Laughlin AFB Fire Emergency Services
Professor, Adler University/Colorado State University–Global Campus/Pima Community College
Laughlin, Texas

Russell McCullar
Senior Instructor
Mississippi State Fire Academy
Jackson, Mississippi

Frank McKinley
Dallas Fire-Rescue Department
Dallas, Texas

Kevin Milan, PhD
South Metro Fire Rescue
Centennial, Colorado

Bill Pfeifer
Training Specialist II
Nebraska State Fire Marshal, Training Division
Grand Island, Nebraska

Jonathan Poganski
Firefighter
UC Davis Fire Department
Davis, California

Michael Powell
Columbus Ohio Division of Fire, Rescue 16
Columbus, Ohio
Ohio Fire Academy
Reynoldsburg, Ohio

Jeff Pugh
PXT President
www.ThePXTeam.org

John W. Ross, Jr.
Lieutenant
City of Aurora Fire Department
Aurora, Illinois

C. W. Sigman
Director
Kanawha County Office of Emergency Management
Kanawha County, West Virginia

Michael Smith
BoronExtrication.com
Wixom Fire Department
Wixom, Michigan

Rodney Smith
Cedar Hill Fire Department
Cedar Hill, Texas

Jody Smyre
Iredell County Emergency Management
Statesville, North Carolina

Jeremy Souza
National Fire Protection Association
Quincy, Massachusetts

Richard Sparks
Adjunct Fire Instructor, Nicolet College
Rhinelander, Wisconsin

Brandon Sy
Valders Fire Department
Valders, Wisconsin

Darin J. Virag
Captain
Charleston Fire Department
Charleston, West Virginia

Photographic Contributors

Jones & Bartlett Learning would like to thank the photographers who contributed their work to this text:

Kevin Bellucy

Jim Dobson

Carlos Eguiluz

Brad Fellers

Florida Department of Transportation

Genesis Rescue Systems

Houston Holcombe

Mike Jachles

Troy Lanza

Bill Larkin

Jeff Lopez

Makita USA, Inc.

Bill McGrath

Edward Monahan

Brad Myers

Paratech Incorporated

Power Hawk Technologies, Inc.

Rescue 42

Mike Smith

David Sweet

Devon Sweet

Chris Xiste

SECTION 1

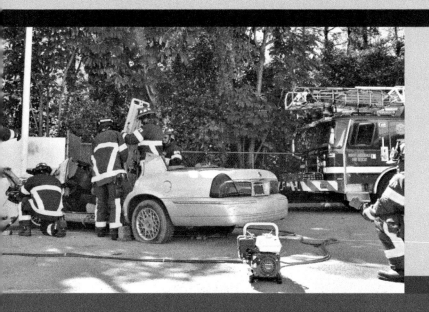

Awareness Level

CHAPTER **1** **Introduction to Vehicle Rescue and Extrication**

CHAPTER **2** **Vehicle Rescue Incident Awareness**

CHAPTER **3** **Tools and Equipment**

CHAPTER 1

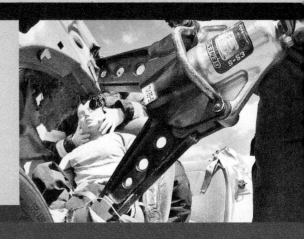

Awareness Level

Introduction to Vehicle Rescue and Extrication

KNOWLEDGE OBJECTIVES

After studying this chapter, you should be able to:
- Explain the need for ongoing and specialized training in vehicle rescue. (pp. 3–4)
- Define the following terms and discuss their role in vehicle rescue incidents:
  - Technical rescue (p. 4)
  - Technical rescuer (p. 4)
  - Extrication (p. 4)
  - Disentanglement (p. 4)
  - Qualification (p. 5)
  - Authority having jurisdiction (AHJ) (p. 5)
- Differentiate standards and laws. (p. 4)
- Identify the NFPA standards covering technical rescue. (pp. 4–5)
- Identify the three primary levels of technical rescuer qualifications outlined in NFPA 1006. (pp. 6–7)
- Describe awareness-level responsibilities under NFPA 1006. (**NFPA 1006: 8.1.2**, p. 6)
- Describe operations-level responsibilities under NFPA 1006. (**NFPA 1006: 8.1.2**, pp. 6–7)
- Describe technician-level responsibilities under NFPA 1006. (**NFPA 1006: 8.1.2**, p. 7)
- List awareness-level organizational tasks outlined in NFPA 1670. (pp. 7–8)
- Identify information that should be gathered on scene to create an incident action plan. (**NFPA 1006: 8.1.2**, p. 12)
- List resources for technical vehicle rescue information and training. (pp. 12–15)

SKILLS OBJECTIVES

There are no skills objectives for this chapter.

You Are the Rescuer

You respond to a multi-vehicle accident with victims trapped. As you approach the scene, your heart is pounding from the rush of adrenaline that's building inside you. You see a twisted ton of metal that resembles a vehicle. You hear screams coming from the wreckage as you step off the rig. Can you handle this call with confidence, knowing that the training you received will produce the most successful outcome? This is a common vehicle rescue and extrication scenario that many technical rescuers encounter daily.

1. Does the current operational level of the crew support this type of incident?
2. Do you have an action plan?
3. What resources do you have?

JONES & BARTLETT LEARNING NAVIGATE — Access Navigate for more practice activities.

Introduction

The 2019 National Highway Traffic Safety Administration (NHTSA) summary of motor vehicle accidents reported a high of 6.7 million motor vehicle collisions in the United States, with 2.74 million people injured in those accidents (NHTSA, 2019) (**FIGURE 1-1**).

These growing figures demonstrate the need for fire rescue and emergency medical service (EMS) organizations across the globe to focus more training on vehicle rescue practice and procedures. With the continual and rapid advancement in vehicle technology, the automotive industry has pushed to make vehicles safer, lighter, stronger, greener (in terms of alternative fuels and propulsion technology), and smarter (with the integration of computer-based artificial intelligence, such as the emergence of self-driving vehicles).

Possessing only a basic skill set and understanding in vehicle rescue is no longer sufficient to successfully manage a motor vehicle accident (MVA) involving the disentanglement and extrication of trapped victims. Proper training and knowledge in the advancement of vehicle technology, tools, equipment, procedures, and techniques to manage vehicle rescue incidents are paramount and are the responsibility of not only the organization but the individual responders as well. Qualifying individual skill levels and providing the appropriate operational response capability for the jurisdiction are not just a great idea or a future goal in an organization's strategic plan but a mandate to provide the best level of service that a community requires and demands of you as a rescuer and/or an organization. The old standard of just "poppin' doors and rippin' roofs" without having the proper qualifications or following structured procedures and a fluid **incident action plan (IAP)** can potentially cause further injury to the victim or injury to you or your crew.

Complacency coupled with a lack of leadership and/or direction is a recipe for disaster. To sit back and think that the training you received years ago is sufficient to carry you or your organization through today's vehicle rescue incidents successfully is irresponsible and a disservice to the community you serve. In today's world of litigations and avoidable rescuer injuries, fire rescue and EMS organizations need to adhere to the goal and sworn oath of providing the best level of care and service that is possible while keeping all emergency personnel safe. In doing so, many organizations turn to agencies such as the National Fire Protection Association (NFPA) or the Occupational

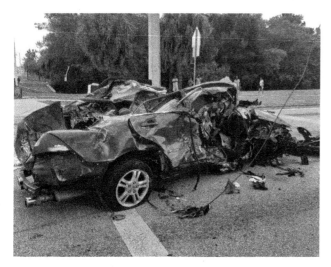

FIGURE 1-1 The number of motor vehicle collisions is on the rise.
Courtesy of David Sweet.

Safety and Health Administration (OSHA) for guidelines, standards, and regulations to follow.

To maintain an optimal level of proficiency and remain current with technical rescue practices and applicable standards, vehicle rescue and extrication training should be scheduled on a continual basis, qualifying each member to the appropriate skill level and demonstrating competency on an annual basis. Qualifying training means using and adopting accredited measurable standards for providing the best level of service and safety to personnel. Proficiency in vehicle rescue and extrication requires continuous training; how you train directly correlates with how you will perform on the street.

According to the NFPA, a **technical rescuer** is a person who is trained to perform or direct the technical rescue. A **technical rescue** is the application of knowledge, skills, and equipment to resolve unique and/or complex rescue situations safely.

In the context of vehicle rescue and extrication, **extrication** is the process of removing a trapped victim from a vehicle. **Disentanglement** refers to the spreading, cutting, or removal of a vehicle away from trapped or injured victims. It is vital for the technical rescuer to fully understand that vehicle rescue and extrication is a step-by-step technical process consisting of three phases: stabilization of the scene, stabilization of the vehicle(s), and then stabilization of the victim(s) (**FIGURE 1-2**).

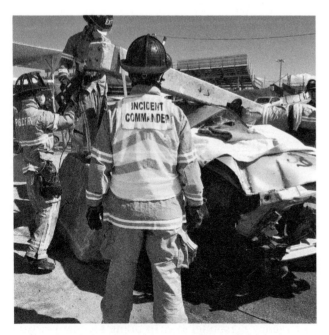

FIGURE 1-2 Organizations must be proficient at the minimum awareness-level capability to conduct operations at a technical rescue incident.
Courtesy of David Sweet.

This text is intended to be used as a training resource that explains the three-step stabilization process in detail. It outlines a no-nonsense street-level perspective on the fundamentals of vehicle rescue and extrication and is guided by NFPA standards for managing a vehicle rescue incident. This text details the operational levels of NFPA 1006 and 1670, separating each level into its own section of the text and thus facilitating this text's use as a training and resource guide.

LISTEN UP!

A technical rescuer is identified by the job-specific discipline performed and the level of qualification (based on job performance requirements [JPRs]) needed to carry out specific tasks for that discipline.

Standards and Qualifications

A **standard** is typically developed to provide guidance on the performance of processes, products, individuals, or organizations. Compliance with standards is considered voluntary, unless the standards are formally adopted by a state, a province, a county, a government municipality, or an organization. Once a standard is adopted, it takes on the force of law. Where not officially adopted, standards can be viewed as generally accepted practice. A common example of such a standard is NFPA 1001, *Standard for Firefighter Professional Qualifications*. Many states have adopted this standard as a requirement for some or all firefighters within their state.

The following standards are addressed in this text:

- NFPA 1001, *Standard for Firefighter Professional Qualifications*, Sections 6.4.1 and 6.4.2
- NFPA 1006, *Standard for Technical Rescue Personnel Professional Qualifications*, Chapter 8 and associated appendices
- NFPA 1670, *Standard on Operations and Training for Technical Search and Rescue Incidents*, Chapter 8 and associated appendices

LISTEN UP!

Organizations and personnel that conduct vehicle rescue operations should be trained at a minimum to the awareness level and demonstrate competency at that level in accordance with NFPA 1670 (organizations) and NFPA 1006 (personnel).

NFPA 1006, *Standard for Technical Rescue Personnel Professional Qualifications*

NFPA 1006 defines the position of technical rescue personnel and establishes the JPRs for technical rescue personnel who perform technical rescue operations, with the intent to ensure that the individuals serving as technical rescue personnel are qualified. The standard mandates that a rescuer remain current in his or her training and "demonstrate competency on an annual basis" (NFPA, 2021, Section 1.2.6).

NFPA 1006 and NFPA 1670 work together to correlate the material so that the standards align with each other. The distinction is that NFPA 1006 focuses on personnel and NFPA 1670 focuses on the organization. The intent of NFPA 1006 is to outline the qualifications and JPRs of technical rescue personnel only. NFPA 1006 does not address the organization or the capability of an organization in reference to technical rescue; this is the intent of NFPA 1670.

JPRs outline specific job tasks, list the knowledge and skills necessary to complete the task, and define measurable or observable outcomes and evaluation areas for the specific task. In NFPA 1006, these JPRs are specific to technical rescue personnel. Each technical rescue discipline covered by NFPA has its own set of specific duties, knowledge, and skills unique to that discipline. These disciplines follow:

- Tower rescue
- Rope rescue
- Structural collapse rescue
- Confined space rescue
- Common passenger vehicle rescue
- Heavy vehicle rescue
- Animal technical rescue
- Wilderness search and rescue
- Trench rescue
- Machinery rescue
- Cave rescue
- Mine and tunnel rescue
- Helicopter rescue
- Surface water rescue
- Swiftwater rescue
- Dive rescue
- Ice rescue
- Surf rescue
- Watercraft rescue
- Floodwater rescue

Technical rescue personnel are identified by their discipline and the level of qualification for that specific discipline. Qualification is when a defined set of skills, conditions, applications, and/or standards has been satisfactorily completed by a person or personnel. NFPA 1006 identifies three operational levels for qualifying technical rescue personnel: awareness, operations, and technician.

Because technical rescue is hazardous and technical rescuer personnel are required to perform rigorous activities in adverse conditions, regional and national safety standards shall be included in agency policies and procedures, as stated in NFPA 1006, Section 1.3.11.

In addition to this, it is the responsibility of the authority having jurisdiction (AHJ) to ensure that all entrance requirements for personnel are met prior to beginning any training or engaging in any technical rescue operations. NFPA 1006 outlines the following entrance requirements as listed in Section 1.3.9 (NFPA, 2021):

- Educational requirements established by the AHJ
- Age requirements established by the AHJ
- Medical requirements established by the AHJ
- Job-related physical performance requirements established by the AHJ
- Emergency medical care performance requirements for entry-level personnel developed and validated by the AHJ
- Minimum requirements for hazardous materials incident and contact control training for entry-level personnel and validated by the AHJ
- Psychological support/education requirements established by the AHJ

Job Performance and General Requirements

The job performance and general requirements for each operational level listed in NFPA 1006 for common passenger vehicle rescue and extrication are designed to be progressive and cumulative, starting with the basic awareness level and then advancing to an operational level and on to the technician level. The hours needed to progress from one level to the next are based on individual state statutes, state or national fire academy guidelines, or the local AHJ operational protocols. This does not by any means allow the AHJ to make up random numbers. The training still has to match or exceed the requirements outlined in NFPA 1006 for each level, but it can and should be tailored to that organization's jurisdictional response needs and resources. One organization may feel that 16 hours of training is sufficient to meet the awareness-level requirements, whereas another organization may say that it will take a minimum of 24 hours of training for personnel to meet the awareness level. As long as the JPR criteria outlined in NFPA 1006 are met, both agencies are correct in their interpretation of the requirements. Note that personnel should be evaluated by an individual other than their instructor when determining the personnel's level of qualification.

Awareness Level. The awareness level represents the minimum requirements or capabilities technical rescue personnel must achieve to perform at a technical rescue incident. Personnel at this level must demonstrate competency in applying operational procedures for the jurisdiction served as well as following and implementing an incident action plan (IAP). An IAP is a strategic plan of operations for an incident and consists of measurable goals and objectives to effectively manage the incident. The IAP can be formal or informal and oral or written, based on the type, duration, size, and complexity of the incident.

Formal incident action plans for large-scale incidents, such as hurricanes, earthquakes, and large forest fires, are written and formulated within an ICS for operational periods that generally run 12 or 24 hours and last from several days to weeks. Formal IAPs can also expand and contract for each operation period and may contain additional components and attachments such as a communications section, a medical section, and resource allocation. Informal incident action plans can be as simple as an engine and rescue company with five or six personnel responding to a motor vehicle accident. Upon arrival of the two units, the company officer on the engine (operations level) mentally starts to formulate the IAP while conducting the size-up and scene survey with the team. After the initial information collection process is complete (generally no more than 30–45 seconds), the company officer explains and directs the plan of action or IAP to the team to safely and effectively mitigate the incident.

Using the IAP, awareness-level personnel must demonstrate a standard approach to operational incidents and training scenarios, including comprehension and application of the incident command system (ICS) and recognition of the complexity of a technical rescue incident, which includes properly identifying the appropriate level of response (operations level or technician level) for the incident.

Awareness-level personnel must have working knowledge of various tools and equipment used on a technical rescue incident. They should also demonstrate competency in scene size-up, scene survey, risk–benefit analysis, hazard recognition, PPE requirements, and basic mitigation of the various types of hazard(s) encountered. Additionally, traffic control is an awareness-level organizational competency in NFPA 1670. Personnel at this level may establish safety zones, perform traffic incident management, and apply defensive apparatus placement procedures. They must also demonstrate efficient information gathering skills pertinent to the incident and be able to relay that information, including status updates, to direct supervisors and/or command.

Operations Level. The operations level represents the capability of individuals to respond to technical search and rescue incidents and to identify hazards, use equipment, and apply limited techniques specified in this standard to support and participate in technical search and rescue incidents. Responders at this level must be able to develop an IAP using the organization's standard operating procedures (SOPs) for operations-level incidents common to the jurisdiction. Using the IAP, operations-level responders must apply a standard approach to operational incidents and training scenarios—implementing the National Incident Management System (NIMS); conducting a scene size-up and scene survey; evaluating needs and requesting additional resources; securing the scene with the assistance of a risk–benefit analysis; recognizing, isolating, and mitigating hazards; implementing fire suppression tactics; recognizing explosion hazards; and implementing necessary safety and protective precautions.

Specific to vehicle rescue and extrication, operations-level responders must be able to recognize the various types, systems, and components of a common passenger vehicle. This includes understanding propulsion systems, alternative fuel sources, various energy sources, beneficial systems, supplemental restraint system (SRS) components, vehicle anatomy, and metallurgical composition. Responders should also understand traffic incident management, vehicle stabilization practices and techniques for common passenger vehicles, and how to recognize and use various tools associated with stabilization.

Tasks at this level include selecting and using incident-specific PPE, developing and implementing both a Plan A and a Plan B for vehicle entry and victim management, and developing and implementing emergency exit strategies for rapid victim removal and personnel safety (including use of emergency evacuation signals). Additionally, traffic incident management and applying defensive apparatus placement procedures are components for the operations-level personnel to understand. Operations-level rescuers must also be able to recognize, select, and apply the various tools needed for entry and disentanglement operations for common passenger vehicles. These tools include non-powered hand tools, powered tools, and stabilization tools.

Operations-level personnel must also use appropriate techniques and follow jurisdictional medical protocols for victim immobilization, packaging, and removal. This includes proper use of immobilization devices and transport protocols. Responders at the operations level must also be competent to terminate a vehicle rescue and extrication operation, including demobilization procedures for units and personnel; evaluation and decontamination procedures of PPE, tools, and equipment; proper disposal of biological hazards; and notification of the proper authority for continued maintenance of existing hazards, such as debris and vehicle removal.

Lastly, operations-level responders are responsible for transferring scene control to responsible parties, collecting information and data for documentation and reporting requirements, conducting an informal postincident analysis (including critical incident stress management [CISM] if needed). If required by the AHJ, these responders may also be required to develop an after-action report and conduct a formal postincident analysis.

Technician Level. The technician level represents those responders who not only identify hazards and use equipment but also apply advanced rescue techniques beyond the operations level to coordinate, perform, and supervise technical search and rescue incidents.

Technician-level personnel must be able to develop an IAP using the organization's SOPs and then use that IAP to apply a standard approach to operational incidents and training scenarios. Elements include ICS implementation; scene size-up; scene survey; needs and requests for additional resources evaluation; scene security (including risk–benefit analysis and hazard recognition, isolation, and mitigation); fire suppression tactics; and explosion hazard recognition, including associated safety and protective precautions. Responders at this level must also recognize types and systems of common passenger vehicles including propulsion systems, alternative fuel sources, beneficial systems, SRS components, common passenger vehicle anatomy, and metallurgical composition.

Technician-level personnel must also understand traffic incident management and apply defensive apparatus placement procedures. They must employ vehicle stabilization practices and techniques common passenger vehicles that have come to rest on their roof, side, or in a configuration or environment where multiple concurrent hazards must be managed to access or remove the occupants. As with operations-level responders, those at the technician level must be capable of selecting and using task- and incident-specific PPE and developing and implementing both a Plan A and a Plan B for vehicle entry and victim management. They must also develop emergency exit strategies for rapid victim removal and personnel safety, including the use of emergency evacuation signals.

Technician-level personnel must be proficient in tool recognition, selection, and application as well as various procedures and techniques for entry and disentanglement operations for common passenger vehicles. These tools include non-powered hand tools, powered tools, and stabilization tools.

Responders at this level must employ appropriate techniques and apply jurisdictional medical protocols for victim immobilization, packaging, and removal, including recognition and application of immobilization devices as well as comprehension of transport protocols for the jurisdiction.

At the technician level, responsibilities also include terminating the rescue operation, including demobilizing units and personnel; evaluating and decontaminating PPE, tools, and equipment; properly disposing of biological hazards; and notifying the proper authority for continued maintenance of existing hazards, including debris and vehicle removal. Lastly, technician-level personnel shall transfer scene control to responsible parties, collect the necessary information and data for documentation and local jurisdictional reporting requirements, and conduct an informal postincident analysis (including CISM if needed). Technician-level personnel may be required by the AHJ to develop an after-action report and conduct a formal postincident analysis.

NFPA 1670, *Standard on Operations and Training for Technical Search and Rescue Incidents*

NFPA 1670 identifies and establishes levels of functional capabilities for rescue organizations to safely and effectively conduct operations at technical rescue incidents, including vehicle rescue and extrication incidents. The requirements outlined in NFPA 1670 apply to *organizations* that provide response to technical search and rescue incidents and are not intended to be applied to individuals and their associated qualifications or skills.

Evaluation

The main purpose of NFPA 1670 is to assist the AHJ in assessing a technical search and rescue hazard within the response area and to identify the level of response capability (awareness, operations, or technician) through risk assessment, current operational level of personnel and established training procedures, and the availability of internal and external resources. In addition, the AHJ is required to establish operational criteria (SOPs) consistent with the identified level of response capability to ensure that the operations at a technical rescue incident are performed consistently, effectively, and safely to minimize threats and harm to rescue personnel and others.

A hazard and risk assessment of the jurisdictional response area to determine response capability requirements should include a study of the environmental, physical, social, and cultural factors that can have an impact on the scope, frequency, and magnitude of technical search and rescue incidents and any limiting effect these factors may have on the organization's ability to respond to (and operate at) vehicle rescue incidents while minimizing threats to rescue personnel and others at those incidents. Documentation of these assessment findings should be reviewed and updated regularly, and the frequency of vehicle rescue and extrication incidents should be continually evaluated.

An evaluation study includes identifying all internal and external resources that can provide additional support when requested based on the complexity or specialty that may be required at an incident. Internal resources that may be available through an organization's municipality, town, county, or province include, but are not limited to, public utility services; street and ground maintenance services; financial services; human resources; information technology (IT) services; and chaplaincy services for various supportive, physiological, and/or spiritual needs of personnel and others. External resources can provide an area of need that is not included in the organizational structure of the agency or may be outside the jurisdictional response area. To assist the AHJ in identifying potential resources, the resources can be separated into four general categories (keep in mind, however, that this list is not inclusive and does not encompass all resource categories):

- Technical services
- Equipment
- Supplies
- Regional, statewide, and national resources

Once the AHJ identifies appropriate resources to support various technical rescue operations, procurement procedures to acquire, rent, and/or share these resources must be drafted and prearranged with vendors, emergency services organizations, or government agencies. Intra-local agreements and mutual and automatic aid agreements as well as general contracts obtaining external resources are additional options.

When the AHJ completes an evaluation to identify the level of response capability for an organization, it must establish written SOPs for all designated levels before conducting operations at a technical rescue incident in the jurisdictional response area. These procedures include training requirements for maintaining the identified level of response capability. To maintain safety and consistency, operational procedures cannot exceed the identified level of response capability. The organization can never exceed the identified level of response capability unless the proper training, including the evaluation process, has determined that the organization is capable of managing a higher level of operations for a technical rescue incident.

Operational Levels

The operational levels for organizations meeting the response capability outlined in NFPA 1670 are as follows:

- *Awareness level.* This level represents the minimum capability of organizations that provide response to technical search and rescue incidents.
- *Operations level.* This level represents the capability of organizations to respond to technical search and rescue incidents and to identify hazards, use equipment, and apply limited techniques specified in this standard to support and participate in technical search and rescue incidents.
- *Technician level.* This level represents the capability of organizations to respond to technical search and rescue incidents and to identify hazards, use equipment, and apply advanced techniques specified in this standard necessary to coordinate, perform, and supervise technical search and rescue incidents.

Training Requirements

The AHJ must ensure that training programs are scheduled throughout the year and that outlines and procedures are consistent with the requirements for the determined level of response capability. An organization must demonstrate proficiency to at least the awareness level capability to be able to conduct operations at a technical rescue incident. If an organization does not meet the minimum awareness-level requirements or, through hazard recognition and risk assessment, the response criteria change to a more advanced level than the organization is capable of providing, the AHJ must arrange to have mutual or automatic aid agreements in place with organizations that can provide the appropriate predetermined level of response capability. The AHJ must also have a written plan in place to provide training and resources to meet or exceed the identified level of response capability.

To determine whether the current standard of training prepares the organization to perform at the identified operational level under extreme conditions, all training programs should account for abnormal weather conditions, extremely hazardous operational conditions, hostile environments, and various other difficult situations. The AHJ should arrange for and provide training for tools and equipment used by the organization as well as procedures for inventory, accountability, maintenance, and care procedures recommended by the manufacturers.

PPE recognition, application, and proper use and medical protocol training at the minimum of basic life support (BLS) should be incorporated into an organization's training procedures as well. Because of the high potential risk of injury at a technical rescue incident, a trained medical staff member or team capable of providing BLS must be standing by during all operations.

The AHJ must also provide training programs for maintaining the technical rescue capabilities of an organization. These programs should incorporate periodical performance evaluations to ensure that the organization has maintained the capability to provide the established level of response.

SOPs should outline the training, use, and implementation of the incident management system and accountability system in accordance with NFPA 1561.

Safety Procedures

The AHJ must ensure that members are physically, psychologically, and medically capable of performing assigned duties and functions at technical search and rescue incidents and that training exercises meet the relevant requirements of the following chapters and sections of NFPA 1500:

- Chapter 5, Section 5.4: Special Operations Training
- Chapter 7: Protective Clothing and Protective Equipment
- Chapter 8: Emergency Operations
- Chapter 11: Medical and Physical Requirements

All personnel must be trained regarding the hazards and risks associated with technical rescue operations, with special emphasis on safety procedures to minimize threats to rescuers. There must be a written policy stating that all members are required to wear the appropriate level of PPE and fully understand the function and limitations of PPE while operating at a technical rescue incident and training exercise. Breathing apparatus must be provided and worn in accordance with the manufacturer's recommendations where an immediate danger to life and health (IDLH) exists.

The SOPs and IAP must also explain emergency evacuation procedures, including notification methods. These procedures can be modified to fit the type and unique characteristics of variations existing at each incident. Emergency evacuation procedures should be developed immediately after the initial size-up and completion of the scene survey and shall be presented, acknowledged, and strictly adhered to by all personnel operating within the IDLH area at every technical rescue incident and training evolution. Because of the inherent dangers, hazards, and unforeseen and/or unpredictable changes that can occur at technical rescue incidents, safety of personnel and victims must be the top priority when developing the IAP.

Organizations responding to technical rescue incidents must also meet the requirements specified in NFPA 472, *Standard for Competence of Responders to Hazardous Materials/Weapons of Mass Destruction Incidents*. Organizations at the awareness level must meet Chapter 4, *Competencies for Awareness Level Personnel*, and those at the operations level must meet Chapter 5, *Competencies for Operations Level Responders*.

Requirements

To meet the requirements of the awareness level for vehicle rescue and extrication incidents, organizations must be competent in the following tasks:

- Recognizing the need for a vehicle search and rescue
- Identifying the resources necessary to conduct operations
- Initiating the emergency response system for vehicle search and rescue incidents
- Initiating site control and scene management
- Recognizing general hazards associated with vehicle search and rescue incidents
- Initiating traffic control (NFPA 1670, 2017 edition, Section 8.2.3)

To meet the requirements of the operations level for vehicle rescue and extrication incidents, organizations' members must be capable of recognizing hazards, using equipment, and implementing techniques necessary to operate safely and effectively at incidents in which persons are injured or entrapped in a typical vehicle found in the jurisdiction. Requirements include developing and implementing procedures for the following:

- Sizing up existing and potential conditions at vehicle search and rescue incidents
- Identifying probable victim locations and survivability
- Making the search and rescue area safe, including identifying and controlling the hazards presented by the vehicle, its position, or its systems
- Identifying, containing, and stopping fuel release
- Protecting a victim during extrication or disentanglement
- Packaging a victim prior to extrication or disentanglement
- Accessing victims trapped in a typical vehicle commonly found in the jurisdiction
- Performing extrication and disentanglement operations involving packaging, treating, and removing victims trapped in a common passenger vehicle or other types of vehicles as identified by the AHJ as being commonly found in the jurisdiction, through the use of hand and power tools
- Mitigating and managing general and specific hazards associated with vehicle search and rescue incidents that involve common passenger vehicles or other vehicles typically found in the jurisdiction
- Procuring and utilizing the resources necessary to conduct vehicle search and rescue operations
- Maintaining control of traffic at the scene of vehicle search and rescue incidents (NFPA 1670, 2017 edition, Section 8.3.4)

To meet the requirements of the technician level, members of the organization must be able to respond to vehicle rescue and extrication incidents; identify hazards; use equipment; and apply advanced techniques to coordinate, perform, and supervise technical search and rescue incidents. Responsibilities include the following:

- Evaluating existing and potential conditions at vehicle search and rescue incidents
- Performing extrication and disentanglement operations involving packaging, treating, and removing victims injured or trapped in large commercial or industrial vehicles or any vehicles that present unique, complex, exotic, or unfamiliar hazards or extrication challenges
- Stabilizing in advance of technician-level vehicle search and rescue situations
- Using all specialized search and rescue equipment immediately available and in use by the organization
- Using specialized outside resources, including heavy equipment (NFPA 1670, 2017 edition, Section 8.4.2)

Compliance with NFPA 1006 and NFPA 1670

The three operational levels for NFPA 1006 and 1670 are guidelines that outline benchmarks to all emergency services personnel and organizations on what operational qualifications and functional response capability they currently meet. If an organization does not meet any of the three criteria levels, then the AHJ needs to reevaluate the response capability, set attainable goals to train personnel to meet these guidelines, or call for qualified mutual aid to handle any incident that is beyond the department's operational level.

To bring personnel and an organization into compliance with NFPA 1006 and NFPA 1670 for vehicle rescue and extrication, a plan that maximizes efficiency and uses the most appropriate and validated resources should be used. The first step in this plan is to conduct a self-evaluation consisting of a needs assessment for your organization (discussed in Chapter 2, *Vehicle Rescue Incident Awareness*). This evaluation gives an organization a clear picture of the type of incidents common to the jurisdiction, hazards associated with those types of incidents, required level of proficiency, equipment needed for these types of incidents, and what the agency is capable of managing with the current resources available.

At a minimum, all emergency services organizations must have SOPs for managing a vehicle rescue and extrication incident and establishing guidelines that minimize risk and threats and that provide consistency and safety for all personnel to follow. The SOPs become the main body of the IAP, which is the basis for all operations being conducted. Individual motor vehicle accidents may present technical rescue personnel with various challenges beyond the basic concerns, but the IAP evolves around the core principles of the SOPs, adapting and changing based on incident needs, such as type and number of vehicles, level of operational capabilities of personnel, available resources, and environmental conditions. Additional

Voice of Experience

As first responders, we have a commitment to provide a wide range of emergency services to everyone within our jurisdictions. The public depends on our services, at any time, in all weather conditions, and for any scenario they might encounter.

It doesn't matter if your organization serves a major metropolitan area or a small rural community—you as a first responder must be prepared to respond with the skills, courage, and commitment to fulfill your duties. How can this be accomplished? Preparation! Preparation begins with the mindset and a personal commitment to be the best you can be. To accomplish this you must dedicate yourself to participating often in regularly scheduled training classes. Training classes must be conducted by seasoned, knowledgeable professionals who provide the latest up-to-date information and training regarding techniques, equipment, and vehicle construction.

For 15 of my 19 years as a firefighter, I have been honored to serve as a certified instructor in Fire, Rescue and Emergency Medical Services. I have taught numerous classes that included a variety of experienced veterans, journeyman firefighters, and novice recruits. In almost every one of those classes, I can always expect to have one particular question raised. "How do you deal with your personal feelings resulting from traumatic calls involving the loss of life?" Over and over again throughout my career, that question finds its way into my classes. My answer is always the same, simple response each time. "It is never easy to respond to a call where a loss of life has occurred. I feel empathy for the victims involved and their loved ones; however, when I return to the station I know that I can look at myself in the mirror and know that I did everything possible to effect a positive outcome." How can I know that? Because I had prepared myself both physically and mentally to perform my duties. I had extensively dedicated myself to continually train to improve my knowledge and skills.

Through training you will develop your skills and knowledge, learning and practicing techniques that are required to perform your duties safely and effectively. This will allow you to gain invaluable experience and confidence in your own abilities. Through regular training you learn and get to experience the proper use of your equipment and all of its capabilities. Without a thorough knowledge of your equipment and the needed training to use them, you become a liability on the emergency scene and an impediment to the safety of your team. When you look at yourself in the mirror, what do you see? Do you see a trained professional who is prepared, both mentally and physically, to perform at the highest standards? Or do you see a safety liability who is not prepared? You might be able to deceive others, but when you look in the mirror you can't fool yourself.

Vehicle technology is a dynamic field that is constantly evolving and requires constant training—from vehicle construction and advanced safety systems, to the ever-evolving list of vehicle rescue equipment and new extrication techniques. A well-prepared first responder has quite a bit to keep up with. How much has changed in the past 10 years? What will the "standard" passenger vehicle morph into in the next 10 years? As you train for vehicle rescue, ask yourself, "What type of rescuer do I want to be? What type of rescuer would I want to respond to my loved ones when they are in need of emergency assistance?" The choice is up to you!

I wish you all the best, great success, and personal safety through continued training.

Darin J. Virag
Charleston Fire Department
Charleston, West Virginia

factors can influence the shaping of an IAP, which will be decided by the incident commander and/or technical rescue personnel with an operations level or higher qualification.

Obtaining Information Required to Develop an IAP

No two emergency incident responses are the same. Each response will require a different approach to developing a functional IAP. The officer must have the ability to adapt to the ever-changing dynamics an incident presents. As previously stated, the SOPs will be the body of the IAP, which provide the basic parameters to work from, but additional information acquired at the scene is needed to complete the plan. IAPs should be developed using several factors:

- *Scene size-up*: Is there a single car or multiple vehicles? Are the vehicles involved gasoline, diesel, hybrid, or all electric? Are the vehicles positioned upright or on their roof or side? How many victims are involved?
- *Risk assessment*: What types of hazards are present (e.g., fuel, electric lines, gas lines, terrain, or bodies of water)?
- *Resource availability and capability*: What resources can you call to assist?
- *Witness information*: Did anyone leave the scene? What was the direction of travel and approximate speed of the vehicles involved?
- *Reference materials*: Check available references (e.g., the alternative fuel vehicle handbook or *Emergency Response Guidebook*).

Remember that the company officer develops the IAP using the base procedures outlined in the organization's SOPs for an operations-level response to a motor vehicle accident. The company officer then builds off the SOPs, uses the information collected, and presents the IAP's Plan A (vehicle entry plan and tactical assignment), Plan B (victim access and removal plan), and emergency plan (including immediate evacuation procedures for the team and victim[s]). The IAP will be discussed further in Chapter 9, *Victim Access and Management*.

Vehicle Rescue and Extrication Resources

Every chapter in this text stresses the need to maintain and follow all safety guidelines and compliance mandates applicable to local, state, tribal, provincial, or federal regulations and recommendations. Reports, published research studies, and publications issued by independent safety science companies, such as Underwriters Laboratories (UL), and all tool and equipment manufacturer recommendations should also be followed.

Specialists

There are also a number of excellent resources and opportunities for acquiring vehicle rescue and extrication information and training. Local fire academies, training institutes, and contracted training specialists that offer vehicle rescue and extrication programs are excellent options; just ensure that any academy, teaching institution, or specialist is qualified by the represented state to teach NFPA 1006– and NFPA 1670–level programs.

Online Resources

The Internet is probably the most economical and convenient resource for acquiring vehicle rescue and extrication information. Search engines can locate photos from across the globe of vehicle rescue incidents requiring extrication. With a little time and patience, finding and piecing together a motor vehicle accident scene as it evolved can pay off in dividends for the technical rescuer. This is a great opportunity to study a vehicle rescue incident and deduce what you believe to be the positives and negatives of how the incident was handled and then to develop your own IAP for how you would have managed/mitigated the incident based on your organization's SOPs and your training or operational skill level. These incidents can also be the basis for training assignments, such as an inside classroom project using a PowerPoint presentation or an outside, hands-on training scenario in which you set up a reenactment of the incident. There are numerous training articles, outlines, and websites on vehicle rescue practices and technology that can be downloaded and utilized at your convenience; all it takes is time and a few strokes on the keyboard (**FIGURE 1-3**).

Emergency Field Guide

Another available resource tool is the NFPA's *Alternative-Fuel Vehicles Safety Training Program Emergency Field Guide*, which is a great resource for responders to use as a quick vehicle reference system. It details various vehicle types, models, and components, including alternative fuels, hybrid and electric propulsion systems, safety systems consisting of SRS and related components, and electrical hazards. The field reference uses the *Emergency Response Guides* developed by the vehicle manufacturers for

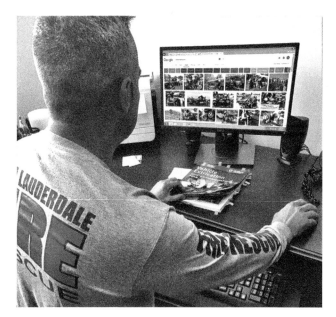

FIGURE 1-3 Training outlines and photos of vehicle rescue incidents requiring extrication can be easily downloaded from the Internet and used to develop a training program.
Courtesy of David Sweet.

each specific vehicle model. Included in these guides is a generalization of procedures for managing vehicle fires, spills, and submersions, and providing basic first aid (**FIGURE 1-4**).

Challenge Events

One of the overall best resources is vehicle rescue competition/challenge events, which are scheduled throughout the year and across the world by several vehicle rescue competition committee organizations. These organizations focus on a common goal: promoting the advancement in education and training in the practice of vehicle rescue management. In the competition/challenge section of these events, teams are measured in three areas that encompass the IAP and overall management of a simulated motor vehicle accident (MVA) using live victims. These components are:

1. Incident command/safety
2. Technical proficiency
3. Medical intervention

Fire rescue organizations and individual personnel do not have to put a team together and compete to be able to attend one of these events. A vast amount of knowledge, information, and general networking is readily available to anyone by just attending one of these events as a spectator and viewing/studying a few of these highly skilled vehicle rescue teams conduct an operation in one of the many assigned MVA scenarios scheduled throughout the day (**FIGURE 1-5**).

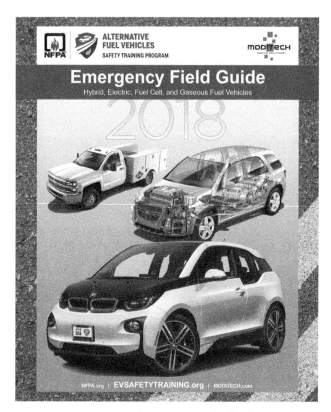

FIGURE 1-4 NFPA's *Alternative-Fuel Vehicles Safety Training Program Emergency Field Guide*.
© NFPA National Fire Protection Association.

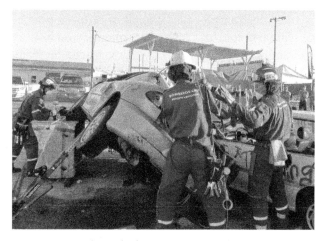

FIGURE 1-5 The Vehicle Rescue Team of Cali Columbia competes in the National Vehicle Rescue and Extrication Challenge.
Courtesy of David Sweet.

The Transportation Emergency Response Committee (TERC), which was first established in 1987, was the catalyst behind the initial movement of training teams using the concept of vehicle rescue management. TERC continues to present vehicle rescue challenges in North America and Canada throughout the year. Another organization is the North American Vehicle Rescue Association (NAVRA), which presents qualifying regional and national vehicle rescue challenge events throughout the year in North America, with top teams advancing to the World Rescue Challenge. NAVRA works hand in hand with the World Rescue Organization (WRO), which is the governing committee organization for the annual World Rescue Challenge.

The World Rescue Challenge hosts fire rescue organizations, medical professionals, instructors, technical rescue specialists, and tool and equipment vendors from across the world to come together to train, compete, and/or share information to advance science, technology, and methodology in vehicle rescue management and trauma casualty care and management. The World Rescue Challenge hosts some of the best vehicle rescue teams and trauma teams to compete in challenge events consisting of realistic scenario-based MVA incident simulations and trauma casualty care and management incidents.

Scenario-Based Training

Fire rescue organizations and/or an AHJ can benefit from using the same scenario-based training template and assessment criteria forms developed by competition committees to coordinate and provide training programs that fulfill the NFPA 1670 requirements (to meet or exceed the level of operational response capability for their jurisdiction) as well as the personnel JPRs outlined by NFPA 1006. An assessment form is an evaluation tool that measures job performance benchmarks for three levels of proficiency on how an operational team manages a vehicle rescue incident. These forms can be modified by a fire rescue organization or an AHJ to meet both the proper skill levels for personnel as outlined in NFPA 1006 and response capability as outlined in NFPA 1670. The three levels of proficiency flow in ascending order where a team can:

1. Complete the operation demonstrating a Basic level of proficiency (substitute/adapt to awareness level)
2. Complete the operation demonstrating an Efficient level of proficiency (substitute/adapt to operations level)
3. Complete the operation demonstrating the highest level of proficiency, which is the Thorough level (substitute/adapt to technician level)

Scenario-based training gives the AHJ and/or instructor the ability to set similar incidents experienced in the jurisdiction that were predetermined through the evaluation process for assessing technical search and rescue hazards within the response area. Scenario-based training also allows for the option to use instructors as interior victims, which understandably can pose a significant safety risk, but the benefit comes from an experienced instructor who is able to provide firsthand information and direction to personnel conducting the operations. Interior victim instructors can offer immediate teaching points on correct technique and placement, proper application of various tools and equipment, and direction in the proper sequence of events for various procedures. Instructors can also provide medical feedback for injuries presented and treatment procedures, express when excessive manipulation of the victim occurs, and identify any possible tool intrusion in areas that can compromise victim and personnel safety. These are valuable lessons to which personnel would otherwise never be exposed if the common standard of practice were to continue the same training routine using a mannequin as the victim or conducting static training with no victim or pressing urgency as experienced at an actual real-life emergency incident. Static type training can be useful when introducing a new tool or demonstrating a technique, a procedure, or an application, but scenario-based training promotes progressive real-life learning that best prepares personnel for managing real-life incidents in their response jurisdiction.

To maintain a safe working environment at all times, it is not recommended for inexperienced instructors or nonqualified personnel to participate as victims. Participation as a victim instructor requires a vast amount of experience, a keen eye, and control to ensure that the highest level of safety is always followed. Technical rescue operations are an inherently dangerous practice, and sometimes, even with established safety procedures being followed and securely in place, unexpected or unforeseen accidents or casualties may occur (**FIGURE 1-6**).

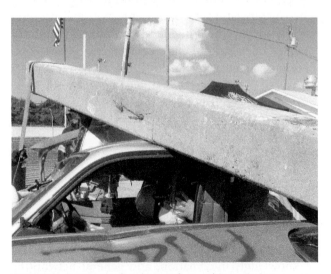

FIGURE 1-6 To maintain a safe working environment, an inexperienced instructor or nonqualified person should not act as a victim. Participation as a victim requires a vast amount of experience to ensure that the highest level of safety is followed.
Courtesy of David Sweet.

To acquire the most benefit from scenario-based training, an organization/AHJ should use three experienced instructors when possible, mirroring the competition/challenge-style format. This offers an opportunity for instructors to teach as well as assess each position simultaneously throughout the evolution. An example of this could be where one instructor monitors/assesses the incident commander position and overall operational management and safety of the scenario, another instructor monitors/assesses the technical position(s) (including tool and equipment application and management), and the third instructor monitors/assesses the medical intervention position by participating as the victim.

Scenario-based training gives the AHJ the ability to evaluate personnel and determine where operational corrections need to be made and also the ability to custom design evolutions that focus on teaching personnel and/or group skills that meet or exceed the JPRs and operational response capability required for the rescue organization. Personnel can be trained and rotated through each of the three operational levels (awareness, operations, technician) for each operational position (incident command, technical, medical).

LISTEN UP!

"See it! Learn it! Master it! Teach it!" is a learning process that combines the benefits of different learning styles to produce maximum understanding and comprehension of a skill. To become proficient at a skill, a person must first *see* the skill demonstrated and then *learn* how to perform the skill by going over it step by step, *master* the skill by continually training on it, and pass the skill along by *teaching* someone else. Following these steps in the cycle of learning should always produce the best results (**FIGURE 1-7**).

See it!

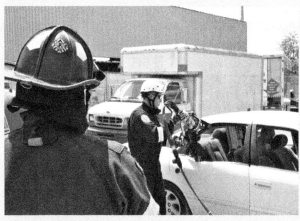

Learn it!

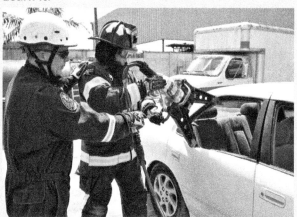

Master it!

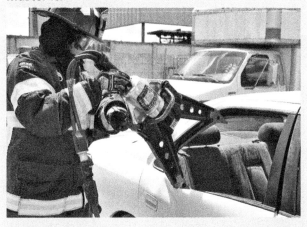

Teach it!

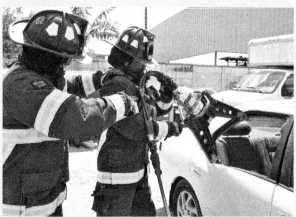

FIGURE 1-7 Maximum learning is best acquired when the four processes in the cycle of learning are followed: "See it! Learn it! Master it! Teach it!"
Courtesy of Edward Monahan.

Continuous Improvement

Training should always be progressive and continuous. Look for ways to stay involved in education and training, and always be open to learning new skills. Sharing resources by organizing vehicle rescue and extrication training events with neighboring fire rescue organizations or contacting a competition committee to host a local extrication competition/challenge together with area fire rescue organizations enables organizations to be engaged and stay active in education and training.

Participating in a team event like a vehicle extrication challenge immediately elevates skills, which then circulate throughout an organization, encouraging each member to improve by wanting to provide a better, more efficient level of service to the community. This desire for improvement occurs because of the sharing of ideas and the viewing of other fire rescue organizations' performance and skills at a competition/challenge. The positive results produced will emphasize the importance of training and motivate others to train.

After-Action REVIEW

IN SUMMARY

- Possessing only a basic skill set and understanding in vehicle rescue is no longer sufficient to successfully manage an MVA involving the disentanglement and extrication of trapped victims.
- Compliance with standards is considered voluntary, unless the standards are formally adopted by a state, a province, a county, a government municipality, or an organization. Once a standard is adopted, it takes on the force of law.
- NFPA 1006 defines the position of technical rescue personnel and establishes the minimum JPRs for technical rescue personnel who perform technical rescue operations, with the intent to ensure that the individuals serving as technical rescue personnel are qualified.
- NFPA 1670 identifies and establishes levels of functional capabilities for rescue organizations to safely and effectively conduct operations at technical rescue incidents, including vehicle rescue and extrication incidents.
- At a minimum, all emergency services organizations must have SOPs for managing a vehicle rescue and extrication incident, which establish guidelines that minimize risk and threats and provide consistency and safety for all personnel to follow.
- There are several safety guidelines and compliance mandates to follow at the local, state, tribal, provincial, and federal levels. Reports, published research studies, and publications issued by independent safety science companies, such as Underwriters Laboratories (UL), and all tool and equipment manufacturer recommendations should also be followed.
- Training should always be progressive and continuous. Look for ways to stay involved in education and training, and always be open to learning new skills.

KEY TERMS

Authority having jurisdiction (AHJ) An organization, office, or individual responsible for enforcing the requirements of a code or standard, or for approving equipment, materials, an installation, or a procedure. (NFPA 1006)

Awareness level (1) This level represents the minimum capability of individuals who provide response to technical search and rescue incidents. (NFPA 1006) (2) This level represents the minimum capability of organizations that provide response to technical search and rescue incidents. (NFPA 1670)

Common passenger vehicle Light or medium duty passenger and commercial vehicles commonly encountered in the jurisdiction and presenting no unusual construction, occupancy, or operational characteristics to rescuers during an extrication event. (NFPA 1006)

Disentanglement The cutting of a vehicle away from trapped or injured victims. (NFPA 1670)

Extrication The removal of trapped victims from a vehicle or machinery. (NFPA 1670)

Formal incident action plans An IAP that is a formally written document and designed within an ICS for operational periods that generally run 12 or 24 hours and last from several days to weeks.

Incident action plan (IAP) A verbal or written plan containing incident objectives reflecting the overall strategy and specific control actions where appropriate for managing an incident or planned event. (NFPA 1026)

Informal incident action plans An IAP that is not a formally written document and is designed for small incidents that are mitigated before an operational period is designated.

NFPA 1006 The standard that establishes the minimum job performance requirements/qualifications necessary for fire service and other emergency response personnel who perform technical rescue. This standard outlines three qualification levels: awareness, operations, and technician.

NFPA 1670 The standard that identifies and qualifies levels of functional capabilities for safely and effectively conducting operations at technical rescue incidents. This standard outlines three operational capability levels: awareness, operations, and technician.

Operations level (1) This level represents the capability of individuals to respond to technical search and rescue incidents and to identify hazards, use equipment, and apply limited techniques specified in this standard to support and participate in technical search and rescue incidents. (NFPA 1006) (2) This level represents the capability of organizations to respond to technical search and rescue incidents and to identify hazards, use equipment, and apply limited techniques specified in this standard to support and participate in technical search and rescue incidents. (NFPA 1670)

Qualification Having satisfactorily completed the requirements of the objectives. (NFPA 1006)

Standard An NFPA Standard, the main text of which contains only mandatory provisions using the word "shall" to indicate requirements and that is in a form generally suitable for mandatory reference by another standard or code or for adoption into law. Nonmandatory provisions are not to be considered a part of the requirements of a standard and shall be located in an appendix, annex, footnote, informational note, or other means as permitted in the NFPA *Manuals of Style*. When used in a generic sense, such as in the phrase "standards development process" or "standards development activities," the term "standards" encompasses all NFPA Standards, including Codes, Standards, Recommended Practices, and Guides. (NFPA 1006)

Technical rescue The application of special knowledge, skills, and equipment to safely resolve unique and/or complex rescue situations. (NFPA 1670)

Technical rescuer A person who is trained to perform or direct the technical rescue. (NFPA 1006)

Technical search and rescue incidents Complex search and/or rescue incidents requiring specialized training of personnel and special equipment to complete the mission. (NFPA 1006)

Technician level (1) This level represents the capability of individuals to respond to technical search and rescue incidents and to identify hazards, use equipment, and apply advanced techniques specified in this standard necessary to coordinate, perform, and supervise technical search and rescue incidents. (NFPA 1006) (2) This level represents the capability of organizations to respond to technical search and rescue incidents and to identify hazards, use equipment, and apply advanced techniques specified in this standard necessary to coordinate, perform, and supervise technical search and rescue incidents. (NFPA 1670)

REFERENCES

National Fire Protection Association. 2017. *NFPA 1670, Standard on Operations and Training for Technical Search and Rescue Incidents*. 2017 ed. Quincy, MA: NFPA.

National Fire Protection Association. 2021. *NFPA 1006, Standard for Technical Rescue Personnel Professional Qualifications*. 2021 ed. Quincy, MA: NFPA.

NHTSA. 2020. National Highway Traffic Safety Administration. Overview of Motor Vehicle Crashes in 2019. https://crashstats.nhtsa.dot.gov/Api/Public/ViewPublication/813060. Accessed February 21, 2021.

On Scene

As a technical rescuer, the only way to become proficient in this specialized field is through continuous training and dedication.

1. The 2019 National Highway Traffic Safety Administration (NHTSA) summary of motor vehicle accidents reported a high of _____ motor vehicle collisions in the United States.
   A. 2.5 million
   B. 3.5 million
   C. 6.7 million
   D. 9.5 million

2. NFPA 1670 outlines three levels of functional capabilities for the technical rescuer; they are awareness level, operations level, and:
   A. special master level.
   B. master level.
   C. superior level.
   D. technician level.

3. The operations level is the minimum level at which all agencies must be able to operate at a technical rescue incident.
   A. True
   B. False

4. The learning process that combines the benefits of different learning styles to produce maximum understanding and comprehension of a skill requires the technical rescuer to See it! Learn it!
   A. Master it! Teach it!
   B. Show it! Copy it!
   C. Teach it! Understand it!
   D. Comprehend it! Forget it!

5. NFPA 1006 identifies the minimum job performance requirements (JPRs) for _____.
   A. technical rescue team
   B. organizations
   C. technical rescue personnel
   D. AHJ

6. Extrication when used as a term in vehicle rescue and extrication is defined as the _____ of removing a trapped victim from a vehicle.
   A. technique
   B. process
   C. intervention
   D. standard of care

7. According to the NFPA, a technical rescuer is a person who is trained to perform or direct a:
   A. situation.
   B. technical extrication.
   C. technical rescue.
   D. scene.

8. An organization, office, or individual responsible for enforcing the requirements of a code or standard, or for approving equipment, materials, an installation, or a procedure, is the definition for the:
   A. code of ethics.
   B. technical rescue procedure.
   C. standard operation procedures.
   D. authority having jurisdiction.

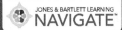

CHAPTER 2

Awareness Level

Vehicle Rescue Incident Awareness

KNOWLEDGE OBJECTIVES

After studying this chapter, you should be able to:
- Define the following terms:
  - Risk assessment (p. 21)
  - Hazard analysis (pp. 21–22)
  - Organizational analysis (pp. 22–23)
  - Risk–benefit analysis (pp. 23–24)
  - Level of response analysis (p. 24)
- Explain how a community assessment is used to determine service level needs. (pp. 21–24)
- Identify the two types of risk–benefit analysis performed at a vehicle rescue incident. (**NFPA 1006: 8.1.3**, pp. 23–24)
- Explain the purpose of a standard operating procedure. (pp. 24–25)
- Identify information necessary to preplan a vehicle rescue response. (pp. 25–26)
- Explain the importance of resource identification and allocation in the preplanning process. (**NFPA 1006 8.1.4**, pp. 25–26)
- Identify jurisdictional authority considerations at a vehicle rescue incident. (p. 26)
- Explain the application of incident command to a technical rescue incident. (**NFPA 1006: 8.1.2**, pp. 28–29)
- Articulate the importance of scene time awareness at a vehicle accident. (pp. 35–36)
- Define the following terms and explain their role in vehicle rescue incidents:
  - Golden Period. (**NFPA 1006: 8.1.3**, pp. 35–36)
  - Defensive apparatus placement. (**NFPA 1006: 8.1.3**, p. 38)
  - Traffic incident management (TIM). (**NFPA 1006: 8.1.3**, p. 38)
- List information to be included in a vehicle extrication scene size-up. (**NFPA 1006: 8.1.1, 8.1.2, 8.1.4**, pp. 42–43)
- Describe the role of the awareness-level responder at the scene, including:
  - The identification of potential hazards. (**NFPA 1006: 8.1.1, 8.1.3, 8.1.4**, pp. 42–43)

SKILLS OBJECTIVES

After studying this chapter, you should be able to:
- Gather information to prepare a preincident plan. (**NFPA 1006: 8.1.2**, pp. 25–26)
- Establish initial incident command at a technical rescue. (**NFPA 1006 8.1.5**, pp. 26–28)
- Communicate information within an established chain of command. (**NFPA 1006: 8.1.5**, pp. 28–32)
- Conduct a scene size-up for a vehicle collision. (**NFPA 1006: 8.1.1, 8.1.3, 8.1.4**, pp. 42–43)

You Are the Rescuer

You are dispatched to a vehicle accident involving a school bus with reported injuries. Your unit is the first of multiple units to arrive on scene. On arrival, you report to dispatch that you have a large C-type school bus on its side with heavy damage and approximately 50 injured students.

1. Does your organization have the appropriate level response capability to manage this type of incident (NFPA 1670)?
2. Will this incident require that an incident command system be used?
3. What resources will be needed to manage this incident?

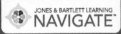

Access Navigate for more practice activities.

Introduction

While conducting rescue and extrication operations at a motor vehicle accident, it is easy to toss the basic fundamentals of vehicle extrication aside and replace them with emotionally driven actions such as *"Just rip the door off and yank the victim out!"* At a vehicle rescue and extrication incident, a rescuer's fight-or-flight response mechanism of the central nervous system will always be active, with emotions running high. This is not an excuse for poor technique or lack of a structured plan. As professionals, we need to be skill driven and follow an **incident action plan (IAP)** based on sound, measurable objectives that reflect the overall strategy for managing the incident (**FIGURE 2-1**). IAPs are discussed in more detail in Chapter 4, *Site Operations*.

In sports, the winning individual or team is usually the one that does the most preparation, follows the game plan, and can execute the basics to perfection. The athlete or team fully understands its challenge or opponent before stepping onto the ball field or into the ring. The great football coach Vince Lombardi based his winning philosophy on focusing and drilling his team on perfecting the basics and building a strong foundation. He believed that if his team mastered the basics, then success would always follow. This philosophy is no different for the technical rescuer, for whom training is directly related to performance; the more preparation, training, and study that are done before the call, the more success you will have.

> **LISTEN UP!**
>
> Vehicle rescue and extrication should never be emotion driven; it should be skill driven.

The fire rescue or emergency services organization must display the ability and skill level to manage an emergency incident effectively, whether large or small. At a minimum, an organization must have the response capability and training to perform awareness-level scene management skills at a technical rescue incident. This chapter discusses the overall planning process for determining an organization's level of operational capability, developing standard operating procedures (SOPs) for the organization, understanding basic operational criteria and preincident planning required for a technical rescue incident, and using the **incident command system (ICS)**.

For a fire rescue organization that has been adequately functioning as an emergency service provider, it is understandable that implementing the requirements and competencies set forth in NFPA 1006, *Standard for Technical Rescuer Professional Qualifications*, and NFPA 1670, *Standard on Operations and Training for Technical Search and Rescue Incidents*, may be met with some resistance if it requires the organization to change the operational structure. With

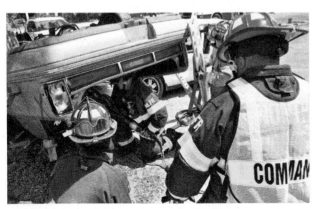

FIGURE 2-1 The incident action plan outlines the objectives that reflect the overall strategy for managing the incident.
Courtesy of David Sweet.

any organizational change, it is important for the authority having jurisdiction (AHJ) and/or the organization not to become overly focused on terminology or chasing titles or tags.

Determining Level of Service

The term *technical rescuer* refers to someone qualified with a particular skill set, in this case vehicle rescue and extrication. You don't have to be on a technical rescue team or squad to be a technical rescuer. NFPA 1006 Section 3.3.198 states that a technical search and rescue incident consists of "complex search and/or rescue incidents requiring specialized training of personnel and special equipment to complete the mission." The goal here is to focus on what level of service (what type of calls you respond to) the fire rescue organization provides for the community or jurisdiction and to identify or match the skills with the action provided based on the operational criteria established in NFPA 1006 and 1670. Most, if not all, fire rescue organizations already provide a level of service to manage complex emergency incidents, such as vehicle rescue and extrication incidents. What level of response capability is the organization currently able to provide? What level is needed to adequately support the community or jurisdiction? To determine the answers to these questions, the AHJ must conduct a risk assessment study of the community and organization.

Risk Assessment

A risk assessment is a process that identifies risks and vulnerabilities to which a community, an organization, or a business is exposed and then determines the actions required to reduce these risks and vulnerabilities. Conducting a community and organizational risk assessment is vital to understanding what level of response capability a fire rescue organization currently has in place and what is going to be required of the organization to reduce the risks and vulnerabilities that the community and/or jurisdiction is exposed to. Four research areas that are used to develop a risk assessment are:

- Hazard analysis
- Organizational analysis
- Risk–benefit analysis
- Level of response analysis

To properly determine the level of response for an organization, the AHJ must acquire the appropriate data identifying the risks. The AHJ cannot just state that because the agency responds to many vehicle accidents that are manged appropriately, it is assumed that the agency is at an operational level. Data must support the function. Developing a community and organizational risk assessment does not require the AHJ to produce a doctoral thesis, but the process should consist of a standard method to come to a factual determination. This is a basic evaluation process that identifies (from an emergency response standpoint) what is actually occurring in the community or general response area.

With this information, the AHJ can determine whether the organization is appropriately equipped to manage these types of incidents as well as actions or steps required to minimize risks associated with those incidents. This analysis in turn will identify and legitimize the current operational response capability of the organization. In addition, this information can provide justification for the AHJ to hire additional personnel; develop the appropriate operating procedures and protocols; provide the appropriate level of training; purchase equipment, including the proper level of personal protective equipment (PPE); procure resource contracts; and negotiate mutual aid agreements.

Hazard Analysis

Hazard analysis is the identification of situations or conditions that have the potential to cause harm and/or injury to the public and personnel, damage to property and the environment, and/or significant economic impact to the community and emergency service providers. In 1993, Hurricane Andrew made landfall in south Florida as a category 5 storm, causing massive widespread devastation to the region. A storm of this strength had not made landfall in the United States in several decades, and in the absence of ever having experienced this type of impact, there was a breakdown in preparation, proper planning, and managing an incident of this magnitude. Any major natural disaster immediately disables and overwhelms local resources and emergency services, but if a thorough risk assessment has been conducted (including a hazard analysis), there is time to set the proper measures and emergency operational procedures in place to account for these losses and to assist in providing the necessary resources to sustain and support the area or region.

Applying a hazard analysis to vehicle rescue and extrication incidents can uncover a multitude of issues that have to be accounted for. Inclement weather can have a major adverse effect on an operation. South Florida in the summertime can have temperatures upwards of 95°F (35°C), which may not seem extreme, but combined with a 100 percent humidity factor will cause personnel to be overcome quickly by heat exhaustion. In contrast, Nebraska has to account for freezing conditions in the winter, which causes such hazards as ice slick roadways and cold exposure injuries. In such cases, the AHJ must provide the appropriate PPE and the proper equipment and training and ensure that rehabilitation policies and procedures are in place to assist in better managing these hazards.

Hazardous conditions may be a consistent known factor for roadway travel with certain topographic features, such as ravines, mountain ranges, and bodies of water. In addition, known seasonal weather changes and increased traffic flow from vacationing visitors occur within the same time span each year. These types of hazards are much easier to predict and plan for, but hazardous conditions that may be a daily, weekly, or monthly event, such as road or lane closures from road construction and general maintenance, can cause havoc to unsuspecting travelers and responding emergency apparatus and increase the likelihood of collisions. Developing an open line of communication with the jurisdiction's public works department or roadway management department by simply asking to be notified prior to any known road closures occurring greatly reduces unexpected hazards and/or response delays. The AHJ needs to determine not only the possibility but, more importantly, the probability of various incidents or conditions occurring within its jurisdiction.

Data research through incident run reports and area surveys can identify the types of incidents that have occurred and are likely to occur within a jurisdiction. This type of research should be conducted at various times throughout the year to account for any crash trends or seasonal increase or decrease in roadway congestion. When conducting a hazard analysis, it is always a good idea to identify and secure your roadways first and then continue to the jurisdictional area. Survey all the major roadways within the jurisdiction, and determine the type of traffic flow: Is the roadway mainly used for residential traffic with an occasional petroleum tanker passing through, or is it mainly used for industrial traffic where hazardous transport cargo travels along with residential flows? What are some ancillary access routes and containment plans that can be set in place?

Another resource to assist the AHJ in predetermining potential roadway hazards is a comprehensive transportation plan developed by the highway, roadway, or transit authority for a municipality, state, or government agency. This plan outlines the multimodal transportation system for a specific geographic or regional location, placing an emphasis on public transportation and roadway traffic flow movement. Identified in the plan are designated emergency evacuation routes; existing peak traffic hours for main roadways; peak direction of travel for roadways; locations of public transit facilities, corridors, or routes such as rail and bus transit, including bicycle; and general walkways. The plan also lists future roadway expansions and general roadway maintenance schedules.

The AHJ may require a traffic incident management class or similar training or even particular safety equipment to manage roadway hazards. Consider whether the organization has the training and equipment to manage a roadway hazardous materials incident properly or whether local resource contracts and/or automatic aid agreements can be obtained from another emergency response organization.

Organizational Analysis

The next area of research in the risk assessment process is an organizational analysis, which seeks to determine what level of response capability is currently in place and whether the organization requires additional training, equipment, personnel, or external resources to meet the required response capability needed for the jurisdiction.

The first step is to look at the personnel requirements. Technical rescue incidents such as motor vehicle accidents can be physically, psychologically, and mentally intensive, requiring the rescuers to perform their duties under stressful conditions. NFPA 1500, *Standard on Fire Department Occupational Safety, Health, and Wellness Program*, Chapters 11 to 13, outline the medical, physical, fitness, and psychological requirements for the performance of duty. NFPA 1500 also references the requirements for establishing a health and wellness program for the organization. Additionally, NFPA 1582, *Standard on Comprehensive Occupational Medical Program for Fire Departments*, presents descriptive requirements for a comprehensive occupational medical program for public, governmental, military, private, and industrial fire departments.

Consider the staffing levels for the organization. Based on past data research, how many responders are required to manage the most common technical rescue incident for the jurisdiction? What type of equipment and PPE are required? Does the organization provide the appropriate apparatus? Does the organization have the financial resources to develop, train for, and maintain the capability as well as purchase the appropriate equipment to support operations?

Training—both initial and ongoing—is a critical component in supporting the appropriate level of response for managing technical rescue incidents within a jurisdiction. Once the level of response capability for the organization is determined or achieving a higher level is deemed necessary, then the required training to meet, maintain, or achieve a higher level must be identified, as should a facility that can provide that level of training. Can the appropriate validated training be acquired locally through a fire training academy or private vendor? What will it cost to obtain and/or maintain the required level of service? Validated technical rescue training programs are state- or federally approved programs that meet or exceed recommended guidelines established through the NFPA and/or Occupational Safety and Health Administration (OSHA).

Training facilities, such as a local fire academy, may provide the technical rescue programs that meet an organization's response needs for its jurisdiction (**FIGURE 2-2**).

Providing technical rescue services can require a significant amount of resources both logistically and financially. Does the organization have the financial resources necessary to support the current or proposed level of response capabilities? Can budgetary adjustments or fire assessment programs be implemented? Are there external funding mechanisms available through local, state, or federal grants? The AHJ needs to determine which resources are available within the jurisdiction and what is available from outside sources, such as mutual aid, local industry, private vendors, and state or federal agencies. Consider the procurement of specialized equipment, tools, consumable supplies, PPE, apparatus, and maintenance contracts/agreements. A list of internal and external resources should be made, updated yearly, and kept available at all times.

Risk–Benefit Analysis

A risk–benefit analysis is the calculation and quantification of whether performing an action will produce a positive or negative outcome. There are two types of risk–benefit analysis that must be performed: a static analysis and an active analysis. A static risk–benefit analysis is conducted in an office setting prior to any incident. This type of analysis is an evaluation and a justification of whether to acquire/support the required level of service needed to manage a technician level technical rescue incident that has the potential to occur or has occurred in the past within the jurisdiction. Two important questions should be considered when conducting a static risk–benefit analysis:

1. Does the organization currently have in place the response capability to manage/mitigate a technician level incident?
2. Is it feasible to acquire, maintain, and support this level of service?

The AHJ and/or organization must determine the capability and feasibility required to manage this type of incident. Does it benefit the jurisdiction, municipality, or town to invest in the training, additional personnel, apparatus, and equipment to support this required level of service when only one or two technician level incidents are likely to occur annually? The financial, environmental, physical, social, and cultural condition of the jurisdiction, municipality, or town must be considered and could pose a financial risk in supporting this level of service. Would the organization be better served to contract out those specialized resources through mutual or automatic aid agreements and maintain a supporting role in a technician level incident?

Every emergency incident that fire rescue personnel respond to poses a certain degree of risk, but some operations have much higher risks than others (**FIGURE 2-3**).

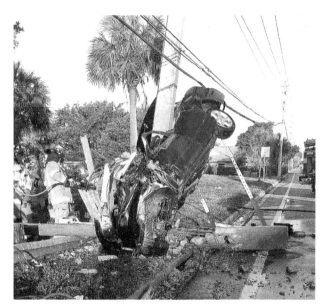

FIGURE 2-3 The high risks associated with some incidents require the scene to be stabilized and the hazards mitigated prior to the performance of the rescue.
Courtesy of Jeff Lopez.

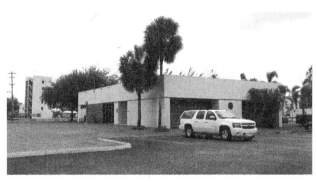

FIGURE 2-2 Training facilities, such as a local fire academy, may provide the technical rescue programs to meet an organization's required response capability.
Courtesy of Edward Monahan.

An **active risk–benefit analysis** occurs during the incident response and/or prior to actively engaging in the operation. This analysis entails an assessment of the risk to personnel and/or victims compared to the benefits that might result from the rescue. Two important questions should be considered when conducting an active risk–benefit analysis:

1. What are the immediate, probable, or possible dangers or harm to personnel?
2. Is the incident a rescue or a recovery operation?

Vehicle rescue and extrication incidents, regardless of the size, require a risk–benefit analysis to be made quickly to determine the safety and necessity of the operation. Will the operation require immediate intervention, or can the operation be delayed based on the viability of the victims or an impending hazard that requires specialized equipment and/or advanced skills beyond the level of response capability? An example would be an underride incident involving a common passenger vehicle colliding with a petroleum tanker, trapping the occupant in the passenger vehicle and causing a tank breach with an active leak. Would this incident be a cause for rushing in and pulling the victim out without assessing the risk to personnel and determining the appropriate action plan to stabilize the scene before entering the hazard zone? Absolutely not! The scene would have to be properly assessed for the risks versus the benefits, and then an action plan would be established and put in place to minimize and/or eliminate those risks.

Level of Response Analysis

One of the AHJ's top priorities should be recognizing the need to provide the appropriate level of service to manage a technical rescue incident for the response jurisdiction. NFPA 1670 states that every organization that responds to technical rescue incidents should have at a minimum the capability of an awareness-level response. Based on the information obtained during the community risk assessment—which includes the hazard analysis, organizational analysis, and risk–benefit analyses—it should be fairly easy to determine the appropriate level of response capability for the organization and to develop a strategic plan of action to either provide that level of service or procure the appropriate resources to assist in providing that level of service.

Organizations with a response area that mainly consists of residential communities may respond only to vehicle rescue and extrication incidents involving common passenger vehicles, with a rare entrapment involving a commercial vehicle. The organization should be trained at an operations or a technician level in heavy vehicle rescue to properly address this type of incident. Performance levels and training are evaluated and documented annually to determine whether the organization and personnel are prepared to manage a potential emergency incident recognized in the community risk assessment. All training must be documented with the data readily available to those who are authorized to view it.

> **LISTEN UP!**
>
> Conducting operations at a technical rescue incident require a consistent approach, regardless of the level of response capability of the organization.

Conducting operations at a technical rescue incident require a consistent approach, regardless of the level of response capability of the organization. Using the ICS and SOPs provides a consistent, step-by-step approach for preparing, assessing, and responding to vehicle rescue and extrication incidents in a safe, effective, and efficient manner. An example of a step-by-step approach may be as follows:

1. Preparation
2. Response
3. Arrival and size-up
4. Stabilization: scene–vehicle–victim
5. Access
6. Disentanglement
7. Removal
8. Transport
9. Incident termination
10. Postincident debriefing and analysis

At the awareness level, responders may be capable of completing only steps 1 through 3 and part of step 4 (stabilization of the scene). The operations- or technician-level responders who have the qualifications to manage the remaining assignments would then complete the operation.

Standard Operating Procedures

A **standard operating procedure (SOP)** is an organizational directive that establishes a standard course of action; in other words, it provides written guidelines that explain what is expected and required of emergency services personnel while performing their job (**FIGURE 2-4**). SOPs are not intended to tell you how to do the job (technical knowledge and skills) but

Anytown Fire Rescue Department

| Policy # SOP OP 8 | Effective Date: 5/22/2018 | Fire Chief's Signature *John Smith* |

Subject: Vehicle Rescue and Extrication Operation Guidelines

FIRE DEPARTMENT REGULATION: OP 8

SUBJECT: Vehicle Rescue and Extrication Operation Guidelines

References: NFPA 1670: *STANDARD ON OPERATIONS AND TRAINING FOR TECHNICAL SEARCH AND RESCUE INCIDENTS*

NFPA 1006: *STANDARD FOR TECHNIC AL RESCUER PROFESS IONAL QUALIFICATIONS*

PURPOSE: To provide a clear understanding of the policy and procedures regarding the safe, efficient, and organized approach to any incident requiring vehicle rescue and extrication.

SCOPE/APPLICATION: To maintain safety and continuity within the organization, these guidelines are applicable to all personnel that respond, train, or otherwise perform vehicle rescue and extrication for the Anytown Fire Rescue Department.

FIGURE 2-4 A section of a sample SOP regarding vehicle rescue and extrication operation guidelines.

rather are designed to describe related considerations (the rules for doing the job), such as safety, evacuation, communication and notification procedures, command structures, and reporting requirements. Technical knowledge and skills, such as how to rappel or operate a specific tool, are obtained through training and technical protocols and are not normally the subject of SOPs. The AHJ shall establish written SOPs consistent with the identified level of operational capability for the jurisdiction to ensure that technical search and rescue operations are performed in a manner that minimizes threats to rescuers and others.

Incident Response Planning

Sound, timely planning provides the foundation for effective incident management. Response planning (preincident planning) is the process of compiling, documenting, and dispersing information that assists the organization should an incident occur at a particular location. Although there are frequently variables in any incident type, preincident response planning provides the framework of the organization's response. The major components of a response plan include the identification of potential problems and issues; resource identification and allocation; and, in some cases, suggested or mandatory procedures. Additional administrative elements include plan authority and approval plus determining who gets a copy of the plan and when the plan is to be implemented and revised (including those with responsibilities outlined in the plan). A system should be in place for making changes or revisions to the plan.

Problem Identification

To write any plan, you must first identify the problem. This is accomplished by conducting the risk assessment, as discussed earlier in this chapter. This assessment, along with the organization's identified operational capability, forms the basis of what the plan will try to accomplish. Whether a single plan or multiple plans are used will depend on the complexity of your organization's involvement in a given rescue incident type.

Resource Identification and Allocation

Response planning is pointless if there are no resources to implement it. The necessary resources (personnel, equipment, and materials) must be identified and must be available in a timely manner. Frequently, this goal is accomplished through the use of mutual aid agreements, although some resources may require other arrangements. For example, agreements may be made with private vendors, such as contractors, for heavy equipment. When possible, these arrangements should be made before the incident occurs and put in writing to try to avoid any confusion.

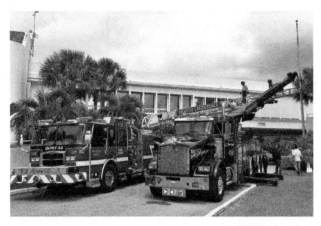

FIGURE 2-5 The preincident plan should include any forms, contracts, or agreements with local resources that might be necessary during the incident.
Courtesy of David Sweet.

Once you have identified these resources, collect the necessary information pertaining to them. This includes procedures for obtaining the needed resource and contact information, such as names and phone numbers. Review this information at least annually to ensure it is still accurate. The preincident plan should also include any forms or agreements that might be necessary during the incident (**FIGURE 2-5**).

Operational Procedures

The preincident plan should identify not only what resources are needed but also how they will be used (deployed). The plan should identify alternative resources in the event that a particular resource is unavailable. It should identify possible scenarios where needed resources may not be available or may be delayed because of response difficulties or responder capabilities. In this event, alternate plans should address the needs of the incident.

Once the preincident plan has been developed, it must be tested to ensure that it will work and accomplish the desired goals. Should any deficiencies be found, revise and retest the plan. Periodic testing is also important because of changing personnel or conditions.

Incident Command System

The success of any operation is dependent on everyone involved, from the awareness level to the technician level, following the same overall IAP. An IAP formulated by an organization or AHJ should be designed following the model of the National Incident Management System (NIMS). The NIMS allows for a standardized approach to incident management by breaking down the incident into controlled or manageable sections and identifying and assigning the appropriate resources for those sections. It is expected that at an awareness level the basics of ICS training will have already occurred prior to reading this chapter.

Jurisdictional Authority

An effective ICS clearly defines the agency that will be in charge of each incident. Although determination of the jurisdiction in charge may never become an issue for a small incident, larger-scale incidents that cross geographic and/or statutory boundaries require coordination with each of those AHJs to maintain a cohesive operation. In addition, other disciplines may need to be involved, such as local, county, or state law enforcement, and therefore must also be factored into the ICS for the operation. When situations arise in which there are overlapping responsibilities, the ICS may employ a unified command. Unified command is often used in multijurisdictional or multiagency incident management. It allows agencies with different legal, geographic, and functional responsibilities to coordinate, plan, and interact effectively. In a unified command structure, multiple agency representatives make command decisions instead of a single incident commander making all decisions on scene. A unified command allows for representatives from each agency participating in the response to share command authority at large, complex emergencies; this power-sharing arrangement helps ensure cooperation, avoids confusion, and guarantees agreement on goals and objectives.

By design, an ICS can and should be used during training and at all types of incidents, including nonemergency events, such as public gatherings (**FIGURE 2-6**). Regular use of the system builds familiarity with standard procedures and terminology.

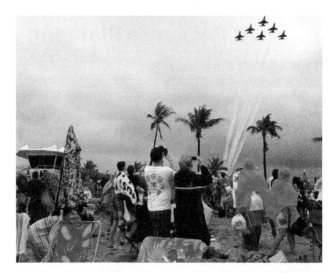

FIGURE 2-6 An ICS can be used for both emergency and nonemergency events.
© PJF Military Collection/Alamy Stock Photo.

Unity of Command

In a properly run ICS, each person working at an incident has only one direct supervisor. All orders and assignments come directly from that supervisor, and all reports are made to the same supervisor. That supervisor then reports to his or her supervisor and so on up the chain of command.

Span of Control

The ICS allows for a manageable span of control of people and resources. In most situations, one person can effectively supervise only three to seven people (with five being the optimal number). In the ICS setting, the incident commander (IC) communicates with and receives information from a maximum of five people rather than assuming responsibility for the assignment of all personnel at the scene. Individual managers of personnel and resources within the ICS are also working within a manageable span of control. The actual span of control depends on the complexity of the incident and the nature of the work being performed.

Modular Organization

An ICS is designed to be modular. Not all components of an ICS need to be used at every incident—only what is appropriate given the incident's nature and size. Additional components can be added or eliminated as needed as the incident unfolds. Some components are used on almost every incident, whereas others apply to only the largest and most complex situations. An example of this would be a motor vehicle accident involving one vehicle and requiring the extrication of one victim. The minimum position that would be established is the IC position, as long as the IC can effectively manage the crews operating on scene and does not exceed the span of control limit of seven personnel.

> **LISTEN UP!**
> Not all components of an ICS need to be used at every incident—only what is appropriate given the incident's nature and size.

Common Terminology

The ICS promotes the use of common terminology both within an organization and among all the agencies involved in emergency incidents. This shared language eliminates confusion about what is intended when different things are called by the same name in different jurisdictions, countries, areas, or departments. For example, a phrase commonly used to identify hydraulically powered rescue tools is "the jaws of life." This phrase was originally established by a hydraulic tool company to describe its hydraulic spreader. The phrase is now inaccurately used by rescue personnel to describe all hydraulic rescue tools. To avoid confusion and with the emergence of electric powered/operated systems, a hydraulic spreader should be referred to as a spreader, a hydraulic cutter should be referred to as a cutter, and a hydraulic ram should be referred to as a ram. Using common terminology as described in NFPA 1936, *Standard on Rescue Tools*, increases the level of understanding among the various response agencies working at an incident site.

Integrated Communications

The ICS must support communication up and down the chain of command at every level. Messages must move efficiently throughout the system. This consideration is especially important because it ensures that control objectives established by the command staff are effectively implemented by task-level resources. Integrated communications are also necessary so that outcomes produced by these task-level units are reported back up the chain of command, allowing progress toward incident goals to be measured as the incident unfolds.

Consolidated IAPs

An ICS ensures that everyone involved in the incident is following the same overall plan. The IAP may be developed by the IC alone on smaller incidents or in collaboration with all agencies involved in larger incidents.

Designated Incident Facilities

Development of a standard terminology for commonly needed operational facilities improves operations because everyone knows what occurs at each facility. Examples of such standard terms include the following:

- Base
- Command post
- Staging area

For incidents that involve only a few vehicles, the command post at a vehicle rescue and extrication incident may be established outside the hazard zone but nearby to maintain control and a visual of the incident. A larger incident may require the command post to be established within a structure with an established base, where logistical and administrative functions, such as traffic control management, are coordinated. A staging area is vital for a large incident and may be used to stage incoming apparatus. The staging area should be established close to the incident, in a location such as a parking lot.

Resource Management

A standard system of assigning and tracking the resources involved in the incident is of critical importance in ensuring accountability and an efficient and safe operation. At small-scale incidents, units and personnel usually respond directly to the scene and receive their assignments there. At large-scale incidents, units are often dispatched to a staging area rather than going directly to the incident scene. Some units are assigned upon arrival, whereas others may be held in reserve, ready to be assigned if needed. A mass casualty incident (MCI) involves casualties that exceed the resources normally available from a local jurisdiction, which places great demand on equipment and personnel and stretches resources beyond their limit (FIGURE 2-7). It is imperative that proper resource management be established in the beginning stages of the incident to ensure any chance of a successful outcome. Delaying the management of resources causes confusion, freelancing, and possible gridlock of incoming units.

Victim Reconnaissance

Victim reconnaissance begins when you are dispatched to the incident. With the information that you receive while responding to the scene, start formulating a plan for the operation. Is this a single vehicle accident with one victim or a school bus with multiple victims? If you are dispatched to an incident that may involve multiple victims, call for additional resources early on rather than waiting until arriving on scene. This action alone can save valuable time. Additional resources can always be canceled if it is determined after arrival that the incident can be managed with the units on scene.

Witnesses to the accident may also assist emergency personnel in confirming how many victims are involved. Witnesses can help establish the location of victims or tell you whether someone walked away from the scene.

ICS Organization

The ICS structure identifies a full range of duties, responsibilities, and functions that are performed at emergency incidents. Its hierarchy is best illustrated by a standard organizational chart that clearly defines the positions within the ICS and the chain of command (FIGURE 2-8).

Incident Commander

The IC is the individual with overall responsibility for the management of all incident operations. The command position is always filled and is initially established by the first unit on the scene. Ultimately, command is likely to be transferred to the senior arriving officer unless organization policy or circumstances dictate that someone else would be more appropriate in this position. During the transfer of command at a vehicle rescue and extrication incident, a brief current situation status report is given to the new IC and includes the following elements:

- *IAP*: Describe what the overall operation encompasses and establish objectives, including what, where, and how resources are allocated.
- *Tactical priorities*: Involve actions that need to be enacted or are presently being performed. For example, personnel may need to mitigate a spill or leak that is preventing operational groups from entering areas to perform the operation.
- *Hazardous or potentially hazardous conditions*: Areas that could potentially jeopardize the safety of personnel on the scene. An example is a petroleum tanker truck leaking fuel.
- *Accomplishments*: Objectives that have been completed at the time of transfer. For example, 15 to 20 victims have been transported from the scene to several area hospitals.
- *Assessment of effectiveness of operations*: May consist of a report that, for example, relays that

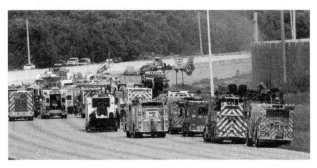

FIGURE 2-7 Mass casualty incidents place great demand on equipment and personnel, often stretching resources to their limit.
Courtesy of Devon Sweet.

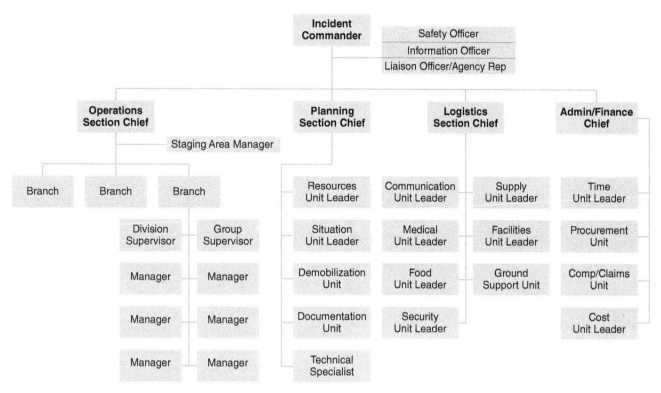

FIGURE 2-8 Incident command organizational chart.

three extrications have been completed and 15 victims have been transported to an area hospital within 20 minutes of the first-arriving apparatus.

- *Current status of resources*: Outlines which resources are allocated and where and how the resources are allocated. This provides information about the units that are in staging ready to deploy and units that may be out of service.

The IC should be thoroughly familiar with the ICS management process for both small and large incidents. At a small vehicle rescue and extrication incident, the IC needs to resist the temptation to get directly involved in the tactical operations. The IC should be nearby (relative to the size and scope of the incident) but apart from the immediate action zone so he or she can oversee and effectively direct the operations. This is not a stationary position; the IC position has to remain active, moving from three to four designated areas around the vehicles and the scene to maintain the best vantage points from which to manage the operation. At incidents that are larger or more complex, the IC should establish a command post that has visual access to the incident and is protected with restricted access so the command staff can function without needless distractions or interruptions.

Command Staff

The IC also communicates directly with command staff:

- Public information officer
- Safety officer
- Liaison officer

Public Information Officer

The **public information officer (PIO)** interfaces with the media and provides a single point of contact for information related to the incident, thereby allowing the IC to focus on managing the incident. The PIO prepares for IC approval any press releases to be issued. Also, prior to any press briefings, the PIO may provide the IC with background information, suggest questions that may be asked, and assist with selection and coordination of photographers.

Safety Officer

The **safety officer (SO)** is responsible for enforcing general safety rules and developing measures for ensuring personnel safety. The SO position should be established at every incident and includes responsibility for the identification, evaluation, and correction of hazards and unsafe practices. The SO can bypass the chain of command when necessary to correct unsafe

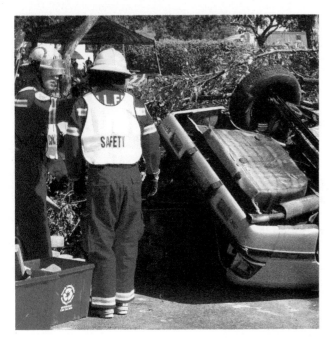

FIGURE 2-9 The safety officer, at a minimum, must be knowledgeable in strategy and tactics, hazardous materials, rescue practices, building construction and collapse potential, departmental SOPs, and departmental safety rules and regulations.
Courtesy of David Sweet.

acts immediately and has the authority to stop or suspend unsafe operations, as is clearly stated in national standards such as NFPA 1500; NFPA 1521, *Standard for Fire Department Safety Officer Professional Qualifications;* and NFPA 1561, *Standard on Emergency Services Incident Management System and Command Safety.* In this event, the SO must immediately report to the IC any action taken that may affect operations (**FIGURE 2-9**).

The SO, at a minimum, must be knowledgeable in the following areas:

- Strategy and tactics
- Departmental safety rules and regulations
- Departmental SOPs
- Hazardous materials
- Rescue practices
- Building construction and collapse potential

More specific responsibilities for vehicle rescue and extrication incidents include:

- Monitoring all hazards and maintaining awareness for potential hazards
- Ensuring personnel working in hazard zones are wearing appropriate PPE
- Conducting an ongoing evaluation of the psychological, physical, and mental state of rescuers
- Ensuring the stability of vehicles is maintained and monitored throughout the incident
- Ensuring best practices regarding safety are followed throughout the incident

The safety officer's role and responsibilities at a vehicle rescue and extrication incident are no different than they are at any other emergency incident. Remember that the main objective is to oversee that the operation is conducted in the safest manner, whether by ensuring that personnel performing their assignment are wearing their protective gear inside a hazard zone or by calling a freeze on an operation because cribbing support on a vehicle shifted when a tool was applied. This is not a stationary position; the safety officer has to remain very active, moving around the vehicles and the scene.

Liaison Officer

The liaison officer (LO) is the IC's point of contact for outside agencies and coordinates information and resources between cooperating and assisting agencies.

ICS Sections

Other than those tasks specifically assigned to the command staff, all activities at an incident can be relegated to one of the following four major ICS sections. Each section can be headed by a section chief or the IC personally, depending on the size and complexity of the incident.

- Operations
- Planning
- Logistics
- Finance/administration

Operations

The operations section is responsible for the development, direction, and coordination of all tactical operations conducted in accordance with an IAP, which outlines strategic objectives and the way in which operations will be conducted. The roles and responsibilities of the operations section chief at a large MCI are to coordinate and disseminate information back and forth through a division or branch manager who oversees the tactical groups, such as an extrication group(s). The number of groups must be no larger than five. An operations section chief can also be established on smaller vehicle rescue and extrication incidents where dialogue is coordinated directly to the tactical group supervisor. Establishing an operations section chief's position at an incident is a great way to manage the on-scene tactical work effectively, keeping the responsibilities of the IC to a manageable level.

Remember, the great thing about the ICS is that it is flexible; it can expand or contract throughout the incident depending on what is required or how the incident evolves.

Under the operations chief, there are functional areas and positions that need to be established at larger incidents to allow for a manageable span of control and to organize resources based on incident needs. The first of these areas is staging. All resources in the staging area are available and should be ready for assignment. This area should not be used for locating out-of-service resources or for performing logistics functions. Staging areas may be relocated as necessary. After a staging area has been designated and named, a **staging area manager** is assigned. The staging area manager reports to the operations section chief (or to the IC if an operations section chief has not been designated).

Divisions, groups, and branches are established when the number of resources exceeds the manageable span of control of the IC and the operations section chief. **Divisions** are established to divide an incident into physical or geographic areas of operation. For example, if a motor vehicle accident involving multiple vehicles and casualties affects two streets, then division 1 might be Street A and division 2 might be Street B. **Groups** are established to divide the incident into functional areas of operation (e.g., extrication group, medical groups, search and rescue groups).

Branches may serve several purposes and be functional or geographical in nature. In general, they are established when the number of divisions or groups exceeds the recommended span of control for the operations section chief or for geographic reasons. Branches are identified by functional name or Roman numerals and are managed by a branch director. They may have deputy positions as required.

Planning

The **planning section** is responsible for drafting the IAP, which includes the collection, evaluation, dissemination, and use of information and intelligence critical to the incident (unless the IC places this function elsewhere). One of the most important functions of the planning section is to look beyond the current and next operational period (generally 12- or 24-hour periods) and anticipate potential problems, events, and logistical needs to execute the upcoming IAP. Other responsibilities include the following:

- Drafting and updating the IAP
- Examining the current situation
- Reviewing available information
- Predicting the probable cause of events
- Preparing recommendations for strategies and tactics
- Maintaining resource status
- Maintaining and displaying situation status
- Providing documentation services

For a smaller MCI requiring the extrication of casualties, a planning section would not have to be created, and the responsibilities would be carried out by the IC. Remember, the IAP can be a formalized written plan, or it can be an informal verbal plan depending on the incident size, complexity, and length of the operational period.

Technical specialists initially report to the planning section and work within that section or are reassigned to another part of the organization. These advisors have the special skills required at the incident. These skills can be in any discipline required—for example, aviation, environment, hazardous materials, and engineering.

Logistics

The **logistics section** is responsible for all support requirements needed to facilitate effective and efficient incident management, including providing supplies, services, facilities, and materials during the incident. Key responsibilities include the following duties:

- Communications
- Medical support to incident personnel
- Food for incident personnel
- Supplies
- Facilities
- Ground support

At a large MCI involving multiple extrication groups and required transports, the logistics section works very closely with all general staff in supplying resources to accomplish and/or satisfy the incident objectives. Are additional powered rescue tools or specialty tools needed? Should heavy equipment, such as large tow units, or operators be allocated? How many transport-capable units are required? Is there a temporary rehabilitation facility that can be established for personnel? Are the communications sufficient to handle the size or complexity of the incident?

Even at a smaller incident, a logistics section can help manage resources, such as by maintaining area coverage while jurisdiction units are operating at the incident. The service branch within the logistics section may include the following units:

- *Communications unit*: Develops plans for the use of incident communications equipment

and facilities and installs, tests, distributes, and maintains communication equipment. This unit also supervises the incident communications center.
- *Medical unit*: Develops the medical plan, obtains medical aid and transportation for injured and ill incident personnel, and prepares reports and records.
- *Food unit*: Supplies the food needs for the incident.

The support branch within the logistics section may include the following units:

- *Supply unit*: Obtains, stores, and maintains inventory of supplies needed for an incident and services supplies and equipment. This unit also orders personnel, equipment, and supplies.
- *Facilities unit*: Is responsible for the layout and use of incident facilities and provides sleeping and sanitation facilities for incident personnel. The facilities unit is also responsible for managing base and camp operations.
- *Ground support unit*: Transports personnel, supplies, food, and equipment and implements the traffic plan for the incident. This unit also fuels, services, maintains, and repairs vehicles and other ground support equipment.

Finance/Administration

The **finance/administration section** is responsible for the accounting and financial aspects of an incident as well as any legal issues that may arise. Although not staffed at most incidents, this position accounts for all activities and ensures that enough money is made available to keep operations running. The following units are contained within the finance/administration section:

- *Time unit*: Is responsible for equipment and personnel time recording.
- *Procurement unit*: Administers all financial matters pertaining to vendor contracts, leases, and fiscal agreements.
- *Compensation/claims unit*: Handles financial concerns resulting from property damage, injuries, or fatalities at the incident.
- *Cost unit*: Tracks costs, analyzes cost data, creates cost estimates, and recommends cost-saving measures.

A finance section is another management asset that can be used regardless of the size of an incident. Even at an MCI on a large interstate highway, the finance section can immediately procure funding to acquire needed equipment that may not be readily available or that may take a lot of time to establish. An incident on a highway during a hot summer day may require additional personnel to be called in to replace or cover for those requiring rehabilitation. This is an unforeseen expenditure that an IC will not have time to negotiate during an incident.

Additional ICS Terminology

Single Resources and Crews

A **single resource** is an individual vehicle and its assigned personnel. A **crew** is a group of personnel working without apparatus and led by a leader or boss.

Task Forces and Strike Teams

Task forces and strike teams are groups of single resources assigned to work together for a specific purpose or for a specific period of time under a single leader. A **task force** is a group of up to five single resources of any type. A **strike team** is a group of five units of the same type working on a common task or function.

Tracking Systems

Personnel Accountability

The accountability system is one of the most important tools an IC can use to ensure safety at an incident and should be implemented at all incidents and large events. Implementing accountability on a vehicle rescue and extrication incident can be as basic as ensuring that personnel operating powered rescue tools or conducting other strenuous tasks be rotated out to rehabilitation on a continual basis to prevent heat-related stress/emergencies.

Training on the implementation of a personnel accountability system should meet the requirements of NFPA 1561. An accountability system tracks the personnel on the scene, including the following information:

- Responders' identities
- Their assignments
- Their locations

This system ensures that only qualified rescuers who have been given specific assignments are operating within the area where the rescue is taking place. By using an accountability system and working within ICS, an IC can track the resources at the scene, delegate the proper personnel assignments, and monitor time expenditure of personnel/assignments. This in turn allows the IC to rotate personnel as needed to prevent stress and fatigue.

Voice of Experience

It is a constant challenge in the world of vehicle extrication to balance the equipment purchased for vehicle rescue with the field members' requests to have tools for every situation. With new vehicle technology and the never-ending situations that can occur on the streets and highways, further consideration must be given to apparatus compartment space and agency budgets.

Late on a summer night, an intoxicated driver drove his 2-door pickup truck at high speed into the back of a large SUV. The impact was substantial; it caused moderate damage to the large SUV but major damage and intrusion to the truck. Upon arrival, the SUV driver was out of the vehicle with minimal injuries. The driver of the truck was trapped by the engine, dashboard and steering wheel. The engine had been pushed back and down, causing the steering wheel to rise to a level above the semi-conscious victim's face. Following an inner and outer circle with stabilization, the plan was made for door and roof removal, and then a dashboard displacement coupled with ongoing medical care. Upon the quick removal of the roof and driver's side door, the dashboard was just a few inches from the victim's chest. As additional stabilization was placed for the pending dashboard displacement, an interior plastic removal effort was made to inspect the victim's feet, which were covered by the interior components of the displaced floorboard.

Following relief cuts to the firewall, a dashboard lift was attempted. As the dashboard started to move, the intoxicated victim screamed out in pain. The lift was immediately stopped, and the victim stopped screaming. The decision was made to make another attempt to lift, and the same victim reaction occurred. The operation was stopped, and manual delayering of the dashboard was undertaken to discover what was making contact with the victim's lower extremities and moving when the dashboard moved. The only tools available for the delayering were wire cutters, tin snips, and other similar hand tools. Power tools were not considered due to the proximity to the victim's body and the unknown location or orientation of the victim's lower extremities. After a lengthy delayering of the dashboard, it was discovered that the emergency brake pedal had been displaced by the engine, causing the pedal to move in an upward direction and imbedding itself inside the victim's left hamstring. No additional dashboard displacement would be possible; every time the dashboard assembly was moved up or forward the brake pedal would move with it, impaling it deeper into the victim's leg. The brake pedal had to be cut to extricate the victim without further harm.

Every tool in the arsenal we had available to us at that time was considered. No options were available that would either fit in the space provided or cause an acceptable amount of movement during the cutting operation. With the mental status of the victim declining and the extended time that we had already been on scene, a rapid option was chosen. The only available tool that would fit into the space was a pneumatic hammer with a long bit to cut the brake pedal shaft in small increments. Once the pedal was successfully cut, the dashboard was lifted and the victim was extracted and taken to the trauma center.

Having a wider variety of small cutting tools, powered and non-powered, is essential for these types of "surgical" disentanglement operations. They are relatively inexpensive and not often used, but invaluable as an option for confined space cutting.

Harris Henbest
Broward Sheriff's Fire Rescue & Emergency Services Dept.
Fort Lauderdale, Florida

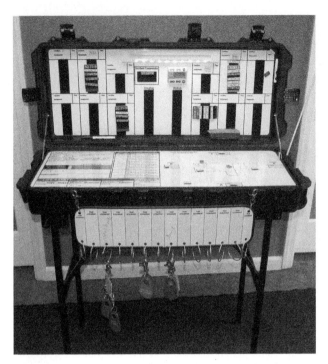

FIGURE 2-10 Accountability systems, such as the accountability tag and the passport system, are available to keep track of personnel at a rescue.
Reproduced with permission from American Trade Mark Co.

A number of accountability systems exist, including lists, boards, tags, badges, T cards, bar-code systems, and radio frequency identification (RFID) tags (**FIGURE 2-10**). Bar-code systems and RFIDs are used with electronic systems, which can give real-time information on personnel, such as qualifications and assignment. This information can even be transmitted to multiple electronic devices so more than one individual or location (such as the safety officer, IC, or even the emergency operations center) can have real-time access to this information.

LISTEN UP!

Radio frequency identification (RFID) tags use radio waves to transmit personnel data. Some models do not need to be within the receiver's line of sight for the equipment to function.

Equipment Inventory and Tracking Systems

In addition to documentation on the purchase, maintenance, and use of equipment, many organizations maintain certain records during an incident (**FIGURE 2-11**). The combination of these records provides a comprehensive resource and accountability system that can be manually or electronically tracked.

Agency	ST	Kind	Type	I.D. No.

Order/ Request No. | Date/time Check In

Home Base

Departure point

Leader Name

Crew I.D. No./Name (For Strike Teams)

No. Personnel | Manifest ☐Yes ☐No | Weight

Method of Travel ☐ Own ☐Bus ☐Air

Other

Destination Point | ETA

Transportation Needs ☐ Own ☐Bus ☐Air

Other

Ordered Date/Time | Confirmed Date/Time

Remarks

Agency	TF	Kind	Type	I.D. No./ Name

Incident Location | Time

Status ☐Assigned ☐O/S REST ☐O/S PERS. ☐Available ☐O/S MECH ☐ ETR

Note

Incident location | Time

Status ☐Assigned ☐O/S REST ☐O/S PERS. ☐Available ☐O/S MECH ☐ ETR

Note

Incident Location | Time

Status ☐Assigned ☐O/S REST ☐O/S PERS. ☐Available ☐O/S MECH ☐ ETR

Note

Incident Location | Time

Status ☐Assigned ☐O/S REST ☐O/S PERS. ☐Available ☐O/S MECH ☐ ETR

Note

FIGURE 2-11 Resource tracking systems are used to keep accurate records during an incident.
Courtesy of NIMS/FEMA.

Manual systems may include lists and sign-out sheets. Computerized or electronic systems may consist of bar-code systems and RFID tags. In some cases, both types of systems may be used simultaneously. Fully integrated systems include all information on all equipment and may use bar codes or RFID tags to identify both the equipment and the personnel signing out that equipment.

Long-Term Operations

Fire rescue personnel are accustomed to incidents that terminate quickly, often within an hour of onset. Many short-term incidents can be effectively directed and controlled using a basic ICS system consisting of an IC, a safety officer, and an operations section chief, with the various group functional assignments being established under the operations section as needed.

By comparison, technical rescue incidents can extend well beyond these relatively short time periods and be much more complex. The IC needs to consider both immediate and anticipated needs for all phases of such an incident. Remember that whichever functions and responsibilities the IC does not assign to others in the ICS stay with the IC. The IC could become overwhelmed easily in a technical rescue incident if he or she attempts to handle all these issues for the duration of the incident.

Use of an expanded ICS can assist the IC with planning and functioning in the long-term incident environment. This should include staffing the planning, logistics, and finance/administration sections.

A rescue team can typically work for up to 24 hours without downtime (depending on the type of rescue) but then must have at least 24 hours for rest and equipment maintenance. If the rescue effort is expected to go beyond 24 hours, plans must be made for long-term operations. This determination can depend on any of the following factors:

- The extent of rescue required
- The training level of the rescue team
- The available resources
- The physical conditions of the rescuers
- The psychological conditions of the rescuers
- Needs supported by other ICS functions

Safety

To all organizations and ICs, the health and safety of their personnel are of the highest importance. Long-term operations or physically demanding incidents can take a debilitating toll on personnel. Injuries can also cause a negative psychological effect on the entire team. Personnel who are injured not only reduce the available personnel by their loss but also can divert other personnel and resources to assist the injured individuals. Work-related stress will be covered in Chapter 11, *Terminating the Incident*.

There are numerous programs and guidelines available on health and safety programs for emergency personnel. NFPA 1500 is one such document that covers topics in health and safety programs within the organization. Contained within this standard are provisions that can be invaluable not only to developing a health and safety program but also in the development of response plans, SOPs and standard operation guidelines (SOGs), and risk assessments. NFPA 1500 in concert with NFPA 1250, *Recommended Practice in Fire and Emergency Service Organization Risk Management*; 1521; and 1561 provides the tools necessary to run a safe and effective organization.

Time Management

At any emergency scene, time is a major factor. Prolonged scene times, combined with insufficient or lack of advance life support procedures, negatively affect your victim's chances of survival. The late Dr. R. Adams Cowley, who founded the R. Adams Cowley Shock Trauma Center in Baltimore, Maryland, theorized that a victim of a critical traumatic injury has the greatest chance of survival if he or she is treated at a trauma facility within 60 minutes from the moment the injury occurs. Dr. Cowley believed that this "Golden Hour" was the difference between life and death—that 60 minutes after receiving a traumatic injury, the body has increasing difficulties in compensating for shock and the associated traumatic injuries. This general guideline was used as a standard of care for trauma victims for many years, but through years of research data, this critical period is now known to vary from one victim to another based on a number of factors and type of traumatic injuries sustained.

Because many injured victims require definitive care in less than an hour, Cowley's concept is now considered a general guide and has morphed into the "Golden Period" without the delineation of a definitive 60-minute time factor. The Golden Period is the time during which treatment of shock and traumatic injuries is most critical and the potential for survival is best accomplished through rapid medical intervention. Victims who have sustained physical traumatic injuries require rapid assessment, treatment, and transport to a trauma-capable facility. Current research cannot conclusively determine that shorter on-scene times equate to higher mortality rates because so many variables can exist, but victims who sustain traumatic injuries demonstrate the best chance for survival when they receive critical care on the street and necessary surgical interventions at a trauma facility.

A basic vehicle extrication involving the assessment, removal, stabilization, and packaging of a victim should take no longer than 20 minutes; this does not include response or transport times. This general guideline is recommended as a tactical benchmark for the operation (**FIGURE 2-12**).

To maintain a realistic scenario, the total incident time should be approximately 45 minutes for agencies located in urban areas. It is understood that some rural agencies responding to vehicle rescue and extrication incidents may well exceed the 60-minute benchmark. The idea is to strive for that 20-minute on-scene extrication benchmark regardless of whether the agency area consists of urban or rural response. For example, a standard 45-minute vehicle rescue and extrication

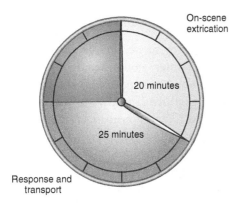

FIGURE 2-12 This general guideline should be used as a tactical benchmark for the operation.

incident for a fire rescue agency in an urban response area can be broken down as follows: Once again, no more than 20 minutes should be dedicated to extrication time. This means that it should take no more than 20 minutes from the moment of apparatus arrival until the victim is extricated from the vehicle and placed on a backboard. This leaves approximately 25 minutes for apparatus response and transport. Although there are complex incidents that require extended extrication time, in general, the goal for the technical rescuer should be no more than 20 minutes for the standard, or basic, one-victim extrication. This on-scene time is monitored by the incident commander (IC) and/or dispatch.

Some dispatching agencies have a standard protocol that automatically notifies the IC at 10-minute intervals until the incident is mitigated. This is known as an incident clock. Check with your local dispatching agency to see if an incident clock is instituted in its protocols. The incident clock is referenced in NFPA 1500.

SAFETY TIP

The technical rescuer should use an incident clock for on-scene time management.

Responding to the Scene

Responding to the scene is a critical component of the overall operation because it should set the stage for how the incident will evolve. Several benchmarks should be followed prior to the incident being dispatched and as the incident is dispatched:

- Maintaining a readiness state where all equipment and personal protective equipment (PPE) are operational and accounted for
- Preincident planning with preassignments for personnel prior to the incident dispatch to alleviate confusion on arrival
- Starting the size-up of the incident as the incident is dispatched, by gathering additional information from dispatchers to better shape the scope of the incident, calling additional resources based on the description for the type and severity of the incident, and checking for electrical hazards by scanning the entire area on approach

Personal Protective Equipment

The rescuer must be operationally ready, not only in the area of mental and physical readiness but particularly in the area of personal protection. NFPA 1500 and NFPA 1951, *Standard on Protective Ensembles for Technical Rescue Incidents*, describe the protective ensemble required to be worn by the technical rescuer at the scene of rescue or recovery operations. NFPA 1951 lists rescue and recovery technical rescue protective ensembles and ensemble elements for technical rescue personnel. These ensembles include coats, trousers, coveralls, helmets, gloves, footwear, and interface components. Respiratory protection may also be necessary if operating in an area with airborne contaminants or in a known or suspected **immediately dangerous to life and health (IDLH)** environment.

To be compliant with NFPA 1951, the protective ensemble must provide protection from exposure to physical, thermal, liquid, and body fluid–borne pathogen hazards. Which specific components of PPE are selected depends on several factors, including, but not limited to, the type of incident, hazards at the scene, the duration of the incident, the type of equipment used, and the weather. A self-contained breathing apparatus (SCBA) is also an important component of PPE because of the necessity of respiratory protection from a hazardous environment or hazardous conditions, such as smoke. The selection of body protection and PPE is made based on the known and potential hazards at the scene of the vehicle rescue and extrication incident as well as what is required by the authority having jurisdiction (AHJ) for the agency.

Dispatch Information

Emergency dispatch centers across the country can vary slightly in terminology, but per the federally mandated National Incident Management System (NIMS), common language is the goal for greater continuity and interoperability between agencies. The following is an example of an incident being dispatched using common language.

A hypothetical call being dispatched may present as follows:

> Dispatch: "Engine 10, Rescue 10, respond to a passenger vehicle rollover with possible entrapment of one victim at the intersection of 12th and Maple. Police are on scene advising to expedite the response."

The technical rescuer needs to dissect the transmission from dispatch and listen for key elements of the call, such as "possible entrapment" and/or "vehicle rollover." The goal is to adhere to common terminology and strive to use plain language whenever possible.

It must be noted that emergency vehicles are not exempt from observing all traffic laws and must manage their response speeds accordingly. NFPA 1500 Section 6.2 and subsequent references require that the agency establish specific rules, regulations, and procedures relating to the operation of fire department vehicles in an emergency mode, including guidelines to establish when emergency response is authorized and when emergency response is not authorized. It is at the discretion of the AHJ to make that determination.

Other important elements to listen for or consider during dispatch may include the time of day; location of the incident; speed of travel (residential roadway vs. major highway); and weather, which can vary greatly in different regions of the country. This key information should motivate the company officer to step into action and reaffirm preassignments for crew members en route to the incident.

Preincident Assignments

Managing resources early on is key to ensuring a successful operation. A useful tool to consider implementing within the organization is the **crew resource management (CRM)** concept. Developed by NASA in the late 1970s, CRM is a crisis management practice that focuses on the officer in charge using all available resources rather than making decisions without any input or assistance from others. CRM is a standard practice in the airline industry and has been recently making headlines in emergency services. Management concepts such as CRM or the race team pit crew management concept are not new management procedures to the fire rescue service; incident management has been used for decades, with origins in the Division of Forestry to manage wildland forest fires NFPA 1500 Section 8.3.1 directs the IC to integrate CRM into the regular functions of the incident command system (ICS). Rescue and extrication competition teams all across the world have always used this same resource management tool with preassigned positions for the use of all personnel on scene to accomplish goals and objectives collectively.

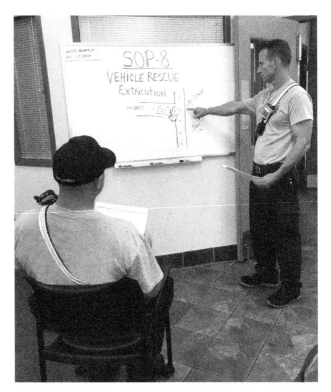

FIGURE 2-13 Crews prepare for an incident by reviewing SOPs and assigning positions prior to the incident being dispatched.
Courtesy of David Sweet.

One of the main objectives of resource management is to delegate assignments early on to minimize being overwhelmed on arrival. Preassigning crew members prior to the incident sets the team in action, preventing freelancing and giving the officer the ability to focus more on the incident and the development of the incident action plan (IAP). Tactical objectives for each assignment should be outlined in the agency's SOPs or standard operating guidelines (SOGs) so there is no confusion regarding what is needed for each assignment (**FIGURE 2-13**). Reviewing departmental SOPs for vehicle rescue and extrication, as well as preassigning personnel prior to an incident being dispatched, will provide consistency and continuity and alleviate confusion when arriving on scene.

An example of a typical preassignment model is as follows:

> *Company officer: Conducts the inner survey and makes sure everyone understands their assignments*
>
> *Rescuer 1: Conducts the outer survey*
>
> *Rescuer 2: Acquires the cribbing and tools off the apparatus and sets up a tool staging area*
>
> *Driver engineer/chauffeur: Blocks traffic, places the apparatus in a defensive position, sets up traffic*

diverting cones and signage, pulls off a minimum 1.75-in. (44-mm) hose line for protection, and assists Rescuer 2 with setting up the tools

This model is only an example, so keep in mind that these assignments can change upon arrival based on the nature and complexity of the incident and the number of personnel available. It is always better to be prepared and have a basic plan in place than to make one up as you go.

Traffic

Traffic incident management for the fire rescue service is a management tool that establishes roadway safety procedures and traffic control measures for emergency operations at a motor vehicle accident. NFPA 1500 Section 9.2 states that "each department shall establish, implement, and enforce SOPs regarding emergency operations involving traffic" (NFPA 2021).

Another excellent resource on traffic safety is the U.S. Department of Transportation's (DOT) *Manual on Uniform Traffic Control Devices (MUTCD)*. MUTCD is a guideline for the safe operation and proper use of traffic control and management devices. This manual seeks to ensure uniformity of traffic control devices and traffic management procedures by providing minimum standards and guidance nationwide on apparatus placement and emergency traffic control devices, such as warning signage and traffic cone types and placements.

Defensive apparatus placement is a component of site operations as well as a requirement of NFPA 1500 (Section 9.4). The main goal is to block and protect the scene from the flow of traffic. Whenever possible, place emergency vehicles in a manner that will ensure safety and not disrupt traffic any more than necessary. It is imperative that these safety measures be strictly followed. On roadway areas with high speed and a heavy volume of traffic, a second apparatus should be dispatched as a roadway blocking unit to protect the scene.

Apparatus placement on incidents should be staged in a defensive position so that it provides a barrier against motorists who fail to heed emergency warning lights. Optimal defensive apparatus placement depends on the flow of traffic in relation to the accident and area maneuverability. Consider whether you can get apparatus around the wreckage to properly stage the units.

As you approach the scene, with the accident in the same direction of travel, position the front of the apparatus facing away (including the wheels turned away) from the scene at a 30- to 45-degree angle to the wreckage, blocking off lanes to guide traffic safely around or divert it away from the designated safety or operational zones (**FIGURE 2-14**). Also, if equipped, attempt

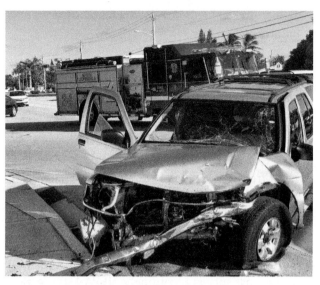

FIGURE 2-14 Many fire departments place an apparatus at a 30- to 45-degree angle to the crash, with the front wheels of the apparatus facing away from the incident.
Courtesy of David Sweet.

to keep a side-mounted pump panel facing toward the incident, away from oncoming traffic, to protect the pump operator/driver engineer. Confirm that the apparatus's wheels face away from the incident scene; this will ensure that the apparatus will not be pushed into the wreckage if struck in the rear by another vehicle. If scene lighting is used, make sure the lights do not shine in the eyes of approaching drivers. Emergency apparatus lights at an incident scene can cause distraction and confusion for passing motorists. Emergency vehicle lighting is not designed for traffic control; these lights provide warning only to alert the motorist of the pending incident. Passing motorists are normally so consumed with getting a view of the wreckage that they do not see you or the apparatus. Having an additional apparatus on scene assigned as a blocking unit provides that extra layer of safety to the crews and victims.

Additionally, the driver must also set up traffic cones or some type of signaling device to warn and divert all oncoming traffic. Most apparatus do not carry the necessary number of cones to divert traffic in a safe and appropriate manner (**FIGURE 2-15**). According to NFPA 1500, properly alerting passing motorists to the incident requires the following:

- At least five 28-in. (71-cm) or greater fluorescent orange traffic cones with double reflective markings that are compliant with the *MUTCD*

- Retro-reflective warning signs compliant with the *MUTCD* (Chapters 3 and 4 of the *Traffic Incident Management Manual* describe the *MUTCD*'s requirements for scene control barriers in further detail)

CHAPTER 2 Vehicle Rescue Incident Awareness

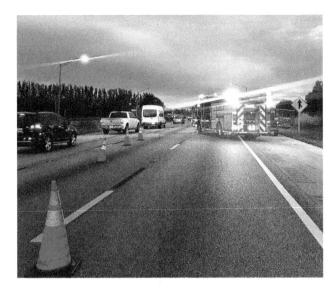

FIGURE 2-15 Traffic cones can be placed to direct motorists away from the crash for scene protection.
Courtesy of Troy Lanza.

It may be necessary to reevaluate the amount carried on each unit based on the response area. Also, if the accident occurs at an intersection with multiple lanes and direction of travel, it is recommended that additional fire rescue apparatus as well as the department of law enforcement (DLE) be dispatched at the onset of the call to assist with lane closures and scene protection. Traffic control measures must be set as a high priority and implemented at every incident. Some agencies have personnel dedicated to the traffic control function, such as fire, police (DLE), or special auxiliary police.

There are numerous reference documents and articles published on the subject of traffic incident management and roadway safety practices, in addition to NFPA 1500 and the MUTCD. The U.S. Fire Administration's Traffic Incident Management Systems is another valuable resource that aims to enhance responder safety and traffic management at roadway emergency scenes.

The DOT's *Emergency Response Guidebook* (ERG) offers guidance for rescuers who may potentially operate at a hazardous materials incident, such as a vehicle accident involving a cargo truck that was transporting hazardous materials (**FIGURE 2-16**). This reference guide is intended to help rescuers decide which

SAFETY TIP

For the safety of all personnel, when placing any advance warning or traffic-diverting devices, such as cones or signs, rescuers should never turn their backs to oncoming traffic; they should always start with the farthest device and work back toward the incident.

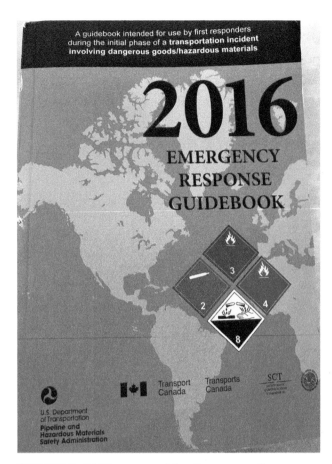

FIGURE 2-16 The cover of the *Emergency Response Guidebook*.
Courtesy of David Sweet.

preliminary actions to take. The guide provides information on approximately 4000 chemicals that may be encountered at an incident scene.

These resources contain an enormous amount of information on traffic control devices, traffic management using the NIMS model, and hazard recognition and mitigation. Some of the topics found in these resources include:

- Incident traffic size-up in determining the scope and magnitude of the incident by categorizing the scene in relation to the estimated elapsed time needed for roadway closures (minor: >30 minutes; intermediate: 30 minutes to 2 hours; major: >2 hours)
- Risk analysis and assessment
- Establishing traffic control zones (different from operational hazard zones, which are labeled cold, warm, and hot)
- Proper traffic cone size and color—must be orange and no less than 18 in. (46 cm) in height for daylight and for low-speed roadways and 28 in. (71 cm) at night or when operating on high-speed highways with the proper type and sizing of retro-reflective material

- Traffic cone spacing requirements—the recommendation being 15-ft (4.6-m) intervals
- Portable electronic message signs and the use of variable message signs that hang over the roadways at various areas in most major highways today
- Stationary pre-warning signs, including proper color, size, lettering, wording (e.g., "Emergency Scene Ahead"), spacing, and distance from the incident
- Flares—incendiary type, chemical light stick type, or light-emitting diode (LED) type
- Directional arrow panels and barricades
- Flagger position—training requirements, equipment types, and role and responsibilities (Any individual who manually directs traffic is known as a flagger.)

Many of these reference materials are readily available through Internet downloads. Technical rescuers must take advantage of these invaluable resources to better prepare and plan operationally for themselves as well as their respective agencies.

SAFETY TIP

For the safety of personnel and victims, it is imperative that traffic control measures be used at every incident.

Crowd Control

Bystanders who act as "Good Samaritans" want to get involved and help, but most often they can be a dangerous liability that can cause havoc or injury to the victim, to themselves, or to the rescue workers. As you arrive on scene, you may see these individuals trying to pull victims from the vehicles. They may also start yelling that the vehicle is going to explode or that the people in the vehicles are dying and you need to move faster. This situation needs to be addressed and mitigated immediately and professionally. Do not get distracted by these individuals and lose focus on the operation. These individuals need to be removed from the scene either voluntarily or by DLE intervention. Call immediately for law enforcement to assist.

Crowd control is an absolute necessity in protecting responders from individuals who might attempt to enter the emergency site. Adequate crowd control provides the necessary space for fire and rescue personnel to operate without being concerned about individuals interfering or bystanders being injured (**FIGURE 2-17**).

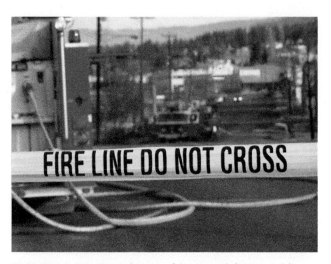

FIGURE 2-17 Crowd control is essential to providing rescuers with adequate space to operate.
© Ron Hilton/Dreamstime.com.

Personnel Resources

The size of an incident determined by the scene size-up dictates whether a large management staff is necessary for oversight and planning. Of course, as an incident grows, the need for additional resources and personnel can grow as well, which is one of the benefits of NIMS. Recognizing the need to bring in additional resources to assist in the incident is a true sign of leadership and proper scene management. A standard rule is to always call for additional support early in the incident; these units can always be canceled or returned if the incident is determined later not to be significant or was mitigated appropriately by your crew alone. Multijurisdictional response incidents may require a unified command system to be established, which incorporates multiple jurisdictions, law enforcement, the DOT, utility companies, and/or public works departments. SOPs should address the levels of response and indicate which positions will be staffed based on the complexity of the incident.

Law Enforcement Personnel

Uncontrolled incident scenes pose serious threats to everyone at the site. DLE should be requested immediately to control crowds and traffic and/or to establish perimeter control (**FIGURE 2-18**). In some agencies, law enforcement is on the same dispatching system as fire rescue, and procedurally, they may receive the notification call before fire rescue is dispatched. The most important point is that there must be clear communication between law enforcement and the fire department/emergency medical services (EMS) agencies; this communication is the key to successful operations and general work cohesiveness. Remember that

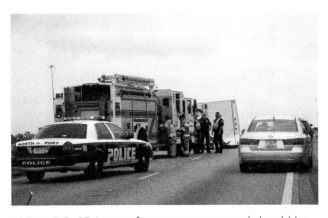

FIGURE 2-18 Law enforcement personnel should be requested for crowd and traffic control at all roadway incidents.
© Peter Titmuss/Alamy Stock Photo.

the overall safety of response personnel is the primary responsibility of the responding agency.

EMS Personnel

Although the common functional description of EMS is prehospital victim care and treatment, in some parts of the country, EMS performs extrication as well as victim care. In other EMS agencies, vehicle extrication, victim access, and disentanglement are handled by another service such as a fire department. Some jurisdictions combine their fire and EMS systems, creating a fire rescue service. Systems vary greatly from one jurisdiction to another, but when using a tiered classification system to identify what these agencies are capable of providing, confusion is alleviated when mutual aid is requested. A tiered fire rescue/EMS–based provider service describes the capability of the agency to provide the response, treatment, and transport of victims. The tier system is basically broken into three levels. A three-tiered system provides three independent types of service, with various agencies or combinations of agencies providing services. A tiered system may consist of the following common components but is not limited to the types of agencies described here:

- Three-tiered system: The fire apparatus responds as a first responder unit to provide basic victim care and support, EMS personnel respond as a separate entity for definitive victim treatment, and a private ambulance service responds for transport of the victim to the designated medical facility.
- Two-tiered system: A two-tiered system consists of the fire apparatus responding as a first responder unit to provide basic victim care and support and EMS personnel responding as a unit capable of treatment and transport.
- Single-tiered system: A single-tiered system consists of one agency responding with a fire apparatus staffed with dual-certified firefighter paramedics and a rescue unit for transport. Some fire apparatus also come equipped with victim transport capabilities. The single-tiered fire rescue system is the optimal level of emergency services from an overall operational viewpoint.

In some jurisdictions, EMS and fire service agencies are separate entities, with basic life support (BLS) being the minimum level of victim care for EMS agencies and emergency medical responder training being the minimum level of victim care for fire service agencies. Alternately, the fire service agency may not provide any medical responsibilities at all, which is considered a two- or three-tiered system, depending on the transport capabilities of the EMS unit. Two- and three-tiered systems may cause confusion and delays when trying to determine the level of care needed on scene. Any delays in treatment could be detrimental to victim survivability. Two- or three-tiered fire service agencies should incorporate EMS (preferably an advanced life support [ALS] unit) and ambulance transport services into their response and operational procedures, including training drills to improve work relations, continuity, and efficiency. ALS is the highest level of care for the victim next to an emergency department physician responding to the incident. In some rural areas, the only medical service available in the district may be a BLS-certified service. This does not mean that the rescuers cannot function, but it does raise the question of whether the injuries the rescuers have identified can be treated by BLS providers or whether ALS support is required; again, causing a potential delay during a critical time. Clearly, the number of victims and types of injuries will help responders make this decision (**FIGURE 2-19**).

For example, if first responders face a scenario in which victims have suffered amputations, crush injuries, severe cervical spine injuries, or other serious trauma, the responders would request ALS units. However, the National Standard Curriculum for emergency medical technicians (EMTs) does outline BLS-level care for these types of injuries; EMTs should provide victim care within their scope of practice and request ALS assistance as appropriate. If necessary, ALS resources may be requested from a neighboring community where a mutual aid agreement has been established. Without question, it is always best practice to obtain ALS medical support as early as possible but remember that not all municipalities and rural areas provide ALS medical services. For this reason,

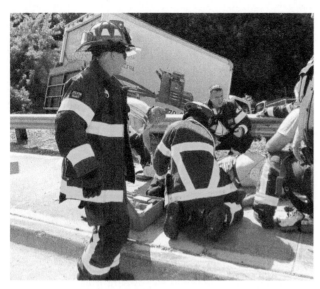

FIGURE 2-19 The number of victims and types of injuries can help you determine whether ALS or BLS providers are needed.
Courtesy of David Sweet.

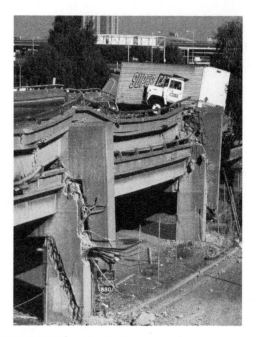

FIGURE 2-20 The Nimitz Freeway after a 6.9-magnitude earthquake struck in 1987.
© Peter Menzel/Science Source.

it is important that BLS service providers be trained to immediately recognize any injuries that require an ALS unit response. ALS units can always be canceled if their services are not needed.

Hazardous Materials Personnel

Hazardous materials incidents could require specialized teams, depending on the complexity of the incident. For example, an accident involving a tanker or semi-truck containing a known or unknown hazardous product would require hazardous materials personnel or a hazardous materials team to respond. In incidents involving hazardous materials, rescuers must allow a proper size-up and evaluation. All too often in incidents involving hazardous materials, rescue personnel are unnecessarily exposed to dangerous agents because they rush into the incident site before they have gathered the necessary information pertaining to the material or agent. Although awareness-level responders' activities are limited in such scenarios, they can certainly assist operations and technician-level responders by looking through a set of binoculars and identifying placards, product labels, numbers, and other information. They can also assist in the response by preventing others from entering the incident site by sealing the site perimeter and referring to the DOT's ERG to identify the product, evacuation distances, the product's flammability and incompatibilities, and other pertinent data.

Additional Personnel Resources

Other valuable resources whose assistance might be requested during major incidents are state and county emergency services, state and county health departments, area hospitals, emergency flight services, and the state's National Guard civil support team. Other resources include K-9 organizations, urban search and rescue (USAR) teams, Federal Emergency Management Agency (FEMA) task force teams, and industry hazardous materials response teams. The mention of these types of resources may seem extreme in regard to vehicle rescue and extrication, but one major disaster—such as the 6.9-magnitude earthquake that struck California in 1987—justifies the discussion of these services in relation to vehicle rescue and extrication. During this major earthquake, the two-tiered elevated Nimitz Freeway, which flows traffic from Oakland into San Francisco, collapsed onto itself, trapping and crushing an estimated 250-plus vehicles (**FIGURE 2-20**). This operation required the deployment of massive resources for the freeway alone, not to mention the rest of the region that also required a response. All of these resources can play a vital role in such incidents.

Scene Size-Up

Scene size-up is the systematic and continual evaluation of information presented in either visual or audible form. It is important to remember that size-up begins at the time the incident is dispatched, not at the time the unit arrives at the scene. Immediately upon arrival, the first company officer sizes up the scene and establishes command. A rapid and accurate visual size-up is needed to avoid placing rescuers in danger and to determine which additional resources if any are needed. Size-up at a vehicle rescue and extrication incident can include the following evaluations:

- Recognition and mitigation of IDLH hazards, such as exposed utilities, water, mechanical hazards, hazardous materials, electrical hazards, and explosives and other hazards, including environmental factors
- Exposure to traffic
- Incident scope and magnitude
- Risk–benefit analysis
- Number, size, and type(s) of vehicles involved (common passenger/commercial vehicle, hybrid vehicle, sport utility vehicle, etc.)
- Number of known or potential victims inside vehicle(s) and ejections
- Identification of witnesses/bystanders
- Stability of vehicles involved
- Access to the scene
- Necessary resources and their availability

With this information, the IAP is set into motion for safe and effective actions to be taken to stabilize the incident. In any event, responders should not rush into the incident scene until an initial assessment can be made of the situation. When conducting a size-up of a motor vehicle collision, follow the steps in (**SKILL DRILL 2-1**).

SKILL DRILL 2-1
Conducting a Size-Up of a Motor Vehicle Collision NFPA 1006: 8.1.1, 8.1.3

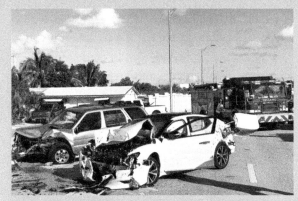

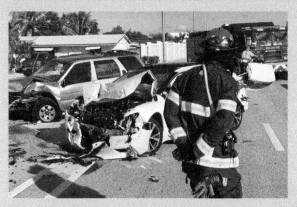

1 Exit the apparatus, and perform the inner and outer surveys, which encompass a 360-degree walk-around of the vehicle(s) and the entire scene. Assess the hazards. Determine the type of vehicle involved and whether the vehicle is running. Identify whether it is a conventional-, commercial-, hybrid-, all electric vehicle-, or alternative-fueled vehicle. Determine the number of victims involved and the severity of their injuries and the level of entrapment. Determine interior hazards, such as supplemental restraint system (SRS) air bag components, including their locations. Assess the resources available, and call for additional units if needed. Provide an updated report. Establish a secure work area with operational zones (hot, warm, cold, and no-entry zones), and establish a staging resource area. Direct the staging/placement of arriving apparatus.

2 Ensure the proper PPE is worn, which may include SCBA depending on the nature of the incident type. Start the size-up process when the incident is dispatched. Position the emergency vehicle so as to protect the scene (defensive apparatus placement). Transmit an initial scene size-up report to dispatch, including the extent of vehicle damage (minor, moderate, or heavy). Establish command if needed. Assign personnel and tasks. Look for obvious IDLH hazards.

Courtesy of David Sweet.

Scene Size-Up Report

As the apparatus arrives on scene, the company officer needs to give a size-up report to dispatch. The main reason for the report is to give an update to the units responding so they can maintain or adjust their response. The units responding should tailor their response to what the report states. This report should be precise and detailed but not lengthy. It should include information such as the number of vehicles involved, type of vehicles, position of the vehicles (upright, on roof, on side, on another car), extent of damage (minor, moderate, heavy), and, if known, victim status and level of entrapment. Chapter 4, *Site Operations*, covers this topic in greater detail.

Inner and Outer Surveys

The inner and outer surveys are 360-degree inspections of the scene that are completed by two or more personnel, depending on the number of vehicles and the size of the incident scene. Rescuers can walk together in the same direction or independently, where one rescuer walks in a clockwise direction around the scene and the other in a counterclockwise direction; either directional choice must ensure that every area within the hot/action zone has been investigated by surveyors. These surveys provide the company officer and crew with additional information about hazards, types of vehicles, the number of victims, possible ejections, the level and type of entrapment, the need for additional resources, and the information necessary to complete an IAP, or objectives for the incident strategy. Lastly, while conducting the inner and outer surveys, if any IDLH hazards are found, then that surveyor needs to call out the hazard immediately, and all members must be ordered to "freeze" until the hazard has been mitigated, or made safe to continue. Chapter 4, *Site Operations*, covers this topic in detail.

Scene Safety Zones

Once the entire area has been surveyed, hazard control zones need to be established and maintained until the incident has been terminated or hazards have been mitigated. NFPA 1500 Section 8.7 recommends that hazard control zones delineate the operational boundaries, which are divided into three areas: hot, warm, and cold. A fourth zone—a no-entry zone—can be added if needed. These zones are designated by the IC prior to position assignments and are strictly enforced by the incident safety officer. The boundaries of the three zones (and the fourth, no-entry, zone if needed) should be established in a manner that ensures the safety of the crews operating within the zones and limits the exposure of personnel outside the zones to any potential hazards or debris. If there are changes to the sizing or location of the zones, these changes must be directed to and acknowledged by all personnel on the scene (**FIGURE 2-21**).

Hazard zones should consist of the following:

- Hot zone: This area, also known as an action zone, is for entry teams and rescue teams only. It immediately surrounds the dangers of the incident, and entry into this zone is restricted to protect personnel outside the zone.
- Warm zone: This area is for properly trained and equipped personnel only. The warm zone is where personnel and equipment decontamination and hot zone support take place, including a debris area for material that is removed from the vehicle(s).

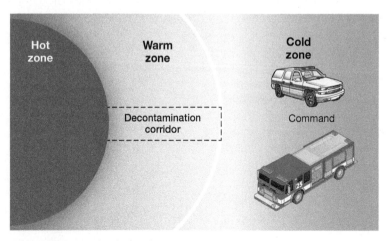

FIGURE 2-21 The hazard zones.

- Cold zone: This area is for staging vehicles and equipment and contains the command post.
- No-entry zone: This is the area at an incident scene where no one is permitted to enter because of an IDLH or the need to preserve the scene for evidence for a postinvestigation team. For crime scene investigations, this zone may be established later in the incident when the initial tactical teams have concluded the operation. This zone may or may not need to be established, based on the type of incident and findings.

The IC assigns personnel or uses law enforcement to establish another perimeter outside the cold zone to keep the public and media out of the operational area. The most common method of establishing the hazard zones for an emergency incident site is to use law enforcement, fire line tape, or barriers. Once the controlled zones have been marked, the IC, incident safety officer, and personnel ensure that the restrictions associated with the various zones of the emergency scene are strictly enforced. Chapter 4, *Site Operations*, covers this topic in greater detail.

After-Action REVIEW

IN SUMMARY

- Vehicle rescue and extrication is a technical process that requires structured successive steps to produce favorable results.
- Most if not all fire rescue organizations already provide a level of service to manage complex emergency incidents, such as vehicle rescue and extrication incidents.
- There are a number of considerations that should be taken into account before committing your organization to providing technical rescue services, including actual need, cost, personnel, and equipment requirements, as well as social and political climate. The components of a risk assessment are hazard, organizational, risk–benefit, and level of response analyses.
- SOPs are designed to describe related considerations (the rules for doing the job), such as safety, evacuation, communication and notification procedures, command structures, and reporting requirements.
- The major components of a response plan include the identification of potential problems and issues; resource identification and allocation; and in some cases, suggested or mandatory procedures.
- An IAP formulated by an organization or AHJ should be designed following the model of the NIMS.
- The ICS is a management structure that provides a standard approach and structure to managing operations. The use of ICS ensures that operations are coordinated, safe, and effective, especially when multiple agencies are working together.
- It is important to have systems in place to keep track of both personnel and equipment on scene.
- Emergency incidents many times extend into long-term operations (greater than a few hours), and consideration must be given to planning for such a possibility.
- The health and safety of members are of the highest importance, and a health and safety program, developed in concert with NFPA 1500, 1250, 1521, and 1561, will provide your organization with the tools necessary to run a safe and effective organization.
- A basic vehicle extrication involving the assessment, removal, stabilization, and packaging of a victim should take no longer than 20 minutes; this does not include response or transport times.
- The selection of body protection and PPE is made based on the known and potential hazards at the scene of the vehicle rescue and extrication incident as well as what is required by the AHJ for the agency.
- The main goal of defensive apparatus placement is to block and protect the scene from the flow of traffic.
- Crowd control is an absolute necessity in protecting responders from individuals who might attempt to enter into the emergency site.
- As an incident grows, the need for additional resources and personnel can grow as well.

KEY TERMS

Active risk–benefit analysis An analysis that entails an on-scene assessment of the risk to personnel and/or victims compared to the benefits that might result from the rescue.

Branches The organizational level having functional, geographical, or jurisdictional responsibility for major aspects of incident operations. (NFPA 1026)

Crew A group of personnel working without apparatus and led by a leader or boss.

Crew resource management (CRM) A program focused on improved situational awareness, sound critical decision-making, effective communication, proper task allocation, and successful teamwork and leadership. (NFPA 1500)

Defensive apparatus placement The positioning of apparatus to block and protect the scene from the flow of traffic.

Division A supervisory level established to divide an incident into geographic areas of operations. (NFPA 1561)

Finance/administration section Section responsible for all costs and financial actions of the incident or planned event, including the time unit, procurement unit, compensation/claims unit, and the cost unit. (NFPA 1026)

Golden Period The time during which treatment of shock and traumatic injuries is most critical and the potential for survival is best accomplished through rapid medical intervention.

Group A supervisory level established to divide the incident into functional areas of operation. (NFPA 1561)

Hazard analysis A documented assessment performed by personnel knowledgeable of the specific hazards of the material or situation and that is acceptable to the AHJ. (NFPA 484)

Immediate danger to life and health (IDLH) Any condition that would do one or more of the following: pose an immediate or delayed threat to life, cause irreversible adverse health effects, or interfere with an individual's ability to escape unaided from a hazardous environment.

Incident action plan (IAP) The objectives reflecting the overall incident strategy, tactics, risk management, and member safety that are developed by the incident commander. Incident action plans are updated throughout the incident. (NFPA 1500)

Incident commander (IC) The individual responsible for all incident activities, including the development of strategies and tactics and the ordering and release of resources. (NFPA 1026)

Incident command system (ICS) A standardized on-scene emergency management construct specifically designed to provide for the adoption of an integrated organizational structure that reflects the complexity and demands of single or multiple incidents, without being hindered by jurisdictional boundaries. (NFPA 1006)

Liaison officer (LO) A member of the command staff, the point of contact for assisting or coordinating agencies. (NFPA 1026)

Logistics section Section responsible for providing facilities, services, and materials for the incident or planned event, including the communications unit, medical unit, and food unit within the service branch and the supply unit, facilities unit, and ground support unit within the support branch. (NFPA 1026)

Mass casualty incident (MCI) An emergency situation that involves more than one victim and that places great demand on equipment or personnel, stretching the system to its limit or beyond.

Operations section Section responsible for all tactical operations at the incident or planned event, including up to 5 branches, 25 divisions/groups, and 125 single resources, task forces, or strike teams. (NFPA 1026)

Organizational analysis A process to determine if it is possible for an organization to establish and maintain a given capability.

Planning section Section responsible for the collection, evaluation, dissemination, and use of information related to the incident situation, resource status, and incident forecast. (NFPA 1026)

Public information officer (PIO) A member of the command staff responsible for interfacing with the public and media or with other agencies with incident-related information requirements. (NFPA 1026)

Response planning (preincident planning) The process of compiling, documenting, and dispersing information that will assist the organization should an incident occur at a particular location.

Risk assessment An assessment of the likelihood, vulnerability, and magnitude of incidents that could result from exposure to hazards. (NFPA 1670)

Risk–benefit analysis An assessment of the risk to the rescuers versus the benefits that can be derived from their intended actions.

Safety officer (SO) An individual appointed by the AHJ as qualified to maintain a safe working environment. (NFPA 1670)

Scene size-up A mental process of evaluating the influencing factors at an incident prior to committing resources to a course of action. (NFPA 1006)

Single resource An individual, a piece of equipment and its personnel, or a crew or team of individuals with an identified supervisor that can be used on an incident or planned event. (NFPA 1026)

Staging area manager ICS position responsible for ensuring that all resources in the staging area are available and ready for assignment.

Standard operating procedure (SOP) A written organizational directive that establishes or prescribes specific operational or administrative methods to be followed routinely for the performance of designated operations or actions. (NFPA 1521)

Static risk–benefit analysis An analysis conducted in an office setting prior to any incident. This type of analysis is an evaluation and justification of whether to acquire/support the required level of service needed to manage a technician level technical rescue incident that has the potential to occur or has occurred in the past within the jurisdiction.

Strike team Specified combinations of the same kind and type of resources, with common communications and a leader. (NFPA 1026)

Task force A group of resources with common communications and a leader that can be pre-established and sent to an incident or planned event or formed at an incident or planned event. (NFPA 1026)

Technical specialists A person with specialized skills, training, and/or certification who can be used anywhere within the incident management system organization where their skills might be required. (NFPA 1561)

Traffic incident management A management tool that establishes roadway safety procedures and traffic control measures for emergency operations at a motor vehicle accident.

Unified command A team effort that allows all agencies with jurisdictional responsibility for an incident or planned event, either geographical or functional, to manage the incident or planned event by establishing a common set of incident objectives and strategies. (NFPA 1026)

REFERENCE

National Fire Protection Association. 2021. NFPA 1006, *Standard for Technical Rescue Personnel Professional Qualifications*. 2021 ed. Quincy, MA: NFPA.

On Scene

Your unit is the first on scene at a multiple vehicle accident. It is apparent that there are several victims. Fluid is noticeably leaking from one of the vehicles, and the odor of gasoline is in the air. Several agencies have already been dispatched to the scene, including law enforcement, fire rescue departments, and transport units from different jurisdictions. A media van is also on scene already, and a crowd is gathering.

1. The first action of the rescuer should be to:
   A. begin crowd control.
   B. initiate victim triage.
   C. conduct size-up and establish command.
   D. identify a staging area.

2. To identify the strategies of the incident, the incident commander should develop a formal or informal:
   A. tactical priority system.
   B. incident action plan.
   C. strategic overview policy.
   D. task assignment method.

(continues)

On Scene Continued

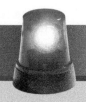

3. The optimal number of individuals within a span of control is:
   A. three.
   B. four.
   C. five.
   D. six.

4. When multiple agencies have responsibility for the incident, it may be advisable to establish a command system that is:
   A. cooperative.
   B. shared.
   C. collaborative.
   D. unified.

5. One member of the command staff is the:
   A. media officer.
   B. medical officer.
   C. logistics officer.
   D. safety officer.

6. The command post should be away from the immediate scene.
   A. True
   B. False

7. In larger incidents, the incident commander may choose to establish a section in charge of:
   A. purchasing.
   B. planning.
   C. performance.
   D. probabilities.

8. The medical unit is responsible for:
   A. triage of victims.
   B. care of responders.
   C. identifying available hospitals.
   D. treating the critical victims.

9. A group of up to five single resources of any type is also known as a:
   A. task force.
   B. strike team.
   C. strike force.
   D. tactical force.

10. One of the things the accountability system is meant to recognize is a responder's:
    A. liability.
    B. experience.
    C. certification.
    D. assignment.

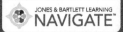

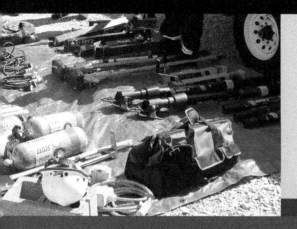

CHAPTER 3

Awareness Level

Tools and Equipment

KNOWLEDGE OBJECTIVES

After studying this chapter, you should be able to:

- Identify the two standards describing protective ensembles for technical rescuers. (p. 50)
- Indicate the primary differences between active and passive hearing protection. (pp. 54–56)
- Articulate the differences between supplied air respirator/breathing apparatus (SAR/SABA) and self-contained breathing apparatus (SCBA). (pp. 56–57)
- Explain advantages and disadvantages of supplied air respirator/breathing apparatus (SAR/SABA) and self-contained breathing apparatus (SCBA) for a vehicle technical rescue. (pp. 56–57)
- Classify hand tools into one of four categories. (pp. 57–66)
- List the types of pneumatic tools and describe their uses at a vehicle rescue incident. (pp. 66–68, 70)
- List the types of air-powered lifting tools and describe their uses at a vehicle rescue incident. (pp. 71–73)
- List the types of electric tools and describe their uses at a vehicle rescue incident. (pp. 74–79)
- List the types of fuel-powered tools and describe their uses at a vehicle rescue incident. (pp. 79–80)
- List the types of hydraulic tools and describe their uses at a vehicle rescue incident. (pp. 80–85)
- List the types of stabilization tools and describe their uses at a vehicle rescue incident. (pp. 85–89)
- Describe the benefits of Class B foam at vehicle rescue incidents and identify the required equipment for its production. (pp. 90–92)
- Identify victim packaging and removal equipment. (p. 93)

SKILLS OBJECTIVES

- Select appropriate PPE for a vehicle rescue. (**NFPA 1006: 8.1.1, 8.1.3, 8.1.5**, pp. 50–57)
- Don appropriate personal protective equipment (PPE) before working with tools. (**NFPA 1006: 8.1.1, 8.1.3**, p. 50)
- Inspect PPE for damage. (pp. 51, 52, 54–57)
- Decontaminate PPE. (p. 54)
- Stage and organize tools at a technical rescue incident. (p. 90)

You Are the Rescuer

You are on the scene of a vehicle rescue and extrication incident, and you are told that one of the hydraulic tools has failed.

1. What alternative tools are available on your apparatus to complete the tasks?
2. Will you need to call for a backup apparatus equipped with hydraulic rescue tools?

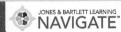 Access Navigate for more practice activities.

Introduction

It's almost inevitable that a technical rescuer will experience some type of tool failure on an incident or in training—whether a seal fails on a hydraulic tool, spewing out all the hydraulic fluid, or a regulator freezes up on an air chisel. The technical rescuer must always be prepared to adapt and overcome obstacles. This is why it is so important for the technical rescuer to have a vast working knowledge of all types of tools used in the field. In the case of a sudden power tool failure, the technical rescuer must be proficient enough to be able to switch that power tool out with a hand/mechanical tool and operate that tool just as effectively without jeopardizing the procedure or prolonging the extrication time.

There are a multitude of types of tools used throughout the world today, some more specialized and geared toward vehicle rescue and extrication and some that cross over to other disciplines and/or professions. It would take an entire book to cover all of these tools, and so this chapter will cover some of the more common tools used in vehicle rescue and extrication today.

Tools for vehicle rescue and extrication purposes can be broken down into five basic categories:

1. Hand tools
2. Pneumatic tools
3. Hydraulic tools
4. Electric- or battery-powered tools (nonhydraulic)
5. Fuel-powered tools

Note that stabilization tools can be classified as a hand, pneumatic, or hydraulic type.

Personal Protective Equipment (PPE)

Before the technical rescuer can start to work with tools, he or she must don full PPE for safety. The National Fire Protection Association (NFPA) has developed two standards describing the protective ensemble technical rescuers must wear at the scene of rescue or recovery operations: NFPA 1500, *Standard on Fire Department Occupational Safety, Health, and Wellness Program,* and NFPA 1951, *Standard on Protective Ensembles for Technical Rescue Incidents.*

NFPA 1951 lists rescue and recovery technical rescue protective ensembles and ensemble elements for technical rescue personnel, including coats; trousers; coveralls; helmets; gloves; footwear; and interface components, which consist of the material that overlaps and meets with another PPE material to provide full protection with no gaps or exposed areas. Respiratory protection may also be necessary if personnel are operating in an area with airborne contaminants or a known and/or suspected immediate danger to life and health (IDLH) environment. To be compliant with NFPA 1951, the protective ensemble must provide protection from exposure to physical, thermal, liquid, and body fluid-borne pathogen hazards. The selection of the specific PPE components will depend on several factors, including the type of incident, hazards at the scene, the duration of the incident, the type of equipment utilized, and the weather.

SAFETY TIP

It should be mandatory for all personnel in the action, or hot, zone at an emergency incident or a training drill to wear all the required protective gear.

Head Protection

The helmet will protect the head and has a minimum of a three-point suspension system, consisting of supports on both sides and the rear of the helmet to maintain the helmet position on the head. Helmets come in several types, including the traditional fire helmet, the lighter urban search and rescue (USAR) helmet, and the Euro-style helmet (**FIGURE 3-1**). Both

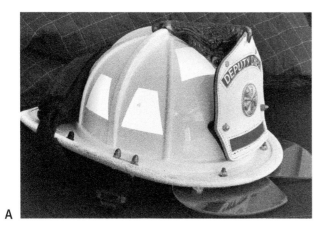

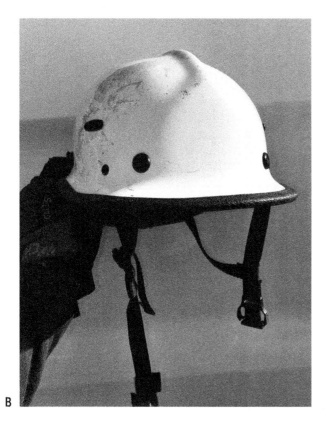

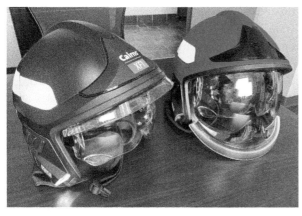

FIGURE 3-1 Head protection. **A.** Firefighter's helmet. **B.** USAR helmet. **C.** Euro-style helmet.
Courtesy of David Sweet.

the traditional and USAR helmets are acceptable; the Euro-style helmet is acceptable if it complies with NFPA 1971, *Standard on Protective Ensembles for Structural Fire Fighting and Proximity Fire Fighting*. Compared to other, traditional helmets, Euro-style helmets offer additional, significant safety features incorporated into the helmet, including integrated eye protection, full face shield, thermal pull-down hood, and head lamp and thermal imaging camera, just to name a few. However, the higher costs and strict maintenance and care policies will have to be considered when deciding whether to use the Euro-style helmet.

Inspect helmets for any signs of damage to the shell, such as cracks, major chips, or gouges. Such flaws could compromise the integrity of the shell; the helmet should be removed from service if these defects are evident. The suspension system, chin strap, and visor should also be inspected for any signs of damage. Inspect helmet liners and hoods for normal and/or unusual wear, tears, or other damage. Keep all head protection clean to facilitate inspection. In addition to these general guidelines, familiarize yourself with any additional recommendations or field maintenance guidance or procedures provided by the manufacturer of the equipment as well the proper equipment required for the position or assignment that has been approved by the authority having jurisdiction (AHJ).

Body Protection

The type of body protection used will depend on the hazards present, the AHJ, and the level of comfort for the wearer while maintaining full protective safety compliance. Protective coveralls or coats/pants protect the upper torso, lower torso, arms, and legs. There are several types that can be worn. Most companies wear full structural firefighting clothing, also known as turnout gear, that meets all related NFPA standards (NFPA 1971, *Standard on Protective Ensembles for Structural Fire Fighting and Proximity Fire Fighting*), but such clothing tends to be bulky and hot. Newer, lightweight turnout gear, offering the same level of protection, is now available. Some companies prefer the coverall or jumpsuit. A fully NFPA 1951 compliant extrication or technical rescue jumpsuit is constructed out of a heavy grade material and may have additional reinforcements sewn on the knee and elbow areas depending on the manufacturer. Extrication jumpsuits are a great alternative to heavier and bulkier turnout gear, providing easier movement and less fatigue from overheating (**FIGURE 3-2**). There are many types of jumpsuits; make sure the suit can offer the extra protection needed to operate safely at an extrication incident. Leave the lightweight mechanic-type jumpsuits

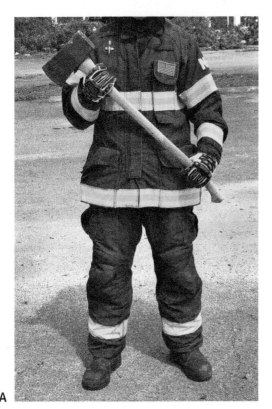 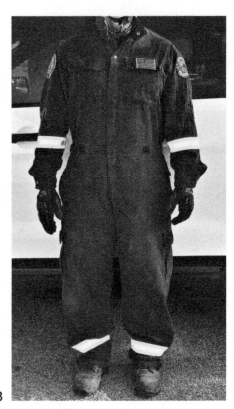

FIGURE 3-2 The technical rescuer must wear a full personal protective ensemble at all rescue or recovery operations. **A.** Structural firefighting clothing. **B.** Extrication jumpsuit.
Courtesy of David Sweet.

at the station; these will offer little or no protection. Remember, the AHJ representing each agency will have the ultimate decision on what will be worn by personnel, but safety should be the driving force for this decision.

In addition to protecting the body from injury, PPE must be bright to help ensure visibility during daylight hours; PPE that is used at night should be equipped with reflective material to increase visibility in the darkness. It is imperative that all personnel wear high-visibility PPE at all motor vehicle collisions and/or when outside the apparatus on unprotected roadway areas. High-visibility garments should meet ANSI 107, *American National Standard for High-Visibility Safety Apparel and Accessories.*

Eye and Face Protection

Exposure to debris, dirt, dust, fumes, bright light, and hazardous fluids can potentially cause temporary or even permanent damage to vision or can enable a point of entry for any bloodborne pathogens (microorganisms in the blood) or other body fluids that can transmit illness and disease in people. NFPA 1500 states that all face and eye protection should meet the requirements of the American National Standards Institute (ANSI) Z87.1 standard, which establishes performance criteria and testing requirements for occupational and educational eye and face protection devices. The various letters, numbers, and symbols associated with the ANSI Z87 marking on the lens will also indicate the following types of lenses.

The impact rating markings are:

- Spectacle lens: +
- All other lenses: Z87+
- Plano frame: Z87+
- Rx frame: Z87-2+

Eye protection can be provided by either goggles or safety glasses certified to ANSI Z87.1+-2015 safety standards in the United States, the European Standards for Eye Protection CE-EN166 in Europe, and the Canadian Standards Association CSA Z94.3-15 in Canada. Each eyewear device has its own set of issues in certain environments. Most safety glasses are not designed to give the wearer a perfect seal and can expose areas on the sides of the lenses, allowing particle debris to enter. Goggle eyewear, on the other hand, provides a tight seal, but this causes heat buildup, condensation, and excessive fogging, which obstructs vision. Newer goggles on the market offer built-in vents and antifogging coatings on the lenses (**FIGURE 3-3**). Face shields normally offer protection from the top of the eyes to the nose area only, leaving an open bottom

CHAPTER 3 Tools and Equipment 53

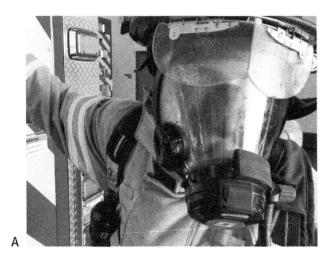

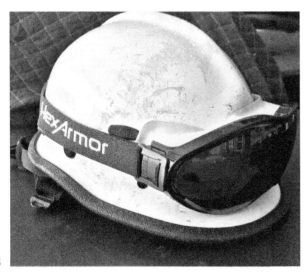

FIGURE 3-3 Eye and face protection. **A.** A respirator face piece provides maximum protection for the eyes and the face. **B.** Rescuers may need specialty eye protection such as a face shield or goggles.
A: Courtesy of Chris Xiste. B: Courtesy of David Sweet.

section where a hazardous substance can enter from underneath the shield and affect the eyes; for this reason, face shields are not considered a primary eye protection device. Safety glasses should include a retainer strap and a side shield or a wraparound design to offer protection to the sides of the eyes.

The inspection of eye protection should focus on looking for broken or missing pieces and scratches or gouges that will impair the vision of the user. In addition to these general guidelines, familiarize yourself with any other recommendations or field maintenance guidance provided by the manufacturer.

Hand Protection

Protective gloves are designed in two parts: the protection area of the glove body, which extends from the tip of the finger to the wrist crease, and the glove

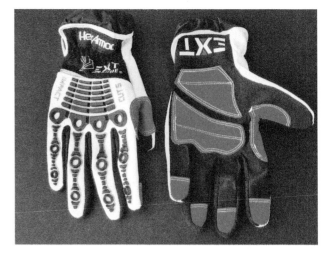

FIGURE 3-4 It is critical that the technical rescuer wear proper gloves; he or she must purchase gloves with maximum dexterity and protection.
Courtesy of David Sweet.

interface component, which is the protection area that extends beyond the wrist crease and is equipped with a closing/cinching mechanism or gauntlet style at the cuff to prevent debris from entering the glove. NFPA 1951 sets glove standards for technical rescue and recovery that measure cut resistance, puncture resistance, abrasion resistance, hand function, grip, and ease of donning.

Gloves are a very important component for the technical rescuer. If the gloves are too bulky, for example, like traditional fire gloves, simple procedures (such as fully depressing the trigger on an air chisel or reciprocating saw) will be extremely difficult and cumbersome. Leather work gloves from the hardware store are not an appropriate choice either; although they provide dexterity, they provide little or no protection for your hands. Gloves designed for vehicle rescue and extrication have special cut resistance and reinforced material in areas that require the most protection—such as fingertips, palms, and knuckles—but do not restrict movement. Gloves that incorporate Kevlar®, Dyneema®, and/or SuperFabric® materials offer the best overall protection (**FIGURE 3-4**).

Even with the strongest material, vehicle rescue and extrication gloves are not impervious to all penetrations; a stray shard of glass or jagged metal could make it through the protective barrier. Still, these gloves offer the best level of protection as compared to other types of gloves. For additional protection, surgical latex gloves can be worn under the extrication gloves to offer an added barrier against any bloodborne pathogens or other biohazards, but remember that latex gloves are not a breathable material and will cause excessive sweating and moisture buildup underneath the glove. It is a general practice to wear medical (latex or nitrile) gloves underneath the working gloves so that when it's time to place hands on the victims, the working gloves can be removed, limiting exposure of the victim to possible contaminants from the gloves, such as glass particles and oils.

SAFETY TIP

Medical gloves can be worn underneath the working gloves so that when it's time to place hands on the victim, the working gloves can be removed, limiting exposure of the victim to possible contaminants from the gloves, such as glass particles and oils.

After each use, gloves should be inspected for rips, tears, weak or missing stitching, and exposure to contaminants. They should be cleaned, decontaminated, sanitized, and dried or discarded according to the manufacturer's instructions, and you should follow any additional recommendations or field maintenance guidance provided by the manufacturer.

Foot Protection

Footwear should consist of boots containing puncture-resistant materials to protect the entire foot, including the sides, sole, and ankle. The boot should also be equipped with an impact- and compression-resistant toecap to prevent crushing injuries to that area of the foot. Most boots used in rescue situations are either firefighters' boots or safety work boots (**FIGURE 3-5**).

When inspecting footwear, look for wear, tears, or holes in the leather or rubber as well as damage or excessive wear to the soles, laces, or zipper. Waterproof boots in accordance with the manufacturer's directions, and follow any additional recommendations or field maintenance guidance provided by the manufacturer.

Hearing Protection

Hearing protection is one of the most underutilized safety items in the emergency service industry. Because rescuers are commonly exposed to high levels of noise from the equipment used to perform vehicle rescue and extrication, hearing protection should be a common PPE item that is consistently worn at every incident or training evolution.

Sound is measured in decibels (dB), with a normal verbal conversation between two individuals measuring at around 60 dB. NFPA 1500 recommends hearing protection for all personnel when the noise threshold is in excess of 90 dB, such as when operating power tools or other motorized equipment. Damage to one's

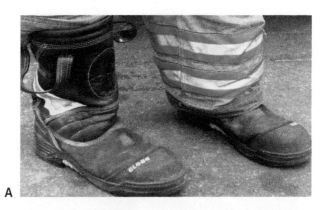

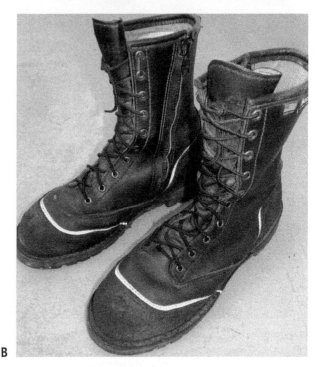

FIGURE 3-5 Boots used in rescues are typically either firefighters' boots or safety work boots. **A.** Firefighters' boots. **B.** Safety work boots.
Courtesy of David Sweet.

hearing and/or hearing loss can occur with prolonged exposure to decibel levels greater than 85 dB. A reciprocating saw measures in the 100 to 105 dB level, and a typical hydraulic engine, depending on the manufacturer's type, can measure 60 to 95 dB. Damage to one's hearing can occur gradually over continual or prolonged exposure; the rescuer may not notice any damage occurring to the eardrum until it is too late (**FIGURE 3-6**). Hearing protection, such as earplugs, earmuffs, and noise-reducing or noise-canceling headphones, is designed to reduce the decibel level that enters the wearer's ear canal.

There are two types of hearing protection recognized by the Occupational Safety and Health Administration (OSHA): passive and active hearing protectors. Passive hearing protectors are hearing protection devices that provide static noise control that cannot be

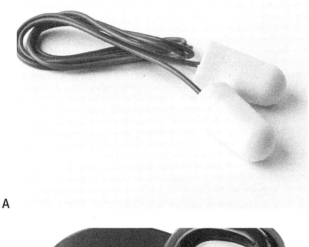

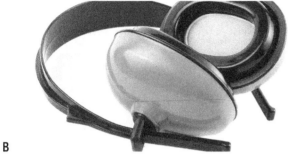

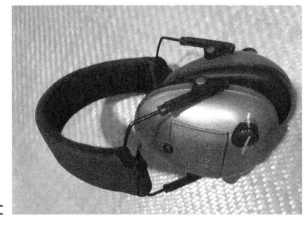

FIGURE 3-6 Hearing protection. **A.** Earplugs. **B.** Earmuffs. **C.** Noise-reducing or Noise-canceling headphones.
A: © niavuli/Shutterstock; B: © Draw/Shutterstock; C: Courtesy of Bill Larkin.

changed or altered, such as standard earplugs. Active hearing protectors use an electronic, intelligent-based design that has the ability to change the attenuation (the strength of a sound signal) of the device based on any sound changes in the surroundings that are deemed potentially harmful. An example of an active hearing protection device is noise-canceling headphones, which recognize damaging decibel levels and automatically create a noise wave that meets the incoming sound, reducing it to a safe level.

The Environmental Protection Agency (EPA) devised a Noise Reduction Rating (NRR) system that rates hearing protection devices based on their attenuation.

This rating system requires manufacturers to use laboratory testing to identify and label the noise reduction capability of all hearing protectors. The NRR is based on a scale of 0 dB to 33 dB. The wearer would subtract the listed device rating from the environment decibel reading to determine the overall decibel effect. For example, if the technical rescuer were operating a hydraulic tool with a noise level of 100 dB and also correctly utilizing a hearing protection device with an NRR of 30, the overall noise level the rescuer would be experiencing would be 70 dB. Although this may work in a perfect world, some situations and environments cannot be accurately reproduced in laboratory testing. For this reason, as a safety measure, OSHA suggests that rescuers cut a listed NRR down by 50 percent to cover any unaccounted variances.

Passive hearing protection devices, such as earplugs, come in a variety of designs. They are manually inserted into the outer ear canal and block damaging high-level sounds from entering. They conform to the shape of the canal and come in disposable or reusable packs. The number one failure of this device is from the wearers not properly seating the device inside the ear canal and/or removing the earplug when someone wants to communicate with them. Earplugs are inexpensive and easy to carry, and some are equipped with a cord so they can hang around the neck when not in use. Today, there are specially designed earplugs that improve safety by blocking hazardous decibel noise levels while maintaining and allowing important lower frequencies through for voice communications and warning signals.

Static earmuffs are another passive hearing protection device. They are generally designed to fit over the head and cup the ears. Earmuffs can be more comfortable than earplugs, with some designed to fit over the head and others designed to be mounted or integrated into the helmet.

Noise-canceling headphones are considered an active hearing protection device because of the ability to change the protection level of the device. Similar to earmuffs, noise-canceling headphones can fit over the wearer's head or, with other models, can be mounted onto or integrated into the helmet. Noise-canceling headphones work by emitting an electronic signal that blocks any high-decibel frequency that can be damaging to the ear. The negative aspects of this type of headphones are the higher cost per unit and that some design features may prevent the rescuer from wearing a helmet during operations unless the helmet comes equipped with a special mounting device.

Inspection of nondisposable hearing protection includes ensuring cleanliness and checking for damage that would reduce the effectiveness of the device.

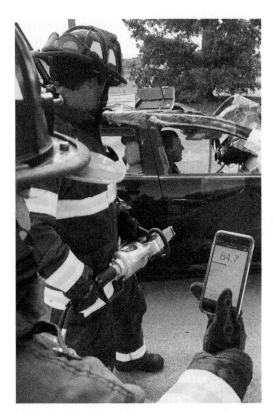

FIGURE 3-7 The NIOSH Sound Level Meter app can assess the decibel levels in real time.
Courtesy of David Sweet.

Another excellent tool that provides real-time decibel levels is the National Institute of Safety and Health (NIOSH) Sound Level Meter mobile app. NIOSH offers this free app (not currently available for Android devices), which continuously measures sound levels in the vicinity, providing the incident commander (IC) or safety officer immediate situational awareness on noise exposure. This can help identify problematic noise levels and allow personnel to take measures to protect their hearing (**FIGURE 3-7**).

It is highly recommended that agencies develop a hearing protection program and/or standard operating procedures (SOPs) on hearing protection that are followed by every member of the department, whether responding to an incident or during training evolutions. Hearing loss is a debilitating but very preventable injury that all emergency personnel, regardless of their specific discipline, should work to prevent.

Respiratory Protection

Potential hazards and respiratory irritants in the air can develop from an incident or from the actions of the technical rescuers at an emergency incident or training session. The selection and use of respiratory protection are of utmost importance, whether it is wearing a simple N-95 face mask or full respiratory protection using a self-contained breathing apparatus (SCBA). Hazards may take the form of chemicals, vapors, fumes, dust, glass particulate/dust, bloodborne pathogens, or oxygen deficiency. NFPA 1500 recommends that emergency agencies develop a respiratory protection program as well as SOPs that address the use of respiratory protection. OSHA describes two types of respiratory protection devices:

- Air filtration respirators, such as masks that utilize filters, canisters, and/or cartridges to filter out the outside air
- Atmosphere-suppling respirators, which use compressed, uncontaminated air stored in bottles to supply a mask or full-face piece

Air-Filtering Face Piece Respirators

Air-filtering devices work by utilizing electrostatic charges in between layers of filter media and fibers, which mimic magnets that attract and contain airborne particles. When choosing an air-filtering device for respiratory protection, utilize masks certified by NIOSH. NIOSH issues a letter designation (N, R, and P) for degradation levels as well as a filtering efficiency number (95, 99, and 100). The letter N means that the filter is not resistant to oils and/or oil aerosols degradation. The letter R means that the filter is resistant to oils and/or oil aerosols degradation but can be used only one time and then must be discarded. The letter P means that the filter is strongly resistant to oils and/or oil aerosols degradation and can be used for longer durations. Filtering efficiency numbers are assigned based on the percentage and size of the airborne particulate matter that is blocked, measured at 0.3 microns or greater in size. For example, a "P-99" rated filtration mask will block out 99 percent of airborne particles 0.3 microns or larger as well as oil-based aerosols. Ninety-five percent (the N-95) is the minimum level of protection NIOSH will qualify for effective filtration protection. This level should be sufficient to protect the technical rescuer from glass particulates and dust but not from any hazardous fumes, which would require full SCBA to be worn. As a general precaution, Nomex hoods pulled over the mouth and nose as well as scarves do not provide sufficient respiratory protection to qualify as air-filtering devices.

Self-Contained Breathing Apparatus

A **self-contained breathing apparatus (SCBA)** is a respirator with an independent air supply, which allows rescuers to enter potentially dangerous atmospheres (**FIGURE 3-8**). SCBA should be compliant with the requirements of NFPA 1981, *Standard on Open-Circuit Self-Contained Breathing Apparatus (SCBA) for*

CHAPTER 3 Tools and Equipment 57

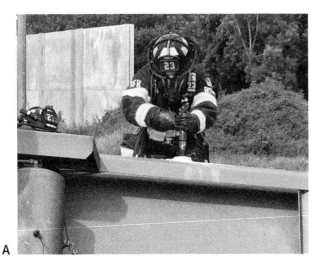

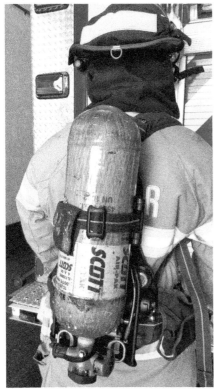

FIGURE 3-8 Self-contained breathing apparatus.
A. Courtesy of Mike Jackles, BSO Fire Rescue. B. Courtesy of Chris Xiste.

Emergency Services. SCBA for rescue, hazardous materials response, tactical law enforcement operations, confined space entry, terrorist incident response, and similar operations should comply with NFPA 1986, *Standard on Respiratory Protection Equipment for Tactical and Technical Operations.* SCBAs are available in 30- to 60-minute versions and protect against almost all airborne contaminants. An SCBA may be a disadvantage in some situations because of the limited air supply. Also, the bulk of the frame that holds the SCBA in place may make working in confined or restricted spaces difficult, and the weight of the unit may cause excessive fatigue during long operations.

Supplied Air Respirator

In a **supplied air respirator/breathing apparatus (SAR/SABA)**, breathing air is supplied by an air line from either a compressor or a stored air (bottle) system located outside the work area. Supplied air respirators should comply with the requirements of NFPA 1986, *Standard on Respiratory Protection Equipment for Tactical and Technical Operations.*

Fit Testing

Mask or face piece fit testing is a process that ensures through quantitative and/or qualitative measuring that the wearer has a proper seal (i.e., the mask fits the wearer's face, and there is no air leakage around the face and the mask), which is set and maintained throughout usage. Each user must undergo a fit test per NFPA 1500 and OSHA Standard 1910.134, *Respiratory Protection.*

Inspection and maintenance of respiratory protection equipment should be performed at regular intervals and after each use. Inspections should include replacement or refill of air cylinders, inspection of system components for signs of excessive wear or damage, and the proper cleaning and sanitation of the face piece. In addition to these general guidelines, familiarize yourself with any other recommendations or field maintenance guidance provided by the manufacturer of the equipment.

Maintenance of PPE

NFPA 1855, *Standard on Selection, Care, and Maintenance of Protective Ensembles for Technical Rescue Incidents*, covers procedures for inspections, cleaning, decontamination, repairs, storage, and record keeping for the following gear components pertaining to technical rescue: garments, helmets, gloves, footwear, and interface components. Every department should create and implement an SOP regarding proper maintenance for all PPE. All gear should be inspected after every incident and at predesignated periodic intervals.

Hand Tools

A **hand tool** is described as any tool or equipment that does not use electric or other motor power but operates from the physical manipulation of human power. The technical rescuer must have a thorough working knowledge of the different types of hand tools that can be utilized at a vehicle rescue and extrication incident. Hand tools are the basis of all working tools; being able to utilize a hand tool effectively or when all other tools fail is an asset the technical rescuer needs to acquire. The first inclination of most rescuers may be to use power tools; however, in some situations, hand tools may be applied faster and be more efficient than power tools. At some point, a technical rescuer will experience a total electrical or mechanical failure of the powered tools he or she is using during an incident. The rescuer will then have to rely on knowledge of hand tools to accomplish the task. Being proficient in knowledge and use of both powered and hand tools is the mark of a skilled professional.

Again, there is a tremendous variety of hand tools for various disciplines, and each individual has personal favorites. This text covers some of the more prominent hand tools common to a vehicle rescue and extrication incident.

Hand tools can be categorized according to how they are applied. There are four basic types common to vehicle rescue and extrication:

1. Striking tools (**FIGURE 3-9**)
2. Leverage/prying/spreading tools (**FIGURE 3-10**)
3. Cutting tools (**FIGURE 3-11**)
4. Lifting/pushing/pulling tools (**FIGURE 3-12**)

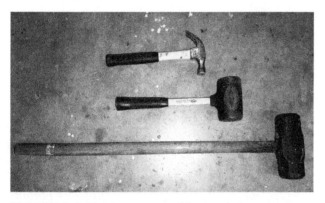

FIGURE 3-9 Hammer-type striking tools (top to bottom): hammer, rubber mallet, and sledgehammer.
Courtesy of David Sweet.

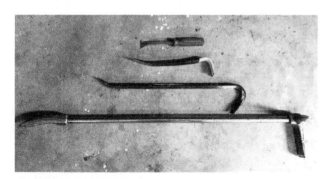

FIGURE 3-10 Leverage/prying/spreading tools (top to bottom): flat-head screwdriver, flat claw tool, pry bar, and Halligan-type tool.
Courtesy of David Sweet.

Striking Tools

Striking tools are used to apply an impact force to an object. Examples of some basic striking tools include a rubber mallet, used to drive a wedge in place; a prying tool, forced into a small opening to create a purchase or access point for another tool; or a center punch, used to break a vehicle window (**FIGURE 3-13**).

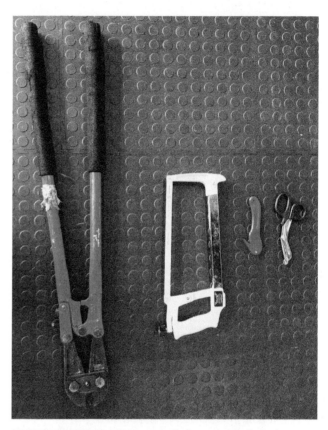

FIGURE 3-11 Cutting tools (left to right): bolt cutters, hacksaw, seat belt cutter, and trauma shears.
Courtesy of David Sweet.

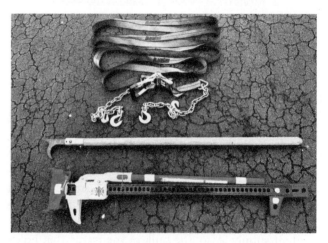

FIGURE 3-12 Lifting/pushing/pulling tools (top to bottom): cargo strap, pike pole, and First Responder Jack.
Courtesy of David Sweet.

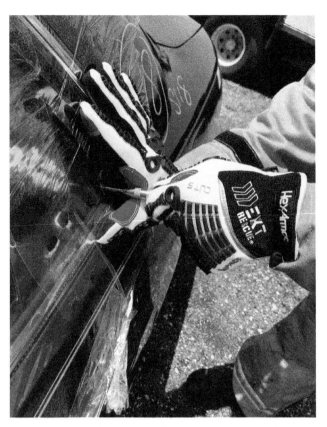

FIGURE 3-13 Center punches are used as striking tools.
Courtesy of David Sweet.

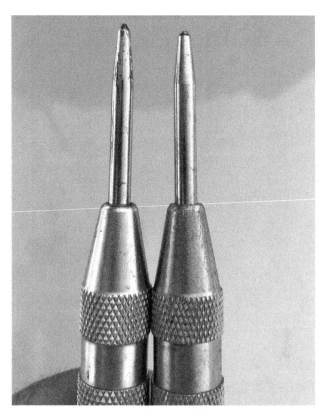

FIGURE 3-14 Examine the tip of your center punch to make sure it is not dull like the center punch depicted on the right in this picture.
Courtesy of David Sweet.

Included in this category are hammers, punches, and some glass saws, which can serve multiple functions of cutting and striking. Hammer-type striking tools have a weighted head with a long handle. Hammer-type tools include the hammer, mallet, sledgehammer, and flat-head axe.

The **spring-loaded center punch** is a glass-breaking tool used only on tempered glass; it is not designed to work on laminated glass. When engaged, the center punch uses a spring-loaded plunger to fire off a steel rod with a sharpened point directly into a pinpoint area of glass, causing the glass to shatter. Two of the biggest flaws of the center punch are that the spring will normally fail from getting water in the chamber, causing it to rust, or the point of the steel rod will dull from repeated use, rendering it useless; you will notice this when the tool fails to break the glass after several attempts (**FIGURE 3-14**). The procedures for breaking tempered glass on a vehicle utilizing a spring-loaded center punch are discussed in the Glass Management section in Chapter 9, *Victim Access and Management*.

Numerous other types of punches are available; some consist of a stationary punch design that has a hardened steel point attached to the end of a knife. There is also the hammer-type punch that consists of a one- or two-sided hardened steel point head. A spring-back–type punch is about the length of a pen; the user must pull back and release a spring in the middle of the device to correctly operate it. All of these glass tools require different operating procedures (**FIGURE 3-15**). Follow the manufacturers' instructions to operate them as they were designed to be used.

An example of a multipurpose tool that is used for cutting and striking is a glass handsaw (**FIGURE 3-16**). The glass handsaw is a manually operated cutting/striking tool used for removing glass. It is an extremely versatile tool with several design applications but is primarily used for removing tempered and laminated vehicle glass.

For breaking tempered glass, the center grip handle of the glass handsaw has a slot where a center punch is stored with the tip facing inward. When ready for use, the center punch sits firmly in the handle and is then positioned with the tip facing outward. The tip of the center punch is placed against the glass with the front guard positioned against a hard surface. Placing the front guard against a hard surface is a safety measure that prevents the tool and the technical rescuer's hand from going through the window when the glass is broken (**FIGURE 3-17**).

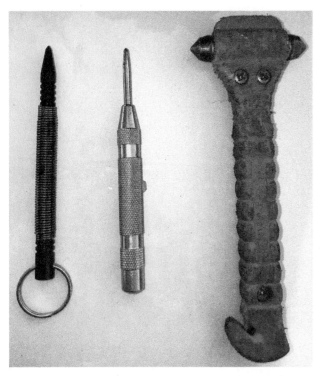

FIGURE 3-15 Various glass breaking tools (left to right): spring-back–type punch, plunger center punch, and glass break hammer.
Courtesy of David Sweet.

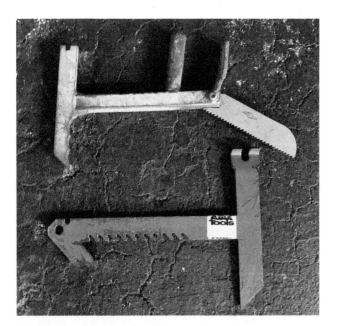

FIGURE 3-16 Glass handsaws.
Courtesy of David Sweet.

Another feature that the glass handsaw offers is a notched section on the end of the tool that fits over the top lip of the glass. When the tool is turned to the side, the glass fractures immediately, which eliminates the possibility of misfires from the use of a center punch. Never attempt to use the point section of the glass tool to break out tempered glass; tempered

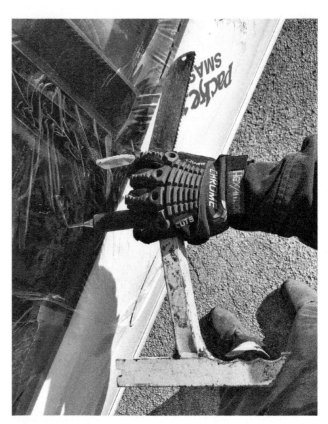

FIGURE 3-17 A glass handsaw is used here to demonstrate the proper technique of breaking tempered glass. The front guard, used against a hard surface, prevents the tool and the technical rescuer's hand from going through the window when the glass is broken.
Courtesy of David Sweet.

glass is designed to resist breaking from impacts such as this. Attempting to break a tempered glass window by striking it with a tool, whether it is a glass tool or a Halligan bar, is not only highly unprofessional but can potentially cause injury to you, the crew, or the victim. Additional glass management tools, such as the Packexe SMASH® self-adhesive film, are discussed in the Glass Management section in Chapter 9. Laminate sheeting can be quickly applied to the glass to prevent shattering, thus keeping the broken glass intact and controllable (**FIGURE 3-18**). This allows the rescuer more flexibility in determining whether the glass should stay in place or be removed. It also provides a safer working environment for the rescuer and victim by limiting glass particles and shards.

Leverage Tools

Leverage tools multiply the force a person can exert to bend, pry, lift, rotate, or spread objects from other objects. Greek mathematician Archimedes of Syracuse (287 BCE) theorized the mechanical advantage of the lever and is quoted with the immortalizing statement

CHAPTER 3 Tools and Equipment

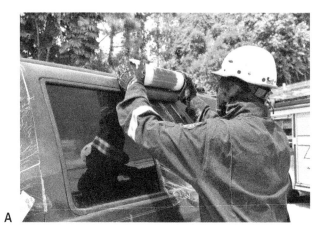

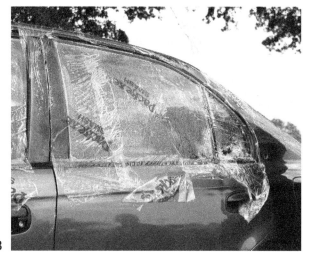

FIGURE 3-18 Self-adhesive film for glass management. **A.** Applying Packexe SMASH® on windows. **B.** Completed Packexe SMASH® on windows.
Courtesy of Edward Monahan.

of "Give me a lever long enough and a place to stand and I will move the world." Leverage tools include rotating, prying/lifting type devices (**FIGURE 3-19**). Rotating tools are designed to turn objects and include wrenches, pliers, and screwdrivers. These types of tools can be used to gain access, expose concealed areas, or disassemble vehicle components.

Simple prying tools act as a lever to separate objects from each other, gain access or create purchase points, and lift/move heavy objects. Common simple hand prying tools include the following equipment:

- Claw bar
- Crowbar
- Flat bar
- Halligan bar
- Kelly tool
- Pry bar

The technical rescuer must be resourceful and adapt when tools are not working or the task becomes

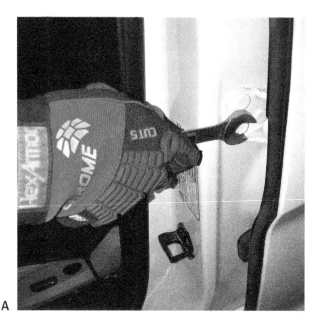

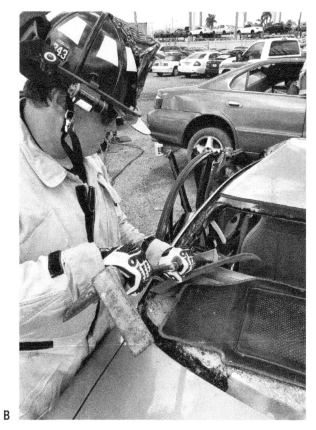

FIGURE 3-19 Leverage tools. **A.** Rotating. **B.** Prying.
Courtesy of Edward Monahan.

SAFETY TIP

Technical rescue personnel are taught to adapt and overcome when presented with a difficult situation. However, modifying a tool to overcome its design limitations is a poor example; such action may go against manufacturer specifications and safety guidelines and could cause injury or harm to you or others.

TABLE 3-1 Cleaning and Inspecting Hand Tools

Metal parts	All metal parts should be clean and dry. Remove rust with steel wool. Do not oil the striking surface of metal tools because this may cause them to slip.
Wood handles	Inspect for damage, such as cracks and splinters. Sand the handle if necessary. Do not paint or varnish; instead, apply a coat of boiled linseed oil. Check to be sure the tool head is tightly fixed to the handle.
Fiberglass handles	Clean with soap and water. Inspect for damage or splintering. Check to be sure the tool head is tightly fixed to the handle.
Cutting edges	Inspect for nicks or other damage. File and sharpen as needed. Power grinding may weaken some tools, and so hand sharpening may be required.

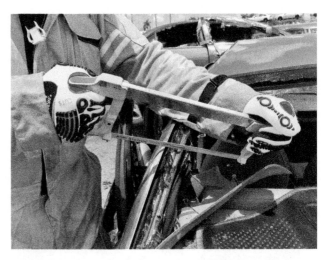

FIGURE 3-20 A firefighter using a hacksaw to cut through a metal A-post of a vehicle roof.
Courtesy of David Sweet.

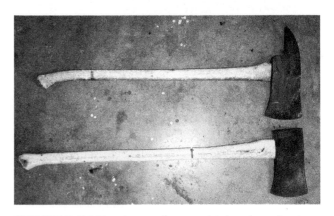

FIGURE 3-21 Two types of axes: pick-head axe (top); flat-head axe (bottom).
Courtesy of David Sweet.

difficult. However, modifying a tool to accomplish a challenging task can compromise the safety guidelines and specifications of the tool, and can put the rescuer or others at risk for harm. For example, a pipe is sometimes used to extend the length of a tool handle; this extension is commonly referred to as a cheater bar. This modification is meant to extend the distance from the fulcrum of the tool to where the force is being applied, thereby increasing the amount of leverage exerted. In doing so, however, the design strength of the tool may be exceeded, ultimately causing its damage or failure. Tools are susceptible to damage, and it is important to take these tools out of service if they show any signs of damage, such as cracks or bends (**TABLE 3-1**).

Cutting Tools

Cutting tools have a sharp edge designed to sever an object. Manual cutting tools range from tools carried in the pockets of turnout coats to larger tools that must be carried to where they are needed. Cutting tools include saws, chopping/snipping shears, trauma scissors or shears, hacksaws, seat belt cutters, knives, chisels, bolt cutters, wire cutters, and axes. Each type of tool is designed to work on certain types of materials and cut in a different manner.

Hacksaws that are used for vehicle rescue and extrication should be the heavy-duty type. They have a thick and durable frame so the technical rescuer can use both hands to push and pull with controlled force for optimum cutting performance. The heavy-duty type also offers the ability to set the blade under high tension, which prevents it from twisting and bending. This setting provides a sturdy and rigid cutting action (**FIGURE 3-20**). Hacksaws are useful when metal needs to be cut under closely controlled conditions or when a powered reciprocating saw cannot be utilized.

Large-tooth saws, such as the bow saw, are effective tools for cutting large timbers or tree branches; as a consequence, they can prove especially useful when a chain saw is not available at a motor vehicle collision. Damaged trees, wood telephone poles, and various loose timbers can become obstructions to the operation and have to be cut down or removed. Wood saw blades with fine teeth are designed for cutting finished lumber and tend to cut the material more slowly. For this reason, they are not usually used in rescue work.

The flat-head axe and the pick-head axe are primarily cutting tools but also can be used as striking tools (**FIGURE 3-21**). These tools consist of a long handle with a weighted head on the end. The head has a sharpened cutting edge that is used to strike the object. These tools should have a semi-sharpened edge so the edge will not chip if it hits an object such as a nail or a stone.

Bolt cutters, cable cutters, insulated wire cutters, sheet metal snips, seat belt cutters, and emergency medical services (EMS) trauma scissors or shears operate on a leverage concept, with the fulcrum being located just behind the cutting edges. This concept allows for a concentration of the cutting force on a small area. Care must always be taken when cutting wires, including ensuring that they are not electrically energized. Seat belt cutters are normally very simple devices that utilize a razor to cut through the material. These razors are prone to dulling and rusting after they have been used a few times. It is advised to purchase seat belt cutting devices designed with blades that can be easily changed out after becoming dull or oxidized. Another cutting tool that is similar to the bolt cutter is a steering wheel ring cutter; this tool uses a ratcheting-type tensioning mechanism that builds pressure to cut through a steel steering wheel ring.

There are several variations of knives used by rescuers (**FIGURE 3-22**). Knives should have a retractable or folding blade that locks when open. Knives should remain sharp to provide for maximum readiness when they are needed.

Hand-operated chisels, which are used to cut wood and metal, are typically operated by striking the chisel with a hammer or mallet. They come in a variety of widths and styles and should be used for cleaving only the material for which they were designed. Metal chisels, sometimes called cold chisels, are used to cut sheet metal or to cut off bolts and other objects.

SAFETY TIP

Safety must always be a priority when cutting wires. Ensure wires are not electrically energized before approaching them.

Lifting/Pushing/Pulling Tools

Lifting, pushing, and pulling tools are the backbone of any vehicle rescue and extrication operation. Pulling tools such as the standard pike pole can be used to extend the reach of the person using them. For example, a ratchet strap can be attached to the hook side of the pike pole and passed under or through a vehicle to a rescuer on the other side.

Manual lifting and pushing tools include mechanical and hand-operated hydraulic jacks (**FIGURE 3-23**). Mechanical jacks can be of the screw, ratchet lever, or cam type. Jacks are used to lift or push heavy objects. The First Responder Jack (FRJ) is a hand-operated tool that works by a mechanical ratcheting system designed to lift, push, pull, and clamp heavy material. This tool is rated at around a 4600-lb (2086.5-kg) working load limit (WLL) and allows the use of chain and sling attachments for easy anchoring and securing. The FRJ can be used exclusively in place of a hydraulic

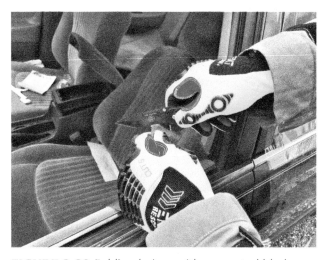

FIGURE 3-22 Folding knives with a serrated blade work well for a variety of fabric materials, such as seat belts, or for cutting through vehicle seat fabric to expose the seat frame during rescue work.
Courtesy of David Sweet.

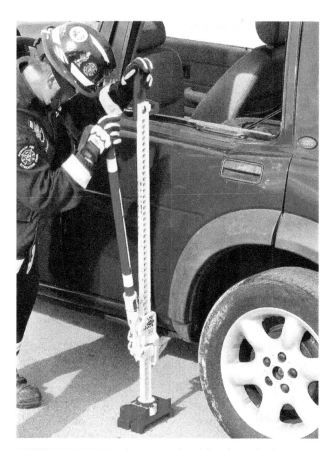

FIGURE 3-23 Hand-operated ratchet lever jack.
Courtesy of Edward Monahan.

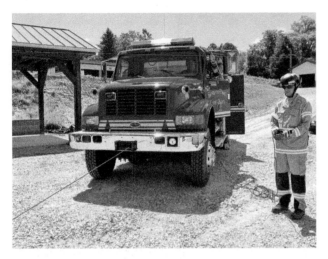

FIGURE 3-24 A winch, or hoist, uses either a rope, a chain, or a cable (wire rope) and is used for pulling or lifting heavy objects.
Courtesy of David Sweet.

spreader and/or ram so that fire and rescue agencies that have limited funding resources to acquire costly hydraulic tool systems can accomplish the same tasks.

Another type of pulling tool is the manual or power-operated winch, or hoist, which uses a cable (wire rope) and is used for pulling, lifting, or stabilizing heavy objects (**FIGURE 3-24**). Winches are used by many rescue organizations for a variety of lifting, pulling, and stabilizing operations. The two varieties of winches are the integrated cable and drum type (come along) and the grip hoist, which is a pass-through cable type.

When inspecting manual winches, look for any damage caused by overloading and friction. Check the winch for warping, bending, or cracking. Examine cables for signs of overloading, such as metal distension, elongation, twisting or separation of stands, cracks, fraying, or flattening of cable. Any damage noted to any part will require the item to be placed out of service immediately and repaired or replaced according to the manufacturer's specifications. Lubricate moving parts properly according to manufacturer specifications, and keep the mechanism free of dust, dirt, and grime.

Electrical winches are discussed later in this chapter.

Grip Hoist

The grip hoist, or TIRFOR®, is a manual winching device that can lift, pull, move, and stabilize heavy materials, such as a standard conventional and/or commercial vehicle. It can be operated in multiple positions and, depending on the model, can pull up to 8000 lb (3629 kg) on a single line using a 1:1 ratio. With the base attached to an anchor point, a wire rope designed for the unit is fed into the back and through the unit, attaching to the object to be pulled. It uses a grip-on-grip locking mechanism, similar to pulling rope in a hand-over-hand motion, that grabs, holds, and moves the wire through the unit. Adding snatch blocks and anchor points can increase the pull to a 3:1 ratio or more depending on the number of blocks and anchor points used. The telescoping handle attaches to the power stroke or reverse lever and has shear pins that will fail and freeze the load if the pull exceeds the limit. The grip hoist, unlike the come along, does not use a ratchet or wire-over-drum mechanism where slippage may occur.

Come Along and Chain Package

The come along is a hand-operated, ratchet lever winching tool that, when used in conjunction with chains and hooks, can provide up to several thousand pounds of pulling force (**FIGURE 3-25**). The standard model used for extrication provides 2000 to 4000 lb (907 to 1814 kg) of pulling force. Used together, the come along and chain package can reap tremendous benefits in safely pulling and stabilizing operations.

The come along operates by ratcheting a wire cable around a drum. It also utilizes mechanical advantage in either a 2:1 ratio by doubling the wire cable around a pulley and then back onto itself or a 1:1 ratio/single line pull. Cable wire is normally 20 to 25 ft (6 to 8 m) in length, so keep in mind that doubling the cable to give you the extra pulling force will cause you to sacrifice the cable by half its length.

Another feature of the come along is the handle. The handle is designed to fail and bend at a certain force well before the tool fails. The failure rating should be listed on the handle (**FIGURE 3-26**). This is an excellent safety feature that gives you full control over the object you are pulling. For example, when lifting a steering wheel assembly off a victim,

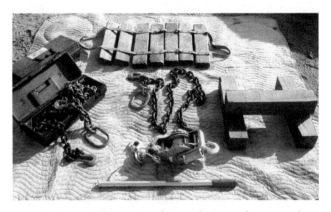

FIGURE 3-25 The come along, chain package, and associated cribbing.
Courtesy of David Sweet.

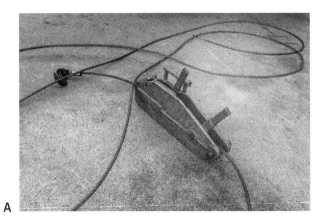

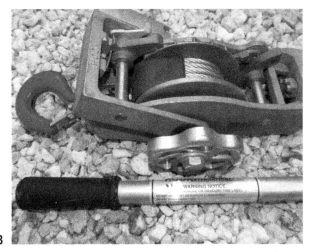

FIGURE 3-26 A. Grip hoist. **B.** Come along.
A: © Chumphon_TH/Shutterstock. B. Courtesy of David Sweet.

the procedure requires very controlled movements whereby the technical rescuer operating the lever can feel the pull. This technique requires extreme caution because of the possibility of the steering assembly becoming dislodged and projecting into the victim or rescuer. With the proper setup and safety checks, and by not overextending the lift, this technique can provide just enough lift clearance to release the entrapment, with the benefit of having full control and feel over the entire length of the pull. This technique can also be accomplished with the FRJ (**FIGURE 3-27**).

> **LISTEN UP!**
>
> Relocation of the steering wheel assembly or a variation of this technique should not be attempted using hydraulics because the operator has no control or feel over the length of the pull; the extreme and rapid force that is applied from the hydraulic tool does not allow for this.

Lifting a steering wheel assembly utilizing the come along and/or FRJ tool is discussed in Chapter 10, *Alternative Extrication Techniques*. Come alongs can also be used for stabilization purposes. For example, if

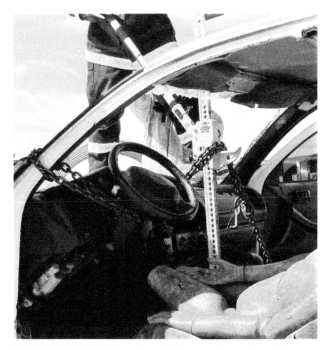

FIGURE 3-27 Relocation of the steering wheel assembly can be accomplished utilizing a First Responder Jack (FRJ).
Courtesy of Edward Monahan.

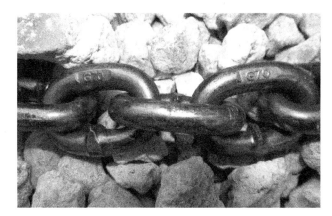

FIGURE 3-28 Load-rating grades, which determine a chain's WLL, are embossed into chain links approximately every 12 to 18 in. (30 to 46 cm). This is a Grade 70 chain.
Courtesy of David Sweet.

a vehicle is on an embankment, it can be secured to a tree, a pole, or an apparatus using a come along. This tool can also be used to pull a vehicle that is wedged up against a road barrier wall (Jersey barrier). Remember to inspect the tool and cable for any signs of damage before and after every use.

The chain package that comes with the come along kit is rated for that system only and should not be used with any other system. Chains must be marked with a grade, which is utilized to determine the chain's WWL or its **working load limit (WLL)** (**FIGURE 3-28**). To determine a product's WLL, the manufacturer utilizes the minimum breaking strength of the device and divides this by a safety or design factor that is predetermined by the manufacturer. The minimum breaking "tensile" strength of a chain is determined by using a formula of dividing the unit of force (Newton) by square millimeter (N/mm^2). For example, the grade 80 chain equals 800 Newton per square millimeters. A manufacturer will determine the minimum breaking strength of their 5/8 grade 80 chain at 72,400 lbs with a 4:1 safety factor, giving the chain a WLL of 18,100 lbs. This WLL is the maximum load determined by the manufacturer that can be applied safely without failure. The WLL is the maximum force that may be applied before failure occurs to an assembly or a component of a device or rope/line/cable in straight tension. Load rating grades are embossed into chain links approximately every 12 to 18 in. (30 to 46 cm). Grade 80 (System 8) and grade 100 (System 10) are the most often used chain types for overhead lifting and rescue.

These chains can come with an assortment of attachments for the various types of anchoring requirements encountered. The assortment of hook attachments can include the master link, which is normally an oblong ring, or O-ring; the slide hook; and the grab hook (the chain shortener) along with the basic towing company attachments, which include the J-hooks (short and long), R-hook, and T-hook. These also come attached together in a cluster package. The cluster attachments are inserted in the various holes or openings found in the undercarriage or frame of the vehicle as anchor points (**FIGURE 3-29**).

Hooks. The slide hook is exactly as its name states. It allows the chain links to pass freely through the throat of the hook to tighten around an object. The slide hook should never be tip loaded by inserting the tip of the hook in a hole or an opening; the hook will bend and possibly dislodge under extreme force. The grab hook is utilized by inserting a link of the chain into the slot of the hook. This is also known as a chain shortener; as the name suggests, it is designed to take up the slack needed to make the chain the appropriate size for the task at hand (see Figure 3-29). The O-ring, or oblong ring, is an attachment designed to join chains together or join a chain to a come along utilizing a hook (see Figure 3-29).

LISTEN UP!

The technical rescuer should never exceed the WLL of chains and cable winching systems.

Pneumatic Tools

Tools utilizing air under pressure to operate are known as pneumatic tools. A wide variety of pneumatic tools are available that can nail, cut, drill, bolt, lift heavy loads, and stabilize. Pneumatic tools the technical rescuer will encounter include air chisels, air impact wrenches, air shores, cut-off tools, and rescue air-lift bags.

The compressed air for pneumatic tools is supplied from air compressors, SCBA cylinders, or vehicle-mounted systems. Most of these tools operate at forces between 90 and 250 psi (621 and 1724 kPa) and use adjustable regulators to provide the proper operating pressure. The standard unit for measuring pressure is pounds per square inch (psi).

Air compressors can be used to provide power to pneumatic tools or to provide breathing air. Those found on rescue units may be portable or fixed (**FIGURE 3-30**). Breathing air compressors are generally larger because of the filtration required to meet ANSI/Compressed Gas Association (CGA) G7.1, *Commodity Specification for Air*, and NFPA 1989, *Standard on Breathing Air Quality for Emergency Services Respiratory Protection*. A minimum air quality of Grade D is used for air-supplying respirators, and a minimum air quality of Grade E is used for dive operations.

Maintenance tasks for air compressors include draining water from the filters and tank and replacing the filter. Oil levels in the compressor (if applicable) and engine fluid levels should be checked after each use. Always familiarize yourself with the manufacturer's provided recommendations, and seek out qualified third-party testing for all annual certifications and quarterly air-quality requirements.

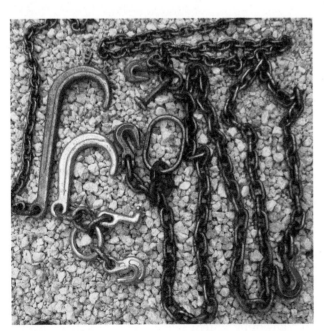

FIGURE 3-29 Various hooks are included with the come along and chain package, including the cluster hook; slide hook; grab hook; and master link, or O-ring.
Courtesy of David Sweet.

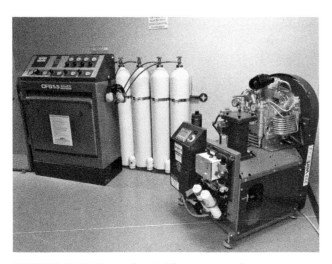

FIGURE 3-30 Cascade air fill system and compressor.
Courtesy of David Sweet.

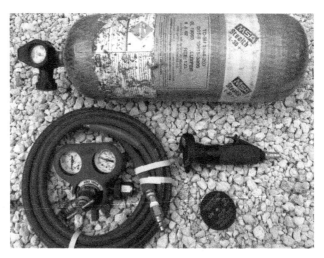

FIGURE 3-31 Pneumatic cut-off tool.
Courtesy of David Sweet.

> **LISTEN UP!**
> Conspicuously label all air tools with the operating pressure so that it is readily known to the user. That way there is no question, especially if a rescuer is not intimately familiar with a given tool.

Pneumatic Cutting Tools

Pneumatic cutting tools include saws, shears, and chisels. The pneumatic saws used in rescue work are either the reciprocating or rotating type. Pneumatic reciprocating saws operate just like the electric variety. Models are available with saw speeds ranging from 1600 to 10,000 rpm. Pneumatic cut-off tools, also known as whizzer saws and die grinders, use a circular, composite cut-off blade that rotates at speeds as high as 25,000 rpm. Such saws are normally used when there is a space limitation, but they can be a problem because of the sparks they generate. The pneumatic cut-off tool is discussed in the following section.

Pneumatic Cut-Off Tool

The **pneumatic cut-off tool**, also called a whizzer tool, uses a small carbide disk, normally 3 in. (8 cm) in diameter, that rotates at high revolutions per minute to cut through most metals (**FIGURE 3-31**). The disk throws off a tremendous number of sparks, but it is a great tool to cut through hardened steel, such as in padlocks, reinforcing bars that are 0.5 in. (1.3 cm) or less, or fence posts. To provide an example of the versatility of this tool, there was an incident where the police department unsuccessfully tried to remove inoperable handcuffs from a prisoner using heavy-duty bolt cutters. After covering the prisoner with a damp blanket to shield him from the sparks and placing a wide, flat crescent wrench under the ring of the

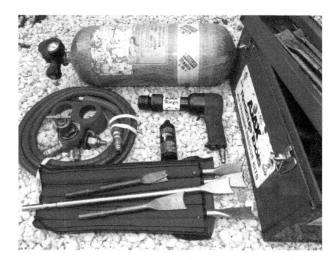

FIGURE 3-32 Pneumatic chisels are used to cut sheet metal or hardened steel.
Courtesy of David Sweet.

handcuff, two sections of the metal handcuff were removed in less than 30 seconds using the pneumatic cut-off tool.

Most models of this tool operate at no greater than 90 psi (621 kPa) and will rapidly deplete an air bottle within minutes. In some models, operating the tool at greater than 90 psi (621 kPa) will potentially damage the tool; always check the manufacturer's specifications for the tool's proper operating pressure. The pneumatic cut-off tool is a great tool to carry on any apparatus; it has many applications and is economical, and it can be stowed almost anywhere because of its small size.

Pneumatic Chisels

Pneumatic chisels, often referred to as air chisels, air hammers, or impact hammers, are used to cut sheet metal and/or hardened steel such as that found in vehicle door hinges (**FIGURE 3-32**).

Voice of Experience

As firefighters and first responders, we have all responded to motor vehicle accidents (MVAs) where mechanical extrication was needed for the entrapped occupants. We have all witnessed these types of calls going well—and not so well. When they don't go well, does your crew, battalion, or department perform an after-action review to understand what went right and what did not? Working as a volunteer and a professional firefighter/officer for over 28 years, as well as an instructor of heavy extrication, I have found that command and control, communications, training, and the right tools for the job can greatly reduce the amount of time involved when performing extrications—resulting in more calls going well.

One MVA where this played out occurred after midnight on a frigid February evening. We arrived to find the vehicles approximately 50 yards from one another with a large debris field from a high-speed, head-on rollover. One was on its wheels, and the other was hanging on its side from the tension cable barrier that separates the east- and west-bound lanes.

After setting up command as well as a large safety zone, we performed our outer- and inner-circle surveys. We quickly determined our extrication plans after confirming one victim, no electrical or other exterior hazards, and the positioning of the vehicle. And then we went to work.

We used both e-draulic tools and hand tools to get the job done. The interior stabilizer (rescuer) determined the door and B-pillar were heavily impacting our victim and needed to be pushed out. Analyzing the use of a hydraulic ram from the inside revealed that there were no viable push points. A B-post push-out, using one of our 48-in. (122-cm) First Responder Jacks, was then called for. We used a hydraulic cutter to move the door and B-pillar away from the victim. It was quick and very effective. While this was being performed, we had a firefighter on the trunk using a 60-in. (152-cm) First Responder Jack for a window tent so the victim could be removed rapidly out the back window and across the trunk.

Working in concert with the other crew members who were performing a complete side removal, and using a combination of e-draulics and a pneumatic chisel, we made excellent headway in a short amount of time. The last maneuver to perform was a seat push-down using the 48-in. (122-cm) First Responder Jack. While our interior stabilizer/rescuer managed the victim off the seat, we slid a backboard in through the rear window tent and prepared for the extrication of the victim. With sharps covered and rescuers in place, we slid the victim through the large rear window tent and onto the trunk lid. We quickly secured the victim before lowering him onto a gurney. The time of extrication from hitting the air brakes to victim removal was 12 minutes. How was this made possible? Through the following:

- Strong size-up and early request for appropriate resources
- Good rig placement with a large, safe working zone
- Rapid plan development with all rescuers on the same page
- Using a combination of hand, pneumatic, and electrical tools
- The proper training

During the after-action report, it was apparent that the hand tools we carried and the appropriate training had made the difference for this victim. What's the moral of this story? Do not place all your eggs in one basket or, in other words, maintain a diverse tool cadre. Having the proper training and power, battery, and pneumatic tools on hand is a must when meeting the international time standards for auto extrication.

Jeff Pugh
Central Pierce Fire & Rescue
Tacoma, Washington
The Puyallup Extrication Team
www.ThePXTeam.org

The tool utilizes an adjustable regulator with a common range setting of 0 to 300 psi (0 to 2068 kPa). The gauge on the regulator displays the bottle pressure and the operating pressure of the air chisel. The regulator can attach to either a 2216- or 4500-psi (15,279- or 31,026-kPa) air bottle, depending on which it is rated for. A high-powered air chisel can have a general operating pressure in the range of 150 to 225 psi (1034 to 1551 kPa). This tool should never be operated at 300 psi (2068 kPa); doing so will potentially damage the tool and cause more blades to break. Check the manufacturer's recommended pressure settings for the various applications encountered.

The pneumatic chisel can be an extremely effective tool in the hands of a skilled technician. It is a precision tool, and proficiency in its use requires a tremendous amount of training. The technical rescuer has to fully understand all the intricacies of the tool and be able to apply this knowledge practically. Some of the intricacies of operating a pneumatic chisel include knowing the proper way to hold the tool and blade, how to maneuver the angle and depth of the cut, how to determine the type of material to cut using the chisel, how to avoid breaking a bit, how to properly dislodge a stuck bit, when to increase and decrease pressure settings, and how to conserve air.

SAFETY TIP

Always place the blade of the air chisel against a solid object when depressing the trigger; free-firing the tool without resistance against the blade can potentially damage the tool's internal mechanism.

There are numerous air chisels available. However, for vehicle rescue and extrication, you want an industrial-duty–rated air chisel that is able to handle the extreme operating conditions of emergency work. Avoid the automotive body shop types; these are commonly underpowered and are not reliable at an emergency incident. Several blade attachments come with the industrialized kits. Some of the more common blades used for vehicle rescue and extrication are the flat blade (long and short shaft), which can be utilized for all cutting requirements, whether cutting hardened steel or lighter sheet metal, and the panel cutter, or T-blade, which is utilized for lighter-gauge steel, such as the sheet metal found in vehicle roofs. If the rescuer is proficient with the flat blade, then the panel cutter, or T-blade, would never have to be used.

In the majority of passenger vehicles or sedans on the road today, vehicle roofs are composed of both light- and heavy-gauge steels, with the outer covering made up of lightweight sheet metal, supported underneath by heavier-gauge steel rib supports. The technical rescuer may be able to cut through the surface of the roof fairly quickly with a panel cutter, or T-blade, but would then have to switch out to a flat blade to cut the remaining steel ribs or framing that supports the roof. This switch would dramatically delay the entry time and possibly cause the rescuer to have to change out air bottles because of the inefficient use and operation of the tool. This is a perfect example of why proficiency training using this tool is critical. When choosing which type of air chisel to carry on the apparatus, keep in mind that not all blades are designed alike; some blades are made of a thicker-gauge high-quality alloy steel that can withstand higher operating pressures and resist accidental breakage of the tip (**FIGURE 3-33**).

The blade retainer is also an important feature to consider when choosing the right tool. The blade retainer prevents the blade from moving and should be

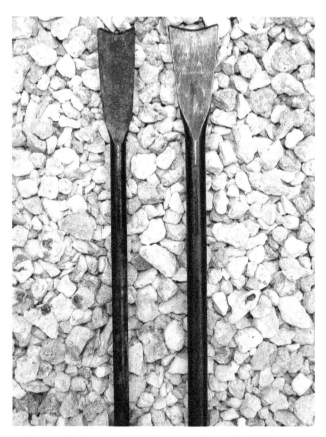

FIGURE 3-33 Not all blades are alike. The blade on the right is a thicker-gauge high-quality alloy steel that can withstand higher operating pressures and resist accidental breakage of the tip. The blade on the left is thinner and has a smaller diameter, making it less forgiving than the thicker blade and prone to breaking at higher pound per square inch settings.
Courtesy of David Sweet.

the quick-change type, where the technical rescuer simply depresses the retainer sleeve to change out a blade. The screw-on type retainers or tools equipped with a collet, which is a sleeve that expands or contracts around the shaft when a retainer is tightened or loosened, are cumbersome and can slow down an operation when a blade change needs to be made quickly. Some blades also come with grooves milled at the insertion point, allowing the technical rescuer to lock the blade in place and prevent it from turning.

> **LISTEN UP!**
>
> When operating the pneumatic chisel using a flat blade, always remember to keep half the blade showing when cutting through a section of metal to avoid burying the tip and jamming the tool.

Pneumatic Rotating Tools
Air Impact Wrench

The **air impact wrench** is a pneumatic rotating tool used to remove nuts and bolts of various sizes, including those found in door hinges, seats, and wheels (**FIGURE 3-34**). The tool has a general air pressure setting of 90 psi (621 kPa) and uses both metric and standard sockets. Remember to always use the sockets that come with the tool set. Never mix hand torque sockets with high-pressure impact sockets; hand torque sockets are not designed to handle the high pressure of an impact wrench and can fail and fragment, possibly causing injury.

Use only impact sockets that are recommended or provided by the manufacturer and are of higher-gauge steel. There are several sizes of impact wrenches, but a 0.5-in. (1.3-cm) drive model with a torque range of 180 to 325 ft-lbs. (244 to 441 Newton-meters) should be adequate to handle most vehicle applications. When dealing with heavier equipment, such as large commercial trucks or buses, a 0.75-in. (19-mm) drive impact wrench will deliver a much higher torque range of 750 to 1200 lb-ft (1017 to 1627 Newton-meters). Using an impact wrench to remove a vehicle door by taking off the hinge bolts is a very fast and easy process, but beware—most doors come equipped with a door-limiting device that limits a door swing and will have to be cut or spread off to fully remove the door.

Pneumatic Lifting Tools
Air Shores

Shoring is used where the vertical distances are too great to use cribbing or the load must be supported horizontally, such as in a trench, or diagonally, such as in a wall shore where a vehicle may have breached a structure and needs temporary structural support (**FIGURE 3-35**). Shoring is defined as the temporary support of structures during activities such as construction, demolition, or reconstruction to provide stability to protect property, workers, and the public. This working definition is obviously related to supporting structural walls but can be used interchangeably with adding structural support to unstable vehicles.

Air shores are a type of strut system that comes in a variety of lengths and may be extended by the use of compressed air. The shoring is then locked in place by pins, notches, and screw collars, with ratchet straps added to the base to add tensioning. Struts and tensioning devices are discussed later in this chapter.

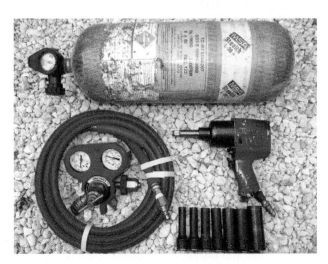

FIGURE 3-34 An air impact wrench.
Courtesy of David Sweet.

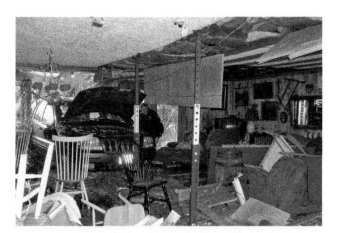

FIGURE 3-35 Shoring is used where the vertical distances are too great to use cribbing or the load must be supported horizontally, such as in a trench, or diagonally, such as in a wall shore where a vehicle may have breached a structure and needs temporary structural support.
Courtesy of Rescue 42, Inc.

SAFETY TIP

Training on maintenance and use must be provided to all personnel to ensure that equipment is operated and maintained in accordance with the manufacturer's recommended guidelines.

Air-Lift Bags

Air-lift bags are pneumatic-filled bladders used to lift an object or spread one or more objects away from each other to assist in freeing a victim (**FIGURE 3-36**). These inflatable devices can move or lift a tremendous amount of weight when inflated. They are commonly composed of rubber with synthetic fiber linings and, depending on the various manufacturers, come in a wide variety of sizes and shapes, each with its own lifting capacity rating. The lifting capacity is measured in metric tonnage, with 1 metric ton equaling 2205 lb.

The lift capacity of a bag is determined by calculating its length × its width × the operating pressure, with a 30-in. (76-cm) length × 30-in. (76-cm) height bag × 115 psi (793 kPa) operating pressure equaling 103,500-lb (47-metric-ton) lift capacity. In a perfect world, this lift capacity number would be great, but in actuality the true lift starts at the center of the bag and spreads out across the entire bag, with the exception of the outside edge or seam area, which cannot be calculated in the lift. Because of this, an inch has to be taken from the length and width, with the true lifting capacity coming from the overall actual surface contact. The 30-in. (76-cm) × 30-in. (76-cm) bag is actually recalculated to 29-in. (74-cm) length × 29-in. (74-cm) height bag × 115 psi (793 kPa) operating pressure equaling 97,715-lb (44-metric-ton) lift capacity.

To achieve an air-lift bag's maximum lifting capacity, the operator must ensure the correct operating pressure is applied and the entire true contact area of the bag is achieved by maintaining maximum contact with the base, maintaining maximum contact with the second stacked bag (if a second bag is used), and maintaining maximum contact with the object to be lifted. Overinflating the bag decreases the surface contact between the bag and the object being lifted. The lift capacity is spread across the entire surface of the bag so that when the surface contact is decreased, the lift capacity decreases as well, as does the overall stability. For example, think of pushing down on two fully inflated footballs stacked on top of one another. The surface-to-surface contact is minimal, with virtually zero stability; this is the same idea as overinflating air-lift bags.

Note that flat-form bags are designed to maintain a flat profile where surface contact is maximized through the lift (**FIGURE 3-37**).

Once a true lift calculation has been determined for each bag, a good practice is to write this true lift capacity on the corners of the bag in a contrasting color that is visible in poor lighting.

Air-lift bags are not used to stabilize a vehicle by themselves; cribbing is always required in conjunction with the bags. Cribbing techniques are discussed in Chapter 8, *Vehicle Stabilization*. There are several air-lift bag classifications used in the field. These include low-pressure bags, medium-pressure bags, high-pressure bags, high-pressure flat-form bags, and multi-cell air-lift bags.

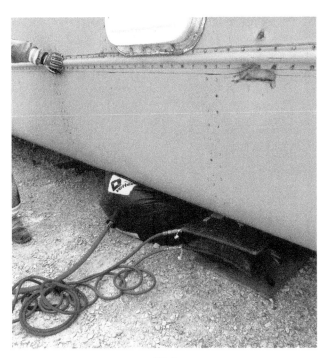

FIGURE 3-36 Rescue air-lift bag.
Courtesy of David Sweet.

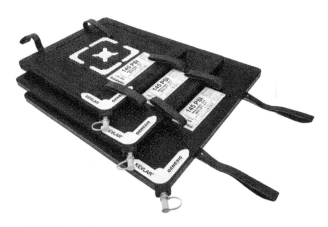

FIGURE 3-37 Flat-form bags.
Courtesy of Genesis Rescue Systems.

General rules when using air-lift bags include the following:

- Do not stack more than two bags because this can cause one or more of the bags to come flying out when inflated, just like a wet seed squeezed between your fingers. (Note: This rule does not pertain to flat-form bag systems or multi-cell systems.) Always refer to the manufacturer's recommendations on stacking operations.
- Always ensure that the valves and hoses are facing outward.
- Never place any objects, such as a thin piece of flat wood or cribbing, on top of or between the bags; doing so will only split the wood, potentially throwing pieces everywhere or causing the entire piece of cribbing to come out under extreme force. Place a piece of plywood below the bag to protect it from the ground.
- Do not overinflate an air-lift bag.
- Do not use an air-lift bag to relocate a steering wheel assembly.
- Do not use an air-lift bag as the sole means to stabilize a vehicle.
- Lift only as high as necessary.
- Always maintain the proper operating pressures. Once the bags have been fully inflated, remember to utilize the shutoff valves on each bag to prevent overinflating or to isolate a bag.

Stacking two bags increases the height of the lift but does not increase the lifting capacity. When stacking bags, always place the larger bag on the bottom, and remember that the lifting capacity is determined by the lower-pressure bag. To maximize each bag's lifting capacity, place the bags next to each other. To better illustrate this, consider trying to lift a 2-ton (1.81-metric ton) cement pole. If you take a 1-ton (0.91-metric ton) bag and then place another 1-ton (0.91-metric ton) bag on top of it and inflate both, the resulting lift capacity will be only 1 ton (0.91 metric ton), and the pole will not move. Now, if you take those same 1-ton (0.91-metric ton) bags and place them side by side and inflate them both, the resulting lift capacity will be the total of both bags, which is 2 tons (1.81 metric tons), thus lifting the cement pole. Remember as a safety measure to always support your lifts with cribbing to compensate for the possibility of a bag failure. Cribbing in place secures a load in the event of any critical failures. The oldest safety rule in the book is "When you lift an inch, you crib an inch."

The basic components of a high-pressure air-lift bag system consist of the following items, with some variations depending on the system, such as a high-pressure multi-cell system, and the manufacturer:

- Cribbing (ample supply of various dimensions and sizes)
- Protective cover (if needed to protect the bag from sharp or heated components)
- Air-lift bag(s)
- In-line/shutoff valves
- High-pressure lines
- Operator controller with dead-man capability (inflation/deflation stops when control valve is released)
- Regulator
- Air cylinder

Low-Pressure Air-Lift Bags. Low-pressure air-lift bags, sometimes called air cushions, provide a very high lift with a maximum working air pressure of approximately 7 psi (48 kPa) (**FIGURE 3-38**). The flat design of the bag when inflated provides a large surface contact and expanded footprint with the item being lifted. These large cushion bags are more commonly found on big tow units because of their ability to upright overturned heavy vehicles, such as semi-trucks and trailers. Disadvantages of some low-pressure air-lift bags are their lower lifting capacities and thinner sidewalls, which can make them less stable when inflating.

Medium-Pressure Air-Lift Bags. Medium-pressure air-lift bags are not as common as the low- and high-pressure rescue air-lift bags; they have a

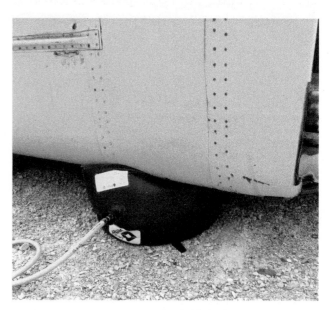

FIGURE 3-38 Low-pressure air-lift bag.
Courtesy of David Sweet.

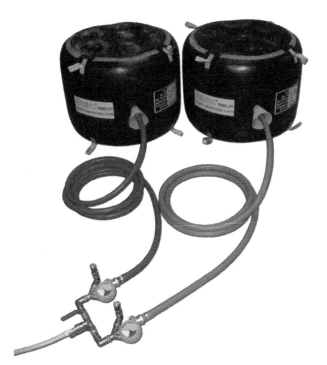

FIGURE 3-39 Medium-pressure air-lift bag.
Courtesy of Savatech Corp.

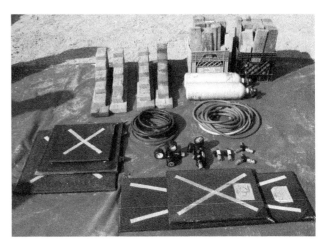

FIGURE 3-40 High-pressure air-lift bag and components.
Courtesy of David Sweet.

more rugged design and use a working air pressure of approximately 15 psi (103 kPa), depending on the manufacturer (**FIGURE 3-39**). Medium-pressure bags commonly have two to three cells and are suitable for aircraft, medium or heavy truck, or bus rescue and recovery work.

High-Pressure Air-Lift Bags. High-pressure air-lift bags are the most commonly used bags among rescue agencies. These bags utilize a working air pressure of approximately 100 to 150 psi (689 to 1034 kPa), depending on the manufacturer (**FIGURE 3-40**). The high-pressure kits come with hoses, a regulator, a master control module, and various other attachments. For safety purposes, a good system comes with hoses of different colors for easy recognition of which bag is in use, a master control module with a dead-man release to prevent overinflating the bag if the control valve is accidentally dropped, and an in-line shutoff/pressure relief valve to isolate a bag and disconnect a line.

An air-lift bag operation will generally require multiple personnel to safely accomplish the task at hand. For example, to safely remove a victim trapped under a vehicle with his or her upper torso and head exposed will require, at a minimum, five personnel to operate safely: one at the head of the victim, two on the sides for cribbing support, one at the controls, and one officer in charge of the lift and overall safety of the operation. Remember the safety rule of thumb, "Lift an inch, crib an inch." Also, remember to lift up equally across the entire vehicle. Lifting on one side forces the opposite side downward, potentially crushing the victim.

High-Pressure Flat-Form Air-Lift Bags. Flat-form air-lift bags are designed to retain their flat profile in the center as they are inflated (see Figure 3-37). This is in direct contrast to the traditional high-pressure bags that round out and decrease surface contact when inflated. The flat design eliminates rolling and shifting and can utilize up to three bags stacked on top of one another. The dimpled surface allows the bags to interlock with one another while side straps assist with alignment and guard against the possibility of a bag ejection. The flat bags vary in operating pressure according to different manufacturers, as well as vary in size and lifting capabilities.

Multi-Cell High-Pressure Air-Lift Bags. Multi-cell high-pressure air-lift bags offer a distinct height advantage over traditional flat bags and utilize a unique lifting system. The most current design is two-cell bags that are joined together and pre-connected. Another version still in use is a round-shaped bag that can be locked together with a threaded connector, creating one bag with multiple cells (**FIGURE 3-41**). The two systems use a working air pressure of approximately 150 or 174 psi (1034 or 1200 kPa) depending on which type is used. Each system has the option of various height adjustments with the attachment of additional bags or inflating a single cell or both cells. With a system that requires the bags to be attached, always reassess the bags before inflation to ensure that they are properly threaded and locked together; these types of systems can detach violently and cause injury or death if not secured correctly.

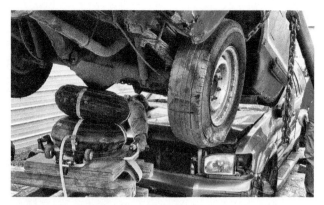

FIGURE 3-41 An example of a multi-cell high-pressure air-lift bag from Paratech.
© Copyright 2018 Paratech.

Electric Tools

Electric-powered tools utilize standard household current or a generator to operate. **Electrical generators** may be portable or fixed and are primarily used to power scene lighting and to run power tools and other electrical equipment (**FIGURE 3-42**). Generators range in capacity from less than 1000 to 75,000 watts (1 to 75 kW) and larger. Depending on the size, they provide output as 120 or 240 volts. Familiarize yourself with any specific recommendations provided by the manufacturer of the equipment, including maintenance instructions. One obvious rule and general disadvantage of portable generator use is that generators cannot be operated inside a structure because of the lethal carbon monoxide gas release and buildup.

Some tools can utilize a battery as an electrical power source. Tools such as reciprocating saws, circular saws, drills, glass cutters, and hydraulics work very well in most applications, but in comparison to an electric-powered or gas-powered system, they do carry certain limitations. Even with the best technology, batteries can sustain only a certain number of amperes per hour (energy) and can quickly drain with continuous use. These tools may not have the reliability of continuous power that a high-amperage tool offers. Reliability is one of the most important features of any tool at an incident where time is critical. Any loss of power or insufficient power has a negative impact on the operation. However, if a generator fails and there is no power to supply a tool, it would be a good idea to have battery-powered options on the apparatus.

A versatile tool that should be on all emergency apparatus is a battery-powered drill set. A battery-powered drill set and charger with an electrical inverter system installed on the apparatus are the best option to maintain constant charge and readiness stage. The ability to use step bits to make quick purchase points for strut insertion, and then quickly

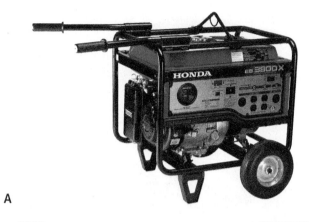

A

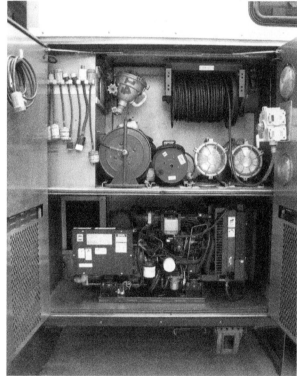

B

FIGURE 3-42 Generators. **A.** Portable. **B.** Fixed.
A: Courtesy of American Honda Motor Co., Inc. **B:** Courtesy of the Berwyn Heights Volunteer Fire Department & Rescue Squad, Berwyn Heights, Maryland.

change out to a laminate glass gutter attachment gives the rescuer multiple uses and quick operational setup for a tool.

There are three types of batteries that have been used in cordless tools over the past several years: nickel–cadmium (NiCd), nickel–metal hydride (NiMH), and lithium-ion (Li-ion) batteries. Li-ion batteries have far surpassed the other two and are widely used as the premier battery type for all cordless operations. If battery-powered tools are used in vehicle rescue and extrication, Li-ion batteries offer the best workload options for heavy operations.

Cordless tools operate from the battery voltage, which gives the tool the power. Amperes per hour (amp-hr/AH) holds the capacity or how fast a battery discharges (**FIGURE 3-43**). The discharge duration also

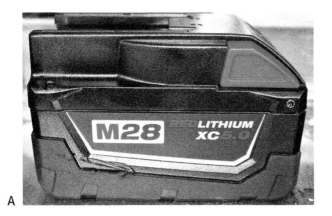

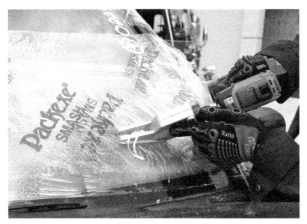

FIGURE 3-43 **A.** Li-ion batteries, along with a higher amperes per hour rating, give the tool the best duration and reliability among battery-powered tools. **B.** Laminate glass cutter attachment on a battery-powered drill.
A. Courtesy of David Sweet. B. Courtesy of Edward Monahan.

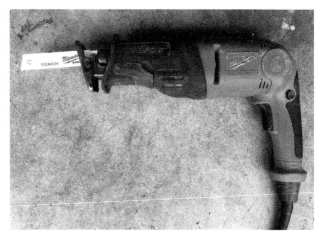

FIGURE 3-44 A reciprocating saw with a handle that bends to a 90-degree angle.
Courtesy of David Sweet.

depends on the efficiency, heat release, and electronic design of the tool as well as the user. Higher voltage can generate more torque, but a high AH with better electronic circuitry management allows that high-power operation for longer.

Adapters may be used to convert a battery-powered tool to a general-current tool. Adapters are a good backup accessory if the batteries run out of power or malfunction.

Electric Cutting Tools

Electric-powered cutting tools include reciprocating saws, metal-cutting circular saws, hydraulic cutters (battery- or electric-driven pumps), and direct current (DC) nonhydraulic cutters as well as specialty items such as plasma cutters.

The plasma cutter is a device with a nozzle that blows inert gas or compressed air at a high speed; at the same time, an electric arc forms within the gas, turning some of the gas to plasma, which is hot enough to easily cut through metal.

Electric Reciprocating Saw

One of the most utilized electric-powered tools common to the extrication incident is the reciprocating saw. The **reciprocating saw** is a type of saw in which the cutting action utilizes a back-and-forth motion (reciprocating), or a push and pull of the blade. Most reciprocating saws come equipped with variable-speed triggers that provide a 1.125- to 1.5-in. (2.9- to 3.8-cm) stroke length and up to 3200 strokes per minute. Electric versions normally range from 6 to 15 amps depending on the manufacturer, with the battery versions normally ranging from 18 to 36 volts depending on whether it is a Li-ion, NiMH, or NiCd battery.

Several operational options are offered by various manufacturers, including the ability to change the angle of a cut to better adapt to a particular situation. Some of the angle features allow the handle to rotate 360 degrees or bend to a 90-degree angle (**FIGURE 3-44**). Another option is an orbital action that forces the blade to lift up and rotate over after it cuts through the material. This is best utilized for wood materials where it is necessary for the wood fragments to be removed to provide a more efficient cutting action. When cutting metal material, it is recommended to disable this orbital feature and maintain a straight cutting action.

When choosing a blade for the reciprocating saw, consider blade type and blade thickness. Will you be cutting wood or metal? Bi-metal blades are the best choice for cutting metals found on vehicles. Bi-metal blades have a high-speed steel cutting edge with hardened teeth welded to tough, thick, flexible spring-back steel. These blades can handle the toughest jobs and can be used multiple times before having to be discarded. The more thinly constructed blades are not designed to perform the high-speed and rigorous applications of vehicle extrication. Thinner blades will heat very quickly, warp, and dull, making the blade useless.

Another consideration when choosing a blade is the TPI rating. The **TPI rating** refers to the number of teeth per inch on the blade (**FIGURE 3-45**). For example, a TPI rating of 18 indicates a large number of small teeth producing a very fine cut, whereas a TPI rating of a 6 indicates much larger teeth producing a very coarse cut. For vehicle rescue and extrication purposes, optimal choices between lengths of 6 to 9 in. (15 to 23 cm) and a TPI rating of 7 to 14 appear to yield the best results, but this depends on the type of material being cut, operating speed, and experience level of the user as well as the preference of the user.

Last, consider the type of metal you will be cutting. Are you dealing with **ferrous metals** (containing iron) or **nonferrous metals** (free of iron)? Why is this important to know? Nonferrous metals such as aluminum melt under the high speed of the blade and cause the aluminum particles to actually weld themselves onto the teeth of the blade, rendering it ineffective. Some of the vehicles constructed today use aluminum in the frame and structure. Reciprocating saw blades, regardless of the type, will have very little or no success cutting through advanced high-strength steel (AHSS) alloys, such as boron or titanium. A better practice is to avoid these types of steels by cutting around them or choosing an alternate method when they are encountered. When in doubt, read the manufacturer's package to determine what the blade is designed to cut.

Reciprocating saw blades generally fail when the tool is operated continuously on the highest speed. This action causes excessive friction, overheating, and melting of the blade. A moderate cut speed with some form of lubrication to cool the blade produces the best result and fastest cut. A spray bottle containing a lubricant (such as soapy water) can be used to spray the blade while cutting. This reduces friction and heat and minimizes degradation of the blade. Keep in mind that the goal of the IC in charge of the operation is to utilize personnel and resources in the most efficient manner.

Be very cautious when changing a blade immediately after using the tool. The blade will be extremely hot. The best method for changing a blade is to face the blade toward the ground and engage the quick-release mechanism, letting the blade fall to the ground without touching it. Keep plenty of blades on hand, and change them as often as needed.

Electric Circular Saw

A **circular saw** moves in a circular motion (**FIGURE 3-46**). These saws come in a variety of sizes and are used primarily for cutting wood, although special blades are available that will cut metal or masonry. These saws come in an AC powered model or an 18- to 20-volt battery-powered metal-cutting circular saw with a 5.5- to 7-in. (14- to 18-cm) diameter carbide tip blade that is designed for the tool, which is excellent for cutting fence post and rebar material that may have become impaled in a victim. The battery-powered option offers the versatility to access tight spaces.

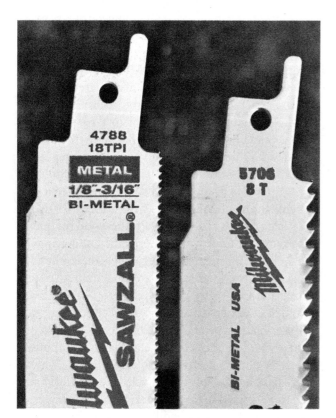

FIGURE 3-45 The TPI rating of a blade indicates how many teeth per inch the blade has. Left blade, 18 TPI. Right blade, 8 TPI.
Courtesy of David Sweet.

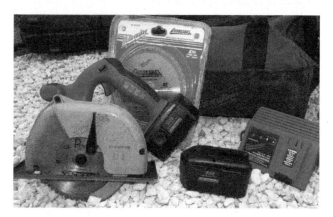

FIGURE 3-46 A metal-cutting circular saw.
Courtesy of David Sweet.

The AC-powered version is a powerful tool that can cut through steel plate up to a 0.75-in. (1.9-cm) thickness depending on the model type. Blade diameters range from 7.25 to 9 in. (18 to 23 cm) depending on the model type. The disadvantage of the AC powered saw compared to the battery version is the weight; the electric saw can weigh from 13 to 20 lb (5.9 to 9.1 kg) depending on the brand, whereas the battery-powered tool can weigh as little as 5 lb (2.3 kg). This may not seem like a big difference, but it matters when you are extending your arm to cut a post and you have to hold either a 5- or a 20-lb (2.3- or 9.1-kg) tool.

The advantage of a metal-cutting circular saw is that there are minimal sparks and vibrations caused when the saw blade passes through the material. It is a very clean and fast cut. In comparison, a reciprocating saw creates significant vibrations, and a hydraulic cutter creates a tremendous amount of torque and twisting of the material.

Electric Lifting and Pulling Tools

Electric-powered lifting and pulling devices include winches and hoists. Winches are used by many rescue organizations for a variety of lifting, pulling, and holding operations. There are two common types of power-driven winches—electrically operated and hydraulically operated. An electric winch is typically driven by an electric motor that draws its power from the vehicle's battery, and a hydraulic winch generally uses a power take-off (PTO) system. The winch uses a wire or a synthetic rope at a minimum of 75 ft (22.9 m) in length and comes in various pulling capacities ranging from 2000 to 12,000 lb (907 to 5443 kg) or more. As a safety precaution, NFPA 1901, *Standard for Automotive Fire Apparatus*, states that a winch should be remotely operated with at least 12 ft (3.7 m) between the winch and the object in an enclosed area.

Any winch is only as strong as what it is attached to, and so winches are normally connected in some fashion to the frame of the vehicle or apparatus (**FIGURE 3-47**). Bumper-type winches are attached in or on the bumper of the vehicle and are mounted permanently. Tow hitch-type winches attach to the tow hitch receiver of a vehicle and are designed to be removed when not in use. All wire rope assembly items, such as hooks, clevises, and snatch blocks, must have a design load rating that is greater than the line pull capacity of the winch.

Winch-pulling capacity should be 1.5 times the gross vehicle weight of the vehicle to be pulled. If the vehicle weighs 8000 lb (3629 kg), the winch capacity should equal 12,000 lb (5443 kg). Never exceed the rated capacity as listed by the manufacturer.

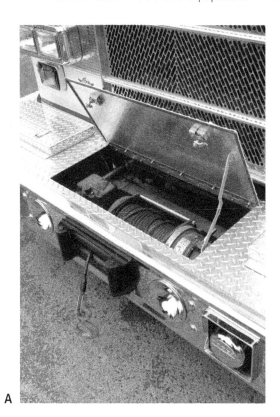

A

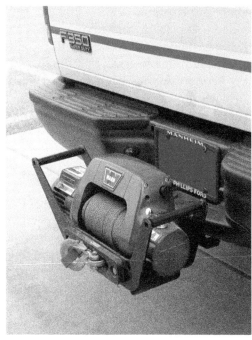

B

FIGURE 3-47 Electric lifting and pulling tools. **A.** Winches can be attached to the bumper of a vehicle. **B.** Winches can also be attached to the tow-hitch receiver.
© Jones & Bartlett Learning. Photographed by Glen E. Ellman.

Unfortunately, the rated capacity of a winch will pull the maximum capacity for only a short duration, normally until the first layer of cable wraps around the drum. After this occurs, the capacity significantly drops because of the change in gear ratios. Electric-driven winches are easy to set up on a vehicle using universal mounting kits, and there are more features available compared to the hydraulic type. Two disadvantages of electric-driven winches are that they are prone to overheating if used for long durations and they can quickly drain an electrical system if the vehicle is not running.

When using a winch, always wear full protective gear, including helmet, eye protection, and gloves, and always operate from a safe distance using the remote controls. To ensure the safest pull, try to keep at least five wraps (not layers) of wire rope around the drum prior to starting the winching operation. Remember that the more layers or wire rope on the drum, the less the pulling power. Some manufacturers recommend placing a heavy blanket on the wire rope at the midpoint between the winch base and the anchor to absorb some of the stored potential energy should the wire rope break. Be aware that there are some possible problems that can occur with this blanket technique; the blanket can move and may be drawn into the winch. Also, setting or removing a blanket can place an added impact load on the line, causing it to fail. Always proceed with caution.

When inspecting a winch, look at the cable, hook, and gears closely for indications of damage or overloading. Periodically inspect the connections to the vehicle frame for rust, bolt tightness, or weld cracks. Periodic lubrication and other inspection/maintenance procedures should be in accordance with any recommendations or field maintenance guidance provided by the manufacturer.

Electric Lighting

Most fire rescue apparatus carry an assortment of portable and mounted scene lighting equipment on the units. Typically ranging from 300 to 1000 watts (0.3 to 1 kW) or more per light, they are found in a variety of styles. Portable lights are meant to provide light where fixed lights cannot. Portable lights are usually adjustable for elevation and have a broad base to prevent them from being tipped over. There are also portable light stands containing one or more lights. These stands are adjustable in height and are useful for providing large-area or higher-height lighting (**FIGURE 3-48**). Hand lights and helmet lights are also used by rescuers.

Fixed lights are mounted on the rescue vehicle and, like portable lights, come in a variety of styles. Some are mounted into the body of the vehicle for perimeter lighting and are not adjustable. Others are mounted so they can be adjusted for direction and elevation, some being a fixed height and some being on adjustable poles. More elaborate systems, referred to as *light*

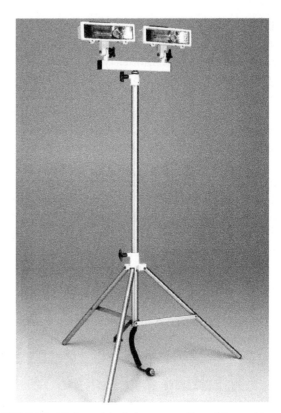

FIGURE 3-48 Portable lights are adjustable and have a broad base to prevent tipping.
Courtesy of Akron Brass Company.

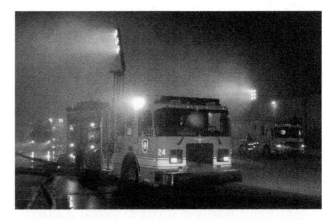

FIGURE 3-49 Light towers mounted to vehicles offer a significant amount of overhead lighting.
© Glen E. Ellman.

towers, consist of telescoping masts with a bank of lights with up to 6000 watts (6 kW) or more of lighting (**FIGURE 3-49**). These masts, which can be vehicle or trailer mounted, can be 30 to 40 ft (9 to 12 m) tall and provide a significant amount of overhead lighting. Because of the height of these towers, it is common to see stabilizers installed on the vehicle or trailer to prevent tipping during high-wind situations.

Make sure the lights you are using do not exceed the rated capacity of the generator supplying the power. Consider not only the possible power usage of the lights but also any other needs you may have. Overloading your generator could cause damage to the generator, lights, or other attached equipment.

After use, check all lights for any physical damage such as wires pulled from the sockets or disfigurement caused by overloading or other injury. Bulbs are susceptible to shock damage and are usually easy to change, so keep a stock for replacement as needed. Never install a bulb with a higher wattage than the light's rating, and never touch one with your bare hands because any residue on your hands may make the bulb fail prematurely. Keep the lens and reflector clean and the lens protector in place to ensure maximum light output. Additionally, familiarize yourself with any additional recommendations or field maintenance guidance provided by the manufacturer.

Light-emitting diodes, better known as LEDs, are the future of lighting for emergency services in the area of scene lighting, apparatus lighting, and personal hand-held lighting. LED lighting draws less current than conventional lights and produces light from passing an electrical current through a semiconductor diode. The advantage of LEDs over halogen lights or regular incandescent lights is that LEDs do not have a filament to heat or gas to ionize; LEDs function in a solid state. Another advantage of LEDs is that they do not contain mercury and are shock resistant. LED lighting ranges from 80 to over 100 lumens per energy watt. Conventional incandescent light bulbs are approximately 15 lumens per energy watt, and halogen lamps are approximately 20 lumens per energy watt. A lumen measures the amount of light reaching a 1 ft^2 (0.09 m^2) area from a 1 candle power source placed 1 ft (0.3 m) away.

LISTEN UP!

Be sure the lights you use do not exceed the rated capacity of the generator supplying the power. Overloading the generator could damage the generator, lights, or other attached equipment.

Fuel-Powered Cutting Tools

Cutting tools include chain saws, rotary saws, cutting torches, and exothermic torches. One of the major advantages of fuel-powered tools is the high power they can generate. Disadvantages include that they can be heavy to carry, depending on the type of tool; some require a fuel mixture of gas and oil (two-stroke engine only); and some can be difficult to start cold. A periodic maintenance schedule and thorough inspection before and after every use are crucial for consistent and reliable operation of fuel-powered tools.

Chain Saws

A fuel-powered chain saw is available for cutting wood, concrete, and even light-gauge steel. Standard steel chains are used to cut wood, carbide-tipped chains can cut wood and light-gauge metal, and diamond chains are used for cutting concrete. Chain saws are a great option to have for an incident where a vehicle has struck a tree and the tree itself or a tree limb is impeding access and has to be removed. The chain saw is the fastest and most efficient tool to get the job done. Always remember to use proper safety procedures when cutting tree branches that are possibly under tension to avoid any spring-back injuries.

All chain saws used by rescue personnel should be equipped with a chain brake (a feature built into the chain saw that stops the blade when manually engaged). Always wear full PPE (including eye protection, hearing protection, and gloves) when working with these tools, and never operate them in enclosed spaces. Wear chaps for lower body protection. Chaps for chain saw use should meet the requirements of the American Society for Testing and Materials (ASTM) F1897, *Standard Specification for Leg Protection for Chain Saw Users*.

Rotary Saws

Fuel-powered rotary saws (K-12 saws) are available for cutting wood, concrete, and metal. There are two types of blades used on rotary saws: a round metal blade with teeth and an abrasive disk. Abrasive disks are made of composite materials and are designed to wear down as they are used. Different styles of disks are available for concrete, asphalt, and metal. It is important to match the appropriate saw blade or saw disk to the material being cut. The application of rotary saws in vehicle extrication would be extremely limited; these saws tend to throw a tremendous number of sparks when cutting through metal and are considered a fire safety hazard. However, if, for example, a concrete pole is impeding access at the incident and must be removed or cut down, the rotary saw would be the best option for this task.

Cutting Torches

Cutting torches produce an extremely high-temperature flame and are capable of heating steel past its melting point, thereby cutting through the object by rapid oxidation. Oxygen fuel/gas base cutting torches combine the correct ratio of fuel—liquid/gas and oxygen—producing an exothermic chemical process that accelerates the oxidation process of the metal. The rapid oxidation process of the metal being cut is based on extremely high temperatures, the speed of the flame (which is determined by the vaporization and expansion of the fuel from liquid to gas), and the BTUs released from the metal being cut. The release of oxygen is controlled by a lever on the outside of the torch body as well as the fuel and oxygen knobs that regulate the percentages. Torches can be used in vehicle rescue and extrication situations where a cutting tool is needed to cut through heavy steel framing or other structural components, such as those found in commercial transit vehicles and other commercial vehicles.

Because these torches produce such high temperatures (5700°F [3149°C] or more), operators must be specially trained before using them. One of the more common types of cutting torch uses oxygen and acetylene, also known as oxyacetylene, to create the flame, but many rescue services have begun to use oxygen/gasoline torches, also known as Petrogen.

Petrogen torches produce a flame temperature range from 5200 to 6400°F (2871 to 3538°C). The oxyacetylene cutting torch produces a flame temperature of 5700°F (3149°C). With the Petrogen cutting torch, the sparks produce little heat and weight, although there can be some molten metal. Other advantages of the Petrogen cutting torch include:

- The gasoline flame is 100 percent oxidizing, producing a clean burn and a cleaner cut; acetylene is only 70 percent oxidizing.
- Gasoline is readily available and is not as volatile as acetylene; with gasoline, there is no potential for a fuel line backflash because the liquid fuel prevents any flame from going back into the torch.
- Petrogen torches use much less fuel by weight, making them more economical.
- Petrogen can cut twice as fast as acetylene when cutting through 2- to 4-in. (5- to 10-cm) steel and up to four times faster than acetylene when cutting through 8- to 10-in. (20- to 25-cm) steel.

An alternative to the Petrogen and oxyacetylene systems is the oxygen/propane torch, which offers a slightly cooler flame temperature (approximately 5112°F [2822°C]). Oxygen/propane is just as economical as Petrogen. Some of the disadvantages of the oxygen/propane torch are that it does not offer the precision cutting that an oxyacetylene torch can and that it throws a tremendous amount of slag when cutting.

Another type of cutting torch is the exothermic torch, which operates by igniting a combustible metal contained within a tube by forcing oxygen down the center of the tube. A benefit of an exothermic cutting torch is that it can burn through almost anything, including ferrous and nonferrous metals, stainless steel, concrete, glass, and cast iron. Although these torches can cut very heavy steel (even underwater), they also produce a tremendous amount of sparks and slag.

Similar to the exothermic cutting torch is the plasma cutter (mentioned previously in the electric cutting tools section). This cutting torch uses inert gas or compressed air that is blown from its nozzle at a high speed. At the same time, an electric arc forms within the gas, turning some of the gas to plasma. This precision cutting tool requires no preheating time (as compared to a Petrogen torch) and comes in a portable power pack for better maneuverability.

Regardless of the type of cutting torch system used, always practice the same safety steps before starting any cutting operations:

- ALWAYS ensure the surroundings, environment, and object/product to be cut are suitable for operating an open flame device.
- ALWAYS thoroughly check your equipment before operating (i.e., fittings, hoses, couplers, regulators, tips, valves, fuel, and oxygen levels).
- ALWAYS check your, your crew's, and the victim's proximity before proceeding with any operation. Full PPE, eye protection, and proper shielding are a priority; remember to account for victim proximity and heat transfer of the metal being cut.
- ALWAYS follow the manufacturer's operating instructions because each system has its own unique settings.

Hydraulic Rescue Tools

Hydraulic rescue tools operate by transferring energy or force from one area to another by compressing a high-density fluid designed for hydraulic rescue tool systems. Hydraulic tools can also be operated by electric and/or battery, gasoline, or pneumatic power; they most commonly operate using a gasoline-powered engine and a hydraulic pump. Many fire rescue apparatuses carry hydraulic pumps used to power a variety of hydraulic rescue tools. The pumps may be powered by the vehicle's engine or have their own engine, which can be mounted or portable (FIGURE 3-50). NFPA 1936, *Standard on Rescue Tools*, outlines the minimum design, performance, testing, and certification requirements of powered rescue tools as well as the specifications for hoses, couplers, and power units.

The major advantage of hydraulic tools over any other tool is the power and speed of operation. Hydraulic tools can be superior to any other tool when

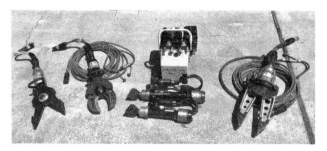

FIGURE 3-51 The four basic types of hydraulic rescue tools used today, left to right: hydraulic combination tool (spreader and cutter), hydraulic cutter, hydraulic ram, and hydraulic spreader.
Courtesy of Kevin Bellucy.

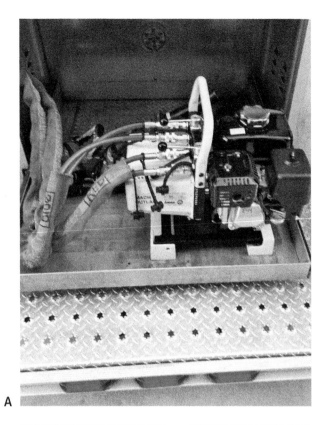

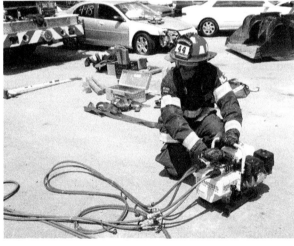

FIGURE 3-50 Hydraulic pumps. **A.** Mounted onto the apparatus. **B.** Portable.
A. Courtesy of David Sweet. B. Courtesy of Edward Monahan.

- Hydraulic combination tool (spreader and cutter)

Hydraulic rescue tools work through a very simple mechanical process: The hydraulic pump, powered by an engine, forces fluid into the cylinder of the particular tool you are operating. The reciprocal movement of the piston within the pump cylinder draws hydraulic fluid from the reservoir and forces the fluid past a discharge check valve into the system, creating increased pressure with each movement. This in turn puts a gradually building pressure on the piston and piston rod inside the tool, forcing the tool to open or close, based on the operator's positioning of the control valve. This is a basic explanation of how a hydraulic system operates; it can get more involved by adding force multiplication factors, such as changing the size of the cylinder and piston, pump capacity, type of system (e.g., single stage and two stage), and so on.

Most power units operate on either a 5000- or 10,500-psi (34,474- or 72,395-kPa) capacity using a two-stage pump system. The first stage of the pump normally operates at a maximum volume flow rate with a lower pressure building up to around 2000 to 3000 psi (13,790 to 20,684 kPa) or greater (this will vary with each manufacturer). A sensing unit then kicks in the second stage, which delivers a maximum pressure for generating a maximum force, which is either 5000 or 10,500 psi (34,474 or 72,395 kPa), depending on the unit you are operating.

Hydraulic rescue tool pumps can come in a variety of sizes, ranging from a single-operation pump, where only one tool can be operated, to multiple-operation pumps, where several tools can be operated at the same time, retaining the same power and speed as a single unit. The more common sized pump is the two-pump system (simo-unit), where two tools can be operated simultaneously. Another feature available with some pumps is the ability to switch the flow of both pumps onto one side, which doubles the speed of one tool but eliminates the ability to operate two

used properly and in the right application. Disadvantages of hydraulic tools are their overall weight and their limited maneuverability in tight spaces. The standard hydraulic tool tends to be very heavy (generally in the range of 35 to 50 lb [16 to 23 kg] for a hydraulic spreader), and the ability to get into very tight spaces is limited because of its relative size. There are generally four types of hydraulic rescue tools used today (**FIGURE 3-51**):

- Hydraulic spreader
- Hydraulic cutter
- Hydraulic ram

tools simultaneously. This feature should be used only by trained professionals who are skilled at using this setting. The increased speed of a tool can catch the novice off guard, potentially causing harm or injury to the operator or others.

There are several types of hydraulic fluid, including mineral (petroleum-based) oil, phosphate ester, water-based ethyl glycol compounds, polyol ester (not to be confused with phosphate ester), and vegetable-based oil. Phosphate ester was the predominant hydraulic fluid until the early 2000s, but since then most companies have been transitioning away from this fluid and moving toward mineral base oil because of the toxicity and skin irritant properties of phosphate ester. Phosphate ester has excellent fire-resistant qualities, but it is considered an irritant, requiring full PPE to be worn by anyone working around it. This fluid burns like pepper spray, requiring a saline flush or a visit to the emergency department for severe exposure (**FIGURE 3-52**).

Mineral base hydraulic fluid, as compared to phosphate ester, is much easier to work with, is less of an irritant, and is more cost effective; it is, however, less fire resistant. When working with a mineral base hydraulic fluid or any other hydraulic fluid, it is recommended that you wear full PPE. Do not wipe your eyes with your gloves after handling a hydraulic rescue tool. This common mistake may occur on a hot summer day when you inadvertently wipe the sweat from your forehead.

It is a requirement of NFPA 1936 that all internal components—including seals, valves, and fittings—of a powered rescue tool system function properly at a maximum hydraulic fluid temperature of 160°F (71°C). NFPA 1936 also lists safety and performance guidelines for powered rescue tools. To be certified to NFPA 1936, rescue tool manufacturers must use third-party certification organizations, such as UL LLC (UL; formerly Underwriters Laboratories Inc.), to conduct safety and performance tests.

SAFETY TIP

Full PPE, including eye protection, is mandatory when operating or servicing hydraulic tools.

NFPA 1936 Section 6.1.1.3 requires powered rescue tools to have a **dead-man control** feature designed to return the operational controls to the neutral position automatically in the event the operational control is released.

The following is an overview of the four common standard hydraulic-powered rescue tools. The definitions of the following hydraulic tools are taken from NFPA 1936.

Hydraulic Spreader

The hydraulic spreader was one of the first hydraulic tools designed to be used as a rescue tool. A **hydraulic spreader** is a powered rescue tool consisting of at least one movable arm that opens to move or spread apart material or to crush or lift material (**FIGURE 3-53**). Spreaders range in size and force, depending on the

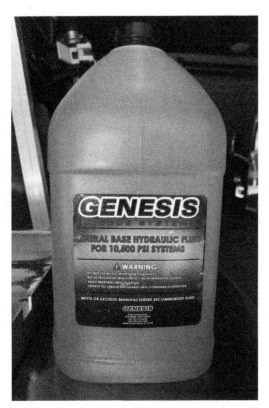

FIGURE 3-52 The two most prevalent fluids utilized in hydraulic rescue tools are phosphate ester and mineral base oil. This photo shows mineral base oil.
Courtesy of Genesis Rescue Systems.

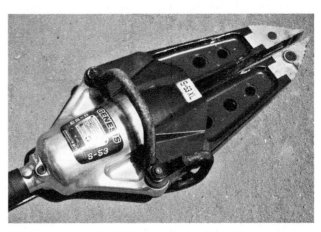

FIGURE 3-53 The hydraulic spreader.
Courtesy of Edward Monahan.

manufacturer and whether the tool is operating at 5000 or 10,500 psi (34,474 or 72,395 kPa). To determine the true usable spreading force exerted from a spreader, NFPA 1936 requires the tool to be measured from the tip area at 10 evenly spaced opening positions, starting from the fully closed position to 95 percent of the fully opened position. This test determines the tool's lowest spreading force (LSF) and highest spreading force (HSF). Using the same 10-point testing system, the spreader is also tested for its pulling force. This test determines the tool's lowest pulling force (LPF) and highest pulling force (HPF).

The LSF is typically the most predominate power feature required from a tool because this is when the tool, in the fully closed position, has to make the initial access opening against virtually no leverage. The HSF is measured when the tool is at 95 percent of being fully opened. A typical (HSF) range of force can measure from 9000 to 25,000 lb (4082 to 11,340 kg) of spreading force. The overall maximum spreading force combining all measurements can be in excess of 100,000 lb, depending on the manufacturer, but this measurement is not a requirement of NFPA 1936.

In general, the higher the overall maximum spreading force of a tool, the heavier the tool. A hydraulic spreader can range in weight from 30 to 59 lb (13.6 to 26.8 kg); the weight of the tool can make a huge difference in maintaining endurance when you are conducting an operation, especially in high temperatures. Newer models are being designed and redesigned each year to create lighter options while maintaining or increasing power. The more power and speed a tool can provide, the better, but a tool's effectiveness ultimately comes down to the individual using it.

Hydraulic Cutter

The **hydraulic cutter** is a powered rescue tool consisting of at least one movable blade used to cut, shear, or sever material (**FIGURE 3-54**). There are two types of blade designs commonly used—the curved, or O, cutter and the straight blade cutter. Each of these blades perform a different cutting action when in operation. Hydraulic cutters do not necessarily cut metal; they are designed to compress the metal until it reaches its fracture point.

The curved blade, when cutting, actually draws material in toward its center; this is where the majority of curved blade cutters carry the most cutting force. The straight blade cutter has a tendency to push material outward as it cuts, but it can give you a deeper cut than the curved blade cutter can.

Another important feature of the blade is the manufacturing of the steel. Blades constructed of

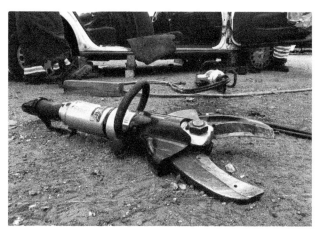

FIGURE 3-54 The hydraulic cutter.
Courtesy of Brad Fellers.

high-grade steel seem to resist breaking or cracking more than those constructed of other types of steel. The quality of a steel depends on the grade process and carbon content, which determines the hardness of the blade and the ability to hold a cutting edge. This is significant when cutting into hardened steel, such as a door latching mechanism or a door hinge. Blades made of low-grade steel can fracture at their weakest point when attempting to cut through hardened steel; this is why some manufacturers do not recommend cutting door latching mechanisms and hinges. Most blades made of high-grade steel do not seem to have these limitations and can cut through most hardened steel with the exception of boron, titanium, and other exotic metals, which require a higher cutting force and special design from the tool itself as well as the blades.

NFPA 1936 devised a series of tests that list nine performance levels or level ratings in measuring the cutting capabilities of a cutter. These tests use five categories of a specific material, which is represented by an alphanumeric label from A to E with various size grades, thickness, and shapes for each material. The materials consist of (A) round bar, (B) flat bar, (C) round pipe, (D) square tube, and (E) angle iron. Each material section is cut in 12 pieces with the largest sized material being represented by the highest numerical performance level or rating of the cutter. Successful severing (one continuous motion) of the largest material section for the first category (A), which consists of a 1.75-in. (4.4-cm) round bar, is given a performance level rating of nine and is represented as A9. If a tool cannot sever a section of material at the minimum performance level in each of the five categories, then the tool does not pass the test.

Cutting forces on high-pressure systems (10,500 psi [72,395 kPa]) can range from 60,000 to 100,000 psi (413,685 to 689,476 kPa) for general cutting requirements to up to almost 400,000 psi (2,757,903 kPa) for

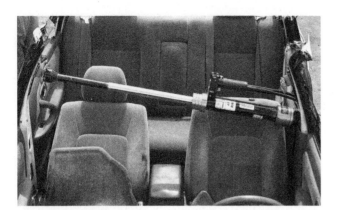

FIGURE 3-55 The telescopic hydraulic ram.
Courtesy of Edward Monahan.

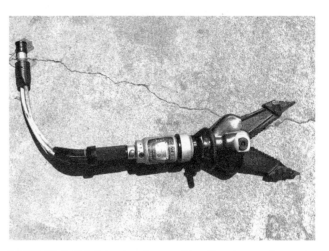

FIGURE 3-56 A hydraulic combination (spreader and cutter) tool.
Courtesy of Kevin Bellucy.

advanced, higher cutting forces required for AHSS alloys. Remember to check with the manufacturer for the cutting force of the tool your organization uses.

Hydraulic Ram

The **hydraulic ram** is a powered rescue tool with a piston or other type of extender that generates extending forces or both extending and retracting forces (**FIGURE 3-55**). Each manufacturer offers various lengths of units, but generally, individual units come in 20 in. (51 cm), 30 in. (76 cm), and 60 in. (152 cm) or in a telescopic type where one unit can extend from 20 to 60 in. (51 to 152 cm). Some manufacturers offer various options such as interchangeable tips or extension bars that screw on.

To evaluate the spreading force a ram is capable of producing, NFPA 1936 requires a ram to be measured from the tip area at three evenly spaced opening and closing positions, from the fully closed position to 95 percent of the fully opened position. This test determines the tool's LSF and HSF. Similarly, to evaluate the pulling force a ram is capable of producing, NFPA 1936 requires a ram to be measured from the tip area at three evenly spaced opening and closing positions, from the fully opened position to 95 percent of the fully closed position, to determine the tool's LPF and HPF.

Hydraulic Combination Tool

A **hydraulic combination tool** is a powered rescue tool capable of spreading and cutting (**FIGURE 3-56**). This tool may not be as effective as a dedicated cutter or spreader because of the limited range it can provide during a cut or a spread, but an advantage of a combination tool is the ability to rapidly apply a spread or a cut on a vehicle without having to switch tools, thus saving valuable time.

To evaluate the spreading force, pulling force, and cutting force a combination tool is capable of producing, NFPA 1936 requires the same testing criteria as an individual spreader and individual cutter as well as the level of performance rating measuring the cutting capability.

Some combi-tool units also come in a hand pump version that has the hydraulics in a self-contained unit that is void of any hoses, combustion engines, or pumps. This is very useful in confined spaces, rapid deployment situations, or areas where the combustion engines cannot be used.

Battery-Powered Hydraulic Rescue Tools

Battery-powered hydraulic rescue tools offer the same spreading, cutting, and ram force as the conventional hydraulic tools but are void of any hoses and have a separate pump, which is self-contained, that produces minimal noise when operated. These tools use a micro-pump and mini hydraulic fluid reservoir built into the tool, which is operated by an electric motor that commonly uses a Li-ion battery ranging from 18 to 28 volts to power the system (**FIGURE 3-57**). Some positive items that can be associated with battery-powered hydraulic tools are that they can be deployed and operated extremely fast with minimal setup time. These tools also operate with minimal noise, which allows for clearer communications. Last, these units are self-contained so there is no concern about attached hydraulic lines, which can rupture, leak, or not reach the incident. Some of the disadvantages that can be associated with battery-powered hydraulic tools are that the basic ergonomics and weight distribution are significantly different from conventional hydraulic tools because these systems have self-contained pumps,

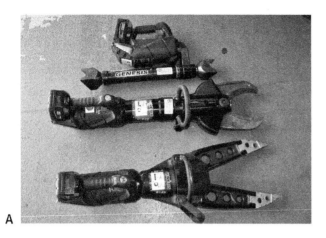

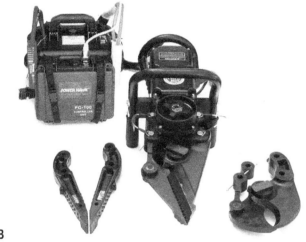

FIGURE 3-57 A. Genesis battery-operated hydraulic tools. **B.** Power Hawk system.
A. Courtesy of Genesis Rescue Systems. B. Courtesy of Power Hawk Technologies, Inc.

fluid reservoirs, and battery packs all designed close together, which can tend to make the tool bulkier or seem off balance. The life cycle of the battery will have a shelf life and will eventually lose power faster as the tool is utilized more often. With battery-powered hydraulic tools, there is no option to double the flow rate of hydraulic fluid onto one tool, which some conventional tools possess. This option equipped on some conventional tools allows two line valves coming off the pump to be switched to one line, which doubles the flow rate and dramatically increases the speed of one tool.

The Power Hawk rescue tool system is a unique self-contained system that does not use hydraulic fluid. This system has incorporated gear technology using an internal 12-volt DC motor to operate the gear and chain drive, which multiplies the force output to produce the cutting, spreading, or ramming power depending on which interchangeable device tips are used.

Whether an agency uses battery-powered tools or conventional-powered tools, maintaining a state of readiness is key to any successful operation. Maintaining the tools in a constant state of readiness, including general maintenance procedures for the hydraulic rescue tools and pumps, includes checking the hydraulic fluid and general operating fluids after every use, checking for leaks, inspecting the equipment for any damaged or improperly functioning parts, and checking all hoses and the fittings for proper operation and cleanliness. It is important to be familiar with the manufacturer's maintenance recommendations and annual service requirements. Some hydraulic tool manufacturers offer service technician classes that certify responders to perform general repair work on the unit and tools. Check with your tool manufacturer to see whether this is an available option; it is a great way to fully understand the inner workings of a hydraulic rescue tool system.

Stabilization Tools

Balance goes hand in hand with stabilization. The main objective in stabilization is to gain a balanced footprint by expanding the vehicle's base and lowering its center of mass prior to performing any work on the vehicle. The goal of vehicle stabilization is to achieve a state of equilibrium or balance. Stabilization consists of two states of equilibrium: stable and unstable.

Mass is what makes up the matter or substance of an object. The mass of an object is always constant; it does not change based on position or location. Weight, by definition, is equal to the force exerted on an object by gravity. The center of a mass of an object is the point where all the weight of the object is concentrated, or the point where the downward force of gravity is at its greatest. The force of gravity is measured through an imaginary straight line passing through the center mass of an object to a ground base of support.

An object is said to be in a state of stable equilibrium when the center of mass or concentrated weight of the object is lowest to the support base and the base is horizontally wider. A vehicle resting on all four tires on level ground is presenting a state of stable equilibrium because its center mass is lowest to the ground base of support and its weight is spread out equally. A vehicle resting on its side, because of its vertical stance and narrowing base, is considered to be in a state of unstable equilibrium. The goal is to lower its center of mass to the support or base level to achieve a state of stable equilibrium. Chapter 8 discusses various scenarios and techniques designed to achieve a state of stable equilibrium for an unstable vehicle.

There are a multitude of tools used to stabilize or shore up a vehicle. This section focuses on stabilization tools that use cribbing, struts, jacks, pneumatic shores, and ratchet straps.

Cribbing

Cribbing consists of short lengths of sturdy timber or composite material—usually 2 in. × 2 in. (5.1 cm × 5.1 cm), 4 in. × 4 in. (10 cm × 10 cm), or 6 in. × 6 in. (15 cm × 15 cm), in lengths of 18 to 24 in. (46 to 61 cm)—used in various configurations to stabilize loads in place. There are several cribbing designs used for extrication, such as step chocks, wedges, shims, and the basic box crib design (**FIGURE 3-58**).

Step chocks are specialized cribbing assemblies made of wood, plastic/composite, or collapsible metal with a successive step design on a platform base. A step chock can easily be inserted to fit under a vehicle to accommodate the differences in height from the base of the vehicle to the ground level, which maintains the maximum contact of the vehicle's underside and the ground.

Wedges are crib sections that are cut at right angles to form triangular sections or incline planes. The wedge is one of the six classic simple machines and is designed to lift a load, but in stabilization of a vehicle it is more commonly used to shore a load that is angled and to fill a void space. Because of the ratio of its length to its slope, the wedge is able to use mechanical advantage to be driven under an object. This allows for various tools to enter tight areas.

Shims are similar in design to wedges but are cut purposely thin and narrow to tighten cribbing sections

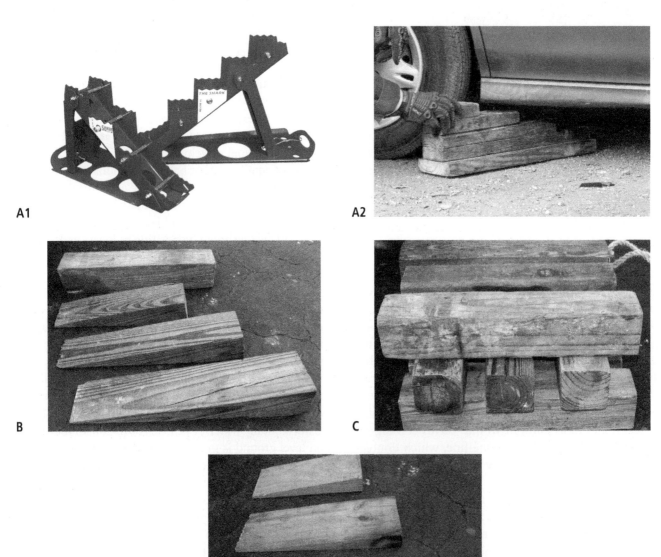

FIGURE 3-58 Cribbing designs. **A1** and **A2**. Step chocks. **B.** Wedges. **C.** Box crib. **D.** Shims.
A1. Reproduced with permission from Rescue 42, Inc. Specializes in reliable vehicle extrication equipment. **A2.** Courtesy of Edward Monahan. **B-D.** Courtesy of David Sweet.

where small crevices or gaps may occur before a load is applied. Unlike a wedge, a shim cannot be driven into a cribbing section or under a load to lift; its thin profile would cause it to break in half or crack at the tip. A wedge and shim should be the same nominal size to maintain continuity with the crib section with which they are being used.

Wood cribbing is the most economical and easy to construct; anyone handy in woodworking can cut up sections and/or put a cribbing set together in a relatively short time. The types of wood commonly used for cribbing are southern yellow pine and Douglas fir, both of which are soft, durable woods. Strength and behavior of wood may be based on the species of wood, moisture content, size and distribution of defects (such as how many knots appear in the board), cracks, grain orientation, and growth rate.

Composite plastic is another material option for cribbing. Composite cribbing comes in several options, such as separate 4-in. × 4-in. (10-cm × 10-cm) sections in various lengths, step chocks, wedges, and various other designs. Composite cribbing costs significantly more up front but lasts much longer than wood because of its resistance to damage from abuse, and exposure to oils and other various substances.

Another option to wood and composite cribbing is metal collapsible step chocks, which can be adjusted to heights from 5 to 16.5 in. (13 to 42 cm) depending on the manufacturer. This multiple adjustment feature is convenient when you are dealing with vehicles such as a sport utility vehicle (SUV) or truck that sits high off the ground. Cribbing techniques are discussed in more detail in Chapter 8.

Struts

Struts are structural supports or shores used as a "buttress" to stabilize and reinforce an object (**FIGURE 3-59**). Struts can be made of steel, aluminum, wood, and composite/Kevlar. Some can also be operated pneumatically or hydraulically. With the exception of the wood type, struts are normally telescopic devices, either tubular or square, that slide to various lengths to accommodate a multitude of stabilization scenarios. The more common lengths used for vehicle stabilization can be anywhere from 3 to 8 ft (0.91 to 2.4 m), with the struts being held in place by supporting pins or locking rings. Struts can vary in support loads, depending on whether they use a single, a double, or a multiple pin system or locking rings and whether they are fully extended or compact. Depending on the manufacturer, most struts can generally support a WLL of 4000 to 18,000 lb (1814 to 8165 kg). This WLL can vary greatly depending on the type of strut system and the design.

Wood struts for vehicle stabilization commonly comprise 4-in. × 4-in. (10-cm × 10-cm) sections in various lengths ranging from 3 to 6 ft (0.91 to 1.8 m) or greater. Wood struts can be used in their simplest form by themselves or with a wood stabilization system, such as a steel ground pad, base, plate, and cap.

Most strut stabilization systems use a strap in a ratchet or jacking device that is either a separate piece independent of the strut or is integrated into the strut, allowing for a rapid application process (**FIGURE 3-60**).

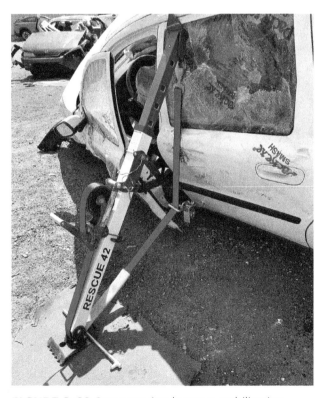

FIGURE 3-60 Some tension buttress stabilization struts come equipped with the ratcheting device, extension sleeves, and locking mechanism built into the system, such as the Rescue 42 TeleCrib® Junior.
Reproduced with permission from Rescue 42, Inc. Specializes in reliable vehicle extrication equipment.

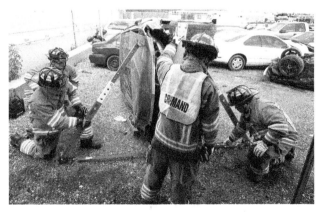

FIGURE 3-59 Struts are used for structural support to stabilize and reinforce a vehicle.
Courtesy of Edward Monahan.

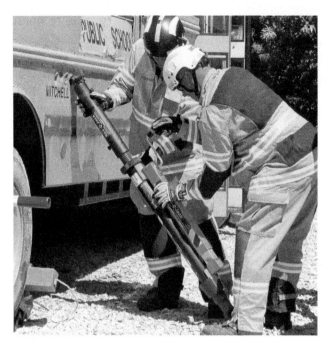

FIGURE 3-61 Some strut systems have the ability to lift the object they are supporting to free a trapped victim, such as the Super-X Strut® from Res-Q-Jack systems.
Courtesy of David Sweet.

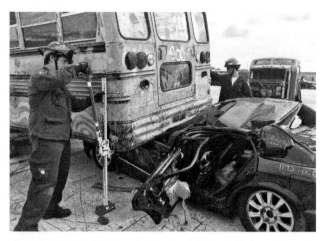

FIGURE 3-62 Ratcheting lever jacks, such as a First Responder Jack, can be used to lift and stabilize large vehicles as long as the WLL of the jack is rated for the task at hand.
Courtesy of David Sweet.

Once attached to the vehicle, the ratcheting device adds tension to the object being stabilized; this method is known as **tension buttress stabilization**. Attaching a strap from the base of the strut to the vehicle and adding tension lock the vehicle in place using a diagonal force that lowers the vehicle's mass point by increasing the vehicle's entire footprint or floor span. This is the same manner in which the outriggers on an aerial apparatus function.

There are multiple variations and applications to the tension buttress stabilization system, with each manufacturer adding various features to enhance its system. Some of these features are interchangeable heads offering different options for the varying penetration or anchoring problems that you will encounter. Some manufacturers provide a jacking device, which can add a lifting option to the strut system (**FIGURE 3-61**). The lifting capacities of each product's jacking device vary, and each product offers its own tip attachments or base attachments, such as a ratchet strap or cam buckle strap. It is best to contact the various manufacturers and physically try all the strut systems in practical training evolutions before purchasing a system.

Jacks

Mechanical jacks and hand-operated hydraulic jacks are excellent lifting and pushing tools that can be used as stabilization devices as well (**FIGURE 3-62**).

The mechanical jacks most commonly used in vehicle rescue are the ratchet lever type and the scissor/screw jack. Ratchet lever jacks, such as the FRJ, consist of a beam and a ratcheted lifting mechanism. This lifting mechanism consists of a long jacking pole or ratchet lever that offers leverage for lifting the vehicle. This lifting mechanism rides on the beam and can be controlled in either direction with a directional latch.

As with any tool, safety and tool familiarization are the most important factors that must be accounted for prior to any operational use on an incident. It's good practice to operate the tool without any load to understand all the movements and components and the mechanism and then to build up to a manageable load or tension gradually to feel how the tool operates under the weight difference. Follow the manufacturer's recommendations for all safety features and operational uses for the tool.

When operating a ratchet lever jack, or any lifting system, never exceed the WLL of the tool. Make sure the load being carried by the jack does not shift because this can cause the jack to tip and fall over. Always stand to the side when jacking or ratcheting the tool under a load. This is especially critical with the jacking pole, which can become extremely hazardous when ratcheting up and even more so when ratcheting down to release a load. If the jack is not released in a safe, controlled manner, the jacking pole can fire up at the rescuer, causing severe injury or death to anyone struck or caught in the path of the pole. Always lock the safety latch and pole upright in place when the proper lifting height is reached.

A scissor/screw jack, such as the sidewinder jack, uses mechanical advantage by a center screw and gear mechanism that, when operated, forces movement of

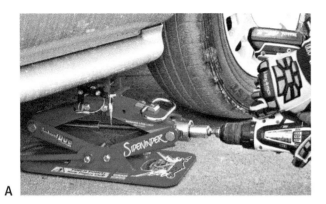

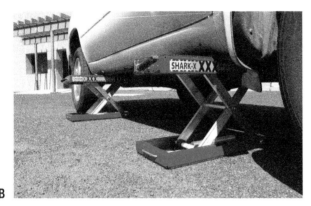

FIGURE 3-63 Scissor/screw jacks, which use mechanical advantage by a center screw and gear mechanism that, when operated, forces movement of the jack's arms toward each other, extending upward from a semi-flat position. **A.** Sidewinder jack. **B.** Shark-X.
A. Courtesy of Edward Monahan. B. Reproduced with permission from Rescue 42, Inc. Specializes in reliable vehicle extrication equipment.

the jack's arms toward each other, extending upward from a semi-flat position. This lifts the vehicle and/or object and also holds it in place via a self-locking screw. The jack uses a hand crank attachment or drill to operate the mechanism up or down. Scissor/screw jacks can also be equipped with an electric motor or powered through hydraulics and are void of a center screw–type manual mechanism (**FIGURE 3-63**).

Ratchet Strap

A **ratchet strap** is a mechanical tensioning device that uses a manual gear-ratcheting drum to put tension on an object, using a webbing material (**FIGURE 3-64**). Ratchet straps are a cost-effective tool designed for cargo or industrial tie-down stabilization and are excellent tools to carry on the apparatus. Ratchet straps are not designed to lift and are best used in locking vehicles together, a technique known as *marrying*. When a vehicle is on top of another vehicle, the objective is to stabilize both vehicles, which is accomplished by marrying the vehicles to form one unit; the proper use of ratchet straps is very effective in meeting this objective. Other uses of ratchet straps include

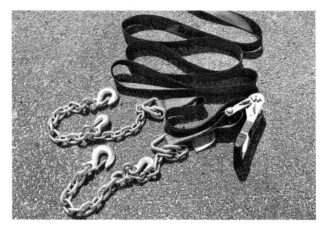

FIGURE 3-64 Ratchet straps are an efficient and cost-effective tool for tie-down stabilization.
Courtesy of Edward Monahan.

tying down objects such as trees and poles on the vehicle or tying down objects that need to be secured to prevent them from entering the area of operation. When operating a ratchet strap, remember to secure both the anchor end and the running end properly and always ratchet or pull the running end toward your base.

Ratchet straps come in lengths of 6, 10, 12, 15, 20, and 30 ft (1.8, 3.0, 3.7, 4.6, 6.1, and 9.1 m). The most commonly used types are composed of nylon or polyester webbing and are available in 1- to 4-in. (2.5- to 10-cm) widths. The 3- and 4-in. (8- and 10-cm) widths can provide breaking strength (stress on the material at the time of rupture) of up to 24,000 lb (10,886 kg) with a WLL of up to 6600 lb (2994 kg). The WLL of a strap is determined by calculating one-third of the break strength, or the weakest component of the system. If the break strength is 15,000 lb, then the WLL would be one-third of that number, or 5000 lb. Some manufacturers offer abrasion-resistant webbing, which dramatically improves wear and tear resistance.

There are several end attachment options that can be added to make it much easier to secure strapping. Some of these options include webbing loops, flat hooks, triangle/delta rings, O-rings, chain anchors with grab hook/chain shorteners, and double wire hooks. The most practical choice may be to custom design an end attachment that can give you several latching options. For example, an O-ring with a double wire hook and a rated chain lead of 2 ft (0.6 m) or a D-ring with a locking gate may be an effective option. To maintain safety and proper rating, attachments should be accomplished through a manufacturer, not your local hardware store. Remember to check with the manufacturer to maintain safety specifications on any of the design options.

Organization of Equipment

Proper organization of equipment includes tool staging at an incident and the proper setup and staging of tools on the apparatus. The proper staging of tools on the scene and on the apparatus can be an incredible benefit to completing the operational tasks more expediently and efficiently.

Tool staging at an incident may involve laying out a tarp at the edge of the secure work area and organizing the tools on the tarp in a manner that allows rescuers to locate the appropriate tools quickly. The location of the tool staging area will depend on the accessibility of the area where the incident occurred. Ensure the entire response team is aware of the location after it has been determined. To maintain control and scene safety, tools and equipment need to be returned to the staging area after usage. The assigned safety officer, while conducting continued walk-around assessments, can retrieve any tools and equipment that have been tossed to the side to avoid these potential trip hazards (**FIGURE 3-65**).

Proper tool staging on the apparatus should ultimately begin at the planning stages for the building and design of the apparatus itself, but it can also be accomplished later, with a little ingenuity and common sense. A simple redesign or rearrangement of the tools in the compartments can consist of several options, such as acquiring hose reels and pre-attaching the tools with one reel dedicated to the cutter and the other reel dedicated to the spreader. This organization allows the rescuer to open the compartment door, pull off the tool, and go. Another option is to place the step chocks and cribbing in a compartment that is readily available, where the rescuer does not have to step up onto the bed of the apparatus or remove other items to retrieve them. Cribbing ends can also be color coded by painting to depict various sizes and types. The proper organization of equipment will be different for each agency based on the type of apparatus and the custom preference of the users. The question to ask is simple: How can the apparatus be set up to improve the overall operations of the department?

> **LISTEN UP!**
>
> After any use, all hand tools and power equipment should be thoroughly inspected and staged in a "ready state" for immediate use at the next incident:
> - The tools should be clean and dry.
> - All fuel tanks should be filled completely with fresh fuel.
> - Any dull or damaged blades should be replaced.
> - Chain saw blades should be inspected for damage or missing teeth. Check the manufacturer's recommendations for the number of teeth allowed to be damaged or missing before total chain replacement is necessary.
> - Belts and chains should be inspected to ensure that they are tight and undamaged.
> - All guards should be securely in place.
> - All hydraulic hoses should be cleaned and inspected.
> - All power cords should be inspected for damage.
> - All hose fittings should be cleaned, inspected, and tested to ensure a tight fit.
> - Tools should be started to ensure that they operate properly.
>
> Tools with damage to the plug or cord should be taken out of service immediately and repaired to avoid any possibility of electrocution. Also, inspect tools for cracked or damaged housings, improperly operating trigger mechanisms, or improperly operating or damaged chucks.
>
> It is very important to read the manufacturer's manual and follow all instructions on the care and inspection of power tools and equipment. It is also important to keep a record of any maintenance performed on power equipment and to repair and report deficiencies with equipment.

Special Equipment

Foam

All foams are not created equal. When incidents such as a significant fuel spill at a motor vehicle collision occur, a Class B Alcohol Resistant Aqueous Film-Forming Foam (AR-AFFF) that is UL listed for flammable liquids (not combustibles) should be used (as per NFPA 11, *Standard for Low-, Medium-, and High-Expansion Foam*). AFFF foam is a major topic of discussion in the fire/rescue service today. The PFAS and PFOA chemicals in the foam have been found to be cancer causing. AFFF foam is slowly being phased out in the service with replacement products without these cancer causing chemicals. All unignited fuel spills should be managed as a polar solvent fuel. Regarding this application, most gasoline is blended

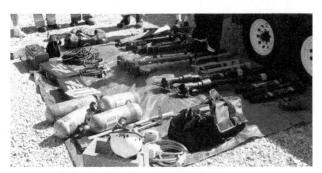

FIGURE 3-65 The proper staging of tools on the scene and on the apparatus can be an incredible benefit to completing the operational tasks more expediently and efficiently.
Courtesy of David Sweet.

to enhance performance and to achieve less environmental impact. The blended fuels are polar and scene security cannot be guaranteed when utilizing a regular Class B Aqueous Film-Forming Foam (AFFF). Note: Class A Foam, Wetting Agents (NFPA 18, *Standard on Wetting Agents*), Mil Spec or regular AFFF, shall not be used for vapor suppression on polar solvents and/or blended gasoline. Although most of these agents do foam, they do not make a polymeric membrane over the fuel that suppresses vapor production like alcohol resistant foam does. The foam blanket they produce will break down immediately on contact with the fuel.

Mil-spec AFFF is the specification of the U.S. Navy and is also used per the Federal Aviation Administration (FAA) at airport authorities in the United States. This foam does not have any vapor suppression characteristics on polar solvent or blended fuels. Use of an Aircraft Rescue and Fire Fighting (ARFF) apparatus, or "crash truck," possibly could overwhelm and extinguish an ignited fuel fire, but there is no scene security after extinguishment.

Foam Equipment

The default foam proportioner for UL is a foam eductor. The foam eductor is a mechanical proportioner that does not require any electronics to operate. All foam eductors require 200 psi (1379 kPa) at the inlet of the eductor to operate accurately. There is a 70 psi (483 kPa) loss through the venturi (area where the pickup tube is connected) to pull the foam concentrate from the foam supply (could be a 5-gal [19-L] pail of foam or onboard foam tank on a fire apparatus). That leaves 130 psi (895 kPa) to operate the hose line. The 95 GPM (6 L/sec) foam eductor will allow enough pressure to operate 200 ft of 1.75-in hose after the foam eductor when utilizing 1.75-in. (44-mm) fire hose. Using this layout, the nozzle typically requires 100 psi (689 kPa), and there is approximately 30 psi (207 kPa) friction loss in the hose. Therefore, there is insufficient pressure remaining to increase hose line length. The foam eductor can be connected to a 2.5-in. (64-mm) discharge of the fire apparatus's pump panel. Installing the eductor behind the pump panel typically results in failure because of lack of maintenance.

Note: Using a low pressure combination nozzle or foam nozzle will allow for more length after the foam eductor. Also, using a larger diameter hose, such as a 2-in. (51-mm) hose, will allow for a longer hose lay after the foam eductor. Keep in mind that the nozzle shall match or be greater than the flow capability of the foam eductor. More than 130 psi (896 kPa) back pressure applied to the foam eductor will result in a proportioning failure. There are also onboard foam systems, which are behind the pump panel of a fire apparatus. These systems can be mechanically operated or run by an electronic system that operates an injection pump that is metered after the discharge of the pump. There are options to have a Class A or a Class B foam used, the choice of which needs to be specified in the purchase of the apparatus. Note: Class A foams should never be mixed with Class B foams.

Class A foam does not have to be aerated unless it is being utilized in an exposure or a wildland/urban interface application. **Class B foam** should be used with a low- or medium-expansion device/nozzle attachment for unignited events/vapor suppression. A combination nozzle will give the foam an expansion of only approximately 3:1, whereas a low-expansion nozzle will be 10:1, and a medium expansion will be approximately 50:1. All use of AR-AFFF should be aspirated (the aeration slows the draindown and allows the polymeric layer to form). UL tests for AR-AFFF Class B foams are typically conducted with the use of a low- or medium-expansion foam nozzle for maximum performance. There are also quick-attack foam systems, such as a PRO/pak system, which are available in a portable package designed for fast deployment and operation (**FIGURE 3-66**).

Signaling Devices

There are many devices available to assist rescuers in getting the job done. For example, portable or fixed communication devices, such as cellular telephones, help rescuers communicate with one another. Marking kits that include paint, chalk, pens/pencils, or crayon may be used to mark a scene and alert other rescuers of a potential hazard. Pickets or stakes may be used to close off the perimeter of the scene to keep bystanders at a safe distance. Preplans and maps help rescuers navigate through or around the scene. Traffic control, or preemption, devices, such as an Opticom system, halt traffic by changing traffic signals to allow emergency vehicles to pass through safely and quickly.

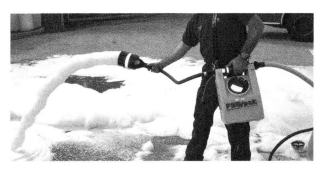

FIGURE 3-66 A PRO/pak is a self-contained foam applicator in a portable package designed for fast deployment and operation.
Courtesy of David Sweet.

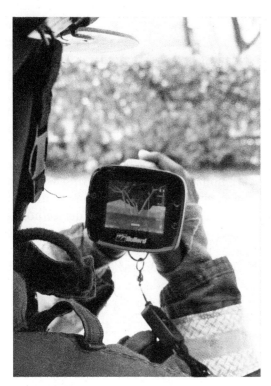

FIGURE 3-67 Thermal imaging cameras can detect body heat at night to scan for possible victims who may have been ejected from a vehicle and cannot be seen because of lack of light, thick brush, or debris.
Courtesy of Edward Monahan.

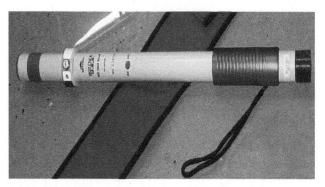

FIGURE 3-68 An AC power locator detects the presence of electrical frequencies below 100 Hz.
Courtesy of HotStick USA, Inc.

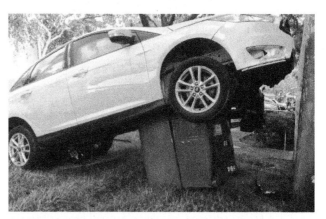

FIGURE 3-69 Car impacted transformer box, exposing live wires under the rear of the vehicle.
Courtesy of Brad Myers.

There are many signaling devices that can be used to your advantage.

Visual Devices

Often, we cannot find the victims we are looking for. Specialized cameras are available to help find victims. The most common of these cameras is the thermal imaging camera (TIC) (**FIGURE 3-67**). Many fire departments carry this camera to detect hidden fire or hot spots, but they are equally useful in detecting victims who have been ejected from a vehicle and now cannot be seen because of lack of light, thick brush, or debris.

TICs are very useful during late-night calls on remote highways where there are no street lights. Victims who have been ejected a distance from the scene and might not otherwise be found can be located immediately using a TIC by scanning the area systematically.

Power Detection

Electrical hazards on a rescue scene are always a concern, and efforts should always be made to identify and isolate any hazards. Because it is often impossible to tell visually whether a wire is energized, every rescue organization should have an AC power locator, such as a hot stick (**FIGURE 3-68**). This tool detects the presence of electrical frequencies below 100 Hz. It does not, however, detect DC power or AC power contained in solid metal enclosures, such as grounded metal conduit. There are other meters available that can detect DC power or provide voltage readings if necessary. These meters are not suitable for emergency response because they require probes to be placed directly on the wire or object to be tested.

At an MVA, if a wire is suspected of being down and resting on the vehicle or in proximity, then the technical rescuer must ensure that the proper jurisdictional power utility company be notified immediately and the proper action taken. This normally consists of shutting down an area grid. Never attempt to see whether a wire is hot, or live, by using a hot stick or pole; always assume that a wire is hot until the power company can determine otherwise. Take the appropriate protective safety measures, and move a safe distance from the area. Live wires are known to jump several feet when energized (**FIGURE 3-69**). What appears dead to the rescuer may suddenly come alive when the power company's computer system automatically, by program, reenergizes the line to detect the break areas. Many utility distribution transformers will attempt three resets via a recloser (not a computer control, nor a break detection method).

Victim Packaging and Removal Equipment

When victims are found, it is important they not be further injured while removing them to definitive medical care. This is accomplished by the use of stretchers and immobilization devices appropriate to the situation. The equipment used is known as victim packaging and removal equipment.

Immobilization Devices

The simplest immobilization devices are the full and half (or short) backboards, which are often used in conjunction with stretchers (**FIGURE 3-70**). The more common victim immobilization tool is the KED (Kendrick extrication device), which consists of a structured but flexible material that is placed on and fitted around the victim. The device can be used in tight spaces and is secured in several areas to maintain victim alignment and movability by rescuers. When inspecting immobilization devices, ensure that there are no cracks, splinters, gouges, worn straps, damaged buckles, or missing pieces.

Stretchers and Litters

Stretchers more commonly used by rescue services when removing victims include collapsible, scoop, and basket stretchers. Each type has advantages and disadvantages. Collapsible and basket stretchers allow for the incorporation of a backboard and may be rigged for vertical lifting. Basket stretchers can also be used for water rescue environments when flotation devices are attached to provide buoyancy. The scoop stretcher is designed to be split into two or four pieces. These sections are fitted around a victim who is lying on the ground or another relatively flat surface. The parts are reconnected, and the victim is lifted and placed on a long backboard or stretcher. This type of stretcher is not designed to be used by itself for immobilization. When inspecting stretchers, ensure that there are no bent rails or supports, cracked welds, rips, tears, damaged buckles, or missing pieces.

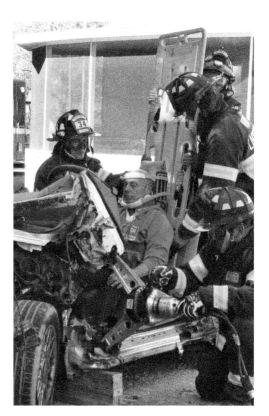

FIGURE 3-70 The KED in conjunction with a long backboard can assist in immobilizing and removing victims from vehicles involved in auto accidents.
Courtesy of Edward Monahan.

Research Tools

The Internet is a research tool readily available to all rescue personnel. The information and research capabilities for vehicle rescue and extrication are endless; the Internet provides an enormous amount of material on vehicle construction and design, locations of key safety and power components, physical tools, tool manufacturers—the list goes on and on. Truly, the greatest tool that a rescue professional possesses is his or her mind. The proverbial saying that "a mind is a terrible thing to waste" speaks volumes in the field of emergency services. It is up to you to take the initiative and apply what was gifted to you by acquiring this information through diligent research and always being open to learning as well as by teaching and sharing what you have learned.

After-Action REVIEW

IN SUMMARY

- A technical rescuer must be proficient with all tools used in the field to adapt and overcome challenges of tool failure that can often arise on an incident or during training.
- There are five basic categories of tools used for vehicle rescue and extrication purposes: hand tools, pneumatic tools, hydraulic tools, electric- or battery-powered tools, and fuel-powered tools.

- The technical rescuer must be fully protected before using any tools. To be compliant with NFPA 1951, the protective ensemble must provide protection from exposure to physical, thermal, liquid, and body fluid-borne pathogen hazards.
- The components of the personal protective equipment (PPE) include protection of the head, body, eye and face, hands, feet, hearing, and the respiratory system.
- A departmental SOP should be implemented for the proper maintenance of all PPE. Setting periodic inspections for all gear, along with inspections after each incident, can help ensure the safety of the individual user.
- A hand tool is any tool or equipment that operates solely from the physical manipulation of human power. There are four basic types of hand tools: striking tools, leverage/prying/spreading tools, cutting tools, and lifting/pushing/pulling tools.
- Working load limit (WLL) is the maximum force that can be applied before failure occurs to an assembly or a component of a device or rope/line/cable in straight tension.
- To determine a product's WLL, the manufacturer utilizes the minimum breaking strength of the device and divides this by a safety or design factor that is predetermined by the manufacturer. The minimum breaking "tensile" strength of a chain is determined by using a formula of dividing the unit of force (Newton) by square millimeter (N/mm^2). For example, the grade 80 chain equals 800 Newton per square millimeters. A manufacturer will determine the minimum breaking strength of their 5/8 grade 80 chain at 72,400 lbs with a 4:1 safety factor, giving the chain a WWL of 18,100 lbs. This WWL is the maximum load determined by the manufacturer that can be applied safely without failure.
- Pneumatic tools utilize air under pressure to operate and include air chisels, air impact wrenches, air shores, cut-off tools, and rescue air-lift bags. Pneumatic tools can be further categorized into cutting tools, rotating tools, and lifting tools.
- Electric-powered tools use standard household current or a generator to operate. Some tools, such as reciprocating saws, circular saws, drills, and glass cutters, use a battery as an electrical power source.
- Fuel-powered cutting tools such as chain saws, rotary saws, cutting torches, and exothermic torches can generate high power. However, they can be heavy to carry, and some require a mixture of gas and oil. Regular inspections before and after use, along with periodic maintenance schedules, are important for reliable operation of these tools.
- Hydraulic rescue tools transfer energy or force from one area to another. They can be operated by electric and/or battery, gasoline, or pneumatic power. The major advantage of hydraulic tools over any other tool is the power and speed of operation. The disadvantages are their weight and the limited maneuverability in tight spaces.
- There are four types of hydraulic rescue tools currently used: hydraulic spreader, hydraulic cutter, hydraulic ram, and a hydraulic combination tool (spreader and cutter).
- There are many tools for stabilizing or shoring up a vehicle, including cribbing, struts, jacks, pneumatic shores, and ratchet straps.
- The proper staging of tools on the scene and on the apparatus is highly beneficial to completing the operational tasks more expediently and efficiently.
- Special equipment used at the scene of vehicle extrication includes Class A and Class B foams, signaling devices, and specialized cameras.
- A thermal imaging camera is one of the most common specialized cameras, detecting body heat in victims not easily seen or detecting hidden fire or hot spots at the scene.
- Victim packaging and removal equipment is used to protect victims from further injury using stretchers and immobilization devices.

KEY TERMS

Adapters Devices used to convert a battery-powered tool to a general-current tool.

Air compressors Equipment used to provide power to pneumatic tools or to provide breathing air.

Air impact wrench A pneumatic tool used to remove bolts/nuts of various sizes.

Air-lift bags Inflatable devices used to lift an object or spread one or more objects away from each other to assist in freeing a victim. They come in various sizes and types, such as low-pressure bags, medium-pressure bags, high-pressure bags, high-pressure flat bags, and multi-cell bags.

Air shores Shores extended by the use of compressed air; shores are used where the vertical distances are too great to use cribbing or the load must be supported horizontally.

Chain saw Gasoline-powered saws capable of cutting wood, concrete, and even light-gauge steel. Standard steel chains are used to cut wood, carbide-tipped chains can cut wood and light-gauge metal, and diamond chains are used for cutting concrete.

Circular saw An electric- or battery-powered saw that moves in a circular motion; these saws come in a variety of sizes and are used primarily for cutting wood, although special blades are available that will cut metal or masonry.

Class A foam Foam for use on fires in Class A fuels. (NFPA 1901)

Class B foam Foam intended for use on Class B fires. (NFPA 1901)

Come along A ratchet lever winching tool that can provide up to several thousand pounds of pulling force, with the standard model for extrication being 2000 to 4000 lb (907 to 1814 kg) of pulling force.

Cribbing Short lengths of timber/composite materials, usually 4 in. × 4 in. (101.60 mm × 101.60 mm) and 18 in. to 24 in. (457.20 to 609.60 mm) long, that are used in various configurations to stabilize loads in place or while a load is moving. (NFPA 1670)

Cutting torches A tool that produces an extremely high-temperature flame capable of heating steel until it melts, burns, and oxidizes, thus cutting through the object. This tool is sometimes used for rescue situations such as cutting through heavy steel objects.

Dead-man control A control feature designed to return the control of the hydraulic tool to the neutral position automatically in the event the control is released.

Electric generators Generators that utilize a general current to operate. Primarily used to power scene lighting and to run power tools and equipment; may be portable or fixed.

Electric-powered tools Tools that utilize a general current or generator to operate.

Ferrous metals Metals that contain iron, cast iron, low- and medium-alloyed steels, and specialty steels, such as tool steels and stainless steels.

Flat-form air-lift bags Pneumatic-filled bladders designed to retain their flat profile in the center as they are inflated to lift an object or spread one or more objects away from each other to assist in freeing a victim.

Grab hook A device designed to take up the slack needed to make a chain the appropriate size for the task at hand; it is utilized by inserting a link of the chain into the slot of the hook. The grab hook may also be referred to as a chain shortener.

Hand tool Any tool or equipment operating from human power.

High-pressure air-lift bags The most commonly used bags among rescue agencies, these bags utilize a working air pressure of approximately 100 to 145 psi (689 to 1000 kPa) to lift an object or spread one or more objects away from each other to assist in freeing a victim. The high-pressure kits come with hoses, a regulator, a master control module, and various other attachments.

Hydraulic combination tool A powered rescue tool capable of both spreading and cutting.

Hydraulic cutter A powered rescue tool consisting of at least one movable blade used to cut, shear, or sever material.

Hydraulic ram A powered rescue tool with a piston or other type of extender that generates extending forces or both extending and retracting forces.

Hydraulic rescue tools Tools that operate by transferring energy or force from one area to another by using a hydraulic fluid such as high-density oil.

Hydraulic spreader A powered rescue tool consisting of at least one movable arm that opens to move or spread apart material or to crush or lift material.

Low-pressure air-lift bags Air bags with a very high lift with a maximum working air pressure of approximately 7 psi (48 kPa); they are used to lift an object or spread one or more objects away from each other to assist in freeing a victim.

Medium-pressure air-lift bags Air bags that have a rugged design and utilize a working air pressure of approximately 15 psi (103 kPa) used to lift an object or spread one or more objects away from each other to assist in freeing a victim. These bags are not as common as the low- and high-pressure rescue air-lift bags.

Multi-cell high-pressure air-lift bags Air bags that offer a distinct height advantage over traditional flat bags and utilize a unique lifting system. The more current design is two-cell bags that are joined together and pre-connected. Another version still in use is a round-shaped bag that can be locked together with a threaded connector, creating one bag with multiple cells.

Nonferrous metals Metals or alloys free of iron, such as aluminum, copper, nickel, lead, zinc, and tin.

O-ring An attachment designed to join chains together or join a chain to a come along utilizing a hook.

Oblong ring See *O-ring*.

Pneumatic chisels Pneumatic tools used to cut through various types and sizes of metal.

Pneumatic cut-off tool A pneumatic tool utilizing a small carbide disk, normally 3 in. (8 mm) in diameter, which rotates at high revolutions per minute to cut through most metals.

Pneumatic tools Tools that use air under pressure to operate.

Protective ensemble Multiple elements of compliant protective clothing and equipment that when worn together provide protection from some risks, but not all risks, of emergency incident operations. (NFPA 1500)

Ratchet strap A mechanical tensioning device with a manual gear-ratcheting drum to put tension on an object, utilizing a webbing material.

Reciprocating saw A power-driven saw in which the cutting action occurs through a back-and-forth motion (reciprocating) of the blade.

Rotary saws Fuel-powered saws capable of cutting wood, concrete, and metal; two types of blades are used on rotary saws: a round metal blade with teeth and an abrasive disk. The application of rotary saws in vehicle extrication is limited.

Self-contained breathing apparatus (SCBA) An atmosphere-supplying respirator that supplies a respirable air atmosphere to the user from a breathing air source that is independent of the ambient environment and designed to be carried by the user. (NFPA 1981)

Shims Objects that are smaller than wedges used to snug loose cribbing under a load or to fill void spaces.

Shoring A stabilization technique used where the vertical distances are too great to use cribbing or the load must be supported horizontally, such as in a trench, or diagonally, such as in a wall shore.

Slide hook A hook that allows chain links to pass freely through the throat of the hook to tighten around an object.

Spring-loaded center punch A glass removal tool used on tempered glass that, when engaged, uses a spring-loaded plunger to fire off a steel rod with a sharpened point directly into a pinpoint area of glass, causing the glass to shatter.

Step chocks Specialized cribbing assemblies made out of wood or plastic blocks in a step configuration. They are typically used to stabilize vehicles.

Struts A compression element used in the support of structures, excavation openings, or other loads. (NFPA 1006)

Supplied air respirator/breathing apparatus (SAR/SABA) A respirator in which breathing air is supplied by an air line from either a compressor or stored air (bottle) system located outside the work area.

Tension buttress stabilization A strut stabilization system that uses a strap in a ratchet or jacking device to add tension to the object being stabilized, locking the vehicle in place by using a diagonal force that lowers the vehicle's center of mass by increasing the vehicle's entire footprint.

TPI rating A rating that indicates how many teeth per inch a blade has.

Wedges Objects used to snug loose cribbing under a load or to fill a void between the crib and the object as it is raised.

Winches Chains or cables used for a variety of lifting, pulling, and holding operations.

Working load limit (WLL) The maximum force that may be applied before failure occurs to an assembly or a component of a device or rope/line/cable in straight tension.

REFERENCES

Occupational Safety and Health Administration. Occupational Noise Exposure. https://www.osha.gov/SLTC/noisehearingconservation/attenuation.html. Accessed November 18, 2020.

Walton, F. R. The Library of History of Diodorus Siculus, Fragments of Book XXVI. In *Loeb Classical Library*; 1957.

On Scene

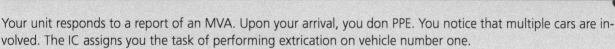

Your unit responds to a report of an MVA. Upon your arrival, you don PPE. You notice that multiple cars are involved. The IC assigns you the task of performing extrication on vehicle number one.

As you perform your size-up of the vehicle, you note that it is a late-model sedan resting on four wheels. The vehicle has suffered major damage from a lateral impact accident. There are two people trapped inside the vehicle, and both will require emergency medical care. After the inner/outer survey has been completed, you confirm you have access from all sides of the vehicle.

1. At this point, what task should you perform first?
    A. Determine whether there are any hazards surrounding the vehicle.
    B. Determine whether the hydraulic hoses will reach the vehicle.
    C. Stabilize the vehicle.
    D. Determine what the weight of the vehicle is.

2. When referring to reciprocating saws, TPI stands for:
    A. total point interaction.
    B. two plus an inch.
    C. teeth per inch.
    D. total percentage of interference.

3. In this scenario, if you were to break the tempered side glass in the vehicle to access the victim, you could use a striking tool such as a:
    A. spring-loaded center punch.
    B. Kelly tool.
    C. steel chisel.
    D. pneumatic window punch.

4. In this scenario, you attempt to manually open the doors and are unsuccessful. You should then:
    A. break out the windows.
    B. use a hydraulic tool.
    C. use bystanders to assist.
    D. utilize a different tool or tactic.

5. The best tool to use to cut through a wide C-post would be a:
    A. hacksaw.
    B. reciprocating saw.
    C. K-12 rotary saw.
    D. bow saw.

6. A come along is designed to be utilized with a rated chain package.
    A. True
    B. False

7. In reference to vehicle rescue and extrication, the acronym WLL stands for:
    A. working leverage limit.
    B. working load limit.
    C. weight load limit.
    D. weight leverage limit.

8. To power pneumatic tools, the rescuer must have a supply of:
    A. compressed fluid.
    B. compressed air.
    C. 220-volt electricity.
    D. rechargeable batteries.

(continues)

On Scene Continued

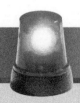

9. Ferrous metals contain:
   A. iron.
   B. aluminum.
   C. tin.
   D. lead.

10. Stabilization of a vehicle on its side should be relative to the vehicle's:
    A. position.
    B. height.
    C. weight.
    D. center of mass.

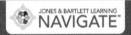

SECTION 2

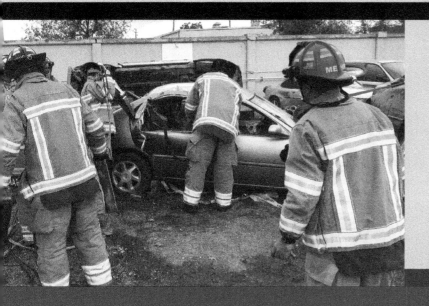

Operations and Technician Levels

CHAPTER **4** **Site Operations**

CHAPTER **5** **Mechanical Energy and Vehicle Anatomy**

CHAPTER **6** **Supplemental Restraint Systems**

CHAPTER **7** **Advanced Vehicle Technology: Alternative-Fuel Vehicles**

CHAPTER **8** **Vehicle Stabilization**

CHAPTER **9** **Victim Access and Management**

CHAPTER **10** **Alternative Extrication Techniques**

CHAPTER **11** **Terminating the Incident**

CHAPTER 4

Operations and Technician Levels

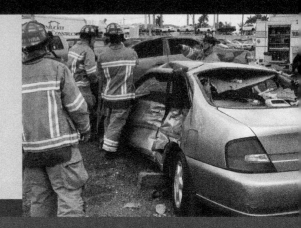

Site Operations

KNOWLEDGE OBJECTIVES

After studying this chapter, you will be able to:
- Describe the three stages of vehicle extrication. (pp. 101, 103)
- Explain the importance of documentation for vehicle extrication incidents. (**NFPA 1006: 8.2.1**, p. 103)
- Communicate fire hazards and rescue objectives to the fire support team. (**NFPA 1006: 8.2.2**, p. 103)
- Compare and contrast vehicle extrication inner and outer surveys. (**NFPA 1006: 8.2.5**, pp. 105–107)
- Compare and contrast formal and informal postincident analysis. (pp. 108–109)
- Identify hazards to rescuer(s) and victim(s) at vehicle extrication incidents. (**NFPA 1006: 8.2.1, 8.3.4**, pp. 111–115)
- Identify fire suppression and safety measures. (**NFPA 1006: 8.2.1, 8.2.2**, pp. 111–113)
- List key elements of landing zone safety. (pp. 115–117)

SKILLS OBJECTIVES

After completing this chapter, you will be able to perform the following skills:
- Stabilize a vehicle accident victim. (**NFPA 1006: 8.2.5**, p. 103)
- Provide expedient rescue while protecting victim(s) and rescuers. (**NFPA 1006: 8.2.6**, pp. 103, 105, 109–113)
- Locate victim(s). (**NFPA 1006: 8.2.5**, pp. 105–108)
- Establish emergency escape route and signals to indicate immediate evacuation. (**NFPA 1006: 8.2.6, 8.3.3, 8.3.6**, pp. 105–108)
- Create access and egress openings in a passenger vehicle for rescue. (**NFPA 1006: 8.2.6**, pp. 105–108)
- Develop an incident action plan (IAP) for a vehicle extrication incident. (**NFPA 1006: 8.2.1, 8.2.8, 8.3.1, 8.3.4, 8.3.7**, pp. 108–109)
- Enforce safety and emergency procedures at a vehicle rescue. (**NFPA 1006: 8.2.5**, pp. 109–111)
- Extinguish a vehicle fire. (**NFPA 1006: 8.2.2**, p. 112)
- Establish a landing zone for a medical helicopter. (pp. 116–117)

You Are the Rescuer

You are the technical rescuer on a vehicle rescue and extrication incident where you arrive as the company officer on scene. Upon arrival, you realize that the first-arriving crew did not follow standard operating procedures (SOPs) and properly stabilize the vehicle. Even from your location, you can see that the vehicle is rocking back and forth as the crew works to extricate the victim. What actions should you take?

1. Should you immediately halt the operation?
2. Should you pull the crew back and have them stabilize the vehicle?
3. Should you allow the crew to continue to extricate the victim?

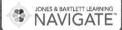
Access Navigate for more practice activities.

Introduction

Vehicle rescue and extrication is a step-by-step technical process consisting of three phases: stabilization of the scene, stabilization of the vehicle(s), and stabilization of the victim(s). This chapter discusses the first phase of the process, stabilizing the scene: site operations (**FIGURE 4-1**).

Safety

Ensuring that proper safety procedures are followed in any operation, whether the operation is responding to an emergency incident, working on an emergency incident, conducting training, or simply checking out or inspecting equipment, is paramount for any organization. SOPs outlining universal safety procedures

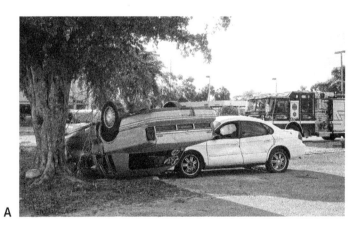
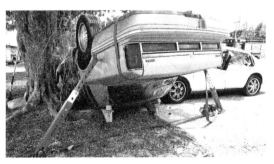
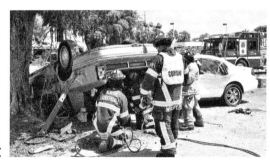

FIGURE 4-1 Vehicle extrication is a technical process that requires structured successive steps to produce favorable results. This chapter will discuss the first phase of this process "Stabilizing the Scene." **A.** Phase 1: Stabilizing the Scene: Site operations—Dispatch, responding to the scene, scene size-up, scene safety zones, hazards, inner and outer surveys, incident action plan. **B.** Phase 2: Stabilize the Vehicle: vehicle safety and stabilization—Vehicle positioning, cribbing/struts, stabilization of vehicles in their normal position, on their side, or resting on their roof or on another object. **C.** Phase 3: Stabilize the victim: victim access and management—Initial access points, using various rescue tools and equipment to gain access, providing initial medical care, packaging and removal.
Courtesy of David Sweet.

and best practice models need to be implemented and followed by every member of every agency. The goal is not to penalize personnel by implementing a rigid policy that is nonflexible but to strive to have voluntary compliance by consistently conducting daily emergency and nonemergency operations in the safest and most efficient manner. An excellent reference in this area of safety is NFPA 1500, *Standard on Fire Department Occupational Safety, Health, and Wellness Program*. The following is an excerpt from NFPA 1500:

> **A.4.3.1** It is the policy of the fire department to provide and to operate with the highest possible levels of safety and health for all members. The prevention and reduction of accidents, injuries, and occupational illnesses are goals of the fire department and shall be primary considerations at all times. This concern for safety and health applies to all members of the fire department and to any other persons who could be involved in fire department activities. (NFPA, 2018, 2021)

This statement on safety is clear and precise and should be adopted by all emergency response agencies regardless of the fact that it was adopted for a fire department. Throughout this text, safety is addressed with every technique and procedure, but it is ultimately the responsibility of personnel to be cognizant of any situation that may occur where safety can and will be jeopardized. All personnel must know how to adjust, adapt, and conform to the best practice model, avoiding or eliminating any and all potential injuries.

Personnel Rehabilitation

Establishing a rehabilitation group is critical in any prolonged vehicle rescue and extrication incident. Weather can be detrimental to personnel operating on scene, whether it is in 100 percent humidity, which occurs on a daily basis in southern Florida, or it is below freezing, which is a frequent occurrence in South Dakota. A properly equipped rehabilitation unit providing shelter and thermal control options should be established early in the incident with personnel rotation mandated by the IC. A great resource for establishing a rehabilitation response protocol is NFPA 1584, *Standard on the Rehabilitation Process for Members During Emergency Operations and Training Exercises*. Some of the issues covered in this guide include:

- Immediate recognition and treatment of heat- or cold-related emergencies, such as frostbite, heat exhaustion, or heatstroke
- Immediate shelter from potentially detrimental climate conditions
- Active or passive cooling/warming techniques based on the type of climate exposure
- Rehydration—basic fluid and electrolyte replacement
- Medical monitoring and base readings
- Personnel accountability with a release from and return to duty procedure/policy
- Transport capabilities

Equipment Resources

When responding to vehicle rescue and extrication incidents, it is vital to know what additional specialized equipment is available to assist in managing the incident. All rescuers realize that these incidents can require a great deal of time on scene, depending on the complexity of the incident and factors involved. Although the availability of specialized equipment sometimes expedites rescue operations, bringing specialized equipment into the operation also adds another layer of safety concerns for the response process. This is a reminder that the need for constant and continual reevaluation of the operation should occur regardless of what specialized equipment is brought in or what the scope or size of the incident is.

Depending on the state's or county's geography, assistance from other resources may be necessary during an incident, such as heavy-equipment providers or operators, portable lighting companies, hardware stores, building suppliers, farm equipment sales, farm equipment mechanics, tow agencies or wrecker services, 18-wheeler operators, physicians, four-wheeler sales, portable generator sales, fast-food restaurants, fire equipment dealers, and rescue equipment dealers (**FIGURE 4-2**). See Chapter 2, *Vehicle Rescue Incident*

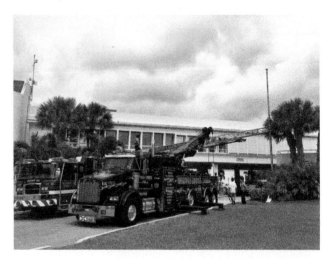

FIGURE 4-2 Assistance from other resources can be crucial during an incident.
Courtesy of David Sweet.

Awareness and Scene Size-Up, for information on hazards and needs assessment for the jurisdiction. All rescuers and other responding agencies should coordinate their training; at a minimum, a meet-and-greet session to open up dialogue and establish a working relationship with each other is valuable. Obviously, training together is the best practice scenario; doing so enhances all parties' equipment familiarity, identifies equipment limitations, and provides for better and more diverse service delivery for those unique or specialized incidents that may occur. Rescuers and other responders should train with the equipment that is available to them and know the equipment's limitations; these training opportunities are more operational tools for the toolbox.

A variety of specialized equipment may be necessary when dealing with vehicle rescue and extrication incidents. In some incidents, more than one wrecker may be required. A heavy-tow unit equipped with an articulating boom may also be useful in lifting, stabilizing, or displacing larger vehicles when necessary.

Chapter 2 discusses the risk/needs assessment and analysis of a jurisdiction's response area, which includes the need for this type of equipment and should be included in the agency's SOPs/SOGs.

Communication and Documentation

Effective communication and documentation are important keys to providing the best level of service to the community. The NIMS dictates the use of plain language and a structured IAP, as described in Chapter 2. Also, using tactical worksheets at large-scale incidents can be the difference for successful outcomes. Tactical worksheets are basically accountability sheets. They identify which engine company or rescue unit is assigned to the particular tactic or group function. For example, Engine 23 may be assigned as extrication group 1 at vehicle 1, and Engine 34 may be assigned as extrication group 2 at vehicle 2.

Proper documentation during site operations always pays dividends for an agency when legal issues, such as lawsuits, occur. Proper documentation also provides justification of service when applying for agency accreditation, such as with the Center for Public Safety Excellence (CPSE), or when old or outdated equipment needs to be replaced or better equipment purchased. Lastly, proper documentation can provide an avenue to improve the agency through recognition of operational deficiencies by incorporating a quality management and assurance program.

Scene Size-Up

As discussed in detail in Chapter 2, *Vehicle Rescue Incident Awareness and Scene Size-Up*, after dispatch and responding to the scene, scene size-up is the systematic and continual evaluation of information presented in either visual or audible form. Size-up begins at the time the incident is dispatched, not at the time the unit arrives at the scene. The technical rescuer needs to start gathering information and formulating and strategizing a plan while en route to the incident. There are many elements to consider in ensuring a safe and successful rescue operation (**TABLE 4-1**).

Immediately upon arrival, the first company officer sizes up the scene and establishes command. A rapid and accurate visual size-up is needed to avoid placing rescuers in danger and to determine which additional resources if any are needed.

With the size-up information, the IAP is set into motion for safe and effective actions to be taken to stabilize the incident. In any event, responders should not rush into the incident scene until an initial assessment can be made of the situation.

TABLE 4-1 Elements of a Rescue Operation

Scene Size-Up	Ongoing Size-Up	Gaining Access to Victims
Appropriately placing apparatus	Controlling associated hazards by stabilizing the scene	Stabilizing the victims by treating and packaging victims
Assessing environmental concerns	Stabilizing the vehicle	Extricating victims
Ensuring appropriate PPE	Creating entry and exit plans: Plan A, Plan B, and emergency escape	Transporting victims
Protecting rescuers with a charged hose line	Dismantling/inspecting equipment	Terminating the incident

Voice of Experience

Truck 6 responded to a single vehicle crash on the expressway. The area is known for high-speed vehicle incidents, and Truck 6 responded to what seemed to be a routine call. The safety-conscious crew approached the scene and defensively parked with the wheels of the truck facing away from the vehicle involved.

The crew activated the flashing directional lights and donned safety vests, and the driver engineer placed reflective safety cones at a significant distance from the approach side of the truck. Recognizing law enforcement was already on scene, we stopped approximately 15 yd (14 m) short of the law enforcement vehicle from the outside shoulder of a divided highway, blocking one of the adjacent lanes.

Medical care was being rendered to the casualty, and bystanders were nearby giving witness accounts of the crash. What seemed to be a routine call soon turned into a near miss and potential fatality of civilians and firefighters.

The posted speed limit on the expressway is 70 mi/h (113 km/h). Within minutes of Truck 6 rendering care, a loud explosion caused by twisted metal and broken glass sent everyone operating at the scene into confusion. Truck 6 was struck on the driver's side by a passenger vehicle traveling at a high speed. The vehicle spun out of control within a short distance from the original crash scene. The teenage driver of the vehicle that struck Truck 6 was emotionally distraught but uninjured. She later advised law enforcement that she drove on the overpass and recognized she was quickly closing on the crash scene. She attempted to move over one lane and accidentally struck the Jersey barrier, causing her to deflect off the barrier and into the side of Truck 6.

This incident was a close call that reminded the responders of the importance of creating a barrier of fire apparatus and law enforcement vehicles to protect the scene from passerby traffic. One risk we cannot control is the speed of vehicles approaching a scene until additional fire apparatus or law enforcement arrives on scene. Each year there are approximately 100 firefighter fatalities in the United States, including those killed at roadway incidents. We should continue to be vigilant about scene safety and incident management to help prevent first responder and civilian fatalities at these incidents.

Jayson Lynn
Hillsborough County Fire Rescue
Tampa, Florida

Scene Size-Up Report

As the apparatus arrives on scene, the company officer needs to give a size-up report to dispatch. The main reason for the report is to give an update to the units responding so they can maintain or adjust their response. The units responding should tailor their response to what the report states. This report should be precise and detailed but not lengthy. It should include information such as the number of vehicles involved, type of vehicles, position of the vehicles (upright, on roof, on side, on another car), extent of damage (minor, moderate, heavy), and, if known, victim status and level of entrapment. A typical size-up report may go as follows:

> "Engine 14 and Rescue 14 arrival. We have two passenger vehicles, one upright and one on its side, with heavy damage to both. We'll advise on injuries."

If extrication or special operations are needed requiring multiple units and/or agencies, the company officer establishes command and requests a tactical or operational channel if available. A tactical or operational channel is a separate working channel designated to the incident so normal air traffic from incoming calls will not interfere with the operation.

After the initial size-up report has been given and a closer evaluation of the scene has been accomplished, an update report can be conveyed to dispatch explaining the level of entrapment. To keep it simple, use the same terminology that was used to describe the damage to the vehicle. There are generally three categories of entrapment: minor, moderate, and heavy (**TABLE 4-2**). These categories are suggested guidelines only; levels of entrapment or terminology may vary from one agency to another. Consistently using the same terms to describe the condition of the vehicle(s) and the level of entrapment conveys a crystal-clear message for incoming units about the severity of the incident. Responding units should act according to this report. Remember that these guidelines are not set in stone; any guideline can be modified to fit your agency's trauma criteria or terminology preference. These entrapment classifications are a simple tool that can be used to keep everyone on the same page when responding to an incident. Once decided upon, entrapment classifications should be considered to be incorporated in departmental response protocols or SOPs.

Inner and Outer Surveys

Both inner and outer surveys should be completed before any operations begin (**FIGURE 4-3**). The inner and outer surveys are 360-degree inspections of the scene that are completed by two or more personnel, depending on the number of vehicles and the size of the incident scene. Rescuers can walk together in the same direction or independently, where one rescuer walks in a clockwise direction around the scene and the other in a counterclockwise direction; either directional choice must ensure that every area within the hot/action zone has been investigated by surveyors. These surveys provide the company officer and crew with additional information about hazards, types of vehicles, the number of victims, possible ejections, the level and type of entrapment, the need for additional resources, and the information necessary to complete an IAP, or objectives for the incident strategy. Lastly, while conducting the inner and outer surveys, if any IDLH hazards are found, then that surveyor needs to call out the hazard immediately, and all members must be ordered to "freeze" until the hazard has been mitigated, or made safe to continue.

TABLE 4-2 Entrapment Classifications

Minor Entrapment	There is no vehicle metal or material that is impinging on the victim. The victim has either no injuries or minor injuries. The extrication process to gain access to the victim would require a basic door release/removal procedure.
Moderate Entrapment	There is some vehicle metal or material that is impinging on the victim. The victim has sustained injuries that require total immobilization. The extrication process to gain access and extricate the victim will involve two or more procedures, such as a door and roof removal.
Heavy Entrapment	There is a large amount of vehicle metal or material impinging on the victim. The victim has sustained substantial trauma and has multiple points of entrapment. The extrication will require an extended time of greater than the standard 20-minute objective. The extrication process to gain access and extricate the victim generally requires three or more procedures, such as a door removal, roof removal, and dash lift.

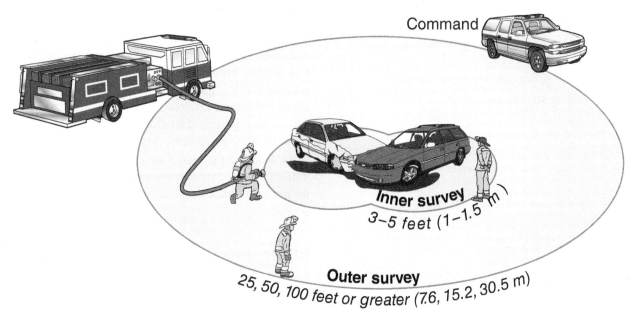

FIGURE 4-3 The inner and outer survey.

The Inner Survey

The **inner survey** is a four-point inspection of the vehicle's front, driver's side, rear, and passenger's side, including the top and undercarriage on all sides. It is recommended that the inner survey be conducted by the first-arriving company officer or the most experienced personnel. Having the company officer conduct the inner survey may be more productive than assigning someone else to do this. The company officer can see firsthand what the incident is presenting and immediately start to formulate an action plan, which will include identifying entry and exit points, victim locations, and victim entrapment type and level as well as vehicle stability for access and removal of the victim(s). Early recognition of the type of entrapment and possible associated injuries of the victim(s) will help direct the officer in the techniques that will be utilized to remove the victim(s), which is Plan B in the overall IAP, described in detail in the succeeding paragraphs.

In addition, any IDLH hazards that are found need to be called out immediately and all members ordered to freeze until the hazard has been mitigated, or made safe to continue.

To begin an inner survey, the company officer must avoid touching the vehicle before clearing any electrical hazards. As an added safety measure, one recommendation is for the officer to lace his or her hands behind his or her back to prevent inadvertently touching the vehicle before clearing any electrical hazards (**FIGURE 4-4**). Obviously, on uneven ground, the rescuer may need the use of his or her hands and

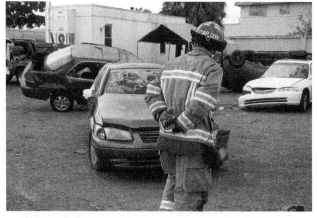

FIGURE 4-4 The company officer must avoid touching the vehicle before clearing any electrical hazards. As an added safety measure, one recommendation is for the officer to lace his or her hands behind his or her back to prevent inadvertently touching the vehicle before clearing any electrical hazards.
Courtesy of David Sweet.

arms for balance and will need to adjust appropriately to the environment that is encountered. The company officer should remain approximately 3 to 5 ft (0.9 to 1.5 m) away from the vehicle in a defensive posture throughout the survey while being cognizant of any sudden forward or rearward lurching of the vehicle. The recommended position and approach to the vehicle is from the front driver's-side corner, but still maintaining that 3- to 5-ft (0.9- to 1.5-m) separation as well as being cognizant of the position of the front wheels, which will determine the direction of travel should the vehicle lurch forward. The company officer should establish immediate verbal contact with the victim with the goal of preventing the victim from moving his or her head or body; victims may immediately track a rescuer's voice, so it is important to tell them to keep still and not to move their head. From a psychological position, if the victim is conscious, he or she will require the reassurance that you are present and going to get him or her out. The moment a victim is located, it is best practice to assign a medical responder immediately to the victim, with contact maintained throughout the incident. Compassion should never be omitted in our role as a public servant.

The entire inner survey is a quick yet thorough survey that should last no longer than 45 seconds with one or two vehicles. The following information should be collected during the inner survey:

- IDLH hazards
- Type of vehicle (conventional/commercial, hybrid, fuel cell, etc.)
- Status of the vehicle (Is it running? Is it in drive or park?)
- Number of victims
- Entrapment
- Entrapment classification type (minor, moderate, heavy)
- Obvious trauma to the victim(s)
- Position and stability of the vehicle
- Activated SRS air bag system—determined by visibly deployed air bags, with the possibility of live nondeployed air bags still present
- Primary access (Plan A - the access plan or initial entry plan), secondary access (Plan B - the removal plan and/or extrication plan), and emergency escape plan

Primary access (Plan A) consists of the existing openings of doors and/or windows that provide a pathway or entry to the trapped and/or injured victim. Secondary access (Plan B) consists of the openings created by rescuers that provide a pathway to remove/extricate trapped and/or injured victims. These two types of access are the basis for establishing the Plan A and Plan B of the IAP; if the team cannot gain entry through existing openings (the established Plan A), then Plan B is implemented to create and gain access. The emergency escape plan is for immediate unexpected hazards that affect the rescuers and/or victim.

The emergency escape plan is established by the officer immediately after the inner/outer survey has been completed. The emergency escape plan is a designated area of temporary refuge that the team can retreat to if an immediate danger to life and health is experienced, such as another vehicle entering the hot zone. The emergency escape plan establishes a safe zone to help provide immediate accountability of all personnel. It is the responsibility of the officer in charge to confirm that all personnel are aware of the designated safe zone area.

Before the incident, emergency evacuation signals should be agreed upon. Signals may be audio (such as an air horn) or visual (such as hand signals). All firefighters should understand the when such a signal is issued, evacuation should begin immediately.

LISTEN UP!

For clear, uninterrupted radio transmissions, ask for a tactical or operational channel if available, and implement NIMS by establishing command. This is a best practice model in establishing scene control and leadership.

If the company officer, upon his or her initial exam of the incident, determines that the victim requires an immediate and rapid extrication for the greatest chance of survival, the company officer may quickly complete the inner and outer surveys with his or her crew, conduct a brief and basic vehicle stabilization, and then take the appropriate action for the safe and rapid extrication of the victim. The risk-versus-benefit scenario can occur at any incident, but it is imperative to remember that safety must never be compromised in any situation. If the vehicle is positioned where stability threatens the safety of the crew, the company officer may proceed with full stabilization of the vehicle and then move on to extricate the victim. The company officer must not put the crew's life in jeopardy by performing a haphazard procedure that can potentially cause harm or serious injury.

In an emergency situation, there is no textbook or template that determines whether a company officer should call for a rapid extrication. The tactical decision for a rapid extrication is a judgment call. This can be one of the hardest decisions to make because of the grave consequences that may occur. One such complication is the potential for paralysis of the victim caused by the lack of proper vehicle stabilization, with further trauma needlessly forced upon him or her because steps were not taken to immobilize and package the victim correctly. This decision has to weigh heavily in favor of benefiting the victim's life. The saying "life over limb" is often used by rescue personnel to justify their actions.

As part of the inner survey, it is important to identify the total number of victims accurately to determine the need for additional resources. While the company officer is conducting the inner survey, another rescuer should perform the outer survey, moving in the opposite or same direction of the company officer around the perimeter of the inner survey. Available personnel, such as DLE officers or medical personnel, who are standing by can interview bystanders to see whether more information on any additional victims can be ascertained.

The Outer Survey

The outer survey is conducted simultaneously with the inner survey. For most incidents, extending from the perimeter of the inner survey position outward is adequate for the outer survey. Note that the rescuer's distance from the vehicle varies with each incident. Generally, a distance of 25 to 50 ft (7.6 to 15.2 m) or the distance of the scattered debris pattern is a good indicator of how far out one should search, but adding in factors such as speed of travel and type of roadway (highway versus residential roadway) could cause the survey to extend as far as 100 ft (30.5 m) or greater. The reasoning behind maintaining these survey areas is simple: the higher the speed of travel, the greater the distances the objects, vehicles, and victims could be thrown from the site of impact. To better illustrate this point, if the vehicle is traveling at 100 mi/h (161 km/h), the occupant is traveling at the same speed as the vehicle; when the vehicle abruptly stops from hitting something, the occupant, unless held in by a seat belt, continues to travel at the original speed. This is why ejections occur. Another suggestion for the rescuer performing the outer survey is to utilize a thermal imaging camera (TIC) as he or she conducts the search. This is an excellent tool that can quickly scan a heat source of a victim who may have been ejected and is now concealed by brush, debris, or darkness.

The rescuer has to use his or her best judgment when determining the proper distance from the vehicle. The recommended position and approach to the vehicle is from the front side, scanning for any of the following:

- IDLH hazards
- Victims who have been ejected
- Walking wounded (victims who were involved in the accident in some way and could have sustained injuries, whether minor or major)
- Additional vehicles
- Infant or adolescent car seats

Again, any IDLH hazards must be called out immediately and all members ordered to freeze until the hazard has been mitigated, or made safe to continue.

The inner and outer surveys should be completed at about the same time, and the rescuers then meet to discuss their findings, compile the information, and formulate an IAP, which includes the primary access (Plan A—access/entry), secondary access (Plan B—removal), and emergency escape plan.

Once the inner and outer surveys have been completed and the scene is deemed safe for operation, a rapid triage of the victims can be implemented. Remember that vehicles must be properly stabilized before entering them, so the primary access (Plan A—access/entry) may be delayed until the vehicle has been made or is deemed safe to enter. The medical responder can also perform a quick assessment or rapid triage of a victim without entering a vehicle, possibly through an open window. Triage is the process of sorting victims based on the severity of each victim's condition. Once all victims have been triaged, rescuers establish treatment and transport priorities. This process helps allocate personnel, equipment, and resources to provide the most effective care to everyone. Chapter 9, *Victim Access and Management*, discusses this process in more detail.

Incident Action Plan

A clear, concise IAP is essential in guiding the initial incident management decision process and continuing collective planning activities of incident management teams, including at incidents where a common passenger vehicle has come to rest on its roof or side. You will need to adjust the IAP based on the vehicle's positioning. An IAP can be developed formally for large-scale or major incidents requiring incident management teams or informally, through a quick mental reference process for smaller incidents (**FIGURE 4-5**). For both the formal and informal processes, the development of an IAP should proceed through five primary phases:

1. Conduct an initial incident size-up.
2. Establish the incident objectives and strategy.
3. Develop the plan.
4. Prepare and disseminate the plan.
5. Evaluate and revise the plan.

Whether dealing with a small- or large-scale incident, the IAP encompasses a complete risk–benefit analysis, including information about hazard mitigation and resource activation and staging as well as confirmation on the incident strategy and tactics. This includes establishing and assigning operational and support tasks. Specific components of a formal IAP and corresponding incident command system

CHAPTER 4 Site Operations

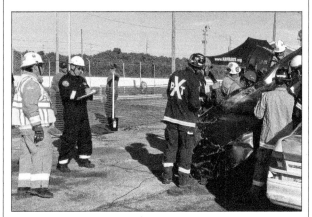

FIGURE 4-5 A sample incident action plan.
Courtesy of Carlos Eguiluz.

TABLE 4-3 IAP Components

Component of IAP	Corresponding ICS Form (if applicable)
Incident objectives	ICS 202
Organization list or chart	ICS 203
Assignment list	ICS 204
Communications plan	ICS 205
Logistics plan	
Responder medical plan	ICS 206
Incident map	
Health and safety plan	

(ICS) forms established through NIMS are found in (**TABLE 4-3**).

Other possible components of a formal IAP may include the following:

- Air operations summary
- Traffic plan
- Decontamination plan
- Waste management or disposal plan
- Demobilization plan
- Operational medical plan
- Evacuation plan
- Site security plan
- Investigative plan
- Evidence recovery plan

Vehicle rescue and extrication in itself is a technical process that requires a plan consisting of structured successive steps to produce favorable results. Almost everything technical in life requires planning with some form of procedures or successive steps to follow to reach a successful outcome. For example, when attempting to build something, you need to follow an outline, a plan, or a formal blueprint, whether it is formulated in your mind or formally drawn up on paper. The first step is to create a solid base, or foundation, and then continue building on that until completion. If steps are skipped or the process is done haphazardly, then a poor product will be the end result. The same holds true for managing a vehicle rescue and extrication incident; the plan needs to start with the basic fundamentals, or foundation, and then continue building in successive steps. By following a detailed plan of action, the technical rescuer is better prepared to mitigate any unforeseen situations when they occur.

Establishing Scene Safety Zones

As previously discussed in Chapter 2, once the entire area has been surveyed, hazard control zones need to be established and maintained until the incident has been terminated or hazards have been mitigated. NFPA 1500 Section 8.7 recommends that hazard control zones delineate the operational boundaries, which are divided into three areas: hot, warm, and cold. A fourth zone—a no-entry zone—can be added if needed. These zones are designated by the IC prior to position assignments and are strictly enforced by the incident safety officer. The boundaries of the three zones (and the fourth, no-entry, zone if needed) should be established in a manner that ensures the safety of the crews operating within the zones and

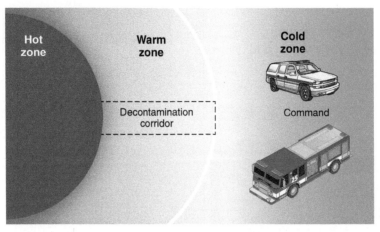

FIGURE 4-6 The area of operation is divided into three safety/operational zones: the hot zone, warm zone, and cold zone.

limits the exposure of personnel outside the zones to any potential hazards or debris. If there are changes to the sizing or location of the zones, these changes must be directed to and acknowledged by all personnel on the scene (**FIGURE 4-6**).

Hazard zones should consist of the following:

- **Hot zone:** This area, also known as an action zone, is for entry teams and rescue teams only. It immediately surrounds the dangers of the incident, and entry into this zone is restricted to protect personnel outside the zone.
- **Warm zone:** This area is for properly trained and equipped personnel only. The warm zone is where personnel and equipment decontamination and hot zone support take place, including a debris area for material that is removed from the vehicle(s).
- **Cold zone:** This area is for staging vehicles and equipment and contains the command post.
- **No-entry zone:** This is the area at an incident scene where no one is permitted to enter because of an IDLH or the need to preserve the scene for evidence for a postinvestigation team. For crime scene investigations, this zone may be established later in the incident when the initial tactical teams have concluded the operation. This zone may or may not need to be established, based on the type of incident and findings.

The IC assigns personnel or uses law enforcement to establish another perimeter outside the cold zone to keep the public and media out of the operational area.

The most common method of establishing the hazard zones for an emergency incident site is to use law enforcement, fire line tape, or barriers. Once the controlled zones have been marked, the IC, incident safety officer, and personnel ensure that the restrictions associated with the various zones of the emergency scene are strictly enforced.

The size of each zone varies depending on the complexity and size of the incident. Anyone who enters the warm or hot zone must be wearing full PPE, without exception. This is strictly enforced to maintain control of the incident and continuity of safety. Senior chief officers may at times enter the scene without wearing any PPE to take a closer look or to give an order; this is jokingly known as the "white wave." If this occurs, treat them with respect and politely ask them to put on some protective gear so they will not be injured by flying debris.

Lockout/tagout systems should be used to secure a safe environment (**FIGURE 4-7**). These are methods of ensuring that systems and equipment have been shut down and/or that switches and valves are locked and cannot be turned on at the incident scene. Lockout/tagout control procedures more commonly are used at hazardous material incidents, machinery entrapment situations, and/or confined-space incidents to eliminate and/or control hazards, such as the flow of fluids, movement of equipment, or the release of stored energy, but they can also be used at vehicle rescue and extrication incidents. For example, during an incident involving an extrication, suppose a hydraulic ram is used to lift the roof of the vehicle off the victim, and it needs to be held in place to prevent it from coming back down. The ram can be locked out in the extended position by disconnecting the hydraulic lines attached to the tool. This action prevents the possibility of the hydraulic ram being accidentally closed or opened by another rescuer.

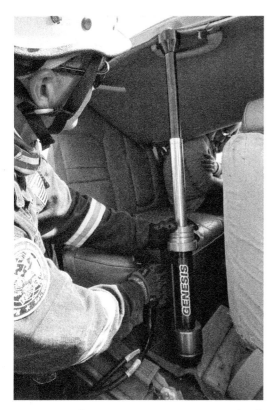

FIGURE 4-7 Lockout/tagout systems are methods of ensuring that systems and equipment have been shut down and that switches and valves are locked and cannot be turned on at the incident scene, such as a hydraulic rescue tool being placed in position and disconnected from its power source.
Courtesy of Edward Monahan.

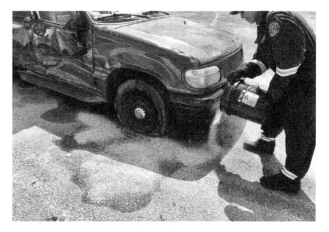

FIGURE 4-8 Decide which absorbent/adsorbent material is best suited for use with the spilled product, and use it to isolate a fuel spill from the area around the damaged vehicle.
Courtesy of Houston Holcomb.

Specific Hazards

Fire Hazards

Because there is a significant risk of spilled fuel in many motor vehicle crashes, a minimum 1.75-in. (44-mm) diameter hose line should be deployed and charged, ready to protect personnel and victims by suppressing any potential fires or hazards that occur. Other forms of protection include an ABC dry chemical portable fire extinguisher; however, the level of protection is greater with a charged hose line in place. Crashes that pose large fire hazards or actual fires may require additional fire suppression resources, which should be requested as soon as possible. Small fuel spills can be handled by using an absorbent or adsorbent material to isolate a fuel spill from the area around the damaged vehicle (**FIGURE 4-8**). The absorbent material can then be removed from the area by a licensed hazardous material agency. Most tow agencies are licensed to remove this type of hazardous substance once the incident has been terminated.

A post-crash fire can occur for many reasons, including a short in the electrical system or sparks created during the crash, igniting spilled fuel. These fires may trap the occupants of the vehicle and require fire suppression. Various fuel types used by vehicles can present a multitude of fire suppression hazards to fire rescue personnel and are discussed in Chapter 7, *Advanced Vehicle Technology: Alternative-Fuel Vehicles*. Additional hazards located in vehicles when on fire pose significant risks to fire rescue personnel. SRS components and associated propellants may rupture when super-heated, launching shrapnel inside and outside the vehicle. Lift assist struts and some bumper assemblies that contain a hydraulic fluid when heated may also expand and rupture when super-heated by fire impingement, potentially launching the piston rod contained inside the strut or suddenly releasing the bumper assembly itself. A minimum 1.75-in. (44-mm) diameter charged hose line should be deployed on all vehicle rescues involving extrication incidents, regardless of whether the vehicle is on fire.

There are times when fire suppression is necessary, and according to NFPA 1006 Section 8.2.2, fire protection must be established for an extrication incident and fire control support so that the potential for fire and explosion is understood and managed. These fire hazards and rescue objectives must also be communicated to the fire support team. A requisite skill in this section is to supply fire protection and manage a fire using various extinguishing devices should a fire occur. Personnel should possess the necessary skills, training, and qualifications before attempting to extinguish a fire. Those with the necessary skills and training know to approach a vehicle fire from an uphill, upwind position, moving in from the side at a 45-degree angle to the vehicle. **SKILL DRILL 4-1** offers a basic overview of how to extinguish a vehicle fire.

SKILL DRILL 4-1
Extinguishing a Vehicle Fire NFPA 1006 8.2.2

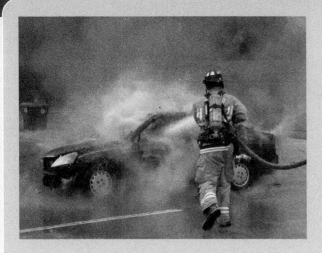

Courtesy of Bill McGrath.

1 Don full PPE. Perform a scene size-up, and give an arrival report. Ensure that apparatus is positioned uphill and upwind and that it protects the scene from traffic. Perform the inner and outer surveys, and protect the crew from hazards. Identify the type of fuel used in the vehicle, and look for fuel leaks. Advance a fire attack line of at least 1.75-in. (44-mm) diameter using water or foam. Beware of the hazards. Suppress the fire using effective water or foam application techniques. Notify command when the fire is under control. Investigate the origin and cause of the fire. Preserve any evidence of arson. Return the equipment and crew to service.

SOPs for vehicle fires may vary between agencies and jurisdictions. To extinguish a vehicle fire, follow the steps in Skill Drill 4-1.

Electrical Hazards

Downed electrical lines present a serious hazard to firefighters and other rescue personnel. Many vehicle collisions occur during the night, which creates problems for emergency response personnel because of the lack of visibility to identify downed electrical lines. In this situation, attention to detail is very important. The technical rescuers must recognize signs dealing with power outages caused by the vehicle. Streetlights that are normally lit may not be functional, or residents or homes in the area may be without lighting. These signs should alert the emergency responders to proceed very slowly into the suspect location.

Once the electrical line has been identified, contact the appropriate utility provider, and isolate the hazard from contact with any personnel or bystanders (**FIGURE 4-9**). Several methods can be used to isolate electrical hazards, such as placing traffic cones around a designated safe-distance perimeter to the electrical line, placing fluorescent snap lights around the safe-distance perimeter, or using barrier tape to tape off the area. Use law enforcement for street or access closures if needed. At no time should a rescuer assume that a downed power line is dead; utility companies

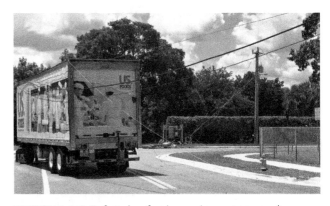

FIGURE 4-9 Safety is of primary importance when dealing with electricity.
Courtesy of Bill McGrath.

are programmed to energize a line several times at various intervals to determine where there is a break in the line. Power lines are known to jump several feet (or meters) when energized, so keep a safe distance, and never attempt to throw anything over a downed line to contain or move it.

Some locations do not have suspended electrical supply lines or electrical transformers; instead, electrical supply lines are buried, and electrical transformers are positioned at ground level. In such a case, the hazards are the same as with suspended lines but a little closer to the responder and surrounding properties. Like overhead electrical lines, those positioned underground are vulnerable to damage from vehicular

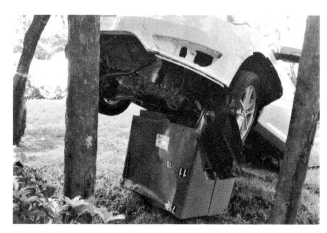

FIGURE 4-10 Electrical transformers positioned at ground or suspended levels may create a number of problems for rescuers.
Courtesy of Brad Myers.

crashes. Similarly, electrical transformers positioned at ground or suspended levels may create a number of problems for rescuers (**FIGURE 4-10**) Such problems include open high voltage, toxic smoke and gas, intense heat, potential for explosion from oil-filled equipment, explosion and flying debris from glass and porcelain insulators, as well as the release of pressurized gas in some systems.

SAFETY TIP

Several methods can be used in isolating electrical hazards, such as placing traffic cones around a designated safe-distance perimeter to the electrical line or using barrier tape to tape off the area.

Fuel Sources

The most common fuel sources today are gasoline and diesel fuel, although the list of alternative fuels is growing. Liquefied petroleum gas (LPG), or propane, continues to be one of the most widely used fuel alternatives to gasoline and diesel on a worldwide basis primarily because of the environmental improvements that use of LPG brings. More than 500,000 vehicles in the United States use propane gas, most of which have spark-ignition engines that can operate on either propane or gasoline.

Gas explosions and leaks normally involve natural gas and propane gas. Natural gas incidents usually involve a ruptured supply line or a line that has failed because of corrosion, surface shift, or human intervention. Rescuers should evaluate any suspected releases with gas and air monitoring devices to determine the actual release point. Once the release point has been located, all buildings in the immediate area should be monitored before the area is considered safe.

In its natural state, propane is odorless, and when it is sent through a distribution system, an odorant is added. If the propane is being transferred by pipeline, however, the odorant may not have been added, creating a major concern for rescuers when incidents involve pipelines. Propane is heavier than air, so it will lie close to the ground surface, seeking an ignition source.

As mentioned, a majority of propane leaks or releases occur from leaking or damaged tanks caused by impacts or overpressurization. One of the concerns in dealing with incidents that involve propane is the potential for a **boiling liquid/expanding vapor explosion (BLEVE)** created when fire impinges on the tank, resulting in temperature and pressure increases within the cylinder. As both temperature and pressure increase, the relief valve activates (opens), allowing the pressure to be released. If the relief valve fails to activate or is overcome, the tank will fail, resulting in a violent explosion. Chapter 7 covers more details on the physical properties and use of the various fuel types used by vehicles.

Fuel Runoff

Fuel runoff can be very dangerous if not controlled by firefighters or rescue personnel. Several concerns arise when dealing with fuel runoff, including the presence of ignition sources, environmental concerns, and reactions of fuels when they mix with each other and other products involved in the incident.

Damming, diverting, diluting, and absorbing are all methods used to control fuel runoff. Fire rescue agencies more commonly use an absorbent product as basic as domesticated feline litter or ground-up corn cobs to soak up oil and/or petroleum products. Or they may use products as advanced as foaming agents to cover, dilute, and/or suppress ignitable fumes. Other tactics include shoveling ground soil to dam up and stop or slow any runoff or placing down a ground absorbent sock (PIG) or float booms for bodies of water.

Ignition Sources

With active fuel leaks, rescuers must be aware of all potential ignition sources when working at a vehicle rescue and extrication incident. It is recommended that some form of atmospheric monitoring, such as a four-gas or multi-gas detection device, be used. Depending on the type of fuel, readings, and proximity to potential ignition sources, all ignition sources should be eliminated if possible, without additional exposure or risk. Additionally, it may be necessary for all apparatus and other vehicles to remain in a staging area upwind beyond the established no-entry zone.

All individuals not associated with the incident must be removed, and no apparatus or portable equipment is to be started until the hazards are identified and/or mitigated.

Hazardous Materials

Responders, no matter what their level of training, must constantly be aware of the complexity, impact, and potential harm that various types of hazardous materials can present. They must also know how to avoid exposure, whether by inhalation, absorption, ingestion, or injection. It is recommended to request from dispatch appropriately trained and equipped personnel to handle any incident involving hazardous materials. Responders must be aware of the threats that such materials pose to health, property, and the environment. In today's world, responders must also be trained to recognize indicators of potential terrorist incidents as a part of their size-up because vehicles are being widely utilized as weapons of attack.

Hazardous materials can come in a variety of forms: solids, liquids, and gas. Such materials can have radioactive, flammable, explosive, toxic, corrosive, biohazardous, oxidizer, asphyxiant, pathogenic, allergenic, or other characteristics that make them hazardous in specific circumstances. Vehicles that carry flammable and nonflammable pressurized gases (e.g., nitrogen, hydrogen, and oxygen) as well as transporters that carry flammable and nonflammable cryogenic liquids, including liquid nitrogen, liquid hydrogen, liquid oxygen (LOX), and liquefied natural gas (LNG), will also occasionally be involved in incidents (**FIGURE 4-11**). Solid materials, including explosives and flammable solids, oxidizers and organic peroxides, and poisons and corrosives, are also sometimes involved in incidents. Common examples are fertilizers, pesticides, caustic powders, water-treatment chemicals, and Class 9 materials, which are especially prevalent around mining or construction activities.

There are three primary NFPA standards and one OSHA regulation that apply to hazardous materials and training for emergency responders:

- NFPA 472, *Standard for Competence of Responders to Hazardous Materials/Weapons of Mass Destruction Incidents*
- NPFA 473, *Standard for Competencies for EMS Personnel Responding to Hazardous Materials/Weapons of Mass Destruction Incidents*
- NFPA 1072, *Standard for Hazardous Materials/Weapons of Mass Destruction Emergency Response Personnel Professional Qualifications*
- 29 CFR 1910.120, Hazardous waste operations and emergency response

The DOT defines hazardous materials as "any substance or material in any form or quantity that poses an unreasonable risk to safety and health and to property when transported in commerce." Rescuers should be aware of these threats and contact the appropriate resources to handle these hazards.

Other Hazards

Environmental conditions can lead to unique hazards at a crash scene. Crashes that occur in rain, sleet, or snow, for example, present an added hazard for rescuers and the victims of the crash. Crashes that occur on elevations, such as a hill or mountainside, pose more challenges than those that occur on level ground.

Be especially alert for the presence of infectious bodily substances. Be prepared for the presence of blood, and follow standard precautions (body substance isolation). Specifically, do not let blood or other bodily fluids come in contact with skin; wear gloves that protect from both contaminated fluids and sharp objects that are present at a crash site. If you or your clothes become contaminated, report the contamination, document it, and then clean and wash the affected clothes and equipment according to the manufacturers' instructions.

Some crash scenes may present threats of violence. Intoxicated motorists or those who are upset with other motorists may pose a threat to you and your crew or to others present at the scene. Be alert for weapons that are carried in civilian vehicles. Law enforcement should always be dispatched on all motor vehicle collision incidents.

Occasionally, animals become a hazard at crash scenes. Dogs and other family pets may be protective

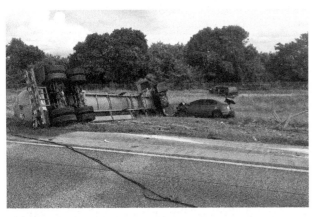

FIGURE 4-11 Cargo tankers can carry hazardous materials, such as chlorine, propane, ammonia, Freon, and butane.
Courtesy of Mike Jachles.

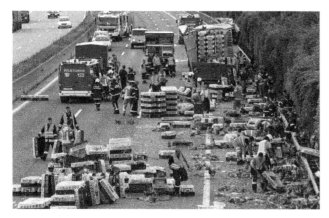

FIGURE 4-12 Vehicles transporting livestock or horses can be involved in a crash, and the animals may need care. You may need to call in specialized resources, such as a large-animal rescue unit or team, to respond to and assist with this type of incident.
© FOTOKERSCHI.AT/AFP/Getty Images.

of their owners and threaten rescuers. Livestock or horses that have been involved in a crash may need care. You may need to call in specialized resources, such as a large-animal rescue unit or team, to respond to and assist with this type of incident (FIGURE 4-12).

Air Medical Operations

Air ambulances are used to evacuate medical and trauma victims. A medical evacuation is commonly known as a medevac and is generally performed by helicopters. Most rural and suburban EMS jurisdictions and many urban systems are capable of performing helicopter medevacs or have mutual aid agreements with other agencies, such as police or hospital-based medevac, to provide such service. They land at or near the scene and transport victims to trauma facilities every day in many areas. There are two basic types of air medical units: fixed wing and rotary wing, otherwise known as helicopters (FIGURE 4-13). Fixed-wing aircraft generally are used for interhospital victim transfers over distances greater than 100 to 150 mi (161 to 241 km). For shorter distances, ground transport or rotary wing aircraft are more efficient.

Rotary wing aircraft have become an important tool in providing emergency medical care. Trauma victim survival is directly related to the time that elapses between injury and definitive treatment. Most air ambulances fly well in excess of 100 mi/h (161 km/h) directly to a hospital helipad without the delays of road or traffic hazards that ground transport units can encounter. The crew may include EMTs, paramedics, flight nurses, or physicians.

Air rescue is a vital component of any emergency operation, regardless of the type of emergency

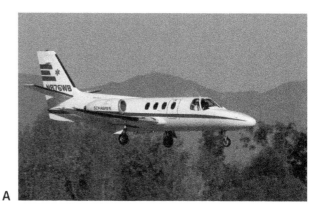

A

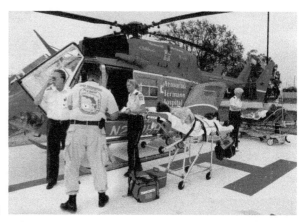

B

FIGURE 4-13 Air ambulances. **A.** Fixed-wing aircraft are generally used to transfer victims from one hospital to another over distances greater than 100 to 150 mi (161 to 241 km). **B.** A rotary wing aircraft, or helicopter, is used to help provide emergency medical care to victims who need to be transported quickly over shorter distances.
A: © Ralph Duenas/Jetwash Images. B: Courtesy of Ed Edahl/FEMA.

response agency. Fire rescue agencies should receive training on the capabilities, protocols, and methods for accessing air ambulances in the response jurisdiction, and departmental SOPs or medical protocols for air rescue should be established. SOPs and/or medical protocols for each response jurisdiction detail specific criteria for the type of victim who may receive air evacuation and how and when to call for an air ambulance. Following are some general guidelines you should be familiar with when considering whether to initiate a helicopter medevac operation.

Establishing a Landing Zone

Establishing a landing zone is the responsibility of the ground crew through a coordinated effort with the flight crew. The landing zone must be agreed upon by both parties. Determining the location involves more than simply looking for a clear space. The ground crew must be prepared to take action to make certain that the flight crew is able to land and take off safely.

To prevent any miscommunication when the request is made for air rescue to respond, the request should include a ground contact radio channel (typically a pre-established operational channel) as well as a call sign of the air rescue unit. Some agencies pre-establish landing zones throughout their jurisdiction and mark them on specialized district maps that are updated quarterly. This type of incident preplanning can be coordinated with air rescue and is a good idea to avoid confusion or conflict that may occur during an incident.

Actions to take when selecting and establishing a landing zone include the following:

- Make sure the area is a hard or grassy level surface that measures 100 × 100 ft (30 × 30 m) (recommended) and no less than 60 × 60 ft (18 × 18 m) (**FIGURE 4-14**). If the site is not level, the flight crew must be notified of the steepness and direction of the slope (**FIGURE 4-15**). Use the local law enforcement department for information on road closures and blockages. Always check with your local air rescue management team for specific landing zone requirements.
- Clear the area of any loose debris that could become airborne and strike either the helicopter or the victim and crew. Such objects include branches, trash bins, flares, accident tape, and medical equipment and supplies.
- Survey the immediate area for any overhead or tall hazards, such as power lines or telephone cables, antennas, and tall or leaning trees. The presence of these hazards must be relayed immediately to the flight crew because an alternate landing site may be required. The flight crew may request that the hazard be marked or illuminated by weighted cones or by positioning an emergency vehicle with its lights turned on next to or under the potential hazard. Treat all downed wires as if they are energized.
- To mark the landing site, use weighted cones, or place lights under these cones for illumination. This procedure is essential during night landings. Never use accident tape or people to mark the site. The use of flares is also not recommended; not only can they become airborne, but they are incendiary devices that can potentially start a fire or cause an explosion. There are products on the market for lighting or marking a landing zone, but always refer to an agency representative on the proper procedures, devices, and/or regulations for marking a landing zone.
- Make sure all nonessential persons and vehicles are moved to a safe distance outside of the landing zone.

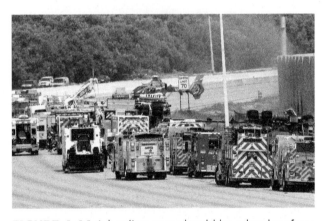

FIGURE 4-14 A landing area should be a level surface measuring 100 ft × 100 ft (30 m × 30 m).
Courtesy of Devon Sweet.

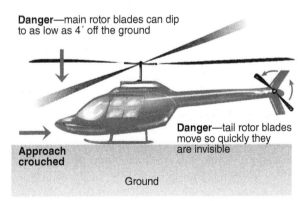

FIGURE 4-15 Approach a helicopter on a grade from the downhill side only.

LISTEN UP!

To prevent any miscommunication, when the request is made for air rescue to respond, the request should include a ground contact radio channel (typically a pre-established operational channel) as well as the call sign of the air rescue unit.

Landing Zone Safety

Helicopter safety is a combination of good sense and a constant awareness of the need for personal safety. You should be sure to do nothing near the helicopter and go only where the pilot or crew member directs you. The most important rule is to keep a safe distance from the aircraft whenever it is on the ground and "hot," which means the helicopter blades are spinning; most of the time the rotor blades will remain running because the flight crew does not expect to remain on the ground for a long time. This means that all personnel should stay outside the landing zone perimeter unless directed to come to the aircraft by the pilot or a member of the flight crew. Usually, the flight crew has its own equipment and does not require any assistance inside the landing zone. If you are asked to enter the landing zone, stay away from the tail rotor; the tips of its blades move so rapidly that they are invisible. Never approach the helicopter from the rear, even if it is not running. If you must move from one side of the helicopter to another, go around the front. Never duck under the body, the tail boom, or the rear section of the helicopter. The pilot cannot see you in these areas.

Another area of concern is the height of the main rotor blade. On many aircraft, it is flexible and may dip as low as 4 ft (1.2 m) from the ground (**FIGURE 4-16**). When you approach the aircraft, walk in a crouched position. Wind gusts can alter the blade height without warning, so be sure to protect equipment as you carry it under the blades. Air turbulence created by the rotor blades can blow off hats and loose equipment. These objects in turn can become a danger to the aircraft and personnel in the area.

SOPs and/or medical protocols must be established for all air operations and landing zone procedures.

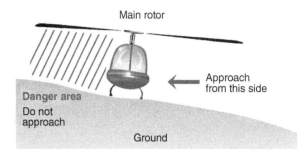

FIGURE 4-16 The main rotor blade of the helicopter is flexible and may dip as low as 4 ft (1.2 m) from the ground.

After-Action REVIEW

IN SUMMARY

- Ensuring that proper safety procedures are followed in any operation, whether it is responding to an emergency incident, working on an emergency incident, conducting training, or simply checking out or inspecting equipment, is paramount for any organization.
- A properly equipped rehabilitation unit providing shelter and thermal control options should be established early during prolonged extrication incidents.
- When responding to vehicle rescue and extrication incidents, it is vital to know what additional specialized equipment is available to assist in managing an incident.
- Proper documentation always pays dividends for an agency when legal issues, such as lawsuits, occur.
- Size-up begins at the time the incident is dispatched, not at the time the unit arrives at the scene.
- A size-up report gives an update to the units responding so they can organize their response.
- There are generally three categories of entrapment: minor, moderate, and heavy.
- The inner and outer surveys are 360-degree inspections of the scene that are completed by two or more personnel.
- An IAP may be formal or informal.
- Scene safety zones or operational zones are divided into hot, warm, and cold zones with a fourth, no-entry, zone established if needed. These zones are strictly enforced by a designated incident safety officer.
- Hazards at vehicle rescue and extrication incidents may include fire hazards, electrical hazards, fuel hazards, ignition sources, and hazardous materials. Personnel should possess the necessary skills, training, and qualifications before attempting to mitigate any of these hazards.
- You should be familiar with the capabilities, protocols, and methods for accessing and landing helicopters in your area.

KEY TERMS

Boiling liquid/expanding vapor explosion (BLEVE) An event that occurs when the temperature of the liquid and vapor (flammable or nonflammable) within a confining tank or vessel is raised by an exposure fire to the point where the increasing internal pressures can no longer be contained and the vessel ruptures and explodes.

Cold zone The control zone of an incident that contains the command post and other support functions deemed necessary to control the incident. (NFPA 1500)

Emergency escape plan A plan for immediate, unexpected hazards that affect the rescuers and/or victim.

Hazard control zones Delineate the operational boundaries, which are divided into three areas: hot, warm, and cold.

Hot zone The control zone immediately surrounding a hazardous area, which extends far enough to prevent adverse effects to personnel outside the zone. (NFPA 1500)

Inner survey A four-point inspection of the vehicle's front, driver's side, rear, and passenger's side, including the roof and undercarriage on all sides of the vehicle. This survey is conducted approximately 3 to 5 ft (0.9 to 1.5 m) from the vehicle and is performed by the first-arriving company officer or experienced personnel.

Lockout/tagout systems Methods of ensuring that systems and equipment have been shut down and that switches and valves are locked and cannot be turned on at the incident scene.

No-entry zone Those areas at an incident scene that no person(s) are allowed to enter, regardless of what personal protective equipment (PPE) they are wearing due to dangerous conditions or crime scene investigation. (NFPA 1500)

Outer survey A survey conducted simultaneously with the inner survey; the rescuer performing the outer survey moves in the same or opposite direction as the rescuer performing the inner survey. Distance from the vehicle will vary with each incident, but it is generally a distance of 25 to 50 ft (7.6 to 15.2 m), starting from the perimeter of the inner survey position outward.

Primary access (Plan A) The existing openings of doors and/or windows that provide a pathway to the trapped and/or injured victim(s). (NFPA 1670)

Secondary access (Plan B) Openings created by rescuers that provide a pathway to trapped and/or injured victims. (NFPA 1670)

Triage The sorting of casualties at an emergency according to the nature and severity of their injuries. (NFPA 1006)

Warm zone The control zone outside the hot zone where personnel and equipment decontamination and hot zone support take place. (NFPA 1500)

REFERENCES

Federal Motor Carrier Safety Administration. n.d. How to Comply with Federal Hazardous Materials Regulations. https://www.fmcsa.dot.gov/regulations/hazardous-materials/how-comply-federal-hazardous-materials-regulations. Updated April 18, 2018. Accessed 2018.

National Fire Protection Association. 2018. *NFPA 1582: Technical Committee on Fire Service Occupational Safety and Health.* 2018 ed. Quincy, MA: NFPA.

National Fire Protection Association. 2021. *NFPA 1500, Standard on Fire Department Occupational Safety, Health, and Wellness Program.* 2021 ed. Quincy, MA: NFPA.

National Fire Protection Association. 2013. *NFPA 1951, Standard on Protective Ensembles for Technical Rescue Incidents.* 2013 ed. Quincy, MA: NFPA.

National Fire Protection Association. 2015. *NFPA 1951, Standard on the Rehabilitation Process for Members During Emergency Operations and Training Exercises.* 2015 ed. Quincy, MA: NFPA.

NFPA Glossary of Terms. 2018. https://www.nfpa.org/-/media/Files/Codes-and-standards/Glossary-of-terms/glossary_of_terms_2018.ashx. Updated January 26, 2018. Accessed 2018.

Occupational Safety and Health Administration. (1996, November 7). Standard Number: 1910.120 Definition of a Hazardous Substance. https://www.osha.gov/laws-regs/standardinterpretations/1996-11-07. Accessed 2018.

U.S. Department of Transportation. *Manual on Uniform Traffic Control Devices (MUTCD).* https://mutcd.fhwa.dot.gov/index.htm. Accessed 2018.

On Scene

Just after dinner, you receive a call for the report of a two-car collision on a busy street at an intersection during rush hour. It is dark outside. You quickly go to your engine and don your PPE. As the engine responds to the incident, you, as the officer, preplan the site operation procedures and assignments with your crew as dispatch updates important information.

1. Stabilizing an incident requires the technical rescuer to manage site operations and stabilize the scene, stabilize the vehicle, and:
   A. stabilize the situation.
   B. stabilize the braking system.
   C. stabilize the victim.
   D. stabilize his or her crew.

2. In compliance with the NIMS, all emergency response personnel are required to utilize _____ for emergency radio communication.
   A. 10-codes
   B. native language
   C. Q-codes
   D. plain language

3. The incident size-up begins at the:
   A. time of dispatch.
   B. arrival of units on scene.
   C. moment all units respond.
   D. time the company officer arrives.

4. Describe the protective ensemble required for a vehicle accident scene on a roadway involving the extrication of a victim.
   A. Helmet, primary eye protection, footwear
   B. Hard hat, ear protection, respiratory protection
   C. Reflective vest, helmet, boots
   D. Body protection, helmet, eye protection, gloves, footwear, and reflective safety vests

5. Once your engine arrives on scene at the busy intersection, what is the best method for protecting the rescuers from traffic flow?
   A. Position apparatus around the corner from the incident.
   B. Position apparatus where the side-mounted pump panel is facing the passing traffic.
   C. Use law enforcement to protect the rescuers.
   D. Position apparatus at a 30- to 45-degree angle to the wreckage with the wheels facing away from the operation.

6. What information does the DOT's *ERG* provide?
   A. Guidance regarding traffic control
   B. Guidance regarding traffic control devices
   C. Guidance to rescuers who may potentially operate at a hazardous material incident
   D. Guidance regarding the positioning of apparatus

7. The inner survey is a _____ inspection of the vehicle.
   A. one-point
   B. two-point
   C. three-point
   D. four-point

8. When conducting the inner survey, the recommended safe distance from the vehicle is approximately:
   A. 6 ft (1.8 m)
   B. 2.5 ft (0.8 m)
   C. 3 to 5 ft (0.9 to 1.5 m)
   D. 30 ft (9.1 m)

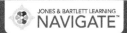

CHAPTER 5

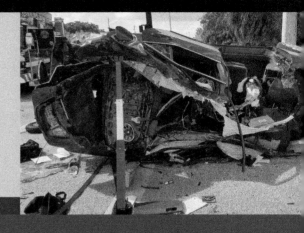

Operations and Technician Levels

Mechanical Energy and Vehicle Anatomy

KNOWLEDGE OBJECTIVES

After studying this chapter, you should be able to:

- Define the following terms and use the terms correctly in discussing vehicle rescue incidents:
  - Energy (p. 121)
  - Kinetic energy (p. 121)
  - Potential energy (p. 121)
  - Work (p. 121)
- Discuss the application of the law of conservation of energy to vehicle crashes. (p. 121)
- Define mechanism of injury (MOI) and discuss the correlation of MOI and injury to the human body. (p. 121)
- Identify air bag deployment and occupant seat belt use at a vehicle crash. (**NFPA 1006: 8.2.4**, pp. 123–124)
- Explain the five general classifications of vehicle collisions. (pp. 124–126)
- Identify common passenger vehicle anatomy and composition. (**NFPA 1006: 8.2.1, 8.3.1, 8.3.4, 8.3.7**, pp. 126–130)
- Describe the implications for vehicle rescue of materials used in vehicle construction including:
  - Metal (p. 127)
  - Carbon (p. 127)
  - Carbon fiber reinforced polymer (CFRP) (p. 127)
  - Magnesium alloy (p. 128)
- Define the following terms and describe their effect on vehicle rescue:
  - High-strength steel (HSS) (p. 129)
  - Advanced high-strength steel (AHSS) (p. 129)
- Identify the three major vehicle frame/construction systems. (**NFPA 1006: 8.2.5, 8.2.6, 8.3.3, 8.3.6**, pp. 130–131).
- Identify common passenger vehicle structural components. (**NFPA 1006: 8.2.1, 8.3.1, 8.3.4, 8.3.7**, pp. 132–136, 138–140)
- Describe two common types of striker plate assemblies in passenger vehicle door construction. (p. 135)
- Identify A-, B-, and C-posts in passenger vehicles. (**NFPA 1006: 8.2.1, 8.3.1, 8.3.4, 8.3.7**, pp. 136, 138–139)
- Discuss the common types of safety glass used in passenger vehicles. (pp. 140–142)
- Identify primary vehicle propulsion systems in passenger vehicles. (**NFPA 1006: 8.2.4**, p. 144)

SKILLS OBJECTIVES

There are no skill objectives for this chapter.

You Are the Rescuer

You are on an extrication training exercise where you have been instructed to perform a roof removal procedure. In the process of removing the roof, you attempt to cut through the B-post and encounter some difficulty with the hydraulic cutters; they cannot cut all the way through the post. You make several attempts to no avail.

1. Is the post composed of advance high-strength steel (AHSS)? Does it contain a boron rod or carbon fiber reinforced polymer insert? Check the make, model, and year of the vehicle.
2. What is the rated cutting force of your hydraulic cutter?
3. Does the hydraulic cutter need servicing? Are the blades separating as you make the cut?

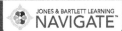

Access Navigate for more practice activities.

Introduction

This chapter explores the application of energy in relation to a motor vehicle collision. This includes applying the law of conservation of energy to vehicle crashes, understanding the mechanism of injury (MOI) as it relates not only to the vehicle collision but also the human body, and exploring the sequence of events in a motor vehicle collision. Additionally, this chapter discusses the anatomy and components of a vehicle system, such as the electrical components, frame systems, vehicle classifications, and vehicle propulsion systems. Understanding these two components of energy and the anatomical parts that make up a vehicle system is integral in the extrication process.

Energy

Merriam-Webster Online Dictionary (2020) defines energy as "a fundamental entity of nature that is transferred between parts of a system in the production of physical change within the system and usually regarded as the capacity for doing work." Energy is all around us; it is a constant force. In fact, the law of conservation of energy states that energy can be neither created nor destroyed; it can only change from one form to another. For example, the forward movement of a vehicle (which is kinetic energy) can be changed into heat energy from the friction caused by the application of the brakes. Energy comes in different forms: electrical, mechanical, heat (thermal), light (radiant), chemical, gravitational, and nuclear. When dealing with the science of a motor vehicle collision, mechanical energy is the driving force behind the dynamics of what actually occurs.

Mechanical energy can be broken down into two types of energy: kinetic and potential. With the combination of work (transfer of energy), a mechanical energy system is produced.

Kinetic energy is the energy of motion, which is based on vehicle mass (weight) and the speed of travel (velocity). Kinetic energy is expressed as follows:

$$\text{Kinetic energy} = \text{mass}/2 \times \text{velocity}^2,$$
$$\text{or } KE = m/2 \times v^2$$

Potential energy is stored energy, or the energy of position. To better illustrate this definition, take two bricks (brick 1 and brick 2), each of equal size and weight. Now, hold brick 1 one inch (2.5 mm) over the top of a glass table, and elevate brick 2 three feet (0.91 m) over the top of the glass table (**FIGURE 5-1**). Which brick, if dropped, has the most energy force, or the *potential*, to cause more damage to the glass table? Brick 2, based on the height, speed of travel, and gravitational force, will have the higher level of stored, or potential, energy. When the brick is actually released, the potential energy is transferred to kinetic energy because the brick is in motion. Once the brick strikes the glass table, a force is applied to stop, displace, or alter the brick's kinetic path of travel. This force is known as *work*.

Work, in its most basic definition, is a mechanism for the transfer of energy. Work is said to be applied to an object when energy is transferred to the object and the object is displaced. Work can be applied in the form of a positive (with the direction of travel) or negative (against the path of travel) force. To better illustrate this, let's look at two vehicles that are the same type, make, weight, and model. Vehicle 1 is traveling in a forward motion at 20 mi/h (32 km/h), and vehicle 2 is coming up from behind vehicle 1 at a speed of 40 mi/h (64 km/h). Vehicle 2 eventually crashes into the rear of vehicle 1. Through the application of work, vehicle 2 has transferred its forward kinetic energy

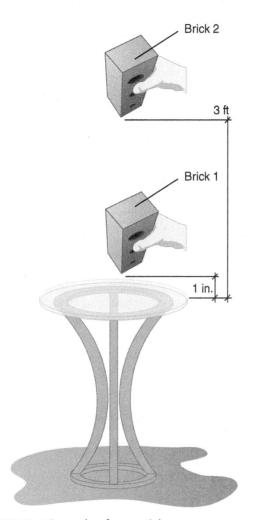

FIGURE 5-1 Example of potential energy.

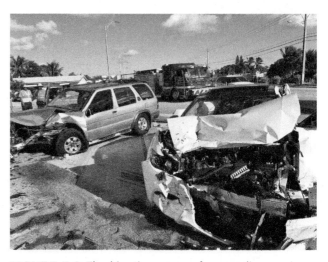

FIGURE 5-2 The kinetic energy of a speeding car is transferred by the work force of stopping the car.
Courtesy of David Sweet.

into vehicle 1, causing a positive work displacement of vehicle 1's path of travel. Vehicle 2 has also experienced a *negative* work force because its path of travel at 40 mi/h (64 km/h) has been displaced by crashing into the rear of vehicle 1, which slowed vehicle 2 or stopped it altogether.

This work, or transfer of energy, can be extreme or lessened based on a number of factors. These factors include the stored potential energy of the vehicles, which is based on the speed of travel, weight of the vehicles, whether the brakes are applied (which would transfer and displace some energy by means of releasing frictional heat when the brakes are applied), and whether the vehicle design is of a unibody type construction (which is designed to collapse and absorb and/or displace energy as a crash occurs) (**FIGURE 5-2**).

Newton's first law of motion states that objects at rest tend to stay at rest and objects in motion tend to stay in motion unless acted on by an outside force. This outside force at the moment of impact is considered the applied work force, which causes displacement. To better illustrate this, if a vehicle in motion crashes into a stationary wall (an outside force containing potential energy and a negative work force, which occurs at the moment of impact), the forward energy from the vehicle (kinetic energy) cannot be destroyed by the wall; the energy changes form and is transferred by work being diverted and distributed throughout the vehicle and its occupants.

The science of a motor vehicle collision through the application of energy can be directly applied to the understanding of how an occupant sustains injuries.

Traumatic injury occurs when the body's tissues are exposed to energy levels beyond their tolerance. The mechanism of injury (MOI) is the way in which traumatic injuries occur; it describes the forces (or energy transmission) acting on the body that cause injury. The same release of energy that occurs during a vehicle collision, on and from the vehicle through the mechanical system of potential energy, kinetic energy, and work, is also applied directly to the human body. The exception to this is that the human body will experience both a positive and negative work force when the internal organs are bounced back and forth against the inside of the human body. The types of injuries that the human body can potentially sustain relate not only to the release of energy on it but also to the type of collision that occurs during the vehicle crash.

Sequence of Events in a Motor Vehicle Collision

The sequence of events that occur during a motor vehicle collision typically consists of three separate collisions. Understanding the sequence of events during each one of these three collisions will help you be alert for certain types of injury patterns. Let's examine the sequence of events involving the three separate collisions that occur during a front impact vehicle collision.

Event 1: Vehicle Impact with Object

The first event is when the vehicle impacts an object, whether the object is stationary or in motion. Depending on the speed of travel, weight of the vehicle, braking distance, and whether the object struck was stationary or in motion, damage to the vehicle is perhaps the most dramatic part of the collision. The amount of damage can provide information about the severity of the collision and the resulting injuries of the occupants (**FIGURE 5-3**). The greater the damage to the car, the greater the release of energy that was involved and, therefore, the greater the potential to cause injury to the victim. By assessing the vehicle that has crashed, you can often determine the mechanism of injury (MOI), which may allow you to predict what injuries may have happened to the passengers at the time of impact according to forces that acted on their bodies. A great amount of force is required to crush and deform a vehicle, cause intrusion into the passenger compartment, tear seats from their mountings, and collapse steering wheels. Such damage suggests the presence of high-energy trauma.

Event 2: Occupant Impact with Vehicle

The second event during the collision is the occupant striking or impacting the interior of the vehicle. Just as the kinetic and potential energy of the vehicle's mass and velocity is converted into the work of bringing the vehicle to a stop, the kinetic and potential energy of the passenger's mass and velocity is converted into the work of stopping his or her body. This work can be greater or less depending on whether the occupants were restrained by a three-point seat belt harness or by an air bag deployment system. Remember Newton's first law of motion, which states that an object in motion will remain in motion until acted upon by an outside force. If the vehicle is traveling at 40 mi/h (64 km/h) at impact, then the occupant's body still travels at 40 mi/h (64 km/h) until his or her impact on the interior of the vehicle stops this forward motion. With the amount of damage to the exterior of the car, the injuries that result are often dramatic and can be immediately apparent during your scene size-up and primary assessment of the occupants.

Common passenger injuries that can occur from this type of impact include lower extremity fractures (knees into the dashboard), flail chest (rib cage into the steering wheel), and head trauma (head into the windshield) (**FIGURE 5-4**). These types of injuries can occur more frequently and be more severe if the passenger is not restrained. However, even when the

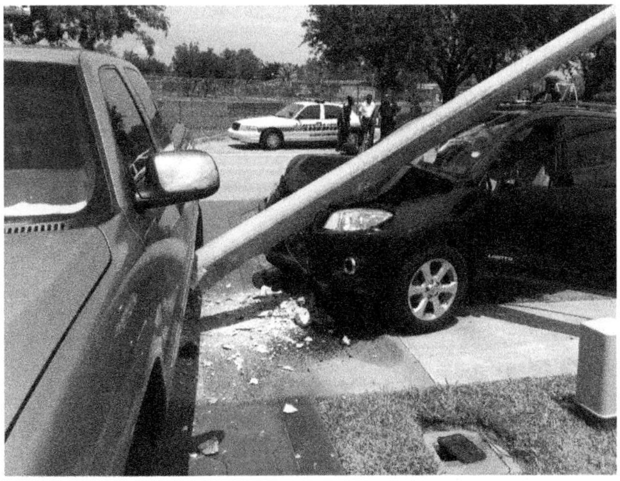

FIGURE 5-3 The first collision in a frontal impact is that of the vehicle against another object, whether the object is stationary or in motion (in this case, a utility pole). The appearance of the vehicle can provide you with critical information about the severity of the crash and can often determine the mechanism of injury (MOI) sustained by the occupants.
Courtesy of Bill McGrath.

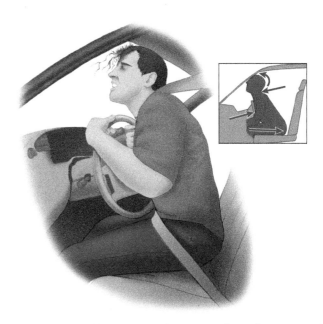

FIGURE 5-4 The second collision in a frontal impact is the occupant striking or impacting the interior of the car.

passenger is restrained with a properly adjusted seat belt, injuries can occur, especially in lateral and rollover impacts.

Event 3: Occupant Organs Impact Solid Structures of the Body

The final event during the collision is the occupant's internal organs striking or impacting the solid internal structures of the body. These organs can impact back and forth several times, depending on when the body's motion finally comes to rest. The injuries that occur during the third collision may not be as obvious as external injuries, but they are often the most life threatening. For example, as the passenger's head hits the windshield, the brain continues to move forward until it comes to rest by striking the inside of the skull (**FIGURE 5-5**). This results in a compression injury (or bruising) to the front of the brain and stretching (or tearing) of the back of the brain. Similarly, in the thoracic cage, the heart may slam into the sternum, which may tear the aorta, the largest artery in the body, and cause fatal hemorrhaging.

Understanding the series of events that occur with these three collisions will help you make the connections between the amount of damage to the exterior of the vehicle and potential injury to the passenger. For example, in a high-speed collision that results in massive damage to the vehicle, you should suspect serious injuries to the passengers, even if the injuries are not readily apparent. A number of potential physical problems may develop as a result of trauma or injuries. Your initial general impression of the victim and the evaluation of the MOI can help direct life-saving care and provide critical information to the appropriate medical facility.

LISTEN UP!

When you are assessing trauma victims at a motor vehicle collision, the MOI is a crucial element to consider for the potential and type of injuries that can be sustained by the occupants. Be alert to the extent of damage to the interior and exterior of the vehicles involved in crashes. Use this observation to paint a picture of the scene in written and verbal communication, especially when consulting with a trauma or medical facility.

Vehicular Collision Classifications

Motor vehicle collisions are classified traditionally by the area of initial impact. They consist of the following: front impact (head-on), including underrides and overrides (discussed later); lateral impact (T-bone, side impact); rear end; rollovers; and rotational (spins), which can also consist of secondary collisions with multiple impacts.

Front Impact Collisions

A front impact collision occurs when the vehicle strikes an object head-on, whether that object is stationary or in motion. With this initial impact, two other events can occur: The vehicle can travel under the object (which is known as an underride collision) or on top of the object (which is known as an override collision). Understanding the MOI after a frontal collision first involves evaluation of the vehicle's restraint systems, which include seat belts (standard three-point harness and a pretensioning system); seat backs, including headrests; and supplemental restraint system (SRS) air bag systems. You should determine whether the occupants were restrained by a full and properly applied standard three-point restraint harness or pretensioning system. In addition, you should determine whether the air bag deployment impacted the occupant, which could cause crushing injuries or burn injuries to the face, arms, and upper torso area from the high temperatures that the air bag generates on deployment. Other MOIs to look for include bent

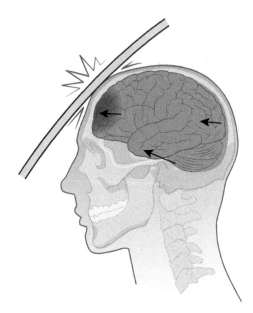

FIGURE 5-5 The third collision in a frontal impact is the occupant's internal organs striking or impacting the solid internal structures of the body. In this illustration, the brain continues its forward motion and strikes the inside of the skull, resulting in a compression injury to the anterior portion of the brain and stretching of the posterior portion.

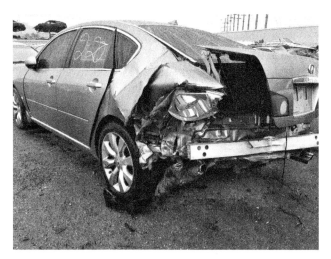

FIGURE 5-6 Rear-end impacts often cause whiplash-type injuries, particularly when the head and/or neck is not restrained by a headrest.
Courtesy of David Sweet.

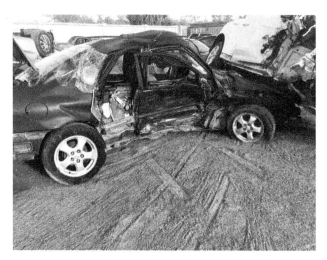

FIGURE 5-7 In a lateral collision, where the vehicle is struck from the side, the impact results in the passenger sustaining a lateral whiplash injury where the movement is to the side and the passenger's shoulders and head whip toward the intruding vehicle.
Courtesy of David Sweet.

or deformed steering wheels and broken or penetrated windshields (imbedded blood, hair, or teeth fragments are all positive confirmation of an impact).

Rear-End Collisions

Rear-end collisions are known to cause whiplash-type injuries, particularly when the passenger's head and/or neck is not restrained by an appropriately placed headrest (**FIGURE 5-6**). On impact, the passenger's body and torso move forward by the transfer of kinetic energy. As the body is propelled forward, the head and neck are left behind because the head is relatively heavy, and they appear to be whipped back relative to the torso. As the vehicle comes to rest, the unrestrained passenger moves forward, striking the dashboard. In this type of collision, the cervical spine and surrounding area may be injured. Because of the anatomical position of the spine, the cervical portion of the spine is less tolerant of damage when it is bent back. Headrests decrease extension of the head and neck during a collision and, therefore, help reduce injury. Other parts of the spine and the pelvis may also be at risk for injury. In addition, the patient may sustain an acceleration-type injury to the brain—that is, the third collision of the brain within the skull. Passengers in the backseat wearing only a lap belt might have a higher incidence of injuries to the thoracic and lumbar spine.

Lateral (Side-Impact) Collisions

Because of the limited protection to the occupants, lateral or side impacts (commonly called T-bone collisions) are a common cause of fatalities associated with motor vehicle crashes. When a vehicle is struck from the side, the impact results in the passenger sustaining a lateral whiplash injury (**FIGURE 5-7**). The movement is to the side, and the passenger's shoulders and head whip toward the intruding vehicle. This action may thrust the shoulder, thorax, upper extremities, and, most importantly, skull against the doorpost or the window. Because of the anatomical position of the spine, the cervical spine has little tolerance for lateral bending.

Rollovers

Certain vehicles, such as large trucks and some sport utility vehicles (SUVs), are more prone to rollover crashes because of their high center of gravity. Injury patterns that are commonly associated with rollover crashes differ depending on whether the passenger was restrained or unrestrained. The most unpredictable types of injuries are caused by rollover crashes in which an unrestrained passenger may have sustained multiple strikes within the interior of the vehicle as it rolled one or more times.

The most common life-threatening event in a rollover is ejection or partial ejection of the passenger from the vehicle (**FIGURE 5-8**). Passengers who have been ejected may have struck the interior of the vehicle many times before ejection. The passenger may also have struck several objects, such as trees, a guardrail, or the vehicle's exterior, before landing. Passengers who have been partially ejected may have struck both the interior and exterior of the vehicle and may have been sandwiched between the exterior of the vehicle

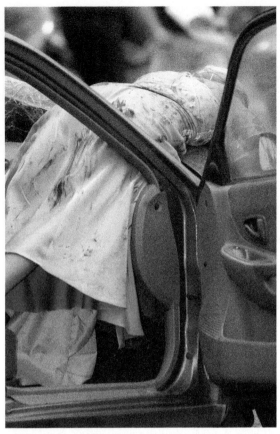

FIGURE 5-8 Passengers who have been ejected or partially ejected may have struck the interior of the car many times before ejection.
© wh1600/iStock/Getty Images Plus/Getty Images.

and the environment as the vehicle rolled. Ejection and partial ejection are significant MOIs; in these cases, you should prepare to care for life-threatening injuries.

Rotational Collisions

Rotational collisions (spins) are conceptually similar to rollovers. The rotation of the vehicle as it spins provides opportunities for the vehicle to experience secondary impacts. For example, as a vehicle spins and strikes a pole on the driver's side, the driver experiences not only the rotational impact and motion but also a secondary lateral impact.

Vehicle Anatomy and Composition

This section discusses the basic anatomy and composition of a vehicle. From the onset of training in the field of vehicle rescue, it is vital for the technical rescuer beginning at the awareness level to establish a solid foundation in understanding the design and structural components that make up a vehicle.

Before a rescuer can properly apply any vehicle rescue and extrication procedures to a vehicle, he or she must understand the inner and outer components that make up a vehicle system. Just as a surgeon thoroughly understands the inner workings of the human body well before making that first incision, the technical rescuer should know the components or basic parts that make up various kinds of vehicles well before starting to extricate. This is why it is so important to establish this knowledge at the awareness level of training. To better illustrate this statement, place yourself on the scene of an extrication incident where the officer in charge tells you to perform a dash-lift technique to gain access to the patient. During this process, you are told to make a relief cut through the upper rail section between the strut tower and firewall. If you do not have a thorough understanding of vehicle anatomy, you will not have any idea where this relief cut needs to be made. This may make you a burden on scene and a hindrance to the operation. Do not try to improvise if you do not understand the technique! Step aside, and pass the tool to a more experienced person.

Electricity

Electrical power in standard conventional-type, internal combustion engine vehicles uses a basic 12-volt battery energy storing system for starting and powering various electrical components within the vehicle. Hybrids, fuel cells, and electric vehicles also use a 12-volt battery system for starting purposes but additionally use an advanced electrical design to provide propulsion to power the vehicle. These types of vehicles are discussed in detail in Chapter 7, *Advanced Vehicle Technology: Alternative-Fuel Vehicles.* There are some larger conventional-type vehicles that use two 12-volt batteries for starting in cold weather climates, for heavy towing assignments, or for operating or assisting in powering additional electrical components; these batteries are normally wired in a parallel-type system and still operate only as a 12-volt system, not 24 volts.

Larger commercial trucks as well as military vehicles use a true 24-volt power electrical system. These batteries are wired in series, with the system being designed to operate at 24 volts. Various vehicle manufacturers have designed voltage parameters using 48 volts for battery systems used to power high power–demand vehicle components, such as electronic pumps, fan motors, and turbo systems to name a few. This 48-volt battery would also work in conjunction with a standard 12-volt lead acid battery, which would still be utilized as a cold-starting mechanism for an external combustion engine. As more and more electrical components are added and advanced computer systems grow, vehicles are requiring greater starting and general operating power than the current 12-volt battery systems allow for.

The 12-volt lead acid battery system, which has been the standard type of battery design used for the past century, consists of six cells in an electrolyte solution of roughly 35 percent sulfuric acid and 65 percent water. Contained inside a polypropylene case, this electrolyte solution causes a chemical reaction with plates of lead and lead dioxide, producing electrons that then flow through conductors, thus generating the power for starting the vehicle. Each cell stores roughly 2.1 volts or more for approximately 12.5 volts. When a 12-volt lead acid battery is overcharged and not properly vented, a by-product can be generated consisting of a highly explosive mixture of hydrogen and oxygen gas.

There are several designs of 12-volt lead acid batteries used in vehicles. The wet cell, or flooded cell, is the standard 12-volt battery that contains an active electrolyte solution. It comes in a serviceable type, where fluid can be added, and in a maintenance-free type. The wet cell must be mounted in the upright position. In the absorbed glass mat (AGM) battery type, a glass mat is used to absorb and hold the electrolyte, preventing it from moving within the battery housing. Each cell contains tightly compressed plates kept under pressure in a fully sealed container and can be stored in multiple positions. The gel cell type uses a silica base additive that firms up the electrolyte in a gel state. The electrons can still move freely, and the battery can be stored in multiple positions without the worry of any leakage. The last is the spiral wound–type battery, which uses lead plates that are tightly wound in a spiral formation within each cell. This type is also sealed and can be mounted in multiple positions.

Other main sources of power in the vehicle are the alternator and voltage regulator. The alternator is basically a belt-driven generator that produces current used to operate various electrical components within the vehicle. A voltage regulator then regulates the flow of electricity coming from the alternator, which keeps the voltage at a safe 12.5 to 14.5 volts.

Metal, Carbon, and Composites

Metal is a classification or group of elements that possess positive ions, such as iron, gold, silver, and copper. Metal can be ferrous (containing iron) or nonferrous (such as aluminum, copper, or zinc). Metal is a good conductor of heat and electricity and is electropositive, which means an element tends to lose electrons and form positive ions in chemical reactions, thus becoming electrically positive. Metal by itself is generally malleable and is alloyed (a combination of two or more elements) with varying amounts and different combinations of metal elements to form an alloyed metal. Alloying metal and nonmetal elements together produces metal products that can be hardened and are resistant to corrosion, lighter, and stronger while maintaining some elasticity.

Carbon is classified as a nonmetallic element. Carbon is one of the most abundant elements in the universe and has the unique ability to bond with multiple elements, making it the foundation for over 95 percent of known chemical compounds. Carbon is the vital composition in the development and design of vehicle components and the overall structure. Carbon is used to produce fossil fuels; plastic polymers, such as carbon fiber reinforced polymer (CFRP); and alloyed metals. When carbon is alloyed with iron ore, the end product is carbon steel, which was once the standard for all structural framing and vehicle components.

New compounds and advanced high-strength steels are being discovered and developed to replace conventional steels. One of the newest compounds, developed in 2004, is a crystalline allotrope of carbon known as graphene. Graphene is the strongest molecular compound known on the planet; yet it is as flexible as rubber. Graphene is 200 to 300 times stronger than steel and harder than a diamond. Because of its unique molecular structure (1 atom thickness), a single square meter sheet of graphene is as thin as a sheet of paper and 1000 times lighter. Through nanotechnology and 3D printing, graphene will one day be possible to mass-produce into any vehicle component, whether it's the frame of the vehicle, structural and mechanical components, body panels, or electrical components. This compound is truly the product of the future.

The Energy Policy and Conservation Act passed by the U.S. Congress in 1975 established the Corporate Average Fuel Economy (CAFE) standards, the sole purpose of which was to reduce energy consumption by increasing the fuel economy of cars and light trucks. With the Energy Independence and Security Act of 2007, CAFE was amended to include fuel economy requirements for passenger cars and light trucks, imposing two phases for new vehicles to be fully compliant by the year 2030. Vehicle manufacturers are on an endless quest to make vehicles more fuel efficient, lighter, stronger, and more crash resistant. The development of strong, crash-resistant vehicles requires engineers and the steel industry to develop stronger and lighter steels to meet these demands. They are using many of

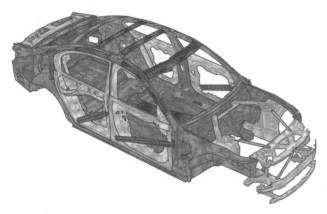

FIGURE 5-9 CFRP is being used to reinforce the structure as an insert section of roof pillars and roof rails, encased in a channel of alloyed steel or aluminum.

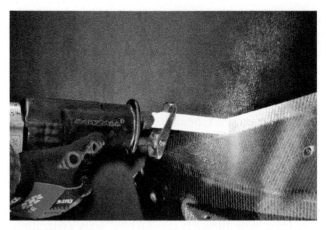

FIGURE 5-10 Cutting into a section of CFRP with a reciprocating saw produces fine particulate matter that can cause respiratory issues. Ensure everyone, including the victims, has respiratory protection.
Courtesy of Edward Monahan.

the same concepts that the race car industry uses, such as incorporating a "safety cage" into the design so the vehicle has reinforced sides, roof, floor panels, rocker panels, and seat structures that are designed to protect occupants from rollovers and various types of impacts. These are just a few of the safety measures of which the technical rescuer must be aware.

Conventional vehicle designs using low- and medium-strength steels are becoming obsolete; unfortunately, these are the vehicles on which most technical rescuers have been or are presently being trained; the junkyards are loaded with them. Today's vehicle manufacturers are using metals and materials such as aluminum, magnesium alloys, and/or CFRP to replace or strengthen the frame, structural components, and/or body parts of the vehicle. CFRP is also being used to reinforce the structure as an insert section of roof pillars and roof rails encased in a channel of alloyed steel or aluminum (**FIGURE 5-9**). Carbon fiber is composed of organic polymers where a crystalline, polyacrylonitrile (PAN) fiber, petroleum pitch, is spun into fine filament strands or fibers and heated to link carbon atoms together. An epoxy resin or thermoplastic is used to bind, reinforce, and shape the final product. CFRP in its highest modulus form can be 5 to 10 times stronger than some steel alloys and up to three times stronger than some aluminum alloys as well as significantly lighter than both metals.

Cutting into a section of CFRP with a reciprocating saw can produce fine particulate matter, which can become airborne and potentially cause respiratory issues, so ensure that everyone—including the victims—have respiratory protection (**FIGURE 5-10**).

Aluminum alloyed metal is a composition of various metals, including pure aluminum, and its main design is to strengthen and lighten the vehicle. The alloyed elements that are added to pure aluminum in various quantities can include magnesium, silicon, zinc, lithium, copper, manganese, and iron. The materials and their quantities determine the resulting metal's strength and rigidity. The strongest grade of alloyed aluminum can be up to two times stronger than some forms of steel at one-third the weight.

Magnesium alloy is a metal that is gaining popularity because of its unique properties and highly sought-after high strength-to-weight characteristics the auto industry requires to meet the CAFE energy standards. Magnesium in its pure form is the lightest structural metal: 33 percent lighter than aluminum, 50 percent lighter than titanium, and 75 percent lighter than steel. Magnesium alloys are the most electrochemically reactive metals. When in contact with dissimilar metals or an electrolyte such as water, magnesium rapidly breaks down from aggressive corrosion unless an anodic protective coating, such as a ceramic oxide, is applied to control the electrode potential and keep the metal in a passive state.

A major concern with magnesium is the danger of fire. The potential for ignition may be prevalent when the melting point (1202°F [650°C]) is exceeded, which can occur from dry cutting through a section with a reciprocating saw as the dust and fragments combined with oxygen and friction ignite. The explosive reaction seen when water is applied to a magnesium fire is the product breakdown of magnesium oxide (MgO) (or magnesium hydroxide, $Mg(OH)_2$, with excess steam) and hydrogen gas. Some vehicle components that may consist of magnesium alloy include the engine block, wheels, steering columns, seats, front consoles, strut cradles, door frames, and hoods.

Steel

Steel in its most basic form is a product of combining iron with a small amount of carbon. This alloyed metal is also known as carbon steel. Steel cannot be labeled as a single component. Steel is a metal product comprising a multitude of varying types of elements based on what is added/alloyed during the processing phase. There are more than 3000 types of steel based on the physical properties and chemical composition of the compound.

Steel is measured by ultimate tensile strength and yield strength, which is identified using the International System of Units (SI) representing pressure, stress, and mass. It is measured in megapascals (MPa) or kilograms per square inch (ksi). One ksi (or 1000 lb of force) on 1 in.^{2} of measurement is equal to 6.89475728 pascals. This conversion factor and terminology are important to understand because of the cutting and spreading force ratings of your hydraulic rescue tools as well as the metals and material with which those tools will engage. If your hydraulic cutter has a cut force rating of 60 ksi and the metal that you are attempting to cut has a tensile and yield force rating of 700 MPa, the rescue tool will not have enough cutting force to cut through that section of metal properly; cutting would require just over 100 ksi. The 60-ksi-rated cutter would be damaged, or the blade movement would stop abruptly midway through the metal.

The **ultimate tensile strength (UTS)** of steel measures the amount of force that is required to tear a section of steel apart. The **yield strength** is the amount of energy absorbed by a material before it fractures or the amount of force or stress that a section of steel can withstand before permanent deformation occurs.

Alloyed steels are composed of a mixture of various metals and elements. They are classified by both their strength range in megapascals and by their metallurgical type designation. The metallurgical type designations can vary throughout the world. Some examples include mild-, low-, and medium-strength steel; high-strength steel (HSS); high-strength low-alloy steel (HSLA) or micro-alloyed steel; ultra-high-strength steel (UHSS); and advanced high-strength steel (AHSS), including dual-phase steel (DP), transformation-induced plasticity (TRIP), twinning-induced plasticity (TWIP), ferritic-bainitic (FB) steel, complex-phase (CP) steel, martensitic (MS) steel, and extremely high-strength steels such as press-hardened steel (PHS). With this many variations, understanding the types of alloyed steels can be quite confusing.

The World Steel Association classifies a **high-strength steel (HSS)** as any steel with an ultimate tensile strength between 39 and 102 ksi (269 and 703 MPa). **Advanced high-strength steel (AHSS)** is classified as any steel with an ultimate tensile strength of 63 to 145 ksi (434 to 1000 MPa). AHSS, unlike other types of steel, can have varying microstructures and element properties that, through multiple types of processing applications, produce different performance factors such as higher strength and elongation and/or plasticity capacity or higher ultimate tensile strength and lower yield strength.

An example of an AHSS-type steel is boron-alloyed steel, which is also recognized as an UHSS. Boron-alloyed steel is produced by alloying very small amounts of boron with steel and other elements through a hot forming and quenching process to gain its unique hardening properties. Because of its high strength, boron-alloyed steel is widely used in the auto industry to improve safety and reinforce specific areas of a vehicle frame that are most subject to impacts from a collision or rollover. This boron reinforcement may come in the form of tailored blanks that are welded/joined onto existing framing (**FIGURE 5-11**). Hot stamped tailored blanks are sections of metal manufactured in various gauges of thickness, sizes, strengths, forms, or coatings to fit perfectly in a specified location; they are welded to the existing frame structure for reinforcement purposes. The boron-alloyed steel used in modern vehicles has a yield point of about 195 to 217 ksi (1344 to 1496 MPa) or greater depending on the processing.

MS steel is rated as one of the highest ultimate tensile strength (130.5 to 246.6 ksi [900 to 1700 MPa]) steels, but it has a very low elongation property. Future third-generation steels (AHSSs) are being developed to include nanoscale particles that produce

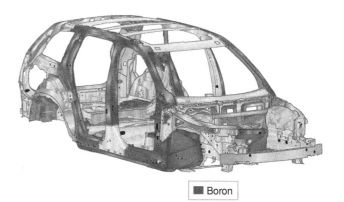

FIGURE 5-11 Boron reinforcement as shown here in the picture of the Volvo XC90 may come in hot stamped tailored blanks, which are sections of metal manufactured in different gauges of thickness, sizes, strengths, forms, or coatings to fit perfectly in a specified location.

a better balance of higher strengthening and elongation properties, increasing strengths up to 246.6 ksi (1700 MPa).

With the auto industry rapidly replacing conventional vehicle designs and structural components with advanced science and technology, so must the world of technical rescue replace the conventional thought processes and procedures to maintain pace with this advancing technology. Becoming adaptive and fluid with techniques and fully understanding the capabilities and limitations of rescue tools in relation to modern body and frame metallurgical elements, such as AHSS, aluminum alloys, magnesium alloys, and CFRP, are imperative for successful technical rescue operations.

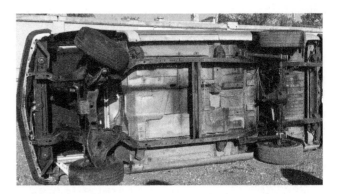

FIGURE 5-12 The cross members are indicative of a ladder-frame design.
Courtesy of David Sweet.

Frame Systems

Two frame systems that are most common in today's vehicles are the body-over-frame construction and the unitized, or unibody, construction. These frames can be composed of steel (most common), aluminum, or CFRP. Another type of frame system is the space frame, which can consist of aluminum, steel CFRP, and some magnesium alloy components. The Audi Corporation has used the space frame–type concept for most of their model vehicles.

Body-over-Frame Construction

The **body-over-frame construction** design is a two-part system: The body of the vehicle is placed onto a frame skeleton, and the frame acts as the foundation for the vehicle. This basic design consists of two large beams tied together by cross member beams. This type of frame is sometimes referred to as a **ladder frame** (**FIGURE 5-12**). Most heavier vehicles, such as a larger pickup truck or SUV, use this type of frame construction. The potential for the body-over-frame design to be split in half with a severe collision is low, but be aware that the force distribution from the impact will be greater on the occupants.

Unibody Construction

The **unibody construction**, or unitized structure, is basically a merged system that joins the body and structure of the vehicle together as one system. The vehicle body is merged with the **chassis**; there is no formal frame structure with the exception of subframe sections in the front and rear of the vehicle. The subframe

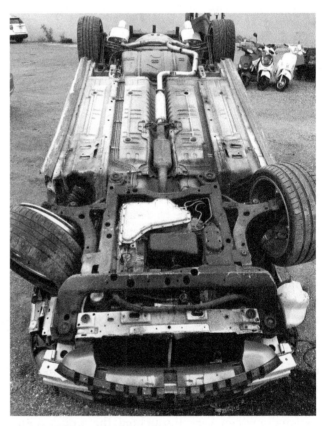

FIGURE 5-13 The unibody design.
Courtesy of David Sweet.

sections consist of two short beams that are attached to the occupant compartment in the front and rear and house the main components of the vehicle such as the suspension system, steering, braking, transmission, and engine (**FIGURE 5-13**). Because there is no solid frame structure on a unibody system, a negative aspect of the construction is the potential for the vehicle to be split in half with a severe collision with another vehicle or with a stationary object, such as a tree or pole (**FIGURE 5-14**).

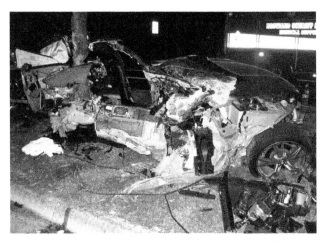

FIGURE 5-14 Because of the design of the unibody system, the vehicle can split in half when involved in a collision.
Courtesy of Jim Dobson.

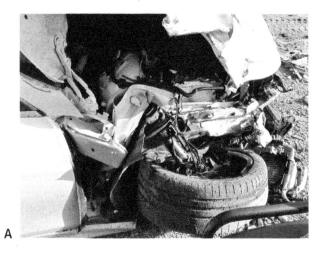

A

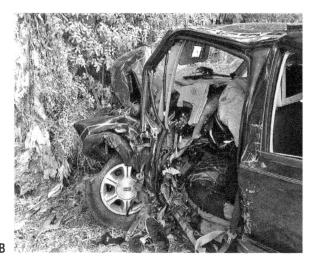

B

FIGURE 5-15 Engineered crumple zones are incorporated into the unibody frame to collapse the framing and absorb and redirect energy away from the occupant compartment during a collision.
A. Courtesy of David Sweet. B. Courtesy of Devon Sweet.

The main difference between the unibody construction and the body-over-frame design is the unibody construction's ability to absorb or redirect energy during a collision. Unibody construction incorporates crumple zones into the front and rear of the vehicle to redirect energy away from the passenger compartment (**FIGURE 5-15**). When an impact occurs, these crumple zones collapse, absorbing and diverting the force or energy of the collision and preventing intrusion into the cab of the vehicle. To fully understand this, you must understand the law of conservation of energy and particularly the mechanical energy system as it relates to the vehicle crash. Understanding the science dealing with the laws and theories related to energy helps clarify what actually occurs during a vehicle crash (explained in the beginning of this chapter).

Space Frame Construction

A true space frame–constructed vehicle was originally designed for the race car industry because of its lighter weight and rigid structure (**FIGURE 5-16**). The traditional body design of the space frame is made of multiple lengths and angles of tubing welded into a rigid, but lighter, web or truss-like structure; the vehicle's outer panels are attached independently to the frame after its completion. The major difference between a space frame–constructed vehicle and the unibody and body-over-frame design is that a traditional space frame can be driven in its skeleton form, void of any body panels. Audi is one manufacturer that uses a modified type of space frame design. Saturn Corporation (no longer in production) also used a space frame construction.

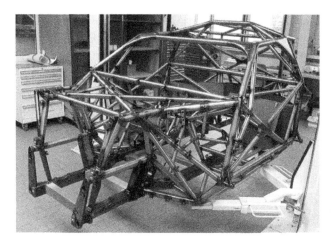

FIGURE 5-16 Space frame design. Construction originally designed for the race car industry.
Courtesy of David Sweet.

Structural Components

Several key components make up the body portion of the vehicle. At the front and rear of the vehicle is the **bumper system**. The bumper system was designed to reduce the damage effect of a vehicle involved in low-speed collisions. The bumper is not designed to be a safety item that minimizes or prevents injury to the occupants. Federal Motor Vehicle Safety Standard (FMVSS) 215 and Code of Federal Regulations (CFR), Title 49, Chapter V, Part 581, *Bumper Standard*, mandate performance standards for bumpers on passenger cars. One of these standards states that the vehicle bumper must be able to absorb a front- or rear-impact collision at a speed of 2.5 mi/h (4 km/h) without sustaining damage to the vehicle body. The federal bumper standard is applied only to passenger vehicles; it does not apply to SUVs, minivans, or pickup trucks. Several types of bumper system designs can be found on passenger vehicles. One bumper system uses a gas strut telescoping-type design where two cylinders reside inside the bumper. These cylinders act as shock absorbers when an impact occurs. One cylinder holds nitrogen gas and the other hydraulic oil or mineral oil. As an impact occurs, the nitrogen gas in the first cylinder compresses and is forced into the second cylinder, which displaces the hydraulic or mineral oil through small valves.

Another more common type of bumper system is composed of polypropylene foam or plastic material that is constructed in a crate-like design. In this type of bumper system, the plastic or foam compresses and absorbs force during an impact.

The **core support**, or radiator support, is a key component of the front end of the vehicle. It is designed to secure the radiator to the engine assembly frame and tie the upper and lower rails together. The core support also houses the lights, horn, and other components while maintaining alignment of the hood with the hood latch.

The **upper rails** are two beams running parallel on both sides of a vehicle's front end. The upper rails are located on the front top section of the vehicle, extending out from the cowl section or upper area of the front passenger compartment (directly in front of the windshield). The rails run to the front bumper area and are connected by the core support. These two beams support the front fenders and hold the hood section in place. They also attach the front wheel strut system to the chassis (**FIGURE 5-17**). Designed within the beams of the upper rail may be the crumple zones, which absorb or divert energy when a direct front-end impact occurs.

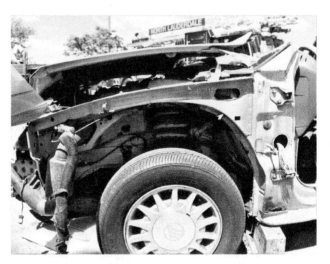

FIGURE 5-17 The upper rail is the main support structure for the front upper section of the vehicle.
Courtesy of Edward Monahan.

An important area of the upper rail section is located between the **strut tower**, which is a structural component of the suspension system, and the dash area. This is a critical relief cut area that is associated with the dash-lift technique, which is discussed in detail in Chapter 9, *Victim Access and Management*. The **engine cradle** is attached to the frame rails. It houses the engine and, in some vehicles, the bolt heads, which lock the engine in place and are designed to shear off on impact to drop the engine under the vehicle instead of into the passenger compartment.

Moving up to the dash area are several support structures that make up the passenger compartment. The **cowl section** is the upper area of the front passenger compartment directly in front of the windshield. Below the cowl section is the **firewall**, or bulkhead, which makes up the front section of the passenger compartment and separates the engine compartment from the passenger compartment. On the outer sections of the bulkhead that bookend the firewall are the hinge pillars, or lower A-post sections, where the front doors are attached. To maintain the crash integrity of the occupant compartment or safety cage, manufacturers reinforce the dash area by installing a metal beam or bar that runs the entire length of the dash or width of the car; this is known as a **dash reinforcement bar** (**FIGURE 5-18**). Attached to the dash bar are two metal brackets. These metal brackets are located in the center console area where the radio, air-conditioning control unit, and various other components are located. The brackets are bolted or welded to the floor pan of the vehicle and are designed to stabilize the dash, thus minimizing movement resulting from an impact (**FIGURE 5-19**).

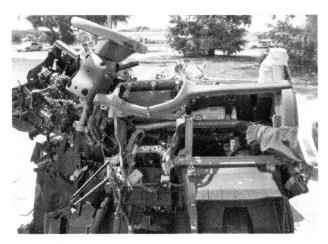

FIGURE 5-18 Dash reinforcement bars are added to give structural support and integrity to the passenger compartment.
Courtesy of Edward Monahan.

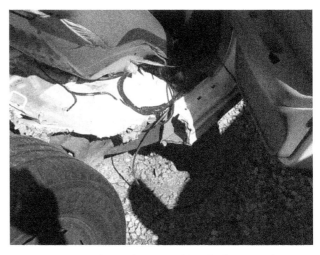

FIGURE 5-20 The rocker panel is a hollow section of metal running along the outermost sections of the floorboard area on both the driver and passenger sides. Various items, such as wiring and fuel lines, and in hybrid vehicles, high-voltage lines, can run underneath or in proximity to it.
Courtesy of David Sweet.

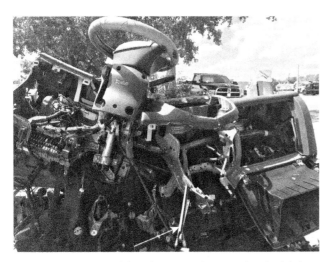

FIGURE 5-19 Steel brackets are designed to hold the dash in place.
Courtesy of Edward Monahan.

When the dash area needs to be displaced to gain victim access, these brackets may need to be cut to create enough space to lift or push the dash section away from the victim. The proper technique for gaining access and cutting through these brackets is discussed in Chapter 9.

Rocker Panel

Running along the outermost sections of the floorboard/floor pan area on both the driver and passenger sides is a channel where the doors rest; this is known as the **rocker panel**. The rocker panel is a hollow section of metal. Various items, such as wiring; fuel lines; and, in hybrid vehicles, high-voltage lines, can run underneath or in proximity to it (**FIGURE 5-20**). There is very little structural support

in this section, so be aware that it will tear or collapse very easily under the force of a hydraulic tool or the impact of a collision.

Doors

There are several key components of a door of which the technical rescuer needs to be aware when gaining access or performing a door removal. The vehicle door is constructed of basically four sections: the inner panel, the outer panel, the hinge and hinge reinforcement plates/panel, and the impact beam. A fifth section can be added to this: the latch and locking assembly. The **door hinge** allows the doors to swing open or closed and is attached to the hinge pillar, or lower A-post, on two-door models. Door hinges come in various sizes as far as thickness and gauge and also in various types. Commonly, there are two hinge designs: a leaf system or a full-body system with hardened steel or other form of AHSS. Some hinges also consist of aluminum alloy (**FIGURE 5-21**). The leaf system has two separate pieces that make up one hinge. One piece is attached to the vehicle door, and the other is attached to the body of the vehicle. The piece attached to the door slips into the center of the other piece that is attached to the vehicle body. It has a pin in the center of it that holds the two pieces together, or holds the door closed. When you look at the two pieces attached together, it looks as if there are two sections of metal on the top (top leaf) and two sections of metal on the bottom (bottom leaf) of the one hinge.

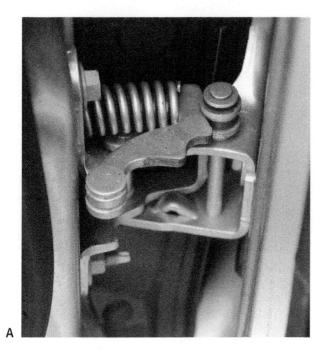

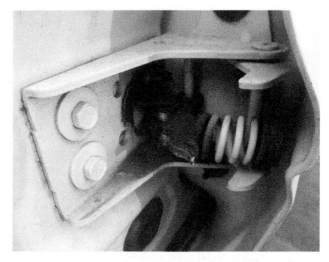

FIGURE 5-22 Door hinges sometimes come equipped with spring attachments that can fire off violently when forced.
Courtesy of David Sweet.

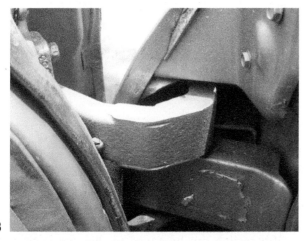

FIGURE 5-21 Common door hinge designs. **A.** Leaf system. **B.** Full-body system.
© Jones & Bartlett Learning. Photographed by Glen E. Ellman.

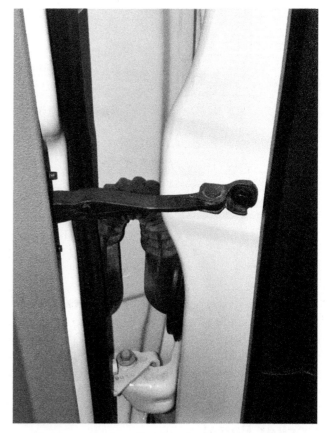

FIGURE 5-23 A door limiting device is designed to limit the opening or overextending of a door.
Courtesy of David Sweet.

The full-body hinge is made of two solid pieces of HSS and has a large pin in the center that holds them together, or holds the door closed. An example may be found on the rear doors of large vans. This hinge design is important to recognize because, if a hydraulic tool is not rated to cut through the hardened steel or HSS, it will fail, sometimes breaking or shattering the blade of the tool. Another important feature that some hinges have is a spring attachment that can come off violently without warning under extreme force, such as when cutting or spreading with hydraulic tools (**FIGURE 5-22**). Full personal protective equipment (PPE) should be worn at all times.

In some vehicles, a **door limiting device**, sometimes coined a "swing bar," can be located between the top and bottom hinge and connects the door to the vehicle body. The door limiting device is designed to stop the motion of the door at a predetermined opening and prevent the door from overextending (**FIGURE 5-23**). The door limiting device can be composed of hardened steel and other alloyed-type metals as well as composite materials. At times, a door limiting device can be very difficult to cut through, but it can be easily detached with very little spreading pressure from a hydraulic tool.

SAFETY TIP

Full PPE should be worn at all times, whether you are training or operating at a vehicle rescue and extrication incident.

The latching and locking assembly on most vehicle doors today has electronically activated systems that are connected to the vehicle's computer and electrical system. The latch and lock mechanisms that the technical rescuer can encounter on a door consist of the latching clasp, or "catcher," located on the door, and the striker plate, located on a post or door housing frame where the door rests when in the closed position. When a door is closed, the latching clasp engages the striker pin or bolt and closes around it, locking or securing the door in place. When the door lock is not set and the door handle from the outside is engaged, the clasp releases off the striker, and the door opens. Two common types of striker plate assemblies are the U-shaped pin and the single striker pin, or latch pin/bolt type, sometimes termed the *Nader pin/bolt* (**FIGURE 5-24**). The **Nader pin/bolt**, which is named after consumer rights advocate Ralph Nader, is composed of heavy-gauge HSS and is round in shape with a cap at the end of it. This is one of the most difficult types of latching mechanisms to cut through or release from the latch mechanism of the door. The **U-shaped striker plate latch pin** is generally made of smaller-gauge steel, which makes it easier to cut through and/or release from the latch mechanism of the door.

Located inside the door is an **impact beam**, which runs the entire length of the door. The impact beam can be located in both the front and rear doors. It is structured to have a very high ultimate tensile strength while remaining ductile so as to absorb the high-impact energy of another vehicle or object and to lessen the intrusion into the passenger compartment. This beam can come in several designs (round, tubular, flat) and various metal alloy types, including PHS; boron alloy; titanium alloy; and, in some instances, aluminum alloy (**FIGURE 5-25**).

An impact beam has one of the highest-rated ultimate tensile strengths of any vehicle component (1000–1500 MPa [145–218 ksi]), making it extremely difficult or unlikely to cut through. Avoid attempting to cut this component if possible, but if the possibility that a front-end collision causes an impact beam (particularly the round tubular type) to breach its outer wall and enter into an adjacent door or panel, locking the doors or door in place, a cutting or spreading procedure may have to be attempted. Check with your

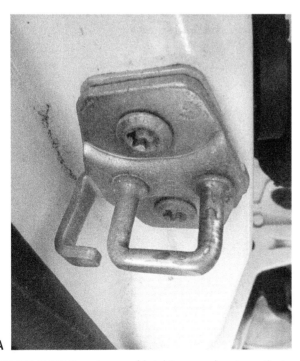

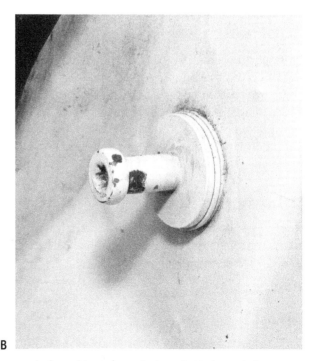

FIGURE 5-24 Two types of latching mechanisms that are commonly found in a door design. **A.** U-shaped door striker latch pin. **B.** Latch pin/bolt.
A: Courtesy of David Sweet; B: © Jones & Bartlett Learning. Photographed by Glen E. Ellman.

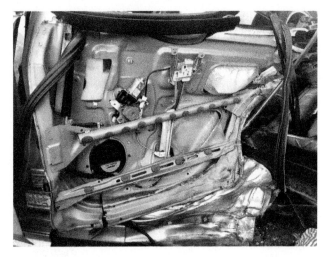

FIGURE 5-25 Door impact beams are structured to absorb the impact energy of another vehicle or object and to lessen the intrusion into the passenger compartment.
Courtesy of David Sweet.

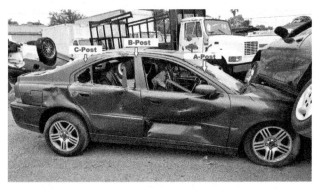

FIGURE 5-26 Roof posts are generally labeled with an alphanumeric-type description (A, B, and C).
Courtesy of David Sweet.

hydraulic tool company to see if your tools are rated to cut this type of metal.

The outer skin or panel of the door is usually composed of light-gauge steel, aluminum, and CFRP. There are still some older vehicles, such as the Saturn, that use a polycarbonate/plastic–type material. These panels can be removed with hand tools when necessary.

Roof Posts

Roof posts/pillars are designed to add vertical support to the roof structure of the vehicle. The posts are generally labeled with an alphanumeric-type description (A, B, and C) (**FIGURE 5-26**).

A-Post

The posts closest to the front windshield are known as the **A-posts/pillars**. The A-post can consist of several layers of steel or aluminum; some manufacturers reinforce them with HSS, thicker-gauge metals, bars, rods, micro-alloy steel sections, CFRP inserts, or tailored blanks. In addition, some manufacturers use a polyurethane or similar type of foam that is either injected or placed in the roof posts and hollow cavities of the vehicle body to give added strength, support, and energy-absorbing qualities when exposed to a collision or rollover type of impact. The structural foam is designed to withstand compression and limit the vehicle body frame from folding on collision.

The technical rescuer may experience difficulties in cutting through a post filled with structural foam because the product can impede the cutting action of some low-pressure hydraulic tools by resisting the compression force exerted from the tool's blades. This resistance can also be experienced with pillars that have CFRP inserts.

The Insurance Institute for Highway Safety establishes crash safety ratings for vehicles through a series of active evaluative tests. One set evaluation is the overlap offset crash that exposes occupant compartment intrusion vulnerabilities in vehicle design and structures. To comply with this evaluation, manufacturers are increasing the design and strength of the lower A-post/hinge pillar and firewall area. This area was easy to cut on a standard conventional vehicle when setting up for a dash lift but is now heavily reinforced or widened or includes additional reinforcement sections that extend to the upper rail area, making this cut and technique extremely difficult (**FIGURE 5-27**).

The technical rescuer must also be prepared for the possibility of air bag cylinders installed in any section of the A-post. All posts, including the roof rail, need to be exposed and examined for SRS components by removing interior liners prior to cutting. SRS components are discussed further in Chapter 6, *Supplemental Restraint Systems*.

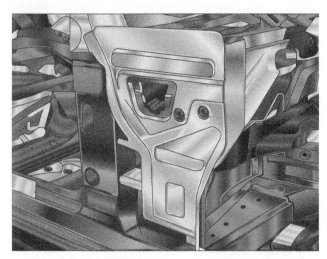

FIGURE 5-27 Manufacturers are increasing the design and strength of the lower A-post/hinge pillar and firewall area.

Voice of Experience

It is vitally important for the rescuer to have a working knowledge of vehicle anatomy. Not only of passenger vehicles, but of all the various types of vehicles that we are exposed to. As the vehicle is transformed by the transfer of mechanical energy during a collision, its anatomy is transformed because of the dissipation of said energy. With proper understanding of vehicle anatomy, a rescuer can determine how a wrecked vehicle will respond as its components are displaced to make room for the rescue. An improper understanding of this concept can put the victim in incredible danger due to the inability to understand how a vehicle will respond to a given technique.

This concept was really driven home for me on an extrication that involved a box truck. We were called to an extrication located in a parking lot in a commercial area. En route to the call we suspected that we might be turned around as a truck was already on scene and had commenced extrication of the victim. Upon arrival, we realized that the victim had driven the truck at low speed into a steel beam that was mounted on two posts. This beam was intended to keep taller vehicles out of the parking lot and the driver was unable to see it as he pulled into the lot. When the truck hit the beam, it rolled it forward onto the hood. As the truck came to a stop, the beam came to rest on the A-post, stopping within inches of the driver's head. During the initial scene assessment it appeared that the only issue was a crushed A-post. Paratech struts and hydro fusions were used to lift the beam. Once it was secured, the attempt was made to cut the A-post. Two issues related to the unique anatomy of the box truck came into play at this point. First, the truck had a large amount of structural reinforcement to the A-post. Because of this it took multiple attempts to cut through the post. The second issue was that due to the way that firewall was constructed, the vehicle had been deformed in an atypical manner. The firewall had buckled, and due to the location of the damage, the responders were required to use rams, spreaders, and a pair of cutters to stabilize the area around the driver while creating enough space to extricate the driver.

Without a working understanding of the anatomy of a box truck, this extrication could have put the driver in grave danger due to the shifting of vehicle components during the extrication. Since the rescuers had a proper understanding of the anatomy of the vehicle, the victim was safely extricated with no further injuries. Understanding the anatomy of a vehicle enables the rescuer to effectively manage an incident with a vehicle that they have had no prior experience with. To be a professional rescuer we must be prepared for any situation that we may be presented with.

Hudson Babler
Dallas Fire Rescue
Dallas, Texas

> **LISTEN UP!**
> All posts, including the roof rail, need to be exposed and examined for SRS components by removing interior liners prior to cutting.

B-Post

Most side-impact collisions occur at the B-post area. In four-door vehicles, the **B-posts** are located between the front and rear doors of a vehicle. Because this area is frequently impacted in a collision, more and more manufacturers are reinforcing sections of the B-post from the rocker panel to the roof rail using AHSS, such as boron or other types of AHSS and CFRP. These reinforced sections can come in the form of plates, bars, channel inserts, rods, tailored blanks, or multiple-layered sheets of steel. This reinforced section of the post, including the lower post area, poses difficult challenges to the technical rescuer when performing a side-out technique. Several alternating cuts have to be made throughout the spreading or separating of the lower B-post from the rocker panel because the spreading force required to accomplish this task is not enough to overcome the tensile and yield strength of the AHSS that has been added to reinforce the structure.

The technical rescuer can encounter several types of seat belt mechanisms within the B-post. The most common seat belt mechanisms are the standard seat belt harness, the pretensioner seat belt system, and the automatic seat belt system.

As a collision occurs, the forward movements of the vehicle and the passenger are independent of each other. Without the seat belt, the force that impacted the vehicle, from either another car or striking a pole, stops the forward movement of that vehicle, but the passenger keeps traveling forward at the rate of vehicle speed prior to the impact. The seat belt is designed to merge the passenger and vehicle, combining the forward energy of the vehicle and passenger into one, using the vehicle to distribute most of the force.

The **standard seat belt harness** includes a shoulder and lap belt, known as a three-point harness system. This system helps distribute the energy of a collision over larger areas of the body, such as the chest, pelvis, and shoulders. The three-point belt mechanism uses a retractor gear that locks in place when activated.

The **pretensioner seat belt system** is designed to pull back and tighten when activated by a collision. The more common pretensioner seat belt system uses a pyrotechnic propulsion device to engage a retractor gear, which pulls back on the belt. The pretensioning seat belt system is normally tied in with the SRS air bag system, using the same crash impact sensors to activate that SRS air bags use when a collision occurs.

The **automatic seat belt system** uses a shoulder harness that automatically slides on a steel or aluminum track system on the door window frame. When the door is closed, the shoulder harness automatically slides into place. The lap section of the harness must be manually engaged.

All seat belts have an anchoring device that is most commonly attached in two areas, the top of the B-post and either the floorboard or the bottom of the B-post. Be aware that these areas around the anchors are reinforced with heavier-gauge steel, so try to avoid cutting into these areas if possible (**FIGURE 5-28**).

Some manufacturers install a height-adjusting anchor at the upper section of the B-post. The anchor is attached to a slide track that adjusts the seat belt to the height of the occupant. This slide track is normally heavy-gauge steel or HSS, which can cover several inches in the upper section of the B-post; this will cause cutting problems with low-pressure hydraulic tools or reciprocating saws (**FIGURE 5-29**).

C-Post

The **C-post** in most standard two- and four-door vehicles is the rear post, with the exception of larger vehicles, such as an SUV or a wagon-type vehicle, which may have numerous roof posts. In these larger vehicles, the midposts, between the B-post and the rear post, can contain the same components and materials as described for the previous roof posts.

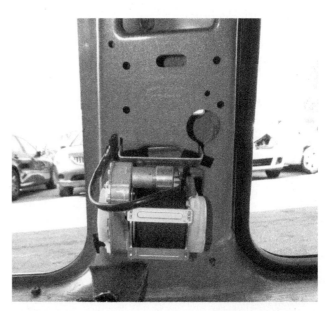

FIGURE 5-28 The areas around the seat belt anchoring devices are reinforced with heavier gauge steel to add support. Avoid cutting into this area whenever possible.
Courtesy of David Sweet.

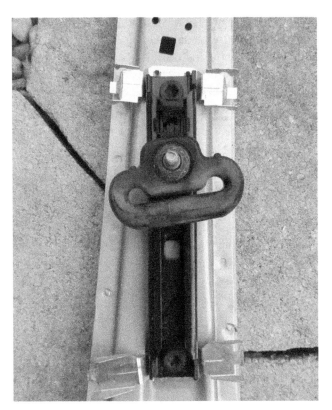

FIGURE 5-29 Heavy-gauge steel slide tracks for a seat belt anchoring device can extend down a post, causing cutting problems for low-pressure hydraulic tools or reciprocating saws.
Courtesy of David Sweet.

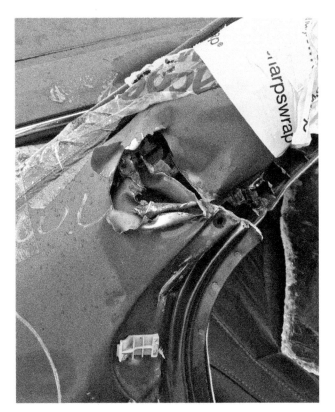

FIGURE 5-30 Wide posts are generally two separate sections of metal that are molded together.
Courtesy of David Sweet.

Be aware that every vehicle manufacturer and vehicle design are different. Most have the same layout, with the A-, B-, and C-posts, but one manufacturer may place a steel rod in the B-post for safety, and another manufacturer may put one in the A-post or add an air bag cylinder. It is very difficult to keep up with all the safety upgrades and design changes from one vehicle to the next. You need to be cognizant of the potential to encounter one or more of these safety features anytime you cut into a vehicle. Oftentimes, these added safety features are reported by technical rescuers who discover the safety features while engaged in an extrication incident; they may have cut into a post, had problems with the post, and eventually found that they were dealing with some type of HSS, CFRP, boron rod, or other AHSS.

Rear posts can be wide or narrow, depending on the make and model of the vehicle. The wide posts are generally two separate sections of metal that are welded together. This forms a hollow pocket that manufacturers may use to insert structural foam, speakers, wires, or various other items (**FIGURE 5-30**). Air bag cylinders can be present in almost any area of the vehicle, so always remember to expose every post, roof rail, or area prior to any cutting or spreading.

The rear end of the vehicle consists of the trunk/hatchback, rear suspension, rear quarter panels, and rear deck/shelf, or package tray, which is a panel behind the rear seat and in front of the rear window. This panel can be composed of CFRP, magnesium, aluminum, or other form and grade strength of metal. The rear section area of the vehicle is discussed further in Chapter 9.

Piston Struts

Hydraulic or gas-filled piston struts are becoming common in passenger vehicles, SUVs, and small trucks. Piston struts are used to assist in the lifting and support of vehicle components, such as hatchbacks, hoods, trunks, hard tonneau truck bed covers, tailgates, toolboxes, vehicle seatbacks, or doors (**FIGURE 5-31**). Hydraulic or gas-filled piston struts are designed with a basic theory of compression: Nitrogen gas or a petroleum-based or mineral-type hydraulic fluid is placed in a steel or aluminum tubular cylinder. A steel rod is inserted in the cylinder with seals and compression fittings to support the movable rod from being fully ejected. The cylinder has a smaller chamber inside with small holes designed to bleed out the fluid or gas slowly into this chamber when the piston is compressed. Pressure is naturally built up inside

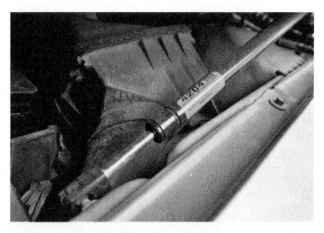

FIGURE 5-31 Gas-filled piston struts are commonly utilized in vehicles to assist in the lifting and opening of the engine compartment hood.
Courtesy of Edward Monahan.

the cylinder through the compression of the hydraulic fluid or nitrogen gas when the steel rod is pushed into the cylinder. This can be noticed when a hatchback is placed in the closed position. The pressure is now against the rod inside the cylinder; once the hatchback is released from the latching mechanism, the fluid or gas fills the chamber again and pushes against the rod, forcing it open, either rapidly or gradually, based on the design of the piston strut. The hatchback in the open position is now supported by the extended piston rod from the pressure release of the previously compressed fluid or gas.

The location of piston struts varies with each manufacturer; they can be in clear view or hidden within the contour of a roof post or upper rail section of the engine compartment hood. These are areas that are normally cut with hydraulic cutters when performing certain techniques; these areas must be exposed prior to cutting and the piston strut dealt with accordingly. Some types of struts utilize a nylon ball joint to connect the base of the cylinder to one of the sections (normally the nonmovable section) of the vehicle. The ball joints can be easily separated from their housing with a pry tool, such as a Halligan bar, with very little leveraging pressure applied under the rod closest to the area of attachment. It is advised that the piston strut be removed in this fashion or cut with a hydraulic cutter at the area of attachment; avoid cutting into the pressure-filled cylinder. Accidentally cutting the cylinder section of the piston strut with a hydraulic cutter will cause a rapid release of pressure or hydraulic fluid, which can possibly cause the piston rod or a section of the piston rod to fire out of the housing unit. Proper removal of these devices is discussed in Chapter 9.

Another area of concern when dealing with piston struts is vehicle fires. Fire that impinges on a piston strut will cause rapid pressure buildup and expansion of the cylinder walls, causing the cylinder wall to breach and possibly separate or fire the piston rod out of the cylinder housing unit. It has been documented that some piston rods have penetrated through vehicle bodies and impaled walls or rescuers. Extreme caution and proper procedures must be observed when dealing with vehicle fires.

Federal Safety Standards and Regulations

An excellent research tool to better understand vehicle structures, frames, and components is the Federal Motor Vehicle Safety Standards (FMVSS) and regulations. These are federal safety compliance regulations that outline the minimum safety performance requirements for motor vehicles or items of motor vehicle equipment. Vehicle manufacturers design and redesign vehicle frames, structures, and components based on these federally issued regulations. Under Title 49 of the United States Code, Chapter 301: Motor Vehicle Safety, the National Highway Traffic Safety Administration (NHTSA) issues all FMVSS and regulations. The first standard (FMVSS 209: Seat Belt Assemblies) became effective on March 1, 1967. Since then, many FMVSS have been adopted to protect the public against the risk of death or injury from vehicular crashes occurring as a result of the design, construction, or performance of motor vehicles.

Vehicle Glass and Glazing

Glass management is the process of controlling the voluntary or involuntary fragmentation of glass by applying proper removal techniques and/or securing the glass in place. Properly managing glass from the onset of the rescue increases proficiency, speed, and overall safety not only for the rescuer but also for the victims. Glass management is discussed further in Chapter 9. There are several types of glass and glazing that the technical rescuer can encounter in a vehicle, including laminated safety glass (LSG), tempered safety glass (TSG), polycarbonate, and ballistic-type glass.

Laminated Safety Glass

Laminated safety glass (LSG) is created by bonding two layers of glass with clear resin film of polyvinyl butyral between them. This process holds the two pieces of glass together and prevents big shards of glass from flying in on the vehicle occupant. It also prevents occupants from being ejected from the vehicle (**FIGURE 5-32**). Window spidering is an effect caused

CHAPTER 5 Mechanical Energy and Vehicle Anatomy

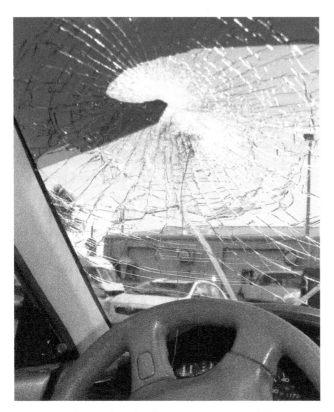

FIGURE 5-32 When broken, LSG prevents big shards of glass from flying at vehicle occupants and also prevents occupants from being ejected from the vehicle.
Courtesy of David Sweet.

when an object breaks the laminated safety glass and causes spiraling rings at the area of impact, resembling a spider's web. Windshield LSG has a thickness of approximately 5 to 6 mm (0.20 to 0.24 in.) and is designed to resist impacts from small projectiles. New products in the lamination process are being developed to make the windshield thinner as well as stronger.

FMVSS 226: Ejection Mitigation, which took effect in September 2013, increases the safety standards and design for vehicles sustaining a side impact. The goal of the standard is to keep passengers from being ejected (or partially ejected) from a vehicle during a side impact or rollover. This rule is designed with the intention of manufacturers increasing the size, inflation duration, and strength of side air bags. As an additional compliance measure, some vehicle manufacturers are adding LSG primarily on side and rear windows because of its ability to retain a passenger's body/extremities inside the vehicle as well as the additional benefits of added security and soundproofing qualities.

Gorilla® Glass

Gorilla® Glass, developed by Corning®, uses a three-layer fusion process to make laminate glass that is compatible to use in vehicles. The inner layer is the thin layer of prioritized Gorilla Glass, measuring about 0.5 mm (0.02 in.); the center layer is a thermoplastic material to bond the inner and outer layers together; and the outer layer is standard plate, or sheet, glass. This product reduces the overall weight of the laminated section as much as 40 percent compared to traditional laminates. The process begins when raw materials are blended into a glass composition, which is melted and conditioned. The composition of Corning Gorilla Glass enables a deep layer of chemical strengthening through an ion-exchange process in which large ions are incorporated deep into the glass surface, creating a state of high compression. This layer of compression creates a surface that is more resistant to fractures.

Tempered Safety Glass

Tempered safety glass (TSG) undergoes a process in which the glass is heated and then cooled; this process of heating, quenching, expanding, and contracting the glass increases the tensile and yield strength of the glass, making it 5 to 10 times stronger. Tempering gives the glass its strength and resistance to impacts. When tempered glass is fractured, the energy of the tensile and yield strength holding the glass together is suddenly released, and the glass breaks into small, dull-edged pieces. Conversely, standard nontempered glass can produce sharp, long shards and small airborne fragments when fractured.

Polycarbonate

Polycarbonate is a clear plastic material that is very strong and can endure impacts without breaking. The big advantage of polycarbonate is that it is very pliable on impact, with the flexibility to conform to the impact rather than shattering, as glass would. Polycarbonates can also be up to 50 percent lighter than regular glass, providing better fuel economy and safety features.

Lexan™ and Makrolon® are two of the brand names used to label polycarbonate material. Until recently, polycarbonate had limited use in vehicle window design because of several problems with the material itself; it was not scratch resistant, nor could it overcome the noise vibrations from wind and basic driving that regular glass provided. In addition, polycarbonate materials used for vehicle windows could not pass all of the strict safety standards established by the NHTSA. Some manufacturers are now using polycarbonate in sunroofs and side-panel windows.

Newer technological advances include a system that adds a glazing layer over the polycarbonate material, thus reducing the scratch potential and giving the material rigidity to reduce noise and vibration problems.

This material poses some difficult access problems for the technical rescuer. It is designed to resist breaking from impact; therefore, forcible entry tools will only bounce off because of the flexibility of the plastic. The tool could then rebound out of your hands, causing possible injury to yourself or someone else. Cutting into the material with a tool, such as a reciprocating saw, can, at times, cause the cut to reseal itself because of the heat generated from the blade.

The better technique to handle polycarbonate material is to treat it as a part of the vehicle body and leave it in place, removing the entire section as one, whether it is an entire roof or door structure. If there happens to be a purchase-point section caused by a vehicle's crash deformity, you may be able to place the tips of a hydraulic spreader into the opening and release the section containing the polycarbonate material from its casing. A **purchase point** is an access area where you can insert and better position a tool for operation. Using the hydraulic spreader correctly to create an opening eliminates the need for some of the traditional techniques that are taught using hand tools. The process of creating a purchase point is described in Chapter 9.

Beware that any polycarbonate material that has a bend or some type of deformity caused by an impact can potentially be loaded and can release from its casing suddenly on its own or from the force of a tool. It is designed to conform back to its original shape. Chapter 9 discusses techniques in detail.

Ballistic Glass

Ballistic glass for vehicles can be composed of several types of materials and/or glazing and can vary in thickness, depending on the level of protection needed. The U.S. Department of Justice National Institute of Justice (NIJ) is one of several entities that establish the minimum performance requirements and methods of testing for levels of protection against ballistic-type weaponry. NIJ Standard 0108.01, *Ballistic Resistant Protective Materials*, establishes five armor classifications based on the munitions size and type. Ballistic, or bullet-resistant, types of glass utilize multiple layers of tempered glass, laminate material, and polycarbonate thermoplastics, all sandwiched together to the desired thickness. The weight and thickness of the glass increase depending on each increased level of protection, which can be as high as 3 in. (7.6 cm) or more. Any attempts to remove or cut into this type of material are not advised; this type of glass should be handled just as the polycarbonate material, by treating it as a part of the vehicle body and leaving it in place. When removing an entire section or part of the vehicle with ballistic-rated, or bullet-resistant, glass, the area should be viewed as one unit, whether it is an entire roof or a door structure.

The future of vehicle glass is rapidly expanding, with new smart technology being the driving force. Various glazing and embedding techniques through nanotechnology allow glass to have several enhanced features, such as electrochromic, suspended-particle heads-up display; self-tinting; self-cleaning; side and rear view monitor viewing; auto-temperature adjustments; and solar-energy absorption/production. Laminates, thermoplastics, and other glazing materials are also being incorporated in areas such as curved/extended rooflines (sometimes called a "Cielo" roof) and panoramic-type wraparound styles.

Vehicle Classifications

Vehicles can be classified in several ways. The Department of Transportation (DOT) classifies vehicles based on whether the vehicle transports passengers or commodities, with a non-passenger vehicle being further classified by the number of axles and unit attachments it has. A **passenger vehicle** is defined by the DOT as all sedans, coupes, and station wagons manufactured primarily for the purpose of carrying passengers, including vehicles pulling recreational or other light trailers.

The Department of Energy (DOE) classifies vehicles by size using a cubic-foot system (passenger and cargo volume) and a gross-weight system. A type of passenger vehicle that is termed a *sedan*, for example, is classified or known as a sedan based on the cubic feet of space it has for passengers or cargo. Sedan types, according to the DOE, range in size from less than 85 ft^3 (2.4 m^3) to up to 130 ft^3 (3.7 m^3), depending on whether the sedan is minicompact, subcompact, compact, midsize, or large. **TABLE 5-1** describes the classifications of vehicles based on size and weight.

Vehicle Identification Numbers

A vehicle identification number (VIN) is a unique identification system composed of a 17-character sequence containing both numbers and letters, with the exclusion of the letters *I*, *O*, and *Q* to avoid confusion with the numbers 1 and 0. In 1981, the United States enacted the VIN system under CFR, Title 49, Chapter V, Part 565, *Vehicle Identification Number (VIN) Requirements*, which mandated that every passenger

TABLE 5-1 Vehicle Classifications

CARS

Class		Passenger and Cargo Volume in ft^3 (m^3)
Two-seaters		Any (cars designed to seat only two adults)
Sedans	Minicompact	< 85 (< 2.40)
	Subcompact	85–99 (2.40–2.80)
	Compact	100–109 (2.83–3.09)
	Midsize	110–119 (3.11–3.34)
	Large	≥ 120 (≥ 3.40)
Station wagons	Small	< 130 (< 3.68)
	Midsize	130–159 (3.68–4.50)
	Large	≥ 160 (≥ 4.53)

TRUCKS

Class	Gross Vehicle Weight Rating (GVWR) in lb (kg)	
Pickup trucks	Through Model Year 2007	Beginning Model Year 2008
Small	< 4500 (2041)	< 6000 (2722)
Standard	4500–8500 (2041–3856)	6000–8500 (2722–3856)

Vans

Passenger	< 8500 (< 3856)
Cargo	< 8500 (< 3856)
Minivans	< 8500 (< 3856)
Sport utility vehicles (SUVs)	< 8500 (< 3856)
Special purpose vehicles	< 8500 (< 3856)

Modified from U.S. Environmental Protection Agency. Vehicle Size Classes Used in the Fuel Economy Guide [http://www.fueleconomy.gov/feg/info.shtml]. Accessed February 11, 2011. Courtesy of U.S. Department of Energy.

vehicle, SUV, truck, or trailer manufactured be identified and tracked using the VIN system. A VIN is affixed to every type of vehicle manufactured in the United States and many other countries. The VIN is normally etched on a plate and attached to or embossed on the driver's-side dashboard, labeled on the driver's-side vehicle door, or affixed to the inside of the glove compartment. The VIN is also listed in vehicle documents such as insurance and registration documents. Each alphanumeric designation of a VIN has a specific meaning, such as the type and make of the vehicle, country of origin where the vehicle was manufactured, and year of manufacturing.

Vehicle Propulsion Systems

A propulsion system is a type of machine that generates force to move an object. For vehicles, there are two types of propulsion systems that are utilized today, the internal combustion engine and the electric motor. The following paragraphs are an overview of these propulsion systems. Alternative-powered vehicles and fuel systems are discussed in depth in Chapter 7.

Conventional Vehicles

The overwhelming majority of vehicles on the road today are **conventional-type vehicles**; these vehicles use internal combustion engines for power. An **internal combustion engine (ICE)** can be designed to burn many petroleum-based fuels and alternative fuels, with gasoline and diesel fuel being the most common. Fuel tanks for conventional-type vehicles are more commonly constructed of steel or aluminum, but high-density plastic fuel tanks are also used because they are lighter than the steel or aluminum designs. There has also been a rise in the use of compressed gas systems that use high-pressure storage tanks composed of steel, aluminum, or a combination of both with a carbon fiber or fiberglass wrapping. These tanks can range in pressures from 3500 to 10,000 psi (24,132 to 68,948 kPa), depending on the type of gas being stored. **Pounds per square inch (psi)** is a unit of measure to describe pressure; it is the amount of force exerted on an area equaling 1 in.^{2} Alternative-fueled vehicles and fuel systems are discussed in depth in Chapter 7.

Hybrid Electric Vehicles

A **hybrid vehicle** is defined as a vehicle that combines two or more power sources for propulsion. This combination of power sources generally consists of generated electricity through a high-voltage electrical system and a petroleum-based fuel or alternative-fuel system through the process of an internal combustion engine. This is known as a hybrid electric vehicle (HEV).

LISTEN UP!
The basic components of an HEV system consist of an electric motor, generator, internal combustion engine, and battery pack.

Hydrogen Fuel Cell Vehicles

A hydrogen fuel cell is an electrochemical device that uses a catalyst-facilitated chemical reaction of hydrogen and oxygen to create electricity that is then used to power an electric motor. A fuel cell vehicle by definition is a hybrid vehicle system in which two separate sources of power are used or combined as a propulsion mechanism for the vehicle. The first fuel cell was developed in 1839.

LISTEN UP!
Hydrogen fuel cell vehicles have the potential to be two to three times more efficient than conventional vehicles, emitting little to no greenhouse gas.

Electric-Powered Vehicles

Electric-powered vehicles use an electric motor for propulsion and are powered by batteries in a rechargeable battery pack. Also known as electric vehicles (EVs), many can travel an average distance of 100 to 200 mi (161 to 322 km) between recharging. Recharging can be accomplished through dedicated charging stations or a general plug-in house current (120/240 volts).

After-Action REVIEW

IN SUMMARY

- Three concepts of energy are typically associated with injury: potential energy, kinetic energy, and work.
- Motor vehicle collisions are classified traditionally by the area of initial impact: front impact (head-on), lateral impact (T-bone or side impact), rear end, rotational (spins), and rollovers.
- In every crash, three collisions occur:
  - The collision of the vehicle against an object

- The collision of the passenger against the interior of the vehicle
- The collision of the passenger's internal organs against the solid structures of the body
- Before a rescuer can properly apply any vehicle rescue and extrication procedures to a vehicle, he or she must understand the inner and outer components that make up a vehicle system.
- The DOT classifies vehicles based on whether the vehicle transports passengers or commodities, with a non-passenger vehicle being further classified by the number of axles and unit attachments it has.
- The DOE classifies vehicles by size, utilizing a cubic foot system (passenger and cargo volume) and gross weight system.
- Most vehicles on the road today are conventional-type vehicles; these types of vehicles utilize ICEs for power. Other types of vehicles include hybrid electric vehicles, hydrogen fuel cell vehicles, and electric-powered vehicles.
- Electrical power in conventional-type vehicles with ICEs is supplied by a basic 12-volt lead acid battery system. In hybrids, fuel cell vehicles, and electric vehicles, a different, advanced electrical design is used.
- The development of strong, crash-resistant vehicles requires engineers and the steel industry to develop stronger and lighter steels to meet demands.
- There are two frame systems that are most common in today's vehicles: body-over-frame construction and unitized, or unibody, construction. These frames can be composed of steel (most common), aluminum, or carbon fiber/composite. Another type of frame system that is less common today is the space frame, which can consist of aluminum, steel CFRP, and some magnesium alloy components.
- Several key components make up the body portion of the vehicle.
- The technical rescuer can encounter several types of glass in a vehicle, including LSG, TSG, polycarbonate, and ballistic glass.

KEY TERMS

Absorbed glass matt (AGM) A type of battery in which a glass mat is used to absorb and hold the electrolyte, preventing it from moving within the battery.

Advanced high-strength steel (AHSS) Steel with a minimum tensile strength of 63 to 145 ksi (434 to 1000 MPa).

Alloyed Created by combining two or more elements.

Alloyed steels Materials composed of steel and a mixture of various metals and elements. They are classified by both their strength range in megapascals and by their metallurgical type designation.

Aluminum alloyed metal A composition of various metals, including pure aluminum; its main design is to strengthen and lighten the vehicle.

A-posts/pillars Vertical support members located closest to the front windshield of a vehicle.

Automatic seat belt system A seat belt system that uses a shoulder harness that automatically slides on a steel or aluminum track system on the door window frame. When the door is closed, the shoulder harness automatically slides into place. The lap section of the harness has to be manually engaged.

Ballistic glass Glass that uses multiple layers of tempered glass, laminate material, and polycarbonate thermoplastics, all sandwiched together to the desired thickness. The weight and thickness of the glass increase depending on each increased level of protection, which can be as high as 3 in. (76 mm).

Body-over-frame construction Vehicle design in which the body of the vehicle is placed onto a frame skeleton and the frame acts as the foundation for the vehicle. The design consists of two large beams tied together by cross member beams.

B-posts Vertical support members located between the front and rear doors of a vehicle.

Bumper system Front and rear vehicle frame attachment system designed to reduce the damage effect of a vehicle involved in low-speed collisions.

Carbon One of the most abundant elements in the universe, classified as a nonmetallic element. It has the unique ability to bond with multiple elements.

Carbon fiber reinforced polymer (CFRP) An extremely strong and light fiber-reinforced plastic that contains carbon fibers.

Chassis The basic operating motor vehicle including the engine, frame, and other essential structural and mechanical parts but exclusive of the body and all appurtenances for the accommodation of driver, property, passengers, appliances, or equipment related to other than control. Common usage might, but need not, include a cab (or cowl). (NFPA 1911)

Conventional-type vehicles Vehicles that use an internal combustion engine (ICE) for power.

Core support A key component of the front end of the vehicle, designed to secure the radiator to the engine assembly frame and tie the upper and lower rails together. It also houses the lights, horn, and other components while maintaining alignment of the hood with the hood latch.

Cowl section Upper area of the front passenger compartment directly in front of the windshield.

C-post A vertical support member located behind the rear doors of a vehicle.

Crumple zones Engineered collapsible zones that are incorporated into the frame of a vehicle to absorb energy during a collision.

Dash reinforcement bar A metal beam or bar that runs the entire width of the dash.

Door hinge A mechanism that provides the opening and closing movements for a door. Door hinges commonly range from 8- to 15-gauge metal and can be a full-body or layered-leaf system.

Door limiting device A hardened section of steel or composite material that is designed to assist the door in opening and closing. It can be located between the top and bottom hinge.

Electropositive Electrically positive.

Energy A fundamental entity of nature that is transferred between parts of a system in the production of physical change within the system and is usually regarded as the capacity for doing work.

Engine cradle Attached to the frame rails and houses the engine and, in some vehicles, the bolt heads, which lock the engine in place; they are designed to shear off on impact to drop the engine under the vehicle instead of into the passenger compartment.

Firewall Also known as the bulkhead; this makes up the front section of the passenger compartment, separating the engine compartment from the passenger compartment.

Gel cell A type of battery that uses a silica base additive that firms up the electrolyte in a gel state.

Glass management The process of controlling the voluntary or involuntary fragmentation of glass by applying proper removal techniques and/or securing glass in place.

Graphene Strongest molecular compound known on the planet; flexible as rubber.

High-strength steel (HSS) Steel with an ultimate tensile strength between 39 and 102 ksi (269 and 703 MPa).

Hybrid vehicle A vehicle that combines two or more power sources for propulsion, generally consisting of generated electricity through a high-voltage electrical system and a petroleum-based fuel or alternative-fuel system through the process of an internal combustion engine.

Impact beam A steel section located within a door frame designed to absorb the impact energy of another vehicle or object and lessen the intrusion into the passenger compartment.

Internal combustion engine (ICE) Any engine in which the working medium consists of the products of combustion of the air and fuel supplied. (NFPA 20)

Kinetic energy The energy of motion, which is based on vehicle mass (weight) and the speed of travel (velocity).

Ladder frame Body-over-frame construction whose cross members and beams resemble a ladder.

Laminated safety glass (LSG) Glass that contains a layer of clear plastic film between two layers of glass.

Law of conservation of energy A law of physics stating that energy can be neither created nor destroyed; it can only change from one form to another.

Law of motion A law of physics describing momentum, acceleration, and action/reaction.

Magnesium alloy A metal that is gaining popularity because of its unique properties and highly sought-after high strength-to-weight characteristics the auto industry requires.

Mechanism of injury (MOI) The way in which traumatic injuries occur; it describes the forces (or energy transmission) acting on the body that cause injury.

Metal A classification or group of elements that possess positive ions, such as iron, gold, silver, and copper; can be ferrous or nonferrous.

Nader pin/bolt A door striker latch pin or bolt composed of heavy-gauge metal that is round in shape with a cap at the end of it. It is a section of the latching mechanism; named after consumer rights advocate Ralph Nader.

Passenger vehicle All sedans, coupes, and station wagons manufactured primarily for the purpose of carrying passengers, including those passenger cars pulling recreational or other light trailers.

Polycarbonate A clear thermoplastic material that is very strong and can endure impacts without breaking.

Potential energy Stored energy or the energy of position.

Pounds per square inch (psi) A unit of measure used to describe pressure; it is the amount of force that is exerted on an area equaling 1 in.^{2}

Pretensioner seat belt system A seat belt system designed to pull back and tighten when activated by a collision. The most common pretensioner seat belt system uses a pyrotechnic propulsion device to engage a gear that pulls back on the belt.

Purchase point The location at which access can best be gained.

Rear deck/shelf Also known as package tray; a panel behind the rear seat and in front of the rear window.

Rocker panel A hollow section of metal running along the outer sections of the floorboard on the driver and passenger sides.

Roof posts/pillars Posts/pillars that are designed to add vertical support to the roof structure of the vehicle. These are generally labeled with an alphanumeric type description (A, B, and C), starting with the post closest to the front windshield, which is known as the A-post.

Space frame A frame made up of multiple lengths and angles of tubing welded into a rigid, but light, web or truss-like structure; the vehicle's outer panels are attached independently to the frame after its completion.

Spiral wound A type of battery that uses lead plates that are tightly wound in a spiral formation within each cell.

Standard seat belt harness A seat belt system that helps distribute the energy of a collision over larger areas of the body, such as the chest, pelvis, and shoulders. The three-point belt mechanism uses a retractor gear that locks in place when activated. Also known as a three-point harness system.

Strut tower A structural component of the suspension system that normally has both a coil spring and shock absorber. Its main function is to resist compression.

Tempered safety glass (TSG) A type of glass that has been heated and then quickly cooled; this process gives the glass its strength and resistance to impact.

Ultimate tensile strength (UTS) A measurement of the amount of force required to tear a section of steel apart.

Unibody construction A vehicle with a frame and body that are constructed as a single assembly that does not have a separate frame on which the body is mounted. (NFPA 58)

Upper rails Two side beams located in the front of the vehicle that hold the hood in place and attach the front wheel strut system to the chassis.

U-shaped striker plate latch pin A latch mechanism generally made of smaller-gauge steel, which makes it easier to cut through and/or release from the latch mechanism of the door.

Wet cell (Flooded cell) The standard 12-volt battery that contains active electrolyte solution; must be mounted in an upright position.

Window spidering An effect caused when an object breaks laminated glass and causes spiraling rings at the area of impact resembling a spider's web.

Work A mechanism for the transfer of energy.

Yield strength The amount of force or stress that a section of steel can withstand before permanent deformation occurs.

REFERENCES

Corning. Corning Gorilla Glass for Automative Glazing. Accessed November 18, 2020. https://www.corning.com/microsites/csm/gorillaglass/PI_Sheets/PI_Sheet_Automoitive_Glazing.pdf.

Merriam-Webster Online Dictionary, s.v. "energy." Accessed May 2020. https://www.merriam-webster.com/dictionary/energy.

On Scene

You have arrived on the scene of a motor vehicle accident. You begin your size-up and note that the vehicle is upright but has landed on the side of an embankment, approximately 25 feet from the roadway. The car has front-end damage and a spidered windshield. You find an unrestrained driver sitting in the driver's seat. The frame looks as though it is a unibody construction, and the hood is no longer on the vehicle.

1. What type of collision was this?
   A. Rear-end collision
   B. Rollover crash
   C. Frontal collision
   D. Both B and C

2. There are two frame systems that are most common in today's vehicles; they are the unibody construction and the _____ construction.
   A. ladder-type
   B. aluminum
   C. body-over-frame
   D. synthetic wrapped frame

3. You know the unibody frame:
   A. has the ability to absorb or redirect energy during a collision.
   B. has a formal frame structure.
   C. consists of two large beams tied together by cross member beams.
   D. is sometimes referred to as a ladder frame.

4. Kinetic energy is:
   A. the energy of motion.
   B. the force times the speed.
   C. the body in motion remaining in motion.
   D. the energy that can neither be created nor destroyed.

5. Window spidering occurs with which type of glass?
   A. Polycarbonate
   B. Laminated safety glass
   C. Tempered safety glass
   D. Plate glass

6. The hood is off the vehicle. What is the main structural component that assists in holding the hood in place?
   A. B-post
   B. Console area
   C. Dash area
   D. Upper rail

7. Roof posts, also known as roof pillars, are designed to add vertical support to the roof of the vehicle. The posts are generally labeled with:
   A. a color-coding system of red, green, and blue.
   B. a basic numbering system of 1, 2, and 3.
   C. an alpha system of A, B, and C.
   D. There is no system of identification.

8. The door limiting device located on a vehicle door is designed to:
   A. limit the opening or overextending of the door.
   B. retain the door in place.
   C. keep the door locked.
   D. be used in two door models.

9. Boron is alloyed with steel during processing for its unique:
   A. welding properties.
   B. hardening properties.
   C. stress resistance.
   D. ability to remain flexible.

10. Crumple zones are found in what type of vehicle frame?
    A. Unibody construction
    B. Ladder frame structure
    C. Monocoque-type frame
    D. Aluminum frame

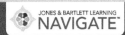 Access Navigate for more activities.

CHAPTER 6

Operations and Technician Levels

Supplemental Restraint Systems

KNOWLEDGE OBJECTIVES

After studying this chapter, you will be able to:
- Define the following terms and explain their role in vehicle rescue incidents:
  - Accelerometer (p. 152)
  - Air bag control unit (ACU) (p. 154)
  - Deployment zone (pp. 156)
  - Distancing (p. 163)
  - Electronic control unit (ECU) (p. 154)
  - Initiator (p. 154)
- Identify the differences between active and passive vehicle restraint systems. (pp. 158–159)
- List the steps in the air bag deployment process. (p. 152)
- Identify the basic components of an air bag system. (pp. 152–158)
- List the types and locations of air bags present in passenger vehicles. (pp. 152–158)
- Explain the importance of expose and cut. (**NFPA 1006: 8.2.4**, pp. 163–164)
- Describe seat belt pretensioning systems and explain their activation. (pp. 158–159)
- Explain safety precautions to protect rescuers in extrication from vehicles with air bag systems. (**NFPA 1006: 8.2.4**, pp. 161–164)

SKILL OBJECTIVE

After studying this chapter, you will be able to perform the following skill:
- Disconnect a vehicle battery to de-energize and disable an air bag or a rollover protection system. (**NFPA 1006: 8.2.4**, pp. 161–162)

You Are the Rescuer

You are on the scene of a vehicle accident that requires the occupants to be extricated. As you and your crew prepare to remove the roof, the rescuer inside the vehicle advises you that there are multiple undeployed air bags throughout the vehicle.

1. As the technical rescuer, what actions will you take?
2. Why should you determine whether the vehicle has electric seats before disconnecting the 12-volt DC battery?
3. Did you and your crew thoroughly expose the inside of the roof posts and roof rails?

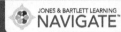

Access Navigate for more practice activities.

Introduction

In 1967, the National Highway Traffic Safety Administration (NHTSA) issued **Federal Motor Vehicle Safety Standards (FMVSS)**. FMVSS were enacted to protect the public from unreasonable risk of crashes, injury, or death resulting from the design, construction, or performance of a motor vehicle. The first of many subsequent regulations that outlined minimum safety requirements for motor vehicles mandating compliance from vehicle manufacturers was FMVSS 209, *Seat Belt Assemblies*. FMVSS 209 includes requirements for the straps, buckles, hardware, and fasteners of seat belt assemblies. FMVSS 208, *Occupant Crash Protection*, was adopted later and specified the type of occupant restraints, seat belts, and air bags required.

FMVSS 214, *Side Impact Protection*, was then established, requiring vehicle manufacturers to reinforce vehicle doors to minimize side-impact intrusions into the occupant areas. Because of this rule, vehicle manufacturers started to reinforce intrusion bars located in the door frames and introduced side air bags in the doors, seats, and roof rails. In January 2011, NHTSA established FMVSS 226, *Ejection Mitigation*, which went into effect in September 2013 with full compliance in 2017. It is based on side-impact crashes and vehicle rollovers and aims to minimize the potential for partial and full occupant ejections through side windows. To meet this standard, vehicle manufacturers had to improve several design features of side air bags, including the following:

- Maintaining the inflation rate for longer periods (6–8 seconds) to account for the extended amount of time the crash is sustained in vehicle rollovers
- Covering more of the window opening to minimize occupant head and extremity ejections
- Incorporating retaining or tether straps to keep the bag inside the vehicle and in the correct position

Manufacturers also considered adding enhanced glazing on side windows to change from a tempered glass, which is easily penetrated by an ejection, to a laminate-type glass, which would flex and retain an occupant inside the vehicle for longer periods. Not all manufacturers do this because this is not a requirement of the FMVSS standard.

Air Bags

In the early 1970s, fatalities from vehicle accidents started to increase dramatically; this was largely caused by the occupants failing to wear seat belts while driving. To counter the growing problem of consumers disregarding the importance of proper seat belt usage, the auto industry introduced the air cushion restraint system. The air cushion restraint system was an air bag device that, at the time, was considered a replacement option to the seat belt, offering occupant protection in head-on collisions. Unfortunately, this theory did not work out as planned because the number of vehicle accident fatalities started mounting. As time passed, the air cushion restraint system faded away, and seat belt education and enforcement started to increase. In the 1980s, a system similar to the air cushion restraint, the **air bag**, emerged as a supplement to the seat belt. By working in conjunction with the seat belt, the air bag became known as a **supplemental restraint system (SRS)** (**FIGURE 6-1**).

Manual seat belts are classified as an **active restraint device** because the occupant has to activate the system by engaging the seat belt mechanism into the anchor unit. A vehicle air bag is classified as a **passive restraint device** because the occupant does not have to activate the device to make it function; the system

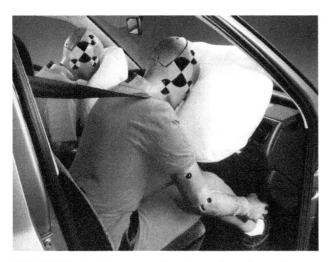

FIGURE 6-1 Air bags working in conjunction with seat belts are known as supplemental restraint systems.
© fStop Images - Caspar Benson/Brand X Pictures/Getty Images.

is automatically activated when power is applied to the vehicle.

As the demand for vehicle air bags grew, new and stricter regulation coincided. In 1984, FMVSS 208 was amended to mandate that motor vehicles manufactured after April 1989 be equipped with a passive restraint system; this included air bags and automatic seat belts. At the time, most vehicles offered only a single-stage air bag system. In this first-generation air bag system, the mechanism would fire at a preset discharge rate and pressure. This inflation rate, pressure, and velocity were tested and measured to protect an average-size adult male; children, women, or smaller-statured individuals were not factored into the equation. The test results determined that to deploy the air bag in approximately 40 to 45 ms, the velocity and pressure needed would be an inflation speed of 150 to 200 mi/h (241 to 322 km/h). Because of the power exerted, out-of-position or unbelted occupants who made contact at the inflation stage would be subject to a crushing force, sometimes causing fatalities and multiple injuries (fractures, contusions, lacerations, soft-tissue injuries, hearing impairment, burns). This resulted in further amendment of FMVSS 208 in 1998.

Air bags became the main focus of the 1998 FMVSS 208 amendment. The revised regulation mandated that air bags be depowered and a deactivation switch be added to passenger-side air bags for vehicles, such as light-duty trucks, that had no rear seating. These depowered air bags, also known as second-generation air bags, were now designed to inflate at a lesser force. The industry and the NHTSA believed that this correction would significantly reduce the casualties caused by its predecessor.

In 1996, the NHTSA proposed changes to the federal air bag requirement to encourage the introduction of smart air bag systems. These changes would not be implemented until 2000. In 2000, FMVSS 208 was amended again. The revision outlined the requirements of advanced frontal, or third-generation, air bag systems, to be phased in for all passenger vehicles and light-duty trucks by 2004, with full compliance for all passenger vehicles manufactured after September 1, 2006. These advanced smart air bag systems use adaptive response features that automatically adjust the pressure in the air bag through multistage inflators and basing the deployment force on a number of calculated factors, such as crash severity, occupant's weight, proximity to the air bag, seat belt usage, and seat position. To obtain the crash severity threshold, a vehicle was crashed into a stationary barrier at 14 mi/h (23 km/h) or greater. The 14 mi/h (23 km/h) was determined to be the minimum cutoff speed for air bag activation (**FIGURE 6-2**).

These new requirements addressed several specific advanced features to protect occupants from air bag injuries:

- *Dual-stage or multistage inflation process*: The inflation process incorporates a full-force deployment and a reduced or multistage reduced force deployment option. The first feature of this revised FMVSS 208 regulation requires the system to be equipped with a reduced deployment option when an occupant is too close to the deployment zone.

- *Suppression system*: The suppression system shuts down the air bag if an occupant classification system detects a child in the air bag deployment zone or if one of the many sensors detects a high-risk potential

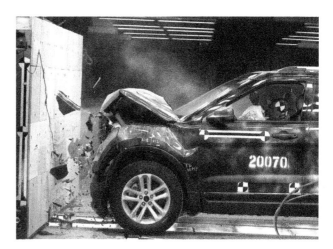

FIGURE 6-2 A barrier crash test is regularly performed by vehicle manufacturers and various testing facilities.
© Bill Pugliano/Stringer/Getty Images News/Getty Images.

by acquiring the occupant's weight, height, proximity to the air bag, seat belt usage, and seat position. The system sends this information to the electronic control unit, which will then shut off the air bag if a high risk to the occupant is determined.

Air Bag Deployment Process

A four-stage process occurs when an air bag is deployed in a crash sequence:

1. The crash itself
2. The crash sensor detecting deceleration
3. The air bag deploying and inflating
4. The occupant moving forward and striking the bag as deflation occurs

The crash sequence for an unbelted occupant would be as follows. The *first stage* is the crash itself, which occurs when the vehicle strikes an object or is struck by an object. The *second stage* occurs when the crash sensor, or **accelerometer**, detects an immediate deceleration of the vehicle, sending the information to the electronic control unit, which then determines the severity of the crash. If the electronic control unit detects a deceleration equivalent to a stationary barrier crash at 14 mi/h (23 km/h) or greater, *stage three* occurs. During stage three, the air bag deploys, and the occupant, still traveling forward at the vehicle speed prior to the impact, is making contact with a fully inflated bag. *Stage four* occurs with the bag deflating as the occupant, still moving forward, bottoms out the bag, causing the gas in the bag to be forced out of the small vent holes on its sides. Certain factors can change some of these crash sequence dynamics, such as seat belt system, size and seated distance of the occupant, and severity of the crash itself.

A vehicle crash is measured in milliseconds, with 1000 ms equaling 1 s. The entire vehicle crash process, which involves dissipating all the kinetic energy of the vehicle, takes approximately 100 to 125 ms, occurring faster than the blink of an eye, which takes approximately 300 to 400 ms. To understand how an occupant's body reacts inside a vehicle as the vehicle strikes an object and causes it to rapidly decelerate, we need to look at Newton's first law of motion. It states that an object in motion will remain in motion until it is disrupted by an external force. If a vehicle traveling at 50 mi/h (80 km/h) suddenly stops, the vehicle may stop, but the objects inside the vehicle that are not attached continue to travel at that speed until something stops their forward motion, such as the steering wheel, dash, or windshield. The air bag is engineered to absorb the force of the occupant's body, accelerating at 50 mi/h (80 km/h) and then gradually dissipating as the gas is pushed out of the bag through its vent holes. The gas inside the air bag must be precisely set with the correct volume to prevent the occupant from bottoming out and striking the steering wheel or dash.

Air Bag Components

Several components make up an air bag system, including the following (**FIGURE 6-3**):

- Air bag
- Initiator
- Air bag control unit
- Propellant
- Inflator
- Sensors

Air Bag

The air bag itself typically consists of a strong, durable nylon or blended material that is folded in a certain manner to facilitate inflation. The bag itself can be coated with a silicone base or use a powdered substance (e.g., talcum, chalk, or cornstarch) to assist in deployment ease and prevent cracking degradation. Once the air bag has deployed, the powdered residue—combined with nitrogen gas, alkaline by-products (sodium carbonate [Na_2CO_3]), small amounts of sodium hydroxide (NaOH), and metallic oxides—visibly floats in the air and may be a mild irritant to individuals with respiratory ailments. Burns have been noted to occupants caused by either thermal (super-heated gas) or chemical (alkaline) material. The air bag also comes equipped with several tethers, which are designed to manage the speed of the deployment. The outer air bag cover for the driver- and passenger-side air bags is composed of a

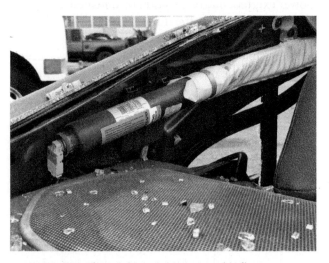

FIGURE 6-3 The air bag, initiator, and inflator.
Courtesy of David Sweet.

plastic material that is scored and designed to tear apart and separate when the air bag inflates.

The size of the bag will vary depending on the manufacturer's specifications, vehicle design, type of bag (driver, passenger, or side air bag), or location of the bag (whether on the driver or passenger side). Vehicles with convertible and/or removable roof systems may combine the side-impact air bags in the doors or seat backs into one larger bag to provide protection for the passenger's head and torso; such vehicles may also incorporate a rear seat air bag system along with a deployable rollover protection system, described later in this chapter. Air bag manufacturers are continuously researching and developing better ways to protect vehicle occupants, and this technology is always evolving; it is up to you as a technical rescuer to keep current with these changes.

The most common air bags are the driver and front-passenger air bags, which are mandatory in all vehicles. Other variations of air bags located within a vehicle include, but are not limited to, the following:

- *Side-impact air bag*: There are several types of **side-impact air bags** designed to protect the following areas of the occupant: the head, the chest/upper torso, and a combination of the head and chest/upper torso. Side-impact air bags are designed to activate immediately (10–20 ms) upon impact because of the proximity of the occupant to the door. Side-impact air bags can be found in the door, seat backs, roof posts, or roof rails. These bags may be labeled HPS (head protection system), IC (inflatable curtain), SIPS (side-impact protection system), or ROI (rollover inflator air bag). With the implementation of FMVSS 226, side-impact air bags are designed to maintain inflation for a few seconds to help protect the occupant in secondary impacts or rollovers (**FIGURE 6-4**).

- *Center air bag*: A center air bag is designed to protect the occupants from secondary impacts of striking a passenger after the side impact of another vehicle or object has occurred. It also protects the occupants from side impacts that occur on the opposite side of the driver or passenger. A center air bag deploys in an upward and forward position between the front and the rear two seats, with the actual bag being located inside the driver right-side front seat and another bag located in the right side of the rear driver-side seat.

- *Knee air bag*: A knee air bag, sometimes referred to as a *knee bolster bag*, is designed to protect the occupant's abdomen, pelvis, and lower extremities, preventing the occupant from being pulled under the dash area. Knee bags are generally designed for the driver side, with the possibility of a second bag positioned for the passenger sides of the vehicle depending on the vehicle manufacturer. These bags incorporate a bladder-type system positioned just behind and integrated into plastic molding. The plastic molding makes contact with the occupant rather than tearing away at a seam like the steering-wheel and passenger-side air bags (**FIGURE 6-5**). Knee bolster bags are designed to prevent the occupant from being pulled under the dash during a front-end collision.

- *Seat belt air bag*: This type of air bag is designed to protect the occupant's upper torso area as well as the pelvic area. These air bag systems can be combined to work in conjunction with a **seat belt pretensioning system**, which can reduce

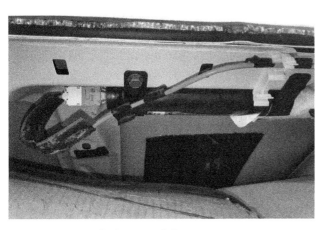

FIGURE 6-4 Side-impact air bags.
Courtesy of David Sweet.

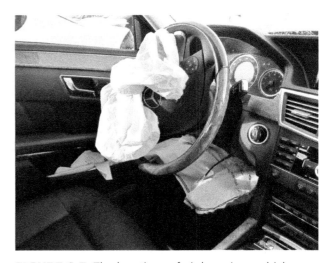

FIGURE 6-5 The locations of air bags in a vehicle will vary, depending on the manufacturer. This photo shows a knee air bag.
Courtesy of David Sweet.

the sudden tensioning or "clothesline effect" that can occur from the automatic engagement of a standard or pretensioning belt system.

- *Seat cushion air bag*: This type of air bag is positioned just under the front section of the seat cushion and is designed to raise the hip and knee area of the occupant, which in turn controls the upper body by reducing the forward movement of the chest and abdomen.
- *Rear seat deployment air bag system*: This type of air bag can be deployed from the center roof area, seat belt, door, roof post, or headrest depending on where manufacturers have placed them.
- *Outside pedestrian protection system*: This air bag system can be deployed from just under the rear section of the engine compartment hood closest to the windshield. A redesign of the hinges allows that rear section of the hood to rise a few inches when deployed and release the air bag, which extends out and upward, covering most of the windshield and A-pillars in the areas a pedestrian is most likely to impact.

With the exception of the driver-side and front passenger-side air bag, there are no standardized locations of vehicle air bags or inflation cylinders. Vehicle manufacturers install air bags in any location they believe provides the best occupant protection for a specific design of vehicle and is the most economically feasible. Most manufacturers offer these unique air bags as upgrades or options to purchase by the consumer.

> **LISTEN UP!**
>
> There are excellent resources the technical rescuer can use in the field or study, such as the *NFPA Emergency Field Guide for Electric and Hybrid Vehicles*, which is offered in hard copy or as an application to download onto cell phones and tablets. This resource uses specific vehicle diagrams, designed by the company Moditech Rescue Solutions, that depict air bag and inflator locations as well as other important and relevant information on vehicle technology and emergency procedures.

Initiator

Air bag systems may use an **initiator** device, such as a **squib**, which is a miniature explosive device, to ignite the propellant that produces the nitrogen or other inert gas that fills the nylon air bag (**FIGURE 6-6**).

Air Bag Control Unit

The **air bag control unit (ACU)** is a computerized control component of the air bag system, which is part

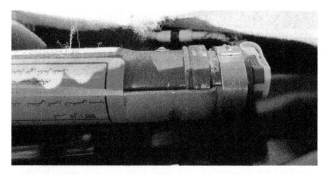

FIGURE 6-6 An initiator device, such as a squib, is used to activate an air bag.
Courtesy of David Sweet.

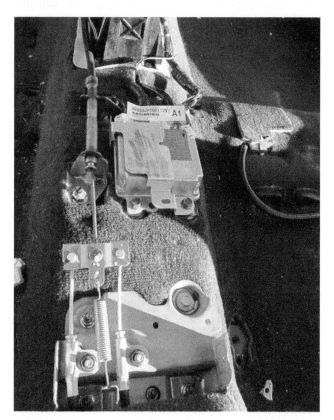

FIGURE 6-7 The electronic control unit (ECU), also known as the air bag control unit (ACU), is the brains of an air bag system.
Courtesy of David Sweet.

of the overall active vehicle safety system within the **electronic control unit (ECU)**, or the master brains of the vehicle (**FIGURE 6-7**). This device is a small processing unit that is generally located in the center of the vehicle under and/or between the seats, but it may be located in other areas depending on the vehicle manufacturer's preference or vehicle design. In advanced air bag systems, this processor is preset with multiple crash algorithms, which calculate the deployment level needed to protect the occupants. Three basic deployment levels are common with advanced air bag systems, each determined by the algorithmic factors. They are no deployment, low deployment, and full deployment. In each scenario, the vehicle crash sensor must first detect a crash and then instantly (within milliseconds) send a signal to the ECU. The ECU determines whether the speed of the deceleration exceeds the crash threshold level of approximately 14 mi/h (23 km/h).

The ECU is designed to limit unnecessary deployments that occurred in first-generation air bag systems. The ECU works in conjunction with multiple sensors located throughout the vehicle, continuously monitoring changes in information. Within milliseconds, this information is sent back to the ECU. The ECU also contains an energy capacitor that acts as a backup system in lieu of any power disruption, such as a battery disconnect. The amount of time that the energy capacitor holds power varies by manufacturer, ranging from 30 s up to 30 min. The energy capacitor is a very important component because it holds power when the vehicle's 12-volt DC battery has been disconnected, thus ensuring that all the power sources have not been eliminated. An ECU can also simultaneously activate a seat belt pretension system, along with an air bag, to give added protection. Some ECUs have a feature that records and stores information from accidents that have occurred, acting similar to a flight recorder. This can provide valuable information to manufacturers for quality improvement measures and for crash investigation teams in determining what occurred during the crash.

Inflator/Propellant

One of the most critical design features for an air bag is the ability to fill up the bag instantaneously, in milliseconds, from the onset of the collision. This is accomplished via three types of inflation systems—a stored compressed-gas system, a pyrotechnic propellant gas-generation system, and/or a hybrid type consisting of both a gas-generation pyrotechnic propellant and compressed gas. These high-pressure inflators are critical considerations of the technical rescuer because they are generally positioned in the cut zone areas, such as roof posts/pillars or roof rails. Exposing areas before any cutting or spreading operation begins is vital to the safety of the rescuer as well as the victims. The techniques and skill drills discussed in this text include precautions and procedures in exposing and operating around these inflators. Just remember to always *"Inspect before you dissect"* and *"If an air bag cylinder is found then cut around."*

A **stored compressed gas system** can comprise a single-stage or multistage inflation process. These types of systems commonly use an inert gas, such as argon or helium, or another type of gas such as nitrous. The gas is stored in a steel or aluminum cylinder and can be pressurized from 2500 to 3500 psi (17,237 to 24,132 kPa), but these pressures may be greater in some designs, depending on the size and use of the bag and the manufacturer's preference or vehicle design. The igniter, or squib, sets off a burst, or rupture, disk that acts as a seal, holding back the compressed gas. When activated, the disk breaks open, releasing the gas from the chamber, which expands and instantly fills the bag. The rapid release of the compressed gas in the ambient air could cause the cylinder to freeze, resulting in variable bag inflation. To prevent this, a heating element keeps the temperature of the gas constant to maintain the proper inflation ratio of the bag.

Multiple gas storage cylinders may be located in various areas of the vehicle depending on the manufacturer. It is difficult to explain or list all of these cylinder locations because there can be such a variance between manufacturers, and this technology is always evolving. The best practice model for the technical rescuer in dealing with cylinder/inflator locations is to always expose the area to be cut and/or spread if it can be exposed before any operation begins. A phrase that is consistently used in this text is "expose and cut." This is not a suggestion but an action that must be implemented at every vehicle rescue and extrication incident to best provide protection to the rescuers and occupant(s) (**FIGURE 6-8**).

Multistage inflators are cylinders that can comprise two separate chambers of compressed gas—one with a large amount and the other with a smaller amount of product. Both chambers have initiators that can fire independently or together. Depending on the severity of the crash (>14 mi/h [23 km/h] and < 25 mi/h [40 km/h]); weight, height, and proximity of the occupant; and whether the occupant is wearing a seat belt, the ECU may tell the inflator to release the smaller chamber, or 50 to 75 percent of the gas product. If the ECU determines that a full deployment is needed (crash is > 25 mi/h [40 km/h]), both chambers will fire simultaneously, filling the air bag to the appropriate inflation ratio to protect the occupant.

A **gas-generation system** uses a chemical reaction that rapidly produces the gas, most commonly nitrogen gas. The gas instantly fills the bag at a rate of approximately 200 to 250 mi/h (322 to 402 km/h), completely filling the bag in approximately 30 to 40 ms. The most common solid fuel used for the nitrogen gas generation is sodium azide. Sodium azide is a very volatile substance; when mixed with water, it rapidly changes to hydrazoic acid in both a toxic gas and a liquid state. In the air bag system, sodium azide, in pellet form, is detonated by the igniter or squib, which rapidly and completely decomposes the product

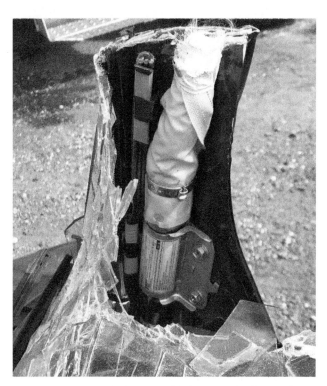

FIGURE 6-8 Multiple gas cylinders can be located in various areas within the vehicle, depending on the manufacturer. This air bag cylinder pictured is located in the lower section of the A-post and dash area.
Courtesy of David Sweet.

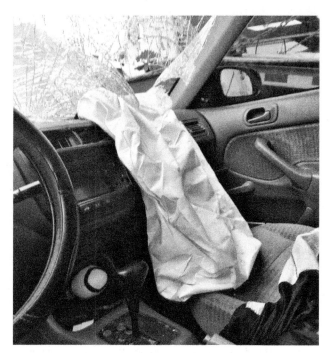

FIGURE 6-9 A fractured windshield is commonly caused by the passenger-side air bag deflecting off of it during deployment.
Courtesy of David Sweet.

through the combustion process and chemical chain reaction. This produces the inert nitrogen gas and a small amount of the by-product sodium hydroxide, an alkaline substrate also known as lye. Additional chemicals are added to neutralize the sodium hydroxide. Most of the other by-products that are produced after the chemical reaction are contained by filters.

Common driver-side air bag housing units that are found in most vehicles can contain approximately 2 oz (57 g) of sodium azide, depending on the size and use of the bag. Because of its volatility and hazardous nature, sodium azide is used in pellet form for easier product containment. A driver-side air bag must produce enough gas to inflate the air bag approximately 10 in. (25 cm) into the compartment space of the front driver area. The deployment zone is measured to 10 in. (25 cm), which is the estimated safe distance that an occupant should be seated from the steering wheel. A common passenger-side air bag housing unit can contain approximately 7 oz (198 g) of sodium azide because of the additional deployment space as compared to a driver-side air bag; the air bag has to inflate big enough to fill the front passenger area. The deployment zone area is measured to 20 in. (51 cm), which is the estimated safe distance that an occupant should be seated from the dash area. Also, most passenger-side air bags are designed to strike and deflect off the front windshield upon deployment, slowing the speed considerably. The technical rescuer should be aware that the fractured windshield or spider effect resulting from the air bag striking it can be mistaken for the occupant striking the windshield (**FIGURE 6-9**).

Because of the toxicity and volatility of sodium azide, some manufacturers have been using non-azide propellants, such as ammonium nitrate, guanidine nitrate, and tetrazole-based energetic materials, to generate enough gas to fill the bags. Ammonium nitrate is a highly unstable chemical used as an explosive for the military and as a vegetation fertilizer base for the farming industry. Ammonium nitrate was the cause of several highly documented explosions, including one of the worst industrial accidents in U.S. history that occurred in 1947 at a Texas shipyard as well as the explosion that killed six Kansas City firefighters in 1988. Several air bag inflators equipped with ammonium nitrate as a propellant have been the cause of documented containment failures causing fragmentation of metal to fire through the occupant compartment, killing and severely injuring several passengers. Air bag inflators using ammonium nitrate start to degrade over time, through exposure to environmental moisture and fluctuations of temperature inside the vehicle from hot to cold or vice versa. The NHTSA issued a national recall of air bag systems equipped with ammonium nitrate with many of these systems still on the road today.

Another type of inflation system is the **hybrid-type inflator**, which consists of both a gas-generation pyrotechnic propellant and compressed gas. This device is composed of two chambers. The first-stage chamber uses a small amount of a pyrotechnic gas-producing propellant, such as sodium azide, guanidine nitrate, tetrazole, or ammonium nitrate. The second-stage chamber is filled with a compressed inert gas, such as argon or helium, or another type of gas such as nitrous. In combination, each chamber produces and/or releases the correct amount of gas to inflate the bag. Hybrid-type inflators are common to side-impact air bags, such as roof rails, seats, doors, or roof posts.

Side-impact air bags located in the roof rail, seats, doors, or roof posts are designed to react and deploy at a much faster rate because of the minimal distance/proximity of the occupant to the impact. A typical side-impact air bag must inflate within 10 to 15 ms as compared to the standard front driver and passenger air bag, which has an inflation range of 30 to 40 ms.

The common estimated elapsed time from bag deployment to bag deflation is approximately 100 to 150 ms. Some advanced inflators are designed to keep the bags inflated for longer to assist with secondary crashes and rollovers. These systems are currently designed for side-impact air bags where the inflators use compressed helium gas, releasing it in a cold state as opposed to using the heating element. This cold state allows the expanded gas to maintain its inflation ratio for longer durations to protect the occupant in the event of a rollover, which can occur several minutes after the initial impact.

> **LISTEN UP!**
>
> Keep in mind that a side-impact air bag has a faster reaction time because of the minimal distance/proximity of the occupant to the impact. A typical side-impact air bag must inflate within 10 to 15 ms as compared to the standard front driver and passenger air bag, which has an inflation range of 30 to 40 ms.

Sensors

Sensors in a vehicle air bag system are designed to measure variances in preset factors and are based on an open-and-closed-circuit electrical system. The sensors send information back to the ECU, which determines whether to deploy the air bags. Sensors are located throughout the vehicle, depending on their type and use (**FIGURE 6-10**). First-generation air bag crash detection sensors commonly used an electromechanical or magnetic sensing device, such as a magnetic bias sensor, or a Rolamite sensor, which consists of a metal roller or spring-loaded weight. The magnetic bias

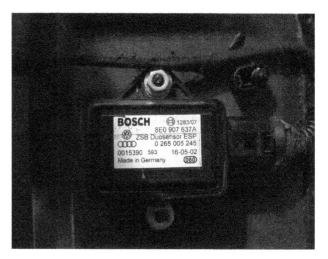

FIGURE 6-10 Several types of sensors can be located in a vehicle.
Courtesy of David Sweet.

sensor consists of a sensing mass steel ball in a tube where the steel ball is held in place by a spring or bias magnet. When the vehicle detected an impact deceleration at a predetermined rate, it would jar the ball, which would move it through the tube, thus completing and closing the electrical circuit and sending the signal to initiate an air bag deployment. Manufacturers would also include a **safing sensor** to prevent false deployments that might occur from jarring the vehicle by driving into a pothole or over an object that would strike the undercarriage. This type of sensor has a deceleration setting lower than the crash-type sensor, and both the crash sensor and safing sensor had to be activated at the same time for the air bag to deploy.

Impact or crash sensors today are designed to detect a rapid deceleration of the vehicle through the use of a microelectromechanical system (MEMS) accelerometer and electronic satellite sensors. The electronic satellite sensor is an acceleration-based sensor that identifies various crash pulses when they occur and sends the data back to the ECU to determine the type of air bag deployment needed in a multistage system that best protects the occupant. A MEMS accelerometer is constructed of small circuits integrated with micromechanical elements. When a crash is detected through a rapid deceleration of the vehicle, the microscopic mechanical element moves. The movement is detected by the circuit board, which sends a signal back to the ECU telling it that a deployment threshold has been reached. Again, this process occurs in milliseconds.

Vehicles will rely increasingly on advanced active safety systems, which incorporate a combination of multiple electronic and environmental crash and pre-crash recognition sensors that serve various functions and are designed to report a constant stream of information back to the ECU. These devices include distancing wave radar sensors, laser radars, and monocular and stereo cameras that detect objects regardless of their size or shape.

Occupant Classification System. An occupant classification system normally consists of three types of sensors, including a suppression system that uses the following sensors for automatic deactivation:

- *Seat position sensor*: Detects the proximity of the occupant to the air bag
- *Seat belt sensor*: Detects whether the occupant seat belt is engaged and locked in the housing unit
- *Occupant weight sensor*: Measures the weight of the occupant, determining whether the occupant has met a preset weight threshold limit

If an occupant measures below the preset threshold limit, such as when a child car seat is placed in the seat, then the air bag will be turned off. This is critical to the technical rescuer because the system constantly monitors the weight in the seat. When the rescuer enters the vehicle and places his or her weight on the seat, the sensor will measure that weight and send the information back to the ECU, thus arming it for possible deployment. There will also be an air bag status indication light located somewhere on the dashboard panel, which will display that the air bag for that area has been shut off or disabled. This varies with each manufacturer. Some vehicles are equipped with a manual on/off switch that is designed to disable the front passenger-side air bag, but again, this feature varies with each manufacturer.

> **LISTEN UP!**
>
> With an occupant classification system, as the rescuer enters the vehicle and places his or her weight on the seat, the sensor measures that weight and sends the information back to the ECU, thus arming it for a possible full deployment.

Rollover Protection System

A **rollover protection system (ROPS)** was initially designed for convertible vehicles to protect occupants in vehicle rollover incidents by means of a deployable roll bar (**FIGURE 6-11**). Unlike fixed roll bars, these deployable roll bars are concealed until activated. They have a reaction time of less than 0.3 seconds and are activated by a sensor detector consisting of an **inclinometer sensor**, or tilt sensor, which detects vehicle inclination or tilt with lateral acceleration (detects how fast the vehicle's tilt is changing). A **gravitational acceleration sensor (G-sensor)** detects a vehicle's weightlessness,

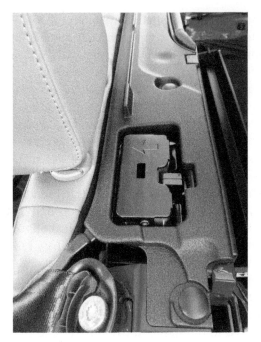

FIGURE 6-11 A deployable roll bar is an automatic rollover protection system.
Courtesy of Bill Larkin.

such as that experienced in a free fall, when the vehicle starts to roll and come down.

To activate the ROPS, the sensors must detect a significant vehicle tilt with lateral acceleration, including a sustained G-force; the ECU of the ROPS then determines when to deploy the roll bars. The roll bars can extend up to 20 in. (51 cm) in some models. Exercise caution when operating around a vehicle containing an undeployed roll bar. Avoid placing any parts of the body over an undeployed roll bar. For instance, if spinal immobilization is used on a victim in the backseat, do not lean across the back of the vehicle to access the victim.

When encountering a ROPS, the technical rescuer must follow the same safety guidelines and electrical disconnection procedures that are established for vehicle air bag systems, as discussed in this chapter.

Seat Belt Systems

Seat belts, also known as safety belts, are active restraint systems designed to maintain the position of the occupant when a force from a sudden acceleration or deceleration is applied. By design, the seat belt webbing material stretches and absorbs the force of the occupant's body weight controlling against the potential impact that can occur from the occupant slamming into a component of the interior. Seat belts designed for automobiles have a tensile strength of over 6000 lb and can be anchored in two points with the standard lap belt or a three-point anchor system incorporating the shoulder harness with the lap belt. There are also four-point harness systems, such as those found in child safety seats and auto race vehicles.

Seat Belt Types

Seat belts can be retractable or nonretractable. The retractable type has the webbing wound up in a gear housing under a tensioned spring mechanism. When the belt is pulled out, the spring winds against itself and automatically takes up slack when the belt is released. The nonretractable type of seat belts, such as the airplane passenger seat belts or the older school bus lap belts, remain static with slack being taken up manually. A locking mechanism web clamp through a weighted pendulum cam or clutch system is built into the retractable seat belt. It engages the spool when a sudden force, such as a rapid weight transfer of the occupant onto the belt, is applied, preventing any further release of the webbing.

A **load limiting device** is a safety design feature that reduces the force applied by the seat belt when it locks in place from the sudden force applied to it. A load limiter can be incorporated in the webbing material of the belt or in a torsion bar attached to the retractor gear. Within the seat belt, a fold is stitched in that is set to tear when a preset amount of force is applied. This prevents the belt from locking up, gradually releasing the tension that can cause injuries to the occupant. The torsion bar has the same concept of elongating by twisting when a preset amount of force is applied and then gradually releasing tension on the belt.

Pretensioning Systems

Pretensioning systems are designed to retract automatically through a mechanical or electrical/pyrotechnical mechanism. They can be activated in conjunction with the vehicle air bags from the ECU or act independently. A seat belt pretensioner can be set up to operate at the belt buckle/latching attachment or to operate at the retractor spool. The belt buckle operates by pulling down and/or back on the buckle itself by means of a cable attachment or piston rod. This type of system is commonly activated by a small pyrotechnic charge or firing mechanism and gas chamber, which draws back on the cable by forcing a piston attachment through the release of the expanding inert gas generated by a small amount of propellants, such as ammonium nitrate, guanidine nitrate, or tetrazole. The pretensioning system that activates at the retractor spool also uses a pyrotechnic charge and gas-generation system where it forces a rack gear to engage the pinion gear connected to the retractor

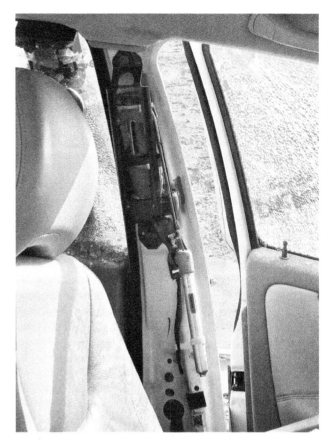

FIGURE 6-12 A seat belt pretensioning system is designed to automatically tighten, or take up slack, in a seat belt when a crash is detected.
Courtesy of David Sweet.

spool mechanism, rapidly winding up the webbing when activated (**FIGURE 6-12**).

Mechanical pretensioning systems use a torsion spring that is pretensioned and operates by means of a pendulum. When the pendulum is offset by a crash, the spring is released and draws back on the retractor that rapidly spools the webbing. Other types of pretensioning systems use a series of steel balls in a chamber tube that, once activated through pyrotechnic and gas generation, is forced through a cog wheel–type mechanism that engages the retractor that spools the webbing and locks the retractor once the slack is removed from the belt. Seat belt retractor assemblies and pretensioning gas chambers can be housed in the lower section of the post or column, on the lower side of the seat, under the seats, or in the center console area. When cutting through a post at the bottom section, the molding must be removed to reveal the possibility of a pretensioning system in order to cut around the device.

The concept of dissection underlies the processes discussed in this chapter. As professionals, our job is not to rip or tear the vehicle apart; it is to dissect it section by section, fully comprehending the action taken,

Voice of Experience

Vehicle extrication involves a specific understanding of automotive restraints systems, and if improperly compromised can cause extensive injury or death to a victim. The type of vehicle involved in an accident can have a tremendous influence on the method and techniques used to remove a trapped victim from the wreckage. The automotive industry has placed great emphasis on the development and installation of safety features in their vehicles, designed to provide the highest level of protection for passengers. Firefighters and other first responders must have a general understanding of the safety system and how it can easily be engaged during extrication activities. There are several resources that can be used to quickly obtain specific information about different types of vehicles before initiating actions.

Several years ago, my truck company responded to a motor vehicle collision that required us to extricate a trapped victim from a car that was severely damaged. The automobile involved was a modern hybrid vehicle, of which I wasn't very familiar. My immediate concern was safely removing the victim without activating any of the sensors to the vehicle's air bag system, which could have caused severe injuries to the firefighters and caused further injuries to the victim. Before giving directions to cut, pry, or breach the vehicle, I instructed firefighters to remove the car's interior encasements to visually locate the cylinders. I then gathered additional information to make myself more familiar with the vehicle's supplemental restraint system. I utilized a smartphone application I became familiar with as an instructor at Tarrant County College. It assisted us in quickly identifying the location of the car's air bag actuators, which helped prevent the unintentional deployment of the air bag system. It also provided the location of the main battery used by this hybrid vehicle, which allowed us to successfully de-energize the car. After the victim was successfully extricated from the car, properly packaged, and transported to a local hospital, our truck company continued making ourselves more familiar with several of the supplemental restraint features of the hybrid vehicle involved in the collision.

Regardless of your individual experience and knowledge of supplemental restraint systems, it can be beneficial to have access to additional resources to reference when encountered with uncertainty. There are several different types of applications that provide details about the supplemental restraint systems in most modern vehicles that can be a tremendous resource for first responders. The associated dangers of vehicle extrication can have severe consequences, including death. Resource familiarization is a critical component in the effective and timely initiation of rescue and mitigation actions. When using smartphone applications or any other type of resource, be thoroughly familiar with it to quickly access the needed information so it can be communicated to rescue personnel.

There are multiple ways to familiarize yourself with vehicle supplemental restraint systems, but I recommend taking formal courses when available to establish a solid foundation in vehicle extrication. Additionally, reading fire-service periodicals helps responders to remain current with the automotive innovations that pertain to the vehicle safety systems. Lastly, share information with your station or department to increase situational awareness in response to incidents involving vehicle extrication.

Frank McKinley
Dallas Fire-Rescue Department
Dallas, Texas

just as a surgeon would operate on a patient. Vehicle extrication is a step-by-step technical process, requiring continuous training to become proficient.

Emergency Procedures

Never assume that an air bag is dead just because the power has been disconnected, regardless of the amount of time that has elapsed. As discussed, a vehicle air bag system comes equipped with an energy capacitor, which has varying power-storing durations, with some models storing power for up to 30 min. Air bag inflators are always "live" until deployed, and even then, they can be a multistage unit with one chamber still containing compressed gas. The best defense is recognition, identification, disconnecting the power supply, and proper distancing. Attempting to disable the inflator can potentially cause the air bags to deploy. Vehicle air bag installation, repair, and removal procedures are to be performed by licensed or certified repair technicians only.

Disconnecting Power

Several things can be done to ensure that power is disconnected from the air bag system and the system is powering down. The first thing to remember is that there is a backup energy system with storage capacitors so that, even when the 12-volt battery is disconnected, there may be a storage capacitor that holds power for a predetermined length of time depending on the manufacturer. One problem that can be encountered when the power is disconnected from the vehicle is the inability to adjust the seats if power seats or other electrical systems are installed in the vehicle. These electrical systems, which include, but are not limited to, the power seats, power windows, and power adjustable tilt steering, are known as **beneficial systems**. The ability to move a seat back in certain instances or move up a steering wheel can greatly assist rescue efforts. The rescuer should be aware of this prior to disconnecting the power. To disconnect the power on a vehicle to initiate the depowering of an air bag system, follow the steps in **SKILL DRILL 6-1**.

SKILL DRILL 6-1
Disconnect a Vehicle Battery to De-energize and Disable an Air Bag or a Rollover Protection System NFPA 1006 8.2.4

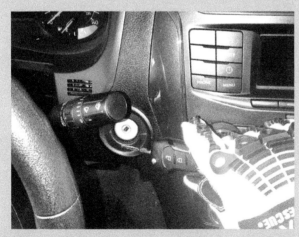

1. Remove the key from the ignition or the smart key from the vicinity. Manually activate (turn on) an electrical component of the vehicle, such as the emergency warning flashers, turn signal, or radio, to indicate to the rescuers whether the power is still connected. If the vehicle has beneficial systems, determine whether these components can be adjusted to provide better access before disconnecting power.

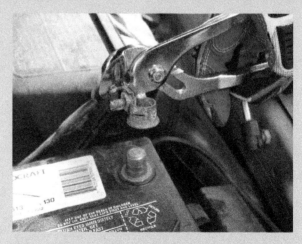

2. Remove or cut the battery cables, starting with the negative side. Fold the cables back onto themselves, and cover the open end to avoid the cables reconnecting with a terminal or the vehicle frame. Verify that this is the only battery in the vehicle.

(continues)

SKILL DRILL 6-1 Continued
Disconnect a Vehicle Battery to De-energize and Disable an Air Bag or a Rollover Protection System NFPA 1006 8.2.4

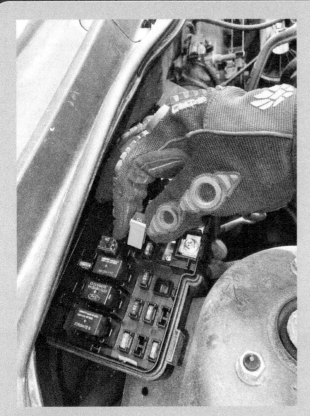

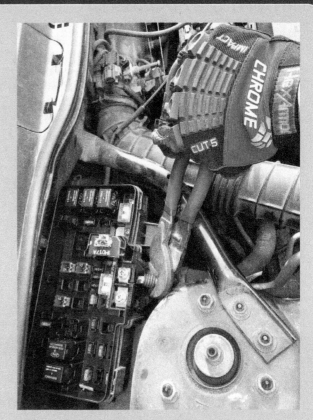

3 Some vehicle manufacturers and emergency response guides recommend removing the main fuses as an additional safety step, but location and time expended must be considered.

4 If removing individual fuses proves to be difficult or time consuming, consider cutting the cable connecting the power to the fuse box.

Steps 1 and 2: © Jones & Bartlett Learning. Photographed by Glen E. Ellman; Steps 3 and 4: Courtesy of David Sweet.

Recognizing and Identifying Air Bags

Vehicle air bag recognition and identification can be determined by the air bag badging or labeling system. These markings consist of acronyms that are generally located in proximity to the inflator (**FIGURE 6-13**).

Standard air bag acronyms include:

- SRS (supplemental restraint system)
- SIR (supplemental inflatable restraint)
- HPS (head protection system)
- IC (inflatable curtain)
- SIPS (side-impact protection system)
- ROI (rollover inflator)

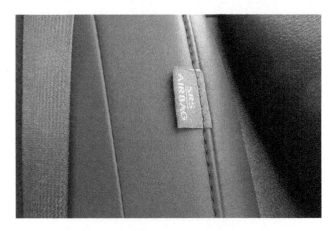

FIGURE 6-13 A labeling system using acronyms is generally used to indicate that an air bag system is present.
Courtesy of David Sweet.

Various other acronyms are used to label vehicle air bags, but the idea here is to recognize the markings and understand that some type of air bag system is located in that general vicinity. These acronyms/letters may be embossed, raised, or sewn into the plastic, cloth, or leather material, depending on the manufacturer's preference. Starting with vehicles manufactured in 1998, all vehicles must contain a driver- and passenger-side air bag. All other air bags will have to be located by the rescuer because there is no standard placement for additional air bags. One of the assignments for the rescuer positioned inside the vehicle is to scan the entire interior of the vehicle for air bag locations. A good practice is that, once the interior rescuer locates an air bag, it should be clearly marked with red tape or other type of marking system, and prior to any cutting or spreading, this area should be exposed and relayed to all technical rescuers on scene.

> **LISTEN UP!**
>
> All vehicles manufactured in 1998 or later must contain a driver- and passenger-side air bag per FMVSS 208. Since 2012, side-impact air bags have also been mandated per FMVSS 214 for side-protection improvements and per FMVSS 226 for ejection mitigation in 2017.

Distancing

Once an air bag location has been identified, the next precaution is to maintain the proper distance from the deployment zone, which depends on the type of air bag system that is installed. The accepted rule of thumb for proper distancing is 10 in. (25 cm) for the driver-side air bag, 20 to 25 in. (51 to 64 cm) for passenger-side air bags, and 5 to 15 in. (13 to 38 cm) for side-impact air bags. These distances are only recommendations and are not guaranteed for safety; each manufacturer has different components and various sizes of air bags installed in the vehicle.

Extrication Precautions

When performing extrication techniques on any vehicle that has a potentially live air bag system, there are certain rules that the technical rescuer must adhere to prior to removal of any sections of the vehicle.

- *Rule 1*: The proper procedures for disconnecting power and proper distancing shall be conducted and maintained.
- *Rule 2*: The technical rescuer should never place anything, such as a backboard or other hard protection, between the victim and an undeployed air bag. Doing so can cause the object to be thrust violently into the victim or rescuer if the air bag deploys.
- *Rule 3*: The technical rescuer should never try to contain the air bag by tying it up with webbing or some type of bag-containment system; the shear force of the bag deploying at greater than 200 mi/h (322 km/h) can rip any containment design apart or possibly cause the steering wheel to come apart.
- *Rule 4*: Always inspect before you dissect! Inspection is critical. The technical rescuer must always expose the area that is going to be cut, spread, or pushed for any air bag components, seat belt pretensioning systems, or high-powered wires prior to performing any maneuver. The tendency to succumb to the adrenaline rush that comes with trying to get the victim out of the vehicle immediately must be held in check, and safety must be maintained above all things. Inadvertently cutting into a high-pressure air bag inflator (2500 to 3500 psi [17,237 to 24,131 kPa] or higher) can cause the cylinder to fragment violently, separating into pieces of metal projectiles and potentially causing injury to the victim or rescuer. All of the plastic molding or material coverings for roof posts, roof rail channels/liners, seat backs, and lower door posts must be removed or pulled back and examined for inflators or high-powered wiring that can be encountered with hybrid or fuel cell vehicle systems (**FIGURE 6-14**). Remember the phrase "Expose and cut"! If an inflator is located, cut a few inches in front of or behind the cylinder, avoiding the wires or initiator clips; the actual

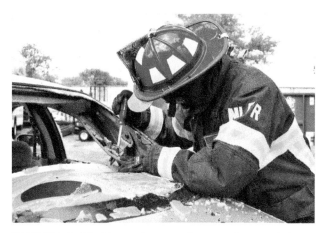

FIGURE 6-14 Always inspect the area for an air bag inflator before committing to cutting into a section of the vehicle.
Courtesy of Edward Monahan.

nylon bag that is attached to the cylinder can be cut into and through without any problem of deployment.

- *Rule 5*: Always consider the location of the ECU anytime you are operating tools along the center console and floorboard area. It can be difficult to pinpoint the exact location of the air bag ECU; each vehicle setup may be different.
- *Rule 6*: Always be cognizant of side-impact sensors before attempting to spread or crush a door. Let's say a vehicle with a full complement of air bag components crashes its front end, causing the driver-side and front passenger-side air bags to deploy. The side-impact air bags do not deploy, and the vehicle framing partially collapses onto itself, causing the vehicle's doors to become jammed in the framing. The moment a hydraulic tool is inserted into the door frame, a side-impact sensor can potentially activate, causing any or all of the side air bags on that side of the vehicle to deploy. One possible solution is to expose the hinges of the door with a wheel well crush technique using a hydraulic spreader or remove a panel section with a pneumatic air chisel and then cut the hinges with the pneumatic air chisel or hydraulic cutter, also removing the attached door limiting device if one exists. Pull back the door, and cut the wires that enter the door frame hole between the hinges. This may disconnect power to the door bag only; when the door is pulled back away from the occupant, there should be enough distance between the occupant and the air bag if a bag is placed inside a door panel. This would be the only time that wires should be cut. Be aware that this is not a foolproof method; there is always the potential for the bag to deploy when the wires are compressed before they shear.

SAFETY TIP

Avoid or be very cautious of using the spreader in the center console area, where the ECU may be located. Several years ago, an educational video was circulating that depicted a live extrication of a victim trapped in a Mitsubishi vehicle. The crew was shown attempting to maneuver the hydraulic spreader next to the center console for better leveraging; they were unaware that the air bag ECU was in the same location. When the tool was engaged, it crushed the housing of the ECU, causing a breach in the circuitry and sending a signal to fire all of the air bags in the vehicle. Both driver- and passenger-side air bags deployed instantaneously, causing serious injuries to two of the fire rescue personnel.

After-Action REVIEW

IN SUMMARY

- In 1967, the NHTSA issued a federal mandate titled FMVSS 209, *Seat Belt Assemblies*. This was the first of many subsequent regulations that outlined minimum safety requirements for motor vehicles mandating compliance from vehicle manufacturers.
- In the 1980s, the air bag became known as an SRS by working in conjunction with the seat belt.
- A four-stage process occurs when an air bag deploys in a crash sequence: the crash itself, the crash sensor detecting deceleration, the air bag deploying and inflating, and the occupant moving forward and striking the bag as deflation occurs.
- Several components make up an air bag, including the air bag, initiator, ECU, propellant, inflator, and sensors.
- ROPS were initially designed for convertible vehicles to protect occupants in vehicle rollover incidents. Roll bars are concealed until activated by sensors.
- Seat belts, also known as safety belts, are active restraint systems designed to maintain the position of the occupant when a force from a sudden acceleration or deceleration is applied.
- Seat belts can be retractable or nonretractable. The retractable type has the webbing wound up in a gear housing under a tensioned spring mechanism that automatically takes up slack when the belt is released. The nonretractable type remains static, with slack being taken up manually.
- Pretensioning systems are designed to retract automatically through a mechanical or electrical/pyrotechnical mechanism. They can be activated in conjunction with the vehicle air bags from the ECU or act independently.

- Never assume that an air bag is dead just because the power has been disconnected; a vehicle air bag system comes equipped with an energy capacitor, which can store power for up to 30 min. in some models.
- Eliminating potential hazards of SRS systems may include disconnecting power, recognizing and identifying air bags, distancing, and taking additional extrication precautions.

KEY TERMS

Accelerometer A sensor that detects a crash.

Active restraint device A device that the occupant must activate; for example, a seat belt is an active device because the occupant has to engage the seat belt mechanism into the anchor unit.

Air bag An inflatable bag that inflates automatically to cushion passengers in the event of a collision. The air bag itself typically consists of a strong, durable nylon or blended material that is folded in a certain manner to facilitate inflation.

Air bag control unit (ACU) See *electronic control unit (ECU)*.

Beneficial systems Auxiliary-powered equipment in motor vehicles or machines that can enhance or facilitate rescues such as electric, pneumatic, or hydraulic seat positioners, door locks, window operating mechanisms, suspension systems, tilt steering wheels, convertible tops, or other devices or systems to facilitate the movement (extension, retraction, raising, lowering, conveyor control) of equipment or machinery. (NFPA 1006)

Electronic control unit (ECU) Also known as the air bag control unit (ACU), this is the brains of an air bag system, consisting of a small processing unit generally located in the center of the vehicle.

Federal Motor Vehicle Safety Standards (FMVSS) Safety standards enacted to protect the public from unreasonable risk of crashes, injury, or death resulting from the design, construction, or performance of a motor vehicle.

Gas-generation system An inflation system that completely fills the air bag to the appropriate inflation ratio to protect the occupant.

Gravitational acceleration sensor (G-sensor) A sensor that detects a vehicle's weightlessness, such as that experienced in a free fall, when the vehicle starts to roll and come down.

Hybrid-type inflator Common to side-impact air bags, this device is composed of two chambers. The first-stage chamber uses a small amount of a pyrotechnic gas-producing propellant, and the second-stage chamber is filled with a compressed inert gas or another type of gas. In combination, each chamber produces and/or releases the correct amount of gas to inflate an air bag.

Inclinometer sensor A tilt sensor that detects vehicle inclination or tilt with lateral acceleration (detects how fast the vehicle's tilt is changing).

Inflators One of the most critical design features for an air bag, which provides the ability to fill up the bag instantaneously in milliseconds from the onset of the collision. There are two basic inflation systems—a stored compressed-gas system and a gas-generation system.

Initiator A device, such as a squib (a pyrotechnic device), that activates the air bag through an electrical current, which becomes instantly hot and ignites the combustible material inside the containment housing or through ignition of a burst disk, which releases compressed gas.

Load limiting device A safety design feature that reduces the force applied by the seat belt when it locks in place from the sudden force applied to it. It can be incorporated in the webbing material of the belt or in a torsion bar attached to the retractor gear.

Multistage inflators Also known as hybrid inflators; cylinders that can comprise two separate chambers of compressed gas—one with a large amount of product and the other with a smaller amount of product.

Occupant classification system A system consisting of three types of sensors: the seat position sensor, which detects the proximity of the occupant to the air bag; the seat belt sensor, which detects whether the occupant's seat belt is engaged and locked in the housing unit; and the occupant weight sensor, which measures the weight of the occupant, determining whether the occupant has met a preset weight threshold limit.

Passive restraint device A device that the occupant does not have to activate for it to function; the system is automatically activated when power is applied to the vehicle.

Rollover protection system (ROPS) A system designed to protect occupants in vehicle rollover incidents by means of a deployable roll bar.

Safing sensor A type of air bag sensor that has a deceleration setting lower than the crash-type sensor. This sensor prevents false deployments.

Seat belt pretensioning system A system designed to automatically tighten, or take up slack, in a seat belt when a crash is detected.

Side-impact air bags Air bags designed to activate immediately upon impact to protect the following areas of the occupant: the head, the chest/upper torso, and a combination of the head and the chest/upper torso. There are three types, and all three types can be found in the door, seat backs, roof posts, or roof rails. These air bags may be labeled HPS (head protection system), IC (inflatable curtain), SIPS (side-impact protection system), or ROI (rollover inflator air bag).

Smart air bag system An air bag system that automatically adjusts the pressure in the air bag by using multistage inflators and basing the deployment force on a number of calculated factors, such as crash severity, occupant's weight, proximity to the air bag, seat belt usage, and seat position.

Squib A pyrotechnic device used to ignite the propellant that produces the gas filling an air bag.

Stored compressed-gas system An inflation system comprising a single-stage or multistage inflation process. The igniter, or squib, sets off a burst, or rupture, disk that acts as a seal, holding back the compressed gas. When activated, the disk breaks open, releasing the gas from the chamber, which expands and instantly fills the air bag.

Supplemental restraint system (SRS) A system that uses supplemental restraint devices, such as air bags, to enhance safety in conjunction with properly applied seat belts. Seat belt pretensioning systems are also considered part of an SRS.

Suppression system A device that shuts down the air bag if an occupant classification system detects a child in the air bag deployment zone or if one of the sensors detects a high-risk potential by acquiring the occupant's weight, height, proximity to the air bag, seat belt usage, and seat position; the system sends this information to the electronic control unit, which will then shut off the air bag if a high risk to the occupant is determined.

On Scene

You arrive on scene at an incident involving two vehicles and two victims. One of the vehicles has rolled over. Because multiple air bags have deployed, you cannot get a good visual of the victims from your vehicle. After performing a scene size-up, you carefully approach and discover that both victims are wearing seat belts and one of the vehicles has a ROPS. All of the information you have learned about SRSs begins to flood your mind.

1. You know that air bags are known as SRSs, which are designed to be a supplement to:
   A. safe driving.
   B. rollover protection system.
   C. being properly positioned in the seat.
   D. wearing a seat belt.

2. Manual seat belts are classified as:
   A. pretensioning.
   B. active restraint devices.
   C. self-activating.
   D. supplemental restraint devices.

3. Air bags are classified as:
   A. pretensioning.
   B. active restraint devices.
   C. self-activating.
   D. passive restraint devices.

4. Before you get any closer, you recall that the technical rescuer's best defense against a live air bag is recognition/identification, disconnecting the power supply, and:
   A. deactivation.
   B. proper distancing.
   C. activation.
   D. pushing the bag out of the way.

5. A vehicle air bag system consists of all of the following except:
   A. the air bag.
   B. the electronic control unit.
   C. the sensor.
   D. the ring clip.

On Scene Continued

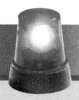

6. The entire vehicle crash process, which involves dissipating all of the kinetic energy of the vehicle, takes approximately:

   A. 100 to 125 ms.
   B. 300 to 425 ms.
   C. 800 to 825 ms.
   D. 2 s.

7. An occupant classification system normally consists of the following sensors except:

   A. a seat position sensor.
   B. a seat belt sensor.
   C. a crash sensor.
   D. an occupant weight sensor.

8. The roll bars in a ROPS can extend up to how many inches in some models?

   A. 10 in.
   B. 15 in.
   C. 12 in.
   D. 20 in.

9. The seat belt pretensioning system can be located in any of the following areas except:

   A. under the seat.
   B. in the B-post column.
   C. under the center console.
   D. in the dashboard.

10. Seat belt pretensioners activate at the belt buckle attachment or the:

    A. anchor attachment using the spool.
    B. webbing section.
    C. door.
    D. ECU.

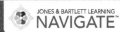

Access Navigate for more activities.

CHAPTER 7

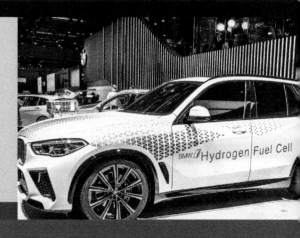

Operations and Technician Levels

Advanced Vehicle Technology: Alternative-Fuel Vehicles

KNOWLEDGE OBJECTIVES

After studying this chapter, you will be able to:

- Describe these alternative-fuel sources and explain the unique extrication hazards they present:
  - Flexible fuel (p. 173)
  - Hybrid electric (p. 188)
  - Electric (p. 193)
  - Natural gas (p. 173)
  - Liquefied petroleum gas (LPG) (p. 173)
  - Biodiesel (pp. 179–180)
  - Hydrogen fuel cell (p. 183)
- Define the following terms and explain their importance in vehicle rescue incidents:
  - *Emergency Response Guide (ERG)* (p. 169)
  - Pressure relief device (PRD) (p. 170)
  - Vehicle identification badge (p. 172)
  - Temperature relief device (TRD) (p. 185)
- Identify dangers common to all alternative-fuel vehicle extrication operations. (**NFPA 1006: 8.2.4**, pp. 169–170)
- List standard safety precautions for alternative vehicle extrication. (**NFPA 1006: 8.2.4**, pp. 170–172)
- Describe the benefits of using the *Emergency Response Guide (ERG)* for alternative-fuel vehicle extrication. (**NFPA 1006: 8.2.4**, pp. 170, 171, 175, 176, 178, 182, 186)
- List classes of hybrid vehicles and explain unique dangers associated with each. (**NFPA 8.3.1**, pp. 188–193)
- Identify typical voltage cable color coding for electric and hybrid vehicles. (pp. 189–190)
- Identify fire suppression and safety measures at an alternative-fuel vehicle extrication incident. (**NFPA 1006: 8.2.1**, pp. 169–170)
- Explain the reasons for using atmospheric monitoring equipment at an alternative-fuel vehicle incident. (pp. 170–171)

SKILLS OBJECTIVES

After studying this chapter, you will be able to perform the following skills:

- Apply universal safety procedures to alternative-fuel vehicle extrication incidents. (**NFPA 1006: 8.2.1, 8.2.2, 8.2.3, 8.2.4**, pp. 170–171)
- Apply emergency procedures to protect victims and rescuers for the following alternative fueled vehicles:
  - Ethanol and Methanol (**NFPA 1006: 8.2.4**, p. 173)
  - Natural Gas (**NFPA 1006: 8.2.4**, pp. 175–177)
  - LPG (**NFPA 1006: 8.2.4**, pp. 178–179)
  - Biodiesel (**NFPA 1006: 8.2.4**, p. 180)
  - Hydrogen (**NPA 1006: 8.2.4**, pp. 181–183)
  - Hydrogen Fuel Cell (**NFPA 1006: 8.2.4**, pp. 186–188)
  - HEV (**NFPA 1006: 8.2.4**, pp. 191–192)
  - EV (**NFPA 1006: 8.2.4**, pp. 193–194)

You Are the Rescuer

You and your crew respond to a vehicle accident involving a hybrid electric vehicle (HEV) that has been severely damaged.

1. Does the vehicle contain hybrid identification labeling or badging on the outside body to confirm that it is an HEV?
2. Is there exposed wiring?
3. Is the vehicle still running?
4. Does the vehicle contain a smart key?

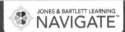

Access Navigate for more practice activities.

Introduction

The world's reliance on petroleum-based fuels has always dominated the auto industry, but the future holds many promises for the development and use of alternative fuels. Many of these alternative fuels are in use today, and rescue personnel are responsible for familiarizing themselves with these fuel types and vehicle systems and the various emergency procedures that are used to manage them.

When responding to incidents involving new technology such as new vehicle design and engineering changes, responders must realize that some safety equipment designed to protect the driver and passengers actually creates additional hazards and extrication issues for the rescuers. Examples of these hazards include multiple batteries; high-voltage power cables; advanced air bag protection systems; various types of alloyed metals, including advanced high-strength steels; a reinforced passenger compartment "safety cage"; and advanced energy management systems for collisions—to name only a few.

The addition of alternative fuels to the vehicle rescue and extrication incident establishes a new set of hazards that emergency personnel must be familiar with, along with how to manage and/or mitigate those hazards. Upon conducting a size-up, the officer must immediately recognize the various types of alternative fuels present and establish safety/hazard control zones based on recommendations from the Department of Transportation's (DOT's) *Emergency Response Guidebook (ERG)*. Additionally, the officer must incorporate the following into the incident action plan (IAP): tactical objectives for the management of these fuels regarding victim treatment and removal, spill containment, potential fire suppression, and/or vapor suppression.

LISTEN UP!

It is important that rescuers be trained to recognize all the hazards associated with alternative-fuel vehicles and how to mitigate or neutralize these hazards before the proper rescue techniques can be applied.

The term "new technology" may be a poor choice of words; given the exponential rate at which technology grows, something labeled "new technology" may very well be obsolete the minute such words are put down on paper. It is a constant challenge to keep current with all the latest advances in the development of vehicle technology. This chapter will discuss several types of alternative fuels, vehicle propulsion systems, and other prominent advancements in vehicle technology to expand the rescuer's knowledge base.

The most common issue in dealing with advanced vehicle technology in vehicle extrication is trying to demystify misinformation that may be circulating around the emergency services community. Misinformation can cause emergency personnel to overreact or not react at all. Knowledge is empowering, and the best way to start acquiring the right information is by visiting a car dealership and asking about the latest hybrid vehicle, alternative-fuel vehicle, or hydrogen fuel-cell vehicle that they have. Most dealerships will go out of their way to accommodate emergency personnel; some will send a vehicle and a technician out to departments to present the information directly. Another important resource for learning about alternative-fuel vehicles and various propulsion systems is the emergency response guide that most vehicle manufacturers offer for emergency personnel; this guide is packed with information about the vehicle and can be accessed free of charge by downloading or contacting the manufacturer. With multiple variations in the types of fuels used today as well as the varying propulsion systems, it is highly recommended that technical rescuers take advantage of these learning opportunities. It is also a good idea to spend time conducting online research.

Using the same emergency procedures on every incident involving one of these advanced vehicle systems is not practical and can be very dangerous; each vehicle system will require some of the steps in its emergency procedures that are unique to the particular type of fuel or propulsion system used. There are some similar steps in emergency procedures that are universal and can be applied to each vehicle type. But remember that the best practice model is to preplan by studying and training so you are better prepared to recognize differences in vehicle types, thus enabling you to adjust and apply your tactics appropriately. After conducting a thorough size-up, if a known immediate danger to life and health (IDLH) hazard is presented with an alternative-fuel vehicle, then set the **hazard control zones** (hot, warm, and cold) appropriate to the type of hazard recognized/confirmed. Use the DOT's ERG to determine the initial zone diameter. Also, look for any visible vapor clouds, and listen for a loud hissing noise, which may indicate product release through a leak or through a **pressure release device (PRD)**.

Depending on the type of fuel encountered, incidents requiring fire suppression may require a large-diameter hose and a master stream device placed in a defensive mode until fire control is established. This will then require a Class B foam for vapor suppression. As described in Chapter 3, *Tools and Equipment*, unignited events, such as fuel spills at motor vehicle accidents, are over 85 percent of the nation's Class B events. When these incidents occur, an alcohol-resistant aqueous film-forming foam (AR-AFFF) Class B foam that is UL listed for flammable liquids (not combustibles) should be used (as per NFPA 11, *Standard for Low-, Medium-, and High-Expansion Foam*). All unignited fuel spills should be managed as polar solvents (water-miscible fuels), requiring a polymeric membrane over the fuel to shut down the vapors. Remember, when applying water or a wetting agent, cryogenic liquids, such as compressed natural gas, can react violently when water is applied. Always refer to the DOT's ERG for fire suppression as well as vapor suppression for the type of fuel encountered. Various chemical characteristics of some of the more common alternative fuels will be discussed further in the following paragraphs.

Safety procedures can be very specific to the type of alternative fuel encountered and must be strictly adhered to, but some safety procedures are universal and can be applied to every vehicle regardless of the type of propulsion system. These safety procedures are defined in **SKILL DRILL 7-1**. Although these basic safety guidelines can be followed for all vehicle types, be aware that various vehicles will have additional or unique emergency procedures that are specific to that particular type of vehicle. Note that some of these steps are not necessarily completed in succession; some can be completed simultaneously depending on the number of personnel on scene who are available to be assigned to the step.

Follow the steps in Skill Drill 7-1 to apply some of the standard safety procedures to a vehicle, regardless of the type of propulsion system the vehicle uses.

SAFETY TIP

Never stand in front of or to the rear of an HEV before determining that the power has been shut off.

Safety

The practice of atmospheric monitoring at vehicle accidents should be considered when dealing with alternative-fuel and fuel-cell vehicles, especially with a heavier-than-air fuel, such as LPG. Unfortunately, not every agency carries the proper equipment to conduct atmospheric monitoring. A multi-gas meter will detect the presence of hazards in the air (**FIGURE 7-1**). Note, some variables may produce inaccurate readings or no reading at all, such as high wind, high humidity, or lack of proper calibration; even so, it still should be considered as a safety measure for ensuring a safe working environment. Additional sensors that detect the presence of hydrogen can be added to some models as an optional feature. Some may say that atmospheric monitoring is unnecessary because high-pressure fuel systems under compression, such as hydrogen, will rapidly empty their contents and disperse upward into the atmosphere before emergency personnel arrive on scene. Nonetheless, atmospheric monitoring is an added safety practice; if you have the equipment on the apparatus, then it should be used. Atmospheric monitoring for combustible gases should be reviewed and decided upon by the agency's authority having jurisdiction (AHJ). If used, it should be incorporated into any emergency procedures for dealing with alterative-fueled or fuel-cell vehicles.

SKILL DRILL 7-1
Applying Standard Safety Procedures to a Vehicle NFPA 1006 8.2.1, 8.2.2, 8.2.3, and 8.2.4

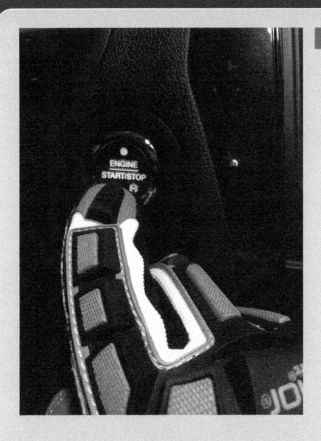

1. Don the appropriate personal protective equipment (PPE), and clear the scene of all hazards and bystanders. Approach the scene using atmospheric monitoring if available. Determine the hazard control zones using the DOT's ERG. Look for any visible vapor clouds, and listen for a loud hissing noise, which may indicate product release through a leak or through a PRD. Stage two charged 1.75-in. (44-mm) hose lines. The first line is for protection of personnel, and the second line if needed is to control the dispersion of escaping vapors. One charged 1.75-in. (44-mm) hose line is the minimum standard of protection for all vehicle extrication incidents, regardless of vehicle type. Make sure the vehicle's transmission is in park. Some vehicles have electrically controlled transmissions and require the ignition to be on to shift gears. Turn off the ignition switch of the vehicle. This turns off the engine and the electric motor(s), preventing the high-voltage electrical current from flowing into the cables and thus shutting down the fuel supply. Then, remove the key so the car cannot be accidentally restarted. Vehicles with a **smart key** will have a start/stop button. Smart keys must be moved out of operational range, a minimum of 20 ft (6 m) from the vehicle.

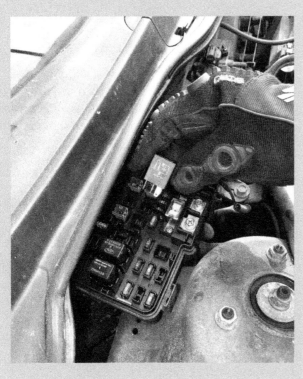

2. Stabilize the vehicle from movement with cribbing. Avoid placing any cribbing under high-voltage wiring, alternative-fuel supply lines or cylinders, and high-voltage battery packs. Location and size of the high-voltage battery pack will affect the center of mass of the vehicle. Engage the parking brake. Some vehicles have transmissions that are electronically controlled by an electric solenoid. Disable the 12-volt direct current (DC) battery by disconnecting the negative and then the positive battery cables. Manufacturers recommend removing the main fuse from the vehicle. Attempt any necessary component adjustments before disabling the power to the vehicle, such as activating the electric parking brake, adjusting power seats, and releasing hatchbacks.

Courtesy of David Sweet.

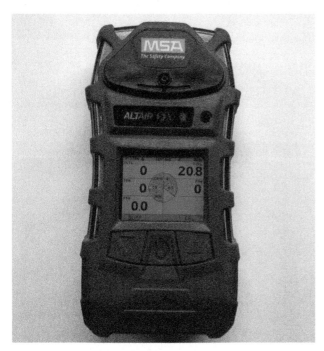

FIGURE 7-1 Multi-gas meters provide information about hazardous atmospheres.
Courtesy of Mike Smith.

SAFETY TIP

Never assume that a vehicle is turned off because it is silent or still. Always turn the ignition switch to the off position and then move the key away from the vehicle.

Alternative Fuels

An **alternative-fuel vehicle** is a motorized vehicle propelled by anything other than gasoline or diesel. These vehicles may be powered by alternative fuels, such as propane, natural gas, methanol, or hydrogen, or by electricity (battery electric vehicles), or they may be a combination of electricity and fuel (HEVs). The Energy Policy Act of 1992 outlines a list of fuels that can be classified as an "alternative fuel" for vehicles:

- Ethanol
- Methanol
- Natural gas
- LPG
- Biodiesel
- Hydrogen
- Electricity

A multitude of alternative-fuel variations are available today. This text outlines a few of the more prevalent alternative fuels and the alternative-fuel vehicles, including transit vehicles such as school buses

LISTEN UP!

Rescue personnel are responsible for situational awareness and notifying command of the type of vehicle or aftermarket products that may be in use, such as nitrous oxide or any other add-ons.

and commercial buses, that are in production. Most vehicle manufacturers will identify the vehicle type or fuel type through a labeling process known as a **vehicle identification badge**. The badges can be found at various locations on the exterior of the vehicle body, with some of the more common symbols presented as a blue triangle with the letters "CNG" for compressed natural gas, a green leaf with the letters "FCV" for fuel-cell vehicle, or simply the word "Hybrid" on the sides or rear of the vehicle (**FIGURE 7-2**). Be aware that badge labeling is not standardized and can vary in design from one manufacturer to another or may not be used at all. For some vehicles, there are NFPA requirements for the use of identification labeling. This will be discussed later in the chapter. It is recommended that the technical rescuer scan the outside of the vehicle for any vehicle identification badges prior to working on the vehicle.

LISTEN UP!

Vehicle identification badges are not standardized and can vary in design from one manufacturer to another or may not be used at all.

Ethanol and Methanol

Ethanol is a fuel composed of an alcohol base that is normally processed from crops, such as corn, sugar, trees, or grasses. Ethanol is also known as a grain alcohol and is denatured to prevent human consumption.

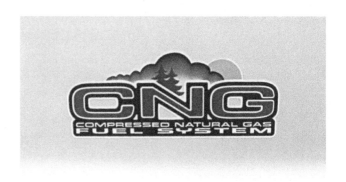

FIGURE 7-2 Most vehicle manufacturers identify the vehicle type or fuel type through a labeling process known as a vehicle identification badge.
Courtesy of David Sweet.

This fuel can be blended in several percentages with other fuels such as gasoline.

E10, better known as gasohol, is a blend of 10 percent ethanol and 90 percent gasoline. This blend is classified by the Environmental Protection Agency (EPA) as "substantially similar" to gasoline and is not considered an alternative fuel. All auto manufacturers approve the use of blends of 10 percent or less in their gasoline vehicles.

Another ethanol option is E85 flex fuel. E85 contains 85 percent ethanol and 15 percent gasoline. E85 is classified as an alternative fuel and is used to fuel E85-capable **flexible fuel vehicles (FFVs)**. FFVs are capable of running on gasoline alone or on the E85 blend of up to 85 percent ethanol and 15 percent gasoline.

Methanol, like ethanol, is an alcohol-based fuel. Methanol is known as a wood alcohol because it is processed from natural wood sources, such as trees and yard clippings. Methanol can also be used as a flex fuel in a ratio of 85 percent methanol and 15 percent gasoline, better known as M85. Since the early 1990s, the use of methanol has dramatically declined in the United States; it is, however, widely used outside of the United States. Methane is the most common gas used to extract or separate the hydrogen gas from within it through a steam-reforming or electrolysis process. This process will be discussed in the hydrogen gas section.

More vehicle manufacturers are offering FFVs, and most label the vehicle with a flex fuel badge on the side or rear of the vehicle (**FIGURE 7-3**); as of 2008, most manufacturers have also started using yellow gas caps to indicate this distinction, but remember that this is not standardized among manufacturers.

Ethanol and Methanol Emergency Procedures

Because both ethanol and methanol are alcohol-based fuels, when their content is greater than 10 percent of the fuel mixture, they require an alcohol-resistant foam as the effective method of fire extinguishment. In the case of a breached fuel tank, vapor suppression and the use of diking procedures may be necessary to contain runoff. Diking is the placement of materials to form a barrier that will keep a liquid hazardous material from entering an area or hold a liquid hazardous material in a given area. Both fuels are also miscible in water and will separate from the gasoline blend when water is applied. With the exception of a vehicle fire, the emergency procedures will be the same as those for a standard conventional vehicle.

Natural Gas

Natural gas is a fossil fuel primarily composed of methane that can be used as compressed natural gas or liquefied natural gas. Although known as one of the cleanest burning alternative fuels, natural gas vehicles are not produced commercially in large numbers but are steadily growing each year.

When natural gas is processed and cooled to a temperature below −260°F (−162°C), it turns into a cryogenic liquid and can be used as liquefied natural gas in vehicles that have been modified to run on this fuel. **Liquefied natural gas (LNG)** is a colorless, odorless, nontoxic gas that floats on water and is lighter than air when released as a vapor. LNG has an expansion vapor ratio that is 600 to 1 and a flammability ratio of 5 to 15 percent. When LNG flows out of a tank from a leak, it will form a liquid pool and then boil off into gas form. Because of its cryogenic state and large expansion ratio, as LNG changes to a gas and releases into the atmosphere, it condenses the dry ambient air surrounding it, causing a visible vapor cloud to appear. This vapor cloud does not necessarily comprise natural gas because the actual gas can travel well ahead of or behind the cloud, depending upon the general wind currents.

Avoid using water on an LNG leak or fire because the warm water will cause the liquid gas to violently react with an instant boil-off, causing a sudden expansion and vaporization of the liquid, which will intensify a fire or cause an explosion. High-expansion foam or dry chemicals are best used for this type of incident in place of water. A hose stream should be directed toward a vapor cloud only to disperse the product; be cognizant of the PRD location, and avoid directing the stream toward this area, which could freeze the device and render it inoperable. PRDs rapidly release product through a small metal tube attachment when they detect excessive amounts of heat at a preset temperature.

The fuel tank needed to store LNG to keep it in its cryogenic liquid state must be double walled and well

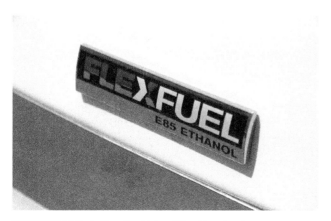

FIGURE 7-3 A flex fuel identification badge.
© David R. Frazier Photolibrary, Inc./Alamy Stock Photo.

insulated to prevent a boil-off. This makes the tanks very bulky, limiting space in a vehicle; these types of tanks are commonly placed in trunks. LNG is stored at low pressures in tanks up to a maximum pressure of 230 psi (1586 kPa) and is regulated back down to an operating pressure up to 120 psi (827 kPa). Remember that LNG is stored as a cryogen, which is a liquid that boils at temperatures below −260°F (−162°C). It is in a constant state of boil-off and is consistently changing into a gas. As a result, there will always be an increase in the tank vessel pressure, which is regulated by a PRD. As the liquid is drawn from the tank to the vehicle's internal combustion engine, it travels through the fuel lines and is heated by a heating mechanism to change it to its useable gaseous state for the internal combustion engine. NFPA 52, *Vehicular Gaseous Fuel Systems Code*, covers all the requirements for fuel storage and use of LNG fuel vehicle systems.

Compressed natural gas (CNG) is a natural lighter-than-air gas compressed for use as a fuel that consists principally of methane in gaseous form plus naturally occurring mixtures of hydrocarbon. It is much more practical and is used primarily as a fuel type for many fleet vehicles found on the roadways today. CNG storage tanks are composed of steel, aluminum, or carbon fiber/composite (**FIGURE 7-4**). According to the DOT, these tanks must go through extensive crash and drop tests to ensure durability. In passenger vehicles, these fuel tanks are normally located behind the rear passenger seat or in the trunk area or under the vehicle in some fleet vehicles.

To achieve the desired pressures for storage, natural gas is compressed to pressures ranging from 3000 to 3600 psi (20,684 to 24,821 kPa) and may have to be stored in several onboard tanks to achieve the same mile range as gasoline (**FIGURE 7-5**). These high storage pressures are regulated at the engine to workable pressures. Stainless steel high-pressure lines run under the vehicle from the tanks to the engine compartment (**FIGURE 7-6**). Several safety features are built into both CNG and LNG fuel systems; these features will vary depending on the manufacturer. One such safety design occurs when the vehicle's ignition is turned off; a sensing unit or valve will turn off the fuel at the tanks, stopping any flow of fuel from escaping. This sensing unit or valve will also engage and shut off the tank when any leak is detected. Depending on the manufacturer, each tank will have its own manual shutoff valve that can be accessed from under the vehicle or through the trunk area if the tank is placed in the trunk (**FIGURE 7-7**). This will cut off all fuel from the tanks to the engine. Another safety feature is the PRD. The PRD is designed to rapidly release all the gas when exposed to high temperatures, such as exposure to fire, which causes an overpressurization of the cylinder and actuates the PRD. PRDs are also

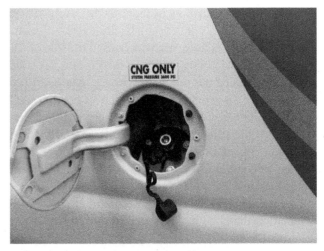

FIGURE 7-5 To achieve the desired pressures for storage, natural gas is compressed to pressures ranging from 3000 to 3600 psi (20,684 to 24,821 kPa) and may have to be stored in several tanks to achieve the same mile range as gasoline.
Courtesy of David Sweet.

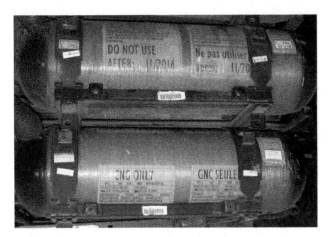

FIGURE 7-4 CNG storage tanks are composed of steel, aluminum, or carbon fiber/composite.
Courtesy of David Sweet.

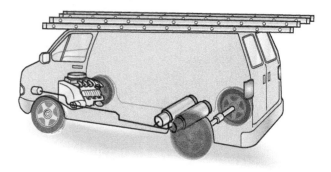

FIGURE 7-6 Stainless steel high-pressure lines run under the vehicle from the tanks to the engine compartment.
Courtesy of Culver Company.

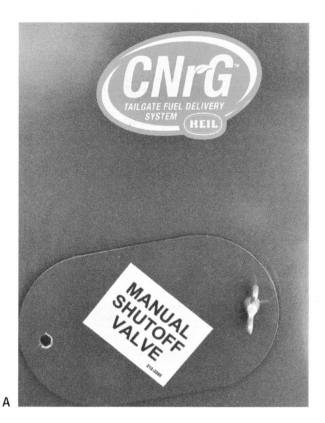

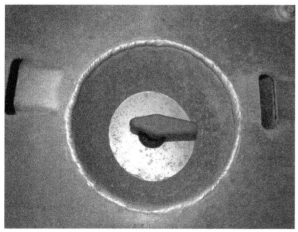

FIGURE 7-7 Depending on the manufacturer, each tank will have its own manual shutoff valve. **A**. The manual shutoff valve can be accessed from under the vehicle or through the trunk area if the tank is placed in the trunk. **B**. A manual shutoff valve.
A: Courtesy of Heil Company. B: Courtesy of David Sweet.

required to be vented to the outside of the vehicle with the relief valve discharge points directed upward or downward within 45 degrees of vertical. Emergency personnel should be aware of these discharge points. Remember, natural gas is lighter than air and will dissipate when released into the atmosphere. As another safety measure for CNG-type fuels, a chemical odorant called ethyl mercaptan is added primarily to detect any potential leaks.

According to NFPA 52, vehicles that use both CNG and LNG as fuels are required to be clearly marked

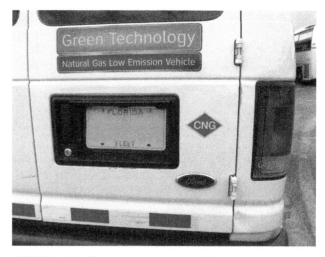

FIGURE 7-8 The natural gas identification label should have a diamond shape with the letters "CNG" or "LNG" in white or silver reflective lettering against a blue or dark background.
Courtesy of David Sweet.

with an identification label adhered to the right lower rear section of the vehicle. This identification label should have a diamond shape with the letters "CNG" or "LNG" in white or silver reflective lettering against a blue or dark background (**FIGURE 7-8**).

Natural Gas Emergency Procedures

It is highly recommended that the technical rescuer review various manufacturers' emergency response guides for dealing with vehicles that use LNG or CNG as a fuel. Also, the DOT's *ERG*, particularly Guide 115, is a great reference for initial planning (**FIGURE 7-9**). Some of the guides recommend steps for mitigating any potential problems or leaks before attempting to extricate any victims. This will be determined by the incident commander (IC); quick hazard and risk analyses will have to be determined prior to taking action. The hazard analysis identifies situations or conditions that may injure people or personnel or may damage property or the environment. The risk analysis assesses the risk to the rescuers compared to the benefits that might come from the rescue. Hazard and risk analyses are continual processes that are reevaluated throughout the entire incident.

General emergency procedures when dealing with CNG or LNG incidents include the following. Note, some of these steps are not necessarily completed in succession; some of them can be completed simultaneously depending on the number of personnel on scene who are available to be assigned to complete each step.

- Don the appropriate PPE, including self-contained breathing apparatus (SCBA) if needed, and clear the scene of all bystanders and hazards.

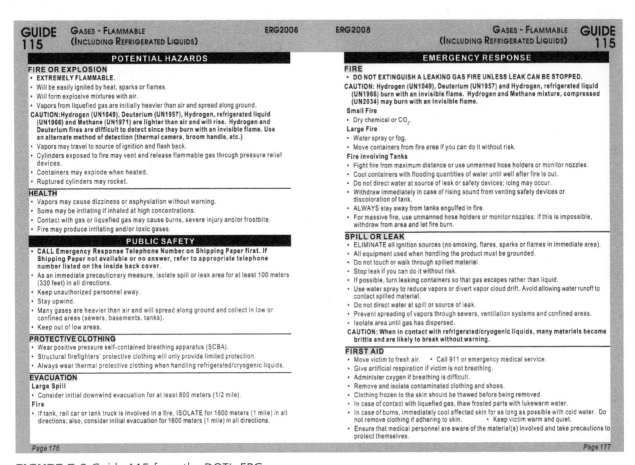

FIGURE 7-9 Guide 115 from the DOT's *ERG*.
Courtesy of the U.S. Department of Transportation.

- Establish hazard control zones (hot, warm, and cold). Use the DOT's *ERG* as a reference guide to determine initial zone sizing.
- Conduct the inner and outer surveys. If possible, approach the vehicle from upwind and uphill and from the sides because the CNG and LNG tanks are commonly stored in the trunk area, behind the rear seat, or under the vehicle. Look for a visible vapor cloud, and listen for a hissing noise, which may indicate product release through a leak or through a PRD.
- A multi-gas meter can identify combustible gases at the accident site, based on the sensors in the unit. If carried on an apparatus, a combustible gas meter is used to pinpoint possible leaks and concentrations of combustible gases or vapors in the surrounding atmosphere. This is a continuous process until the leak has been contained and stopped.
- Look for a vehicle identification badge; in this situation, it may be a blue or dark-colored diamond shape with the letters "CNG" or "LNG" in white or silver.
- Two 1.75-in. (44-mm) charged hose lines should be deployed to protect personnel and disperse any significant release of LNG vapor or CNG product to keep it below the flammable range. Fires involving vehicles utilizing CNG as the fuel source should not be extinguished until the leak can be isolated and eliminated or the fuel tank containing the product can be shut down.
- When the scene is safe, ensure that the vehicle's ignition is turned off, the keys are out of the ignition, and the vehicle is placed in park.
- Stabilize the vehicle from movement with cribbing. Avoid placing any cribbing under high-voltage wiring, alternative-fuel supply lines or cylinders, and high-voltage battery packs. Location and size of the high-voltage battery pack can affect the center of mass of the vehicle.
- Attempt any necessary component adjustments before disabling the power to the vehicle, such as activating the electric parking brake, adjusting power seats, and releasing hatchbacks.

- Disconnect the 12-volt DC battery starting with the negative line first. (Location of the 12-volt DC battery will vary on each model of vehicle.)
- Manually turn off the gas at the tanks utilizing the shutoff valves.
- Manufacturers recommend removal of the main fuse from the vehicle to ensure that the electrical system is disabled. This will be an AHJ's decision because the location of fuses can vary greatly among models.

For CNG to be combustible, it must fall within its flammability range. Flammability range refers to the amount of a gas that must be present in the surrounding air for combustion to occur. For CNG, this amount is 5 to 15 percent. Thus, if an air mixture contains 4 percent CNG, it will not support combustion; likewise, if an air mixture contains 16 percent CNG, it will also not support combustion. The same procedures are to be followed for PRDs that are releasing product with visible flame. Do not extinguish the flame; instead cool the tank, or eliminate the flame impingement, and the PRD will reset and self-extinguish once the tank and product are cooled. The high pressure of CNG tanks, 3000 to 3600 psi (20,684 to 24,821 kPa), should cause the contents to release quickly, and the fire at the point of product release should self-extinguish. Other exposures, such as the vehicle itself, additional vehicles, or surrounding structures, can be protected and/or extinguished with hose streams if needed. Until the leak can be isolated and eliminated, it is safer to let the product burn itself out.

When attempting an extrication technique on a CNG or an LNG fuel vehicle utilizing power or hand tools, it is best practice to ensure that the emergency procedures discussed in Skill Drill 7-1 are followed, which includes wearing full protective gear, including SCBA, to ensure safety. Also, examine the vehicle carefully for fuel line locations before attempting any cutting. The techniques that will require extra caution will be any of the dash displacement techniques where relief cuts are made or tearing will occur when the dash is released or pushed forward. In addition, techniques that involve cutting and dropping the floorboard area under the brake and gas pedals should not be attempted. Such maneuvers could expose high-voltage wires or gas lines running under the rocker panel channel area, which should be avoided regardless of the type of fuel system the vehicle uses or whether the power supply has been secured. Alternative techniques that are safer should be considered.

Liquefied Petroleum Gas

Liquefied petroleum gas (LPG), also known as propane, is a fossil fuel produced from the processing of natural gas and also produced as part of the refining process of crude oil. Propane is the third most widely used fuel source behind gasoline and diesel; it is commonly used with forklifts and other similar work units.

Propane is heavier than air (1.5 times as dense) and will sink and pool at floor level when released into the atmosphere. Propane fuel tanks that are designed for passenger vehicles are built according to the specifications and standards set by the American Society of Mechanical Engineers (ASME) *Boiler and Pressure Vessel Code*.

In compliance with the *Boiler and Pressure Vessel Code* of the ASME, propane vehicle tanks are constructed from carbon steel. These tanks are designed to be 20 times more puncture resistant than a standard gasoline tank. ASME tanks used for passenger vehicles vary in size but cannot exceed 200 gal (757 L) according to NFPA 58, *Liquefied Petroleum Gas Code*. The fill capacity of an ASME tank uses water in gallons as a unit of measurement; this is expressed in the letter markings on the tank normally stenciled in "WC" (water capacity). Because of the high expansion rate of propane (270 parts gas to 1 part liquid, or 270:1), when a tank is filled there is a mandatory 20 percent reduction in product to account for this expansion space. To ensure that the proper expansion space is provided, all tanks are designed with an overfill prevention device that limits a tank to 80 to 85 percent capacity, leaving a 20 percent vapor space just above the fuel line. With the 20 percent reduction, a tank that has a rated WC of 100 gal (379 L) can be filled to hold 80 gal (303 L) of propane. Propane weighs approximately 4.24 lb/gal (0.5 kg/L).

As used with CNG fuels, a chemical odorant called ethyl mercaptan is added to propane as a safety measure to detect any potential leaks. Propane tanks are also equipped with a PRD to release any overpressure caused by high temperature exposure, such as flame impingement. PRDs are also required to be vented to the outside of the vehicle with the relief valve discharge points directed upward or downward within 45 degrees of vertical. Emergency personnel should be aware of these discharge points.

Propane is normally a vapor gas at temperatures above its boiling point (−44°F [−42°C]). When stored under pressure, it is compressed into a liquid state and will remain in a liquid state. When a leak occurs, propane will rapidly convert back to a gaseous state, expanding 270 times its original liquid volume. Rapid release of propane from the tank into the atmosphere will cause frost to accumulate at the liquid level on the outside of the tank. This frost is produced because of the rapid drop in pressure and temperature inside the tank. On an outside tank used to supply fuel to a building or facility, a frost line may be readily visible, but because a tank or cylinder may be concealed in the vehicle, the technical rescuer may not have access to visualize this frost line to determine the amount of remaining product in the tank.

The required working pressure of an ASME tank supplying propane as fuel for passenger vehicles is designed to provide either 250 psi (1724 kPa) if constructed prior to April 1, 2001, or 312 psi (2151 kPa) if constructed on or after April 1, 2001. This is a significant difference from natural gas, which is stored under pressures of 3000 to 3600 psi (20,684 to 24,821 kPa).

Passenger vehicle propane tanks must contain an identification label on the tank itself that displays at a minimum the following information: WC, working pressure, serial number of the tank, and manufacturer.

NFPA 58 also requires that main shutoff valves on a container for liquid or vapor be accessible and operated without the use of any tools or that there be specific equipment provided that can shut off the valve. Also, any LPG container that is permanently installed in a vehicle requires that vehicle to be clearly marked with an identification label adhered to the right lower rear section of the vehicle. This identification label should have a diamond shape with the word "Propane" in white or silver reflective lettering against a black or dark background (**FIGURE 7-10**). Even with this type of labeling requirement in place, because of the inconsistencies that can occur with vehicle identification badging, it is not recommended to rely on these types of identification markings as the only sign that you are dealing with an alternative-fuel vehicle. Always use precaution, and monitor the environment with a gas reading meter to determine whether any flammable vapors exist upon approach.

Proper labeling may be missing from a vehicle that has had aftermarket alterations. The fuel system may have been converted from a gasoline engine to an alternative-fuel engine, such as propane or natural gas. There are some conversion kits that allow the user to run both types of fuel systems; when the gasoline tank runs low, a switch can be flipped so the vehicle runs on propane from an onboard aftermarket-installed tank. These types of propulsion systems will more than likely not have any identification badging on the outside of the vehicle to warn responders.

LPG Emergency Procedures

As just mentioned with natural gas emergency procedures, it is highly recommended that the technical rescuer review emergency response guides pertaining to propane fuel vehicles, which are provided by some vehicle manufacturers. Also, the DOT's *ERG*, particularly Guide 115, is an excellent reference for initial planning. Some of the guides recommend steps for mitigating any potential problems or leaks before attempting to extricate any victims. This will be determined by the IC; quick hazard and risk analyses will have to be determined prior to taking action. Keep in mind again that propane is 1.5 times heavier than air and will accumulate in low-lying areas, such as a ditch or lower road embankment, or can accumulate in confined spaces, such as passenger compartments or truck cargo areas. Propane disperses well beyond its vapor cloud and will seek out ignition sources, which can cause a flashback to the leak.

If there is a substantial breach in the tank, there will be an initial blow-off of product to reduce the overall tank pressure. There can be a freezing of the product with a slower leak.

When dealing with vehicles using LPG as a fuel, general emergency procedures include the actions listed below. Note that some of these actions are not necessarily completed in succession; some of them can be completed simultaneously depending on the number of personnel on scene who are available to be assigned to complete each step.

- Don the appropriate PPE, including SCBA if needed, and clear the scene of all bystanders and hazards.
- Establish hazard control zones (hot, warm, and cold). Use the DOT's *ERG* as a reference guide to determine initial zone sizing.
- Conduct the inner and outer surveys. If possible, approach the vehicle from upwind and uphill

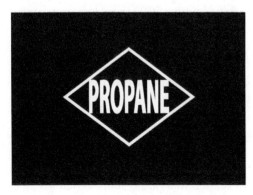

FIGURE 7-10 Any vehicle with a permanently installed LPG container must be clearly marked with a diamond shape with the word "Propane" in white or silver reflective lettering against a black background.

and from the sides because like CNG tanks, LPG tanks may be stored in the trunk area. A loud hissing noise may indicate a leak or the PRD rapidly expelling product from the tank. Unlike CNG and compressed hydrogen gas, which both rise and dissipate quickly, propane is heavier than air and will linger and accumulate in lower areas or confined spaces, causing a flashback to the leak or product release point. The technical rescuer must ensure that the area is safe to work in before attempting to operate on the vehicle.

- If carried on an apparatus, use a combustible gas meter to detect possible leaks and concentrations of combustible gases or vapors in the surrounding atmosphere. This is a continuous process until the leak has been contained and stopped.
- Look for any vehicle identification badging on the outside body of the vehicle, which can indicate LPG on board. This label must have a diamond shape with the word "Propane" in white or silver reflective lettering against a black or dark background.
- Two 1.75-in. (44-mm) charged hose lines should be deployed to protect personnel and disperse any significant release of propane product to keep it below the flammable range.
- When the scene is safe, ensure that the vehicle's ignition is turned off, the keys are removed from the ignition, and the vehicle is placed in park.
- Stabilize the vehicle from movement with cribbing. Avoid placing any cribbing under high-voltage wiring, alternative-fuel supply lines or cylinders, and high-voltage battery packs. Location and size of the high-voltage battery pack will affect the center of mass of the vehicle.
- Attempt any necessary component adjustments before disabling the power to the vehicle, such as activating the electric parking brake, adjusting power seats, and releasing hatchbacks.
- Disconnect the 12-volt DC battery starting with the negative line first. (Location of the 12-volt DC battery will vary on each model of vehicle.)
- Manually turn off the gas at the tanks using the shutoff valve. If the tanks are located in the trunk, remember that there is the potential for a large amount of propane product to accumulate in this space.
- Manufacturers recommend removal of the main fuse from the vehicle to ensure that the electrical system is disabled. This will be an AHJ's decision because the location of fuses can vary greatly among models.

Fires involving vehicles equipped with propane can present unique challenges to the rescuer. For propane to be combustible, it must fall within its flammability range, which is 2.15 to 9.6 percent. Thus, if an air mixture contains only 2 percent propane, it will not support combustion; likewise, if an air mixture contains 10 percent propane, it also will not support combustion. Continuous flame impingement on a tank containing propane will cause the overpressurization and eventual failure of the tank in an explosive reaction known as a **boiling liquid/expanding vapor explosion (BLEVE)**. This reaction occurs when a pressurized liquefied material starts to boil from the flame impingement and releases vapor, which in turn sets off the PRD. When the PRD can no longer compensate for the expanding vapor, which is 270 parts vapor to 1 part liquid (270:1), the tank will start to bulge and eventually fail at its weakest point, releasing a fireball of product and tank pieces. To counter this, hose streams must be directed toward the vapor space of the tank to cool the tank until the PRD is reseated; the fire is then extinguished. If there is a leak with an active fire or the PRD has a flame coming out of it, the fire must not be extinguished, or the product will just be free to release and seek out a new ignition source. The tank must be cooled, the leak must be stopped, or the main shutoff valve must be turned off before the fire is extinguished.

When attempting to extricate on an LPG fuel vehicle utilizing power or hand tools, the same precautions should be used as were described for CNG fuel vehicles. Ensure that the emergency procedures discussed in Skill Drill 7-1 are followed. This includes wearing full protective gear, including SCBA, to ensure safety. Also, examine the vehicle carefully for fuel line locations before attempting any cutting. The techniques that will require extra caution will be any of the dash displacement techniques where relief cuts are made, or tearing will occur when the dash is released or pushed forward. In addition, techniques that involve cutting and dropping the floorboard area under the brake and gas pedals should not be attempted. Such maneuvers could expose high-voltage wires or gas lines running under the rocker panel or channel area. This should be avoided regardless of the type of fuel system the vehicle uses or whether the power supply has been secured. This is not a safe practice.

Biodiesel

Biodiesel is a fuel used solely for diesel engines that is processed from domestic renewable resources, such as plant oils; grease; animal fats; used cooking oil; and, more recently, algae. Biodiesel can be used by itself as a diesel fuel (B100 [100 percent biodiesel]), although B100 is not recommended for use in low temperatures. Biodiesel can also be blended with petroleum diesel at varying percentages—B2 (2 percent biodiesel), B5, and B20. Biodiesel produces fewer air pollutants than petroleum-based diesel and is safe, nontoxic, and biodegradable.

The DOT does not classify biodiesel as a flammable liquid because it has a high flash point (199°F [93°C]). As compared to other fuels, biodiesel has a flash point that is much higher than that of petrodiesel (100°F [38°C]) or gasoline (−45°F [−43°C]). Biodiesel-blended fuels will act as a hydrocarbon-type fuel or a polar solvent depending on the fuel's purity and type of blend. It is best to use an aqueous film-forming foam (AFFF) because this type of foam system can be used on both polar-solvent and hydrocarbon-based fires.

An example of a biodiesel identification badge is shown in **FIGURE 7-11**.

Biodiesel Emergency Procedures

Emergency procedures for vehicles utilizing biodiesel as a fuel are similar to those for a standard conventional vehicle. Because of its high flash point, biodiesel is not considered a flammable liquid. However, it will still burn and require proper emergency procedures for handling a spill, which, again, are similar to those for handling a hydrocarbon spill. Using a foam blanket with an AR-AFFF to suppress vapors is the best practice, including encompassing any diking procedures to control runoff.

> **LISTEN UP!**
> AR-AFFF is best used on a biodiesel or biodiesel-blended fuel spill to suppress vapors from finding any ignition source.

Hydrogen

Hydrogen is one of the most abundant elements on Earth. It is an odorless, colorless, flammable, nontoxic gas that combines easily with other elements. Hydrogen came into the spotlight in 1937 after the tragedy of the Hindenburg airship (**FIGURE 7-12**). The airship used hydrogen gas to create its buoyancy, but during a maneuver to dock the ship, static electricity caught the ship's outer liner on fire. The product used to coat the liner was extremely flammable and ignited, easily consuming the entire vessel. The hydrogen gas in the ship escaped almost immediately once the shell was breached. Hydrogen was proven not to be the culprit in this accident, which was the belief for many decades.

Hydrogen is relatively buoyant, being 14 times lighter than air; it rises and disperses at a rate of 44 mi/h (71 km/h) at approximately 66 ft/s (20 m/s); thus, its contents are quickly emptied and the flammability concentrations dissipated on smaller tanks. Hydrogen has a very wide flammability range, between 4 and 75 percent in air, and its flame burns almost clear, making it very difficult to see when ignited during daylight hours. The dispersion rate of hydrogen is two times faster than helium and six times faster than natural gas. There is no chemical odor additive in hydrogen because the dispersion rate and buoyancy are too great for any odor chemical to keep up with it. The expansion volume ratio of liquid hydrogen into a vapor or gaseous state is 1 part liquid to 848 parts vapor (1:848).

Hydrogen is unique because it can be produced domestically from multiple resources, such as fossil fuels, plants/algae, or water. In the United States, 95 percent of the hydrogen used today is produced from the methane in natural gas using a high-temperature

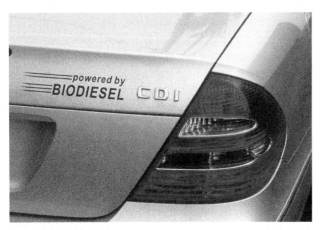

FIGURE 7-11 An example of a biodiesel identification badge.
© Bill Brooks/Alamy Stock Photo.

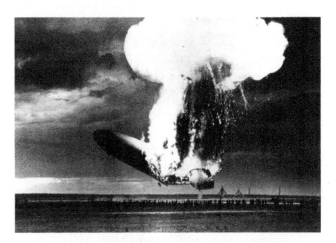

FIGURE 7-12 Hydrogen came into the spotlight in 1937 after the Hindenburg tragedy.
© Photos 12/Alamy Stock Photo.

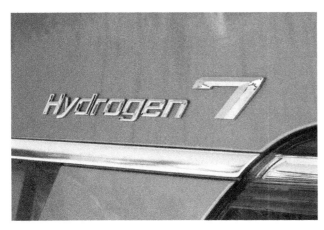

FIGURE 7-13 The identification label for hydrogen may have the word "Hydrogen" in white or silver reflective lettering or may have the word "Hydrogen" somewhere on the vehicle.
© GIPhotoStock Z/Alamy Stock Photo.

steam process called steam methane reforming. This process separates the hydrogen from the methane.

Hydrogen gas can be used directly on a modified internal combustion engine (ICE) or as a catalyst for producing electricity in a fuel cell to run a vehicle. Hydrogen fuel-cell vehicles will be discussed later in this chapter. Vehicles fueled by hydrogen are required to be clearly marked with an identification label adhered to the right lower rear section of the vehicle. Using the same labeling identification markings found with CNG, LNG, and LPG, the identification label for hydrogen may have the word "Hydrogen" in white or silver reflective lettering against a blue or dark background or may have the word "Hydrogen" somewhere on the vehicle (**FIGURE 7-13**).

> **LISTEN UP!**
>
> Hydrogen gas can be used directly on a modified ICE or as a catalyst for producing electricity in a fuel cell to run a vehicle.

Hydrogen Storage Tanks

There are several ways to store hydrogen on a passenger vehicle when used as a fuel:

- Hydrogen can be stored as a liquid but must be cooled to −423°F (−253°C) or it will boil off as a gas.
- Hydrogen can be compressed and stored in high-pressure storage tanks with pressures of 3600, 5000, and 10,000 psi (24,821; 34,474; and 68,948 kPa).
- Hydrogen can be chemically combined in hydride form with certain metals, which can store it more compactly and efficiently than in a gas form.
- Hydrogen can also be stored in the microscopic pores of carbon nanotubes.

Hydrogen storage tanks must conform to several safety standards. Because of its low-molecular structure, hydrogen has very strict storage requirements; hydrogen can cause certain metals to become brittle and fail. Currently, hydrogen storage tanks must meet the federal government's Federal Motor Vehicle Safety Standard (FMVSS) 304 (49 CFR 571.304), *Compressed Natural Gas Fuel Container Integrity*. The International Association for Natural Gas Vehicles lists four pressure cylinder types for various applications and fuel storage, such as CNG, LNG, and hydrogen. These are the various types of fuel tanks that a rescuer can encounter on an alternative-fuel or fuel-cell vehicle.

- *Type 1*: This cylinder type is composed of steel only. Only paint covers the outside of the cylinder. This is the most common type of cylinder.
- *Type 2*: This cylinder type is composed of steel or aluminum with a partial hoop wrap that goes around the cylinder. The wrapping material, which goes over the sidewall, can be made of fiberglass or carbon fiber.
- *Type 3*: This cylinder type is composed of the same material as the Type 2 cylinder; however, the wrapping encompasses the entire tank, including the domes. This type of cylinder has a metal liner, usually made of aluminum.
- *Type 4*: This cylinder type has a nonmetallic liner, usually plastic, and is fully wrapped, including the domes, with the same kind of material used for the Type 2 cylinder.

According to the U.S. Department of Energy and their Alternative Fuel Data Center website, as of August 2020, there were 46 hydrogen fueling stations located throughout the United States, with the majority originating in the state of California. (**FIGURE 7-14**). New standards and codes for hydrogen gas vehicles are currently being developed by the Department of Energy (DOE) because the use of hydrogen as a fuel is relatively new. There are numerous training resources for emergency response personnel provided through the H2 Tools website (n.d.), which is funded by the DOE.

Hydrogen Emergency Procedures

Emergency procedures for vehicles that use hydrogen as a fuel are similar to those for CNG and LNG. It is highly recommended that the technical rescuer review emergency response guides dealing with vehicles that

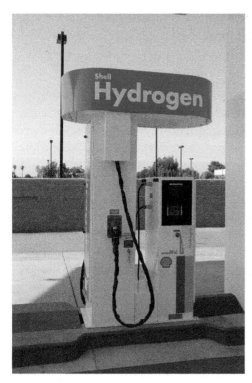

FIGURE 7-14 A hydrogen pump.
Photo courtesy of Michael Penev/NREL.

use hydrogen as a fuel. Also, the DOT's ERG, particularly Guide 115, is a great reference for initial planning. Most guides recommend that any potential problems or leaks be mitigated before attempting to extricate any victims. This will be determined by the IC; quick hazard and risk analyses will have to be determined prior to taking action. The hazard analysis identifies situations or conditions that may injure people or personnel or may damage property or the environment. The risk analysis assesses the risk to the rescuers compared to the benefits that might come from the rescue. Hazard and risk analyses are continual processes that are reevaluated throughout the entire incident.

General emergency procedures when dealing with hydrogen-fueled vehicle incidents include the following. Note, some of these steps are not necessarily completed in succession; some of them can be completed simultaneously depending on the number of personnel on scene who are available to be assigned to complete each step.

- Don the appropriate PPE, including SCBA if needed, and clear the scene of all bystanders and hazards.
- Establish hazard control zones (hot, warm, and cold). Use the DOT's *ERG* as a reference guide to determine initial zone sizing.
- Conduct the inner and outer surveys. If possible, approach the vehicle from upwind and uphill and from the sides because hydrogen tanks can be stored in the trunk area or just below the rear section of the vehicle. Look for any visible vapor clouds, and listen for hissing noises, which indicate product release through a leak or through a PRD.
- If carried on an apparatus, use a hydrogen-specific gas meter to detect possible leaks and concentrations of combustible gases or vapors in the surrounding atmosphere. This is a continuous process until the leak has been contained and stopped.
- Look for a vehicle identification badge; in this situation, it may be the word "Hydrogen" in white or silver reflective lettering against a blue or dark background or may have the word "Hydrogen" somewhere on the vehicle.
- Two 1.75-in. (44-mm) charged hose lines should be deployed to protect personnel and disperse any significant release of vapor from liquid hydrogen or a compressed hydrogen gas product to keep it below the flammable range.
- When the scene is safe, ensure that the vehicle's ignition is turned off, the keys are removed from the ignition, and the vehicle is in park.
- Stabilize the vehicle from movement with cribbing. Avoid placing any cribbing under high-voltage wiring, alternative-fuel supply lines or cylinders, and high-voltage battery packs. Location and size of the high-voltage battery pack will affect the center of mass of the vehicle.
- Attempt any necessary component adjustments before disabling the power to the vehicle, such as activating the electric parking brake, adjusting power seats, and releasing hatchbacks.
- Disconnect the 12-volt DC battery starting with the negative line first. (Location of the 12-volt DC battery will vary on each model of vehicle.)
- Manually turn off the gas at the tanks utilizing the shutoff valves.
- Manufacturers recommend removal of the main fuse from the vehicle to ensure that the electrical system is disabled. This will be an AHJ's decision because the location of fuses can vary greatly among models.
- Some manufacturers recommend using service disconnects as indicated in the manufacturer's emergency response guide for that particular vehicle. This will be an AHJ's decision because the location of service disconnects can vary greatly among models.

Hydrogen burns with a nearly invisible flame that is difficult to see during daylight hours. A thermal imaging camera (TIC) is a useful tool to identify a hydrogen fire if no other material is burning. Fires involving vehicles using hydrogen gas as the fuel source, whether as a compressed gas or a cryogenic liquid, should not be extinguished until the leak can be isolated and eliminated or the fuel tank containing the product can be shut down. The same procedures are to be followed for PRDs that are releasing product with visible flame. Do not extinguish the flame; instead, cool the tank or eliminate the flame impingement, and the PRD will reset and self-extinguish once the tank and product are cooled. Remember that PRDs are also required to be vented to the outside of the vehicle, with the relief valve discharge points directed upward or downward within 45 degrees of vertical. Emergency personnel should be aware of these discharge points. The high pressure of hydrogen storage tanks (3000 to 10,000 psi [20,684 to 68,948 kPa]) causes the contents to release quickly, and the fire at the point of product release should self-extinguish. Other exposures, such as the vehicle itself, additional vehicles, or surrounding structures, can be protected and/or extinguished with hose streams if needed, but until the leak can be isolated and eliminated, it is safer to let the product burn itself out.

Hydrogen Fuel-Cell Vehicles

A fuel cell is an electrochemical device that combines hydrogen and oxygen to produce electricity to power a motor or generator, with the by-products of this process being water and heat. In a vehicle powered by a fuel cell, the electric motor is powered by electricity generated by the fuel cell. The fuel cell uses hydrogen that is stored in an onboard tank combined with the outside oxygen to produce the electricity. According to the California Air Resources Board (n.d.), hydrogen fuel-cell vehicles are potentially two to three times more efficient than conventional vehicles, emitting little or no greenhouse gas emissions. The space industry has used this technology for many years.

The first fuel cell was developed in 1839 by Sir William Grove, who is also known as the "father of the fuel cell." He referred to his invention as the gas voltaic battery, which many years later was changed to the fuel cell. TABLE 7-1 lists a few of the common fuel-cell vehicles.

Four basic elements make up a fuel cell: the anode, the cathode, the electrolyte, and the catalyst (FIGURE 7-15). In a fuel cell, an electrolyte membrane called a polymer exchange membrane (PEM), or proton exchange membrane (PEM), is placed between an anode (negative electrode) and a cathode (positive

TABLE 7-1 Fuel-Cell Vehicles*

Manufacturer	Model	Class	Type
Honda	Clarity FCV	FCV	Sedan
Hyundai	Nexo FCEV	FCV	SUV
Toyota	Mirai	FCV	Sedan

*Note: Fuel-cell vehicles currently have limited availability in the United States.
Data from U.S. Department of Energy. Alternative Fuels Data Center. https://afdc.energy.gov/vehicles/search/data. Accessed November 23, 2020.

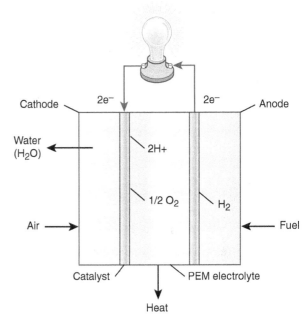

FIGURE 7-15 This diagram explains how a fuel cell works.

electrode). The PEM exchanges positive electrons. The process begins with hydrogen from an onboard storage tank that enters the anode and is split into positive ions and negative electrons. The positive hydrogen ions pass through the PEM, which is permeable only to positive ions, and combine at the cathode with the oxygen supplied from outside air, creating the by-product, which is water. The water is either used in some other area of the vehicle for cooling or omitted out the tailpipe of the vehicle. The negative hydrogen electrons are then used to provide the electrical current to power the vehicle. Heat is also created from the chemical reaction, which requires the use of a coolant (water) to keep the fuel cell at the proper temperature. A separator is used to ensure that the positive and negative elements are routed to the correct paths. This entire process encompasses just one fuel cell. Each cell produces approximately 0.7 to 1.1 volts of electricity.

Voice of Experience

I have often been asked about my experiences with traffic collisions involving hybrid and electric vehicles. In over 20 years in the Fire Service, I have only had a few hybrid collision experiences. The truth is, it's hard to find first responders that have extensive experiences with hybrid or electric vehicles because they are such a small percentage of the overall crashes we respond to. We try to prepare ourselves with knowledge from the manufacturers and training standards, yet these sources of information have struggled to keep up with the rapidly changing technology. Additionally, not all manufacturers provide first responders with the same procedural approaches in emergency response guide books or technical users manuals, and so we are destined to learn the hard way.

There are current and ongoing discussions about the need to standardize the color of high voltage components or provide obvious visual warnings to first responders to prevent injury or death. Would an engine or truck company recognize the floor pan of an electric vehicle that was badly damaged before placing struts? Would the same company recognize or be aware of the "first responder loop" on a Tesla that could be cut as part of the initial stabilization and access phase? Awareness is key, and performing detailed size-ups will promote crew awareness regardless of the type of vehicle.

One example of our approach to wheel resting vehicles is to chock the rear wheels as soon as possible on approach to immobilize the vehicle before cribbing. Chocking the rear wheels first keeps you in a safe position from the side while the medical instructions to the victim are being given from the front quarter panel, offset from the tire's direction. It also allows you the ability to rotate the steering wheel section to the position that, when cut away, will provide the most lap room for the patient. On hybrid and electric vehicles, it is even more important since the element of a running engine is not present to keep you aware. We have found that newer vehicles may have more than one 12-volt system to shut down, and accessing batteries may be very difficult due to the unknown locations.

There are some companies like Moditech Rescue Solutions making apps available on cell phones or hand-held devices that show pertinent information like cut zones or battery locations on hybrids. Companies like Mercedes-Benz have been using scannable QR codes with response guides and cut instructions in the glass and throughout the vehicles. Again, the issue is awareness. Then the situation becomes that of practicality and the image of a first responder looking at his or her phone while a person is trapped during a vehicle extrication. It's up to us to determine what is appropriate and how much technical information we can prepare ourselves with *before* the call goes out.

Jayson Lynn
Hillsboro County Fire Rescue
Tampa, Florida

Hydrogen Fuel-Cell Vehicle Electrical Design

A **fuel-cell vehicle** by definition is a hybrid vehicle system in which two separate sources of power are used individually or combined as a propulsion mechanism for the vehicle. For example, hydrogen fuel compressed as a gas or liquefied and stored in an onboard cylinder and an electrical energy produced from a separate battery pack are examples of two separate sources of power that are used individually or combined to propel the motor.

The basic components of a fuel-cell vehicle system consist of a fuel-cell module pack/stack, electric motor, generator, hydrogen storage system, and battery pack. Multiple fuel cells are stacked together and placed in a series; one complete system for a vehicle can consist of over 300 to 400 individual cells producing over 400 volts of DC electricity. The vehicle will also use a battery pack and/or large storage capacitor (ultracapacitor) for energy reserve to make the vehicle more efficient. The battery packs are configured with the same design as the ones found in the HEV system; they comprise several stacked cells consisting of nickel metal hydride (NiMH) or lithium-ion batteries. These batteries can produce 300 or more volts of DC electricity depending on the number of individual cells used. The vehicle will also be equipped with a standard 12-volt DC lead-acid battery that can be used for the initial starting of the vehicle or can offer auxiliary power for various electrical components. This standard 12-volt DC lead-acid battery is the basic two-pole design with a black negative pole and a red positive pole. The location of the 12-volt DC battery will vary with each model of vehicle. Most fuel-cell vehicles come equipped with a regenerative energy braking system that uses or captures the kinetic energy produced when the vehicle's brakes are applied. The energy produced from the brakes is used to recharge the battery pack or is stored in the onboard energy storage capacitor.

Hydrogen Storage System for a Fuel-Cell Vehicle

A fuel-cell design will normally use a compressed hydrogen gas system comprising several Types 3 or 4 cylinders as opposed to a liquefied hydrogen cryogenic storage system, which requires extreme temperatures (−423°F [−253°C]) to keep the hydrogen in the liquid state. The compressed hydrogen gas storage cylinders come in pressures of 3600, 5000, and 10,000 psi (24,821; 34,474; and 68,948 kPa), which then have to be regulated down to a nominal pressure so the gas can be used as it enters the fuel-cell module. Reinforced framing material is commonly added to

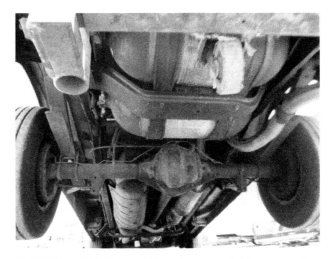

FIGURE 7-16 Reinforced framing material is commonly added to the existing frame to protect the storage cylinders against impacts.
Courtesy of David Sweet.

the existing frame of the vehicle to protect the storage cylinders against impacts (**FIGURE 7-16**).

Hydrogen lines running from the cylinders in the rear of the vehicle to the fuel cells in the front of the vehicle are typically routed underneath the vehicle outside the passenger compartment. Some vehicle models, such as the Toyota Fuel Cell Hybrid Vehicle-Advanced (FCHV-adv), use a red color-coding system on these lines for identification purposes, but this is not a standardized practice among manufacturers.

All hydrogen storage tanks come equipped with a PRD or **temperature relief device (TRD)**, which rapidly releases the product through a small metal tube attachment when detecting excessive amounts of heat at a preset temperature. The hydrogen can take up to several minutes to release all of its contents and is identified by a loud hissing noise when activated. PPE, including SCBA, should be worn when approaching the vehicle; as mentioned earlier in the chapter, hydrogen burns clean with an almost clear flame that is difficult to see. A TIC is a useful tool to identify a hydrogen fire if no other material is burning. A liquid hydrogen release will form a visible vapor cloud because the cryogenic state of the hydrogen temporarily freezes the air around the product as it is rapidly released in the atmosphere. It is not recommended to direct a water stream into this area because of the possibility of freezing/icing the PRD and blocking the product release or the release of pressure from the cylinder. Also, remember never to direct a hose stream into the liquid state of hydrogen because the warmer water will immediately cause a rapid boil-off phase, instantly vaporizing and expanding the liquid hydrogen into its gaseous state. A fog pattern can be directed to disperse any visible vapors.

> **LISTEN UP!**
> Because of the possibility of freezing, it is not recommended to direct a water stream at an activated PRD of a liquid hydrogen storage cylinder that is expelling product.

There are numerous safety features built into the fuel-cell vehicle that vary among models. Some of these features include hydrogen leak detectors placed in strategic locations throughout the vehicle; these sensors, when detecting a leak, will deactivate the hydrogen storage system, stopping the flow of hydrogen gas through the lines. Electronic control units (ECUs), in some models, continuously monitor temperatures and pressures for the entire hydrogen system including its components; any irregularity or leak detected will cause the ECU to shut down the hydrogen system and the medium- to high-voltage electrical system. Most vehicle models incorporate a type of crash detection system that deactivates and shuts down the hydrogen and high-voltage electrical system when a moderate to severe crash is detected; the system uses inertia sensors and activates when any air bag is deployed. Other vehicle models will deactivate and shut down the hydrogen system when the hood release is pulled or the hood is opened. All models deactivate the hydrogen storage system and shut down the gas lines, including the medium- to high-voltage lines, when the ignition key is in the off position and/or the key is removed. Some storage cylinders come equipped with manual shutoff valves that can be accessed from underneath or from the side of the vehicle; research the various models' emergency response guides to find out the type and location of the manual shutoff valves.

Hydrogen fuel-cell vehicles are generally recognizable through vehicle identification badges located on the sides, front hood, and rear of the vehicle. Examples of the letters that may be seen include "FCV," "FCHV," or "FCX" or the words "Fuel Cell Vehicle," "Fuel Cell Hybrid Vehicle," or "Fuel Cell" (**FIGURE 7-17**). To reiterate, these identification badges are not standardized among manufacturers. However, the storage systems must meet the FMVSS for crash safety.

Hydrogen Fuel-Cell Emergency Procedures

Emergency procedures for fuel-cell vehicles that use an onboard storage tank consisting of hydrogen as a catalyst to generate electricity will be similar to the procedures for CNG and LNG systems. It is highly recommended that the technical rescuer review emergency response guides dealing with vehicles that use

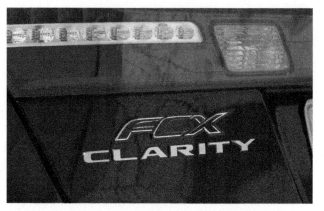

FIGURE 7-17 A vehicle identification badge for a hydrogen fuel-cell vehicle may include the letters "FCV," "FCHV," or "FCX" or the words "Fuel Cell Vehicle," "Fuel Cell Hybrid Vehicle," or "Fuel Cell."
© GIPhotoStock Z/Alamy Stock Photo.

hydrogen because these procedures will vary among models. Also, the DOT's *ERG*, particularly Guide 115, is a good reference for initial planning. Most guides recommend that any potential problems or leaks be mitigated before attempting to extricate any victims. This will be determined by the IC; quick hazard and risk analyses will have to be determined prior to taking action. The hazard analysis identifies situations or conditions that may injure people or personnel or may damage property or the environment. The risk analysis assesses the risk to the rescuers compared to the benefits that might come from the rescue. Hazard and risk analyses are continual processes that are reevaluated throughout the entire incident.

General emergency procedures when dealing with hydrogen fuel-cell vehicle incidents include the following. Note that some of these steps are not necessarily completed in succession; some of them can be completed simultaneously depending on the number of personnel on scene who are available to be assigned to complete each step.

- Don the appropriate PPE, including SCBA if needed, and clear the scene of all bystanders and hazards.
- Establish hazard control zones (hot, warm, and cold). Use the DOT's *ERG* as a reference guide to determine initial zone sizing.
- Conduct the inner and outer surveys. If possible, approach the vehicle from upwind and uphill and from the side or corner of the vehicle because of unexpected lunging or reversing of the vehicle. The vehicle may be silent and appear to be turned off because it is void of an internal combustion engine, which produces the noise we are accustomed to hearing. Remember that the system can still be in an all-electric ready

mode, capable of engaging the drive or reverse motor at any moment. This is similar to an electric golf cart that is always in a ready mode and accelerates when the pedal is depressed. Look for any visible vapor clouds, and listen for loud hissing noises, which indicate product release through a leak or through a PRD.

- If carried on an apparatus, use a hydrogen-specific gas meter to detect possible leaks and concentrations of combustible gases or vapors in the surrounding atmosphere. This is a continuous process until the leak has been contained and stopped.
- Look for a vehicle identification badge; in this situation, it may be the letters "FCV," "FCHV," or "FCX" or the words "Fuel Cell Vehicle," "Fuel Cell Hybrid Vehicle," or "Fuel Cell," or there may be a blue triangle with "Hydrogen" written in white on the rear trunk area.
- Two 1.75-in. (44-mm) charged hose lines should be deployed to protect personnel and disperse any significant release of vapor from liquid hydrogen or compressed hydrogen gas product to keep it below the flammable range.
- Never assume that the vehicle's ignition is turned off because it is silent or still.
- When the scene is safe, manually turn the ignition key to the off position, remove the key, and be sure the vehicle is in park. Various emergency response guides state that smart keys need to be a minimum of 20 ft (6 m) way from the vehicle to remove them from operational range. Place the parking brake on if accessible.
- Stabilize the vehicle from movement with cribbing. Avoid placing any cribbing under high-voltage wiring, alternative-fuel supply lines or cylinders, and high-voltage battery packs. Location and size of the high-voltage battery pack will affect the center of mass of the vehicle.
- Manually engage the hood release device, which in some vehicle models disengages the hydrogen system and the medium- to high-voltage electrical system.
- Attempt any necessary component adjustments before disabling the power to the vehicle, such as activating the electric parking brake, adjusting power seats, and releasing hatchbacks.
- Safely disengage the 12-volt DC battery, which will shut down the flow of hydrogen gas and medium- to high-voltage electricity. Remove or cut the negative cable first, and ensure that the cable does not fall back on the vehicle and make contact with any surrounding metal parts in any way. A 12-volt DC battery can be found in various locations in the vehicle depending on the manufacturer and vehicle model. Traditional locations include under the engine compartment hood, inside one of the wheel wells, under the backseat, or in the trunk. Warning: Energy capacitors in some models can hold power for 5 to 30 minutes after the power has been disengaged.
- Manufacturers recommend removal of the main fuse from the vehicle to ensure that the electrical system is disabled. This will be an AHJ's decision because the location of fuses can vary greatly among models.
- Manually shut off the cylinder tank valve if the cylinder comes equipped with one.
- Some manufacturers recommend using service disconnects as indicated in the manufacturer's emergency response guide for that particular vehicle. This will be an AHJ's decision because the location of service disconnects can vary greatly among models.

In a fuel-cell vehicle, the medium- to high-voltage wires run along the undercarriage of the vehicle, normally on the opposite side of the hydrogen gas lines; this can vary with each vehicle model. These wires are normally protected by some framing material and/or are wrapped in a protective casing. Remember that these wires have ground-fault and short-circuit protection; if there is a break in the line, a relay will kick in and open the circuit, which will isolate and disable the voltage. With various fuel-cell vehicle models, fully discharging the voltage from the capacitor can take from 5 to 10 minutes once a breach in the system has been detected or the power turned off.

When performing various extrication techniques, precaution must be observed when the vehicle is overturned on its roof. If the decision to perform a tunneling technique through the trunk area is considered, remember that the hydrogen storage tanks and battery packs might be placed in the trunk area, under the rear seat section, or under the vehicle, so an alternative method may be safer. Also, when considering a dash displacement technique, such as a dash lift or dash roll, remember that the hydrogen gas lines run along the undercarriage up into the motor/generator compartment and the medium- to high-voltage wires also run on the undercarriage from the battery pack in the rear to the motor/generator compartment located at the front of the vehicle. Opening up the dash area can potentially expose the technical rescuer to the hydrogen gas lines and the medium- and high-voltage wires. The hydrogen system and the power to medium- and high-voltage wires should have been isolated and disconnected prior to performing any extrication, but it is still not recommended to cut into any medium- to high-voltage wire or hydrogen gas lines regardless of whether the power has been neutralized or the hydrogen system has been disconnected. In addition, techniques that involve dropping the floorboard area under the brake and gas pedals should not be attempted; such maneuvers could expose high-voltage wires or gas lines running under the rocker panel/channel area, which should be avoided regardless of the type of fuel system the vehicle uses or whether the power supply has been secured. This is not a safe practice.

Hybrid Electric Vehicles (HEVs)

A hybrid electric vehicle (HEV) is a vehicle that combines two or more power sources for propulsion, one of which is electric power. Several types of vehicles on the roadway today are designed with a propulsion system that uses either a combination of electric power and another type of fuel (such as gasoline) or electric power only. Some of the abbreviations used to label these vehicles include PHEV (plug-in hybrid electric vehicle) and EREV (extended range electric vehicle). For a full list of all alternative fuel vehicles on the market, consult the U.S. Department of Energy's website.

Conventional or alternative fuels can be combined with electric power, which is stored in a battery pack system inside the vehicle. Hybrid technology has been around for over a century. The first U.S. patent issued for a hybrid vehicle was in 1909 by German-born Henri Pieper. Hybrid technology is used to power advanced systems found in submarines (nuclear/electric) and trains (diesel/electric) down to the simplest forms of transportation such as the moped (gasoline/electric). HEVs have the power of conventional vehicles, are economical, and produce lower emissions.

The battery system generally used to supply power to the HEV is an NiMH battery or a Li-ion battery configured in a pack of individual cells (**FIGURE 7-18**). Each battery cell, depending on its size, will produce 1 to 1.5 volts of DC power. These cells are then combined and encased in modules and set in series to produce the specific voltage or DC power depending on the type of HEV system design. The HEV design may use a high-voltage (>60-volt DC) or a medium- to low-voltage system. The NiMH battery carries a small amount of an alkaline base electrolyte composed of

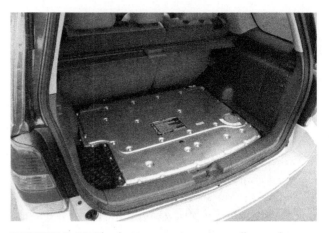

FIGURE 7-18 The battery system generally used to supply power to the HEV is configured in a pack of individual cells.
© Transtock, Inc./Alamy Stock Photo.

sodium and/or potassium hydroxide. This electrolyte is absorbed into the cell plates and should not pose a leak hazard if the case is damaged.

Full and Mild HEV Designs

HEVs are unofficially classified as being full or mild in terms of how they use the electric power that is generated. A full hybrid vehicle can use its electric motor or an ICE or a combination of both to propel itself. In contrast to the full hybrid, the mild hybrid vehicle must use electric power in conjunction with the ICE for vehicle propulsion.

Mild hybrid vehicles can be subdivided into two categories: the start/stop mild hybrid and the integrated motor assist mild hybrid, which is used in Honda vehicles. The start/stop mild hybrid system is not a true hybrid system by definition because the motor/generator is not used to propel the vehicle; it is designed to turn off the vehicle's ICE when the vehicle is idle and turn the vehicle's ICE back on when the accelerator is activated or the brake pedal is released by the driver's foot. The integrated motor assist (IMA) mild hybrid system is also designed to start and stop the HEV's ICE and, in addition, assist the ICE when acceleration is needed. The IMA HEV system will also power electrical devices, such as the air-conditioning, power steering, and various electronics in the vehicle, and it can store and use the vehicle's regenerative braking energy. Some start/stop vehicles have an additional battery located in the trunk (**FIGURE 7-19**).

Mild hybrids generally work off of a low- to medium-voltage range. The voltage for these types of hybrids can range from 36 to 42 volts DC, utilizing a series of NiMH batteries or an advanced lead-acid battery known as a valve-regulated lead-acid battery.

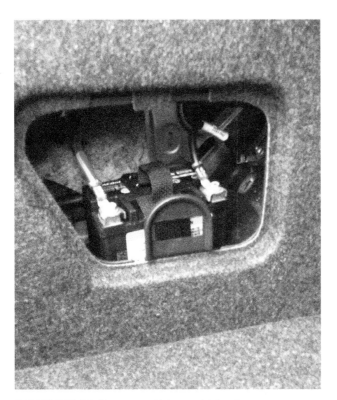

FIGURE 7-19 Some start/stop vehicles have an additional battery located in the trunk.
Courtesy of Mike Smith.

The NiMH battery in the full hybrid produces a high voltage for propulsion and powering various components in the range of 144 to 300 volts DC, with some vehicles using a step-up inverter capable of producing power up to 650 volts DC.

All full and some mild HEVs come equipped with a regenerative energy braking system that uses or captures the kinetic energy produced when the brakes are applied. The energy produced by the braking system is used to recharge the battery pack or is stored in the onboard energy storage capacitor.

All HEVs come equipped with the standard 12-volt DC lead-acid battery that can be used for the initial starting of the vehicle or offering auxiliary power for various electrical components. This standard 12-volt DC lead-acid battery is the basic two-pole design with a black negative pole and a red positive pole. The location of the 12-volt DC battery will vary with each model of vehicle.

Plug-in Hybrid Electric Vehicle (PHEV)

A **plug-in hybrid electric vehicle (PHEV)** is simply a hybrid vehicle with the ability to recharge its battery system using a plug-in cord that can run off general house current in the range of 120 volts, also known as a Level 1 charging system. A 240-volt charging system is known as a Level 2 charging system, which can cut the charging time in half for some models. There is also a Level 3, or DC Fast Charge, system that ranges up to 480 volts, which is generally beyond the household current level and is normally for commercial use only. A Level 1 charging system for a PHEV can take up to 8 hours or longer, depending on the vehicle manufacturer, to fully charge the vehicle. Some Level 3 systems can charge a battery pack to 80 percent capacity in 15 minutes, but again, this depends on the type of system setup and the vehicle manufacturer.

A PHEV gives consumers greater flexibility because the vehicle, when fully charged, can run solely on electric power over short distances. The PHEV has the same components and features as a similar HEV model of vehicle with the exception of a larger battery pack to extend the vehicle's urban driving range on battery power only. There is a potential problem for responders when the vehicle is plugged in and charging from the house current: A rescuer responding to a vehicle fire in the garage of a single-family home must disconnect the power at the vehicle or to the residence to disable the electrical feed to the vehicle before attempting to gain entry into the vehicle to complete any interior extinguishment.

Extended Range Electric Vehicle (EREV)

The **extended range electric vehicle (EREV)** uses a series-type propulsion system that allows the vehicle to run on all-battery or all-electric power until it is near depletion, which occurs in the range of 40 mi or more depending on the manufacturer. An onboard gasoline engine acts as a generator, thus extending the range up to several hundred miles. The EREV can also be plugged into a power grid to fully recharge its high-voltage battery. A popular vehicle in the EREV class is the Chevrolet Volt, which has some unique high-voltage (orange color coding) wiring configurations that can be problematic when there is a need to perform a dash displacement technique. It is vital to ensure that the system is disabled by following the steps recommended in the emergency response guide provided by the manufacturer (**FIGURE 7-20**).

Voltage Color Coding

In some mild hybrid systems, a low- or medium-voltage cable (36 to 42 volts DC) can be identified by a blue cable, and a high-voltage cable is always identified by an orange cable. The color orange for high-voltage cables is an industry standard and required in automotive wiring that contains over 60 volts DC. Currently, there is no industry color standard for medium- or intermediate-voltage cables,

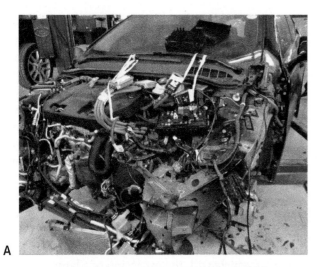

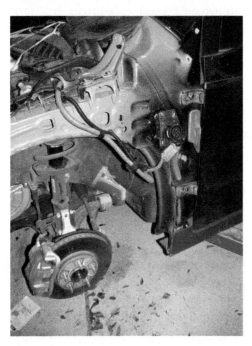

FIGURE 7-20 The Chevrolet Volt has some unique high-voltage (orange color coding) wiring configurations that can be problematic when there is a need to perform a dash displacement technique.
Courtesy of David Sweet.

cable placed before the DC to DC inverter to denote the higher voltage. All cables, regardless of color, must be respected and carefully evaluated for their voltage capacity.

> **LISTEN UP!**
>
> Be aware that some manufacturers may cover exposed voltage cables in a protective casing, thus concealing the blue, yellow, or orange color coding that is used by some manufacturers to identify voltage capacity.

HEV Drive Systems

The basic components of an HEV system consist of an electric motor, generator, ICE, and battery pack. The drive system for a hybrid vehicle can be designed in series or parallel. In a **series drive system**, the electric motor turns the vehicle's transmission to provide propulsion or is used to charge the batteries or store power in a capacitor. The ICE does not provide propulsion to the vehicle as it is designed to do in a conventional vehicle; the ICE supplies power to the electric motor only. The more common **parallel drive system** can use the vehicle's ICE and/or the electric motor to power the vehicle's transmission to provide propulsion. Which propulsion system is used is dependent on the speed of the vehicle and will vary among manufacturers (**FIGURE 7-21**).

HEVs are generally recognizable through vehicle identification badging located on the sides or rear of the vehicle. A green leaf logo, the word "Hybrid," and the letter "H" are some common vehicle badges that the technical rescuer may find, but be aware that there is no standardization of vehicle identification badging among manufacturers (**FIGURE 7-22**).

but they can appear in yellow and/or blue depending on the manufacturer.

One mild hybrid vehicle uses an inverter, which converts the current from 36 volts DC (blue cable in some models) into alternating current (AC), stepping the voltage up to 120 volts DC. This 120-volt DC high-voltage cable is colored orange to denote the higher voltage. Another hybrid vehicle uses a DC to DC inverter, stepping down the high-voltage output to 42 volts DC, which it then uses to power the electric power steering system. This particular manufacturer uses a yellow cable to indicate that the voltage is in the medium range (42 volts DC) along with the orange

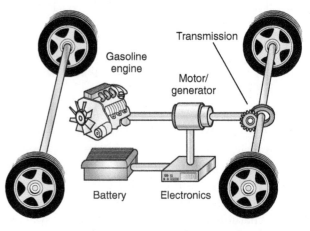

FIGURE 7-21 This picture provides an internal working view of a parallel HEV.

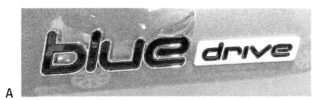

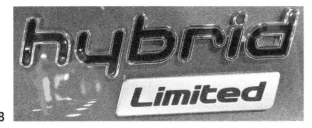

FIGURE 7-22 A. An HEV identification badge may include a green leaf logo. **B.** Standard HEV label.
Courtesy of David Sweet.

HEV Emergency Procedures

With the multitude of HEVs on the roadways today as well as those in future production, it is highly recommended to review the emergency response guides provided by the manufacturers because emergency procedures can vary with each model. All hybrid vehicles have built-in safety features that shut down the medium- and high-voltage lines for various situations, but emergency personnel should always assume that the vehicle is still energized until proven otherwise and emergency procedures are enacted. Safety devices, such as inertia relays, will open when detecting a collision or significant impact, immediately disabling the high-voltage system. Ground faults on each wire will detect any leaks, line breaches, or short circuits and disable the high-voltage service. Thermal detection devices will shut down the high-voltage system if they detect a temperature rise greater than a specific set temperature. The medium- to high-voltage wires run along the undercarriage of the vehicle either in the center or on the sides. They are normally protected by framing material and/or are wrapped in a protective casing. Remember that these wires have ground-fault and short-circuit protection; if there is a break in the line, a relay will kick in and open the circuit, which will isolate and disable the voltage. With various hybrid vehicle models, fully discharging the voltage from the capacitor can take from 5 to 30 minutes once a breach in the system has been detected or the power turned off.

Turning the main engine key in the off position and removing the key is one way to disable the high-voltage system as well as eliminate the vehicle's 12-volt battery. Manufacturers recommend pulling the main fuse, which is another way to disable the high-voltage system. These procedures can be incorporated together to disable the power system. If the main fuse is not recognizable or difficult to locate, then remove all the fuses in the box. There are also manual battery service disconnects that will shut down the high-voltage system, but the service disconnects are specific to each model and sometimes difficult to locate because they are designed for service technicians to access, not emergency responders. Trying to access the battery pack to find a manual disconnect is not a safe or recommended practice for emergency responders. Some models disengage the high-voltage system when the hood to the engine compartment is opened, but again this is not standardized among all HEV models. To ensure a full power down of the HEV, follow the safety procedures that are explained here.

Safety procedures that the technical rescuer can take prior to performing extrication when dealing with an HEV include the following. Note that some of these steps are not necessarily completed in succession; some of them can be completed simultaneously depending on the number of personnel on scene who are available to be assigned to complete each step.

- Don the appropriate PPE, including SCBA if needed, and clear the scene of all bystanders and hazards.
- Establish hazard control zones (hot, warm, and cold).
- Conduct the inner and outer surveys. If possible, approach the vehicle from upwind and uphill and from the side or corner because of the possibility of unexpected lunging or reversing of the vehicle. The vehicle may be silent or appear to be turned off because the ICE has been shut down, but the system can still be in an all-electric ready mode (most vehicle models show this on the vehicle dash display panel), capable of engaging the drive or reverse motor at any moment.
- Look for a vehicle identification badge; in this case, it may be a green leaf logo, the word "Hybrid," or the letter "H."
- One 1.75-in. (44-mm) charged hose line should be deployed for scene and personnel protection.
- Never assume that the vehicle is turned off because it is silent or still.
- When the scene is safe, manually turn the engine key to the off position, make sure the vehicle is in park, and remove the keys. Various emergency response guides state that smart keys need to be a minimum of 20 ft (6 m) away from the vehicle, which removes them from operational range. Place the parking brake on if accessible.

- Stabilize the vehicle from movement with cribbing. Avoid placing any cribbing under high-voltage wiring, alternative-fuel supply lines or cylinders, and high-voltage battery packs. Location and size of the high-voltage battery pack will affect the center of mass of the vehicle. Be aware that some manufacturers may cover exposed voltage cables in a protective casing, thus concealing the blue, yellow, or orange color coding that is used by some manufacturers to identify voltage capacity (**FIGURE 7-23**).
- Attempt any necessary component adjustments before disabling the power to the vehicle, such as activating the electric parking brake, adjusting power seats, and releasing hatchbacks.
- Safely disengage the 12-volt battery, which will shut down the flow of high-voltage electricity. Remove or cut the cable (manufacturers' emergency response guides differ on various models with cutting the negative or positive cable first), and ensure that the cable does not fall back on the vehicle and make contact with any surrounding metal parts. Twelve-volt batteries can be found in various locations in the vehicle depending on the manufacturer and model of the vehicle. The battery may be in the traditional location under the engine compartment hood or inside one of the wheel wells, under the backseat, or in the trunk. Warning: Energy capacitors in some models can hold power for 5 to 30 minutes after the power has been disengaged.
- Manufacturers recommend removal of the main fuse from the vehicle to ensure that the electrical system is disabled. This will be an AHJ's decision because the location of fuses can vary greatly among models.
- Some manufacturers recommend utilizing service disconnects as indicated in the manufacturer's emergency response guide for that particular vehicle. This will be an AHJ's decision because the location of service disconnects can vary greatly among models.

When performing various extrication techniques, precaution must be observed when the vehicle is overturned on its roof. If the decision to perform a tunneling technique through the trunk area is considered, remember that the battery packs can be placed under the rear seat or trunk area, so an alternative method may be safer. Also, when considering a dash displacement technique, such as a dash lift or dash roll, keep in mind that the medium- to high-voltage wires may run along the undercarriage from the battery pack in the rear to the motor/generator located at the front of the vehicle. Opening up the dash area may expose the technical rescuer to the medium- and high-voltage wires below the vehicle. Power to these wires should have been isolated and disconnected prior to performing any extrication; however, medium- to high-voltage wire should never be cut regardless of whether the power has been neutralized. In addition, techniques that involve cutting and dropping the floorboard area under the brake and gas pedals should not be attempted. Such maneuvers could expose the rescuer to high-voltage wires, gas lines running under the rocker panel/channel area, or the battery packs installed in the floor pan area of certain vehicles. This is not a safe

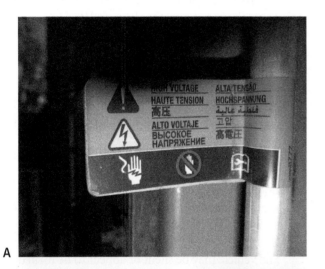

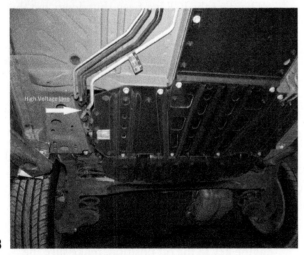

FIGURE 7-23 Be aware that some manufacturers may cover exposed voltage cables in a protective casing, thus concealing the blue, yellow, or orange color coding that is used by some manufacturers to identify voltage capacity.

Courtesy of David Sweet.

practice and should be avoided regardless of the type of fuel system the vehicle uses or whether the power supply has been secured. Alternative techniques that are much safer should be considered.

SAFETY TIP

If the decision to perform a tunneling technique through the trunk area of an HEV is considered, remember that the battery packs are normally placed under or behind the rear seat or in the trunk area, so an alternative method may be safer.

All-Electric Vehicles

The **electric vehicle (EV)**, or battery electric vehicle (BEV), is 100 percent electric and energy efficient and environmentally friendly, emitting no air pollutants. EVs are propelled by one or more electric motors, which are powered by rechargeable battery packs. The EV does not have a tailpipe because it does not emit exhaust.

The Nissan LEAF was one of the first EVs produced by a major auto manufacturer, followed by Tesla, which has become one of the more prominent manufacturers of EVs on the road today (**FIGURE 7-24**). The EV uses regenerative braking to recharge the battery, which is a laminated Li-ion battery with a capacity of 24 kWh. This is a high-voltage battery (approximately 400 volts DC). The vehicle can also be plugged in to be recharged. EVs are most commonly charged from conventional power outlets or charging stations. Fully recharging the battery pack can take up to 20 hours utilizing a Level 1 charging system. The high-voltage battery is encased in steel and located in the undercarriage. A 12-volt DC battery is located under the hood to supply power to the low-voltage devices, such as the lights, horn, and other accessories.

Many EVs can travel 100 to 200 mi (161 to 322 km) without charging. The range of the vehicle may be affected by temperature, speed, topography, driving style, and cargo as well as the manufacturer. As with other advanced vehicles, EVs can be recognized through vehicle identification badging. For example, the Nissan LEAF has two zero-emissions vehicle badges. One is located on the rear of the vehicle, and the other is located on the driver's-side door panel.

A subclass of the EV is the **neighborhood electric vehicle (NEV)** (**FIGURE 7-25**). NEVs are classified as battery-operated low-speed vehicles with a top speed of 25 mi/h (40 km/h) and are approved for street use on public roadways with speeds posted of no greater than 35 mi/h (56 km/h). NEVs can vary on distance traveled on a single charge but generally provide up to 35 mi (56 km) of travel on a full charge. An NEV uses a standard Level 1 charging system, or a 120-volt household outlet, to recharge its battery system.

EV Emergency Procedures

With the emergence of EVs on the roadways today, as well as in future production, it is highly recommended to review the emergency response guides provided by the manufacturers because emergency procedures can vary with each model. All EVs have built-in safety features that shut down the medium- and high-voltage lines for various situations, but emergency personnel should always assume that the vehicle is still energized until proven otherwise and emergency procedures are enacted. During the inner

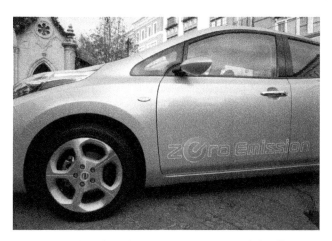

FIGURE 7-24 The Nissan LEAF was one of the first EVs produced by a major auto manufacturer.
© Mike Kahn/Green Stock Media (Agent)/Alamy Stock Photo.

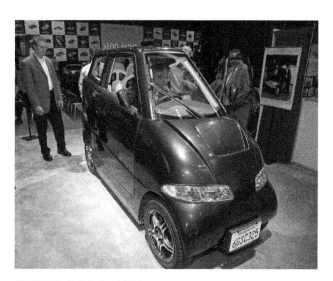

FIGURE 7-25 An NEV.
© Jim West/Alamy Stock Photo.

survey, look for indications that the high-voltage system is on. For example, upon approaching the vehicle, look to see whether the ready indicator is on, the charge indicator is on, the air-conditioning remote timer indicator is on, or the remote-controlled air-conditioning system is active. These are all indications that the high-voltage system of the vehicle is on. Technical rescuers should refer to the manufacturers' emergency response guides for information on how to disable the high-voltage system in various EVs. The high-voltage cables for the Nissan LEAF are located in the undercarriage and under the hood. All high-voltage cables are color coded orange on the Nissan LEAF with a "WARNING" label.

Safety procedures that the technical rescuer can take prior to performing extrication when dealing with an EV include the following. Note that some of these steps are not necessarily completed in succession; some of them can be completed simultaneously depending on the number of personnel on scene who are available to be assigned to complete each step.

- Don the appropriate PPE, including SCBA if needed, and clear the scene of all bystanders and hazards.
- Establish hazard control zones (hot, warm, and cold).
- Conduct the inner and outer surveys. If possible, approach the vehicle from upwind and uphill and from the side or corner because of the possibility of unexpected lunging or reversing of the vehicle. The vehicle may be silent or appear to be turned off, but the system can still be in an all-electric ready mode (most vehicle models show this on the vehicle dash display panel), capable of engaging the drive or reverse motor at any moment.
- Look for a vehicle identification badge; in the case of the Nissan LEAF, it may be a zero-emissions badge.
- One 1.75-in. (44-mm) charged hose line should be deployed for scene and personnel protection.
- Never assume that the vehicle is turned off because it is silent or still.
- When the scene is safe, manually turn the engine key to the off position, make sure the vehicle is in park, and remove the keys (unless it is a push-button start system). Various emergency response guides state that smart keys need to be a minimum of 20 ft (6 m) away from the vehicle, which removes them from operational range. Place the parking brake on if accessible.
- Ensure that the remote heating/air-conditioning system is deactivated.
- Ensure that the charging (electric plug) is disconnected.
- Stabilize the vehicle from movement with cribbing. Avoid placing any cribbing under high-voltage wiring and high-voltage battery packs. Location and size of the high-voltage battery pack will affect the center of mass of the vehicle.
- Attempt any necessary component adjustments before disabling the power to the vehicle, such as activating the electric parking brake, adjusting power seats, and releasing hatchbacks.
- Safely disengage the 12-volt battery, which will shut down the flow of high-voltage electricity. Remove or cut the cable (cutting the negative or positive cable first varies with manufacturers' emergency response guidelines), and ensure that the cable does not fall back on the vehicle and make contact with any surrounding metal parts. A 12-volt battery can be found in various locations in the vehicle depending on the manufacturer and model of the vehicle. The battery may be in the traditional location under the engine compartment hood, inside one of the wheel wells, under the backseat, or in the trunk. Warning: Energy capacitors in some models can hold power for 5 to 10 minutes after the power has been disengaged.
- Manufacturers recommend removal of the main fuse from the vehicle to ensure that the electrical system is disabled. This will be an AHJ's decision because the location of fuses can vary greatly among models.
- Some manufacturers recommend utilizing service disconnects as indicated in the manufacturer's emergency response guide for that particular vehicle. This will be an AHJ's decision because the location of service disconnects can vary greatly among models.

Ongoing Education

The technical rescuer must adapt and change with advancing vehicle technology. Alternative-fuel vehicles, HEVs, EVs, and fuel-cell vehicles will become the dominant forms of transportation in the not-so-distant future. Departmental/organizational standard operating procedures should be developed to reflect the emergency procedures for handling the specific vehicle types discussed in this chapter. Each member in the organization should be trained to at least a basic level of competency in dealing with advanced vehicle technology. Technical rescuers involved in vehicle rescue and extrication practices and procedures have an inherent responsibility to improve their skills and remain on the cutting edge of technology; self-motivation with continual training and education will provide the means to stay focused while always looking for ways to improve. Stay current on the emergence of these vehicles, and download manufacturers' emergency response guides from manufacturers' websites regularly.

After-Action REVIEW

IN SUMMARY

- Alternative-fuel vehicles are vehicles that use fuels other than petroleum or a combination of petroleum and another fuel for power.
- The Energy Policy Act of 1992 outlines a list of fuels that can be classified as alternative fuels for vehicles.
- Most vehicle manufacturers identify the vehicle or fuel type through a label known as a vehicle identification badge. Currently, no standardized labeling system is used to identify hydrogen fuel-cell vehicles.
- Flexible fuel vehicles can run on gasoline alone or use the E85 blend of up to 85 percent ethanol and 15 percent gasoline.
- Natural gas is a fossil fuel primarily composed of methane that can be used as a CNG or LNG.
- A safety feature for high-pressure cylinders is the PRD, which is designed to rapidly release all the gas when exposed to high temperatures, such as during a fire.
- LPG, also known as propane, is produced from the processing of natural gas and is also produced as part of the refining process of crude oil. Propane is the third most common engine fuel today, after gasoline and diesel.
- Biodiesel is a fuel used solely for diesel engines that is processed from domestic renewable resources, such as plant oils; grease; animal fats; used cooking oil; and, more recently, algae. Biodiesel can be used by itself as a diesel fuel or blended with petroleum diesel.
- Hydrogen is one of the most abundant elements on Earth. As a fuel, hydrogen can be compressed and stored in high-pressure storage tanks with pressures of 3600, 5000, and 10,000 psi (24,821; 34,474; and 68,948 kPa). Hydrogen can be chemically combined in hydride form with certain metals, which can store it more compactly and efficiently than in a gas form.
- A fuel cell is an electrochemical device that uses a catalyst-facilitated chemical reaction of hydrogen and oxygen to create electricity, which is then used to power an electric motor. The basic components of a fuel-cell vehicle system are a fuel-cell module pack/stack, electric motor, generator, hydrogen storage system, and battery pack.
- An HEV is a vehicle that combines two or more power sources for propulsion, one of which is electric power. A full hybrid vehicle can use its electric motor or its ICE or both to propel itself. In contrast to the full hybrid, the mild hybrid vehicle cannot propel itself on electric power alone; it must use electric power and the ICE.
- The EV, or BEV, is 100 percent electric and propelled by one or more electric motors, which are powered by rechargeable battery packs. The EV does not have a tailpipe because it does not emit exhaust.

KEY TERMS

Alternative-fuel vehicle A motorized vehicle propelled by anything other than gasoline or diesel.

Biodiesel A safe, nontoxic, biodegradable fuel used solely for diesel engines that is processed from domestic renewable resources, such as plant oils; grease; animal fats; used cooking oil; and, more recently, algae. Biodiesel can be used by itself as a diesel fuel or blended with petroleum diesel at varying percentages.

Boiling liquid/expanding vapor explosion (BLEVE) An event that occurs when the temperature of the liquid and vapor (flammable or nonflammable) within a confining tank or vessel is raised by an exposure fire to the point where the increasing internal pressures can no longer be contained and the vessel ruptures and explodes.

Compressed natural gas (CNG) A natural lighter-than-air gas compressed for use as a fuel that consists principally of methane in gaseous form plus naturally occurring mixtures of hydrocarbon gases. (NFPA 302)

Department of Transportation's (DOT's) *Emergency Response Guidebook (ERG)* A reference book, written in plain language, to guide emergency responders in their initial actions at the incident scene. (NFPA 475)

Electric vehicle (EV) A vehicle that is 100 percent electric, emits no air pollutants, and is propelled by one or more electric motors, which are powered by rechargeable battery packs.

Emergency response guide A booklet prepared by vehicle manufacturers to educate and assist emergency response personnel in responding to emergencies dealing with specific types and models of vehicles, such as hybrid/electric, hydrogen fuel-cell, and alternative-fuel systems.

Ethanol A fuel composed of an alcohol base that is normally processed from crops, such as corn, sugar, trees, or grasses.

Extended range electric vehicle (EREV) A vehicle that use a series-type propulsion system that allows the vehicle to run on all-battery or all-electric power until it is near depletion, which occurs in the range of 40 mi (64 km) or more depending on the manufacturer.

Flexible fuel vehicle (FFV) A vehicle capable of running on gasoline alone or utilizing the E85 blend of up to 85 percent ethanol and 15 percent gasoline.

Fuel cell An electrochemical device that uses a catalyst-facilitated chemical reaction of hydrogen and oxygen to create electricity, which is then used to power an electric motor or generator, with the by-products of this process being water and heat.

Fuel-cell vehicle A hybrid vehicle system in which two separate sources of power are used individually or combined as a propulsion mechanism for the vehicle.

Full hybrid vehicle A vehicle that uses its electric motor or its internal combustion engine or a combination of both to propel itself.

Hazard control zones Delineates the operational boundaries, which are divided into three areas: hot, warm, and cold.

Hybrid electric vehicle (HEV) A vehicle that combines two or more power sources for propulsion, one of which is electric power.

Hydrogen An odorless, colorless, flammable, nontoxic gas that combines easily with other elements.

Integrated motor assist (IMA) mild hybrid system A hybrid system used by Honda that is designed to start and stop the hybrid electric vehicle's internal combustion engine; in addition, it will assist the internal combustion engine when acceleration is needed.

Liquefied natural gas (LNG) A colorless, odorless, nontoxic natural gas that floats on water and is lighter than air when released as a vapor.

Liquefied petroleum gas (LPG) Also known as propane, a fossil fuel produced from the processing of natural gas and also produced as part of the refining process of crude oil. Propane is the third most widely used fuel source behind gasoline and diesel; it is commonly used with forklifts and other similar work units.

Methanol An alcohol-based fuel similar to ethanol. It is also known as a wood alcohol because it is processed from natural wood sources, such as trees and yard clippings. It may be used as a flex fuel in a ratio of 85 percent methanol to 15 percent gasoline, better known as M85.

Mild hybrid vehicle A vehicle that uses electric power in conjunction with an internal combustion engine for vehicle propulsion.

Natural gas A fossil fuel primarily composed of methane that can be used as a compressed natural gas (CNG) or liquefied natural gas (LNG).

Neighborhood electric vehicle (NEV) A vehicle that is classified as a battery-operated low-speed vehicle with a top speed of 25 mi/h (40 km/h) and that is approved for street use on public roadways with speeds posted of no greater than 35 mi/h (56 km/h).

Parallel drive system A system that can use either the vehicle's internal combustion engine or the electric motor to power the vehicle's transmission and provide propulsion.

Plug-in hybrid electric vehicle (PHEV) A hybrid vehicle that can recharge its battery system using a plug-in cord that can run off general house current in the range of 120 volts, also known as a Level 1 charging system.

Polymer exchange membrane (PEM) Also known as a proton exchange membrane, a thin membrane used in a fuel-cell system that is placed between the anode and cathode and through which positive electrons are passed.

Pressure release device (PRD) A safety feature built into high-pressure storage cylinders that is designed to rapidly release gas contents when exposed to high temperatures, such as during a fire.

Series drive system A system that uses the internal combustion engine alone to run an onboard generator, which in turn can either run the electric motor that turns the vehicle's transmission (providing propulsion) or be used to charge the batteries or store power in a capacitor. The internal combustion engine does not provide direct propulsion to the vehicle.

Smart key A device that uses a computerized chip that communicates through radio frequencies to unlock or lock a vehicle as well as start a vehicle remotely without the requirement of traditional keys.

Start/stop mild hybrid system A vehicle that is not a true hybrid system by definition. The motor/generator is not used to propel the vehicle; it is designed to turn off the vehicle's internal combustion engine when the vehicle is idle and turn it back on when the accelerator is activated.

Temperature relief device (TRD) A device that rapidly releases product through a small metal tube attachment when detecting excessive amounts of heat at a preset temperature.

Vehicle identification badge A type of label that vehicle manufacturers use to identify the type of vehicle or the fuel that is used in the vehicle.

REFERENCES

California Air Resources Board. Accessed at https://ww2.arb.ca.gov/homepage.

H2 Tools. Hydrogen Safety Training Materials. Accessed at https://h2tools.org/content/training-materials.

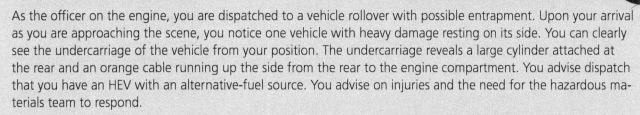

On Scene

As the officer on the engine, you are dispatched to a vehicle rollover with possible entrapment. Upon your arrival as you are approaching the scene, you notice one vehicle with heavy damage resting on its side. You can clearly see the undercarriage of the vehicle from your position. The undercarriage reveals a large cylinder attached at the rear and an orange cable running up the side from the rear to the engine compartment. You advise dispatch that you have an HEV with an alternative-fuel source. You advise on injuries and the need for the hazardous materials team to respond.

1. What can you look for on the vehicle that may indicate the type of alternative fuel in use?
   A. Don't do anything until the hazardous materials team arrives.
   B. There is no way to tell the type of fuel being used.
   C. A product label on the tank.
   D. Notify the vehicle manufacturer to find out.

2. A good source for research and information on auto extrication is the Internet. A lack of information or misinformation can cause rescuers to:
   A. overreact.
   B. fail to act at all.
   C. save more lives.
   D. A and B

3. To use the same emergency procedures on every incident involving one or more advanced vehicle systems is not practical and can be very dangerous. To avoid doing so requires:
   A. an extensive library of vehicle operating manuals of the most popular models.
   B. recognition of all hazards to be mitigated and neutralized before rescue extrication.
   C. preplanning, study, and training.
   D. B and C

4. After approaching the emergency scene from uphill and upwind, the company officer should perform:
   A. a left to right survey.
   B. a north to south survey.
   C. a thorough and ongoing survey.
   D. inner and outer surveys.

(continues)

On Scene Continued

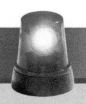

5. When approaching an HEV during an inner survey, the technical rescuer should approach the vehicle from the corner or the:
   A. front.
   B. rear.
   C. side.
   D. center.

6. How many hose lines should be deployed with these operations?
   A. One 1.75-in. hose line
   B. Two 1.75-in. hose lines
   C. One 1.75-in. hose line with a 2A/10BC portable fire extinguisher
   D. One 2.5-in. hose line

7. To prevent accidental ignition, smart keys must be kept a minimum of:
   A. 10 ft (3 m) away from the vehicle.
   B. 12 ft (4 m) away from the vehicle.
   C. 15 ft (4.5 m) away from the vehicle.
   D. 20 ft (6 m) away from the vehicle.

8. When disconnecting a car battery:
   A. cut the negative cable first and then the positive.
   B. cut the positive cable first and then the negative.
   C. cut both cables simultaneously to prevent an electrical arc.
   D. It no longer matters which cable is cut first because advanced vehicle technology has eliminated the hazard.

9. When approaching the emergency scene, look for any visible vapor cloud, and listen for a loud hissing noise; both indicate product release through a leak in the system or through the:
   A. pressure release device (PRD).
   B. pressure regulating valve (PRV).
   C. emergency pressure equalizing unit (EPEU).
   D. a loose fill cap (FC).

10. Most vehicle manufacturers will identify the vehicle type or fuel type through a label known as a vehicle identification badge. Badges can be found at various locations on the vehicle body. Which of the following statements about badges is correct?
    A. Be aware that they are usually found on the exterior right side of the trunk compartment.
    B. Be aware that they are usually found on the driver's-side rear bumper.
    C. Be aware that badge labeling is not standardized and can vary in design from one manufacturer to another.
    D. Be aware that vehicle identification badges have to be placed on both sides of the vehicle similar to the placement of DOT placards.

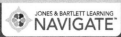 *Access Navigate for more activities.*

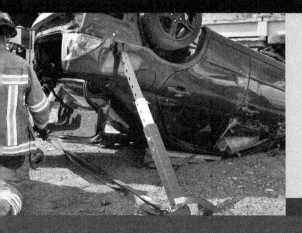

CHAPTER 8

Operations and Technician Levels

Vehicle Stabilization

KNOWLEDGE OBJECTIVES

After studying this chapter, you will be able to:

- Explain how to craft an incident action plan to address the safe removal of victims from a common passenger vehicle. (**NFPA 1006: 8.3.7**, pp. 200, 203–205)
- Create an incident action plan for an incident where a common passenger vehicle has come to rest on its side. (**NFPA 1006: 8.3.4**, pp. 208–209)
- Define the following terms and explain their role in vehicle rescue incidents:
  - Contact point. (p. 202)
  - Tunneling (**NFPA 1006: 8.2.5**, p. 212)
- Explain position and condition effect on a vehicle's equilibrium and stabilization. (pp. 200–201, 203)
- Describe the types and capacities of stabilization devices. (**NFPA 8.2.3, 8.3.2**, pp. 201–203)
- List the five box-cribbing configurations. (pp. 202–203)
- Identify the five directional movements of a vehicle. (p. 203)
- Describe methods for stabilizing vehicles in upright, side, or inverted positions. (**NFPA 1006: 8.2.3, 8.3.5, 8.3.8**, pp. 203–206, 208–212)
- Explain the purpose for marrying vehicles together. (pp. 214–216)
- Select and use stabilization devices in accordance with agency policies and procedures to stabilize a common passenger vehicle. (**NFPA 1006: 8.2.3, 8.3.5, 8.3.8**, pp. 203–206, 208)

SKILLS OBJECTIVES

After completing this chapter, you will be able to perform the following skills:

- Select, operate, and monitor stabilization devices. (**NFPA 1006: 8.2.3**, pp. 201–206, 208–216; **NFPA 1006: 8.3.5, 8.3.8**, pp. 201–206, 208–216)
- Stabilize a vehicle in an upright (normal) position. (**NFPA 1006: 8.2.3**, p. 208)
- Stabilize a vehicle on its side. (**NFPA 1006: 8.2.3**, p. 211)
- Stabilize a vehicle with multiple hazards. (**NFPA 1006: 8.3.8**, pp. 214–215)
- Stabilize a vehicle on its roof. (**NFPA 1006: 8.2.3**, p. 213)
- Marry two vehicles together. (**NFPA 1006: 8.2.3**, p. 215)
- Disable a vehicle electrical system. (**NFPA 1006: 8.2.3, 8.2.4**, p. 218)

You Are the Rescuer

You are on the scene of a vehicle rescue and extrication incident with a car on its side and one victim trapped. The officer asks you and your partner to use the set of struts on the engine. The Incident Commander assigns you and your crew the task of vehicle stabilization.

1. Which technique(s) will you use to accomplish this goal as quickly and as safely as possible?
2. Which section of this vehicle will you crib first?

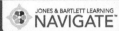

Access Navigate for more practice activities.

Introduction

This chapter focuses on the second step of the vehicle rescue and extrication process: vehicle stabilization (**FIGURE 8-1**).

To review the first step of the vehicle rescue and extrication process, including crafting an incident action plan, see Chapter 2, *Vehicle Rescue and Incident Awareness*.

Unstable vehicles pose serious challenges and risks to rescuers as well as to the victims involved in motor vehicle accidents (MVAs). The shape, size, and resting positions of vehicles after a collision can have a profound effect on the complexity and time spent on an incident. Following the proper steps and procedures to stabilizing vehicles involved in collisions (where victims require medical intervention and/or extrication) provides a solid foundation from which to work and thus ensures safety for the emergency personnel as well as the victims (**FIGURE 8-2**).

Balance goes hand in hand with stabilization. The main objective in stabilization is to gain a balanced footprint by expanding the vehicle's base and lowering its center of mass prior to performing any work on the vehicle. The goal of vehicle stabilization is to achieve a state of equilibrium or balance. Stabilization consists of two states of equilibrium: stable and unstable.

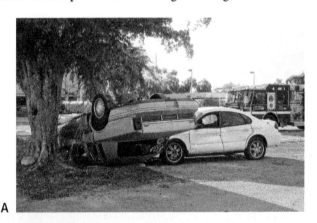

A

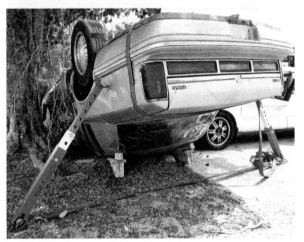

B

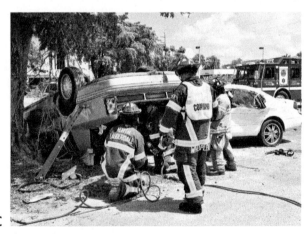

C

FIGURE 8-1 Vehicle extrication is a technical process that requires structured successive steps to produce favorable results. This chapter will discuss the second phase of this process "Stabilize the Vehicle." **A**. Phase 1: Stabilizing the Scene: Site operations—Dispatch, responding to the scene, scene size-up, scene safety zones, hazards, inner and outer surveys, incident action plan. **B**. Phase 2: Stabilize the Vehicle: vehicle safety and stabilization—Vehicle positioning, cribbing/struts, stabilization of vehicles in its normal position, on its side, or resting on its roof or on another object. **C**. Phase 3: Stabilize the victim: victim access and management—Initial access points, using various rescue tools and equipment to gain access, providing initial medical care, packaging and removal.
Courtesy of Edward Monahan.

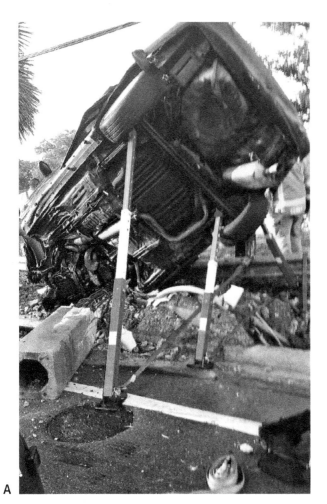 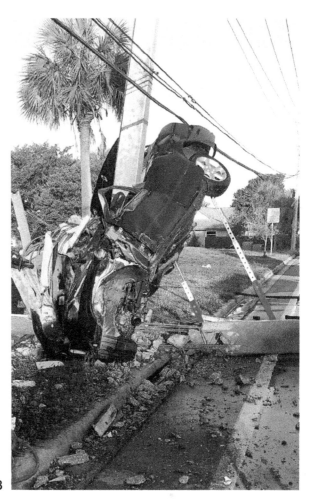

FIGURE 8-2 Ensure vehicles are stabilized before performing any operational techniques on the vehicles.
Courtesy of Jeff Lopez.

Mass is what makes up the matter or substance of an object. The mass of an object is always constant; it does not change based on position or location. Weight, by definition, is equal to the force exerted on an object by gravity. The center of mass of an object is the point where all the weight of the object is concentrated or the point where the downward force of gravity is at its greatest. The force of gravity is measured through an imaginary straight line passing through the center of mass of an object to a ground base of support.

An object is said to be in a state of stable equilibrium when the center of mass or concentrated weight of the object is lowest to the support base and the base is horizontally wider. A vehicle resting on all four tires on level ground is presenting a state of stable equilibrium because its center mass is lowest to the ground base of support and its weight is spread out equally. A vehicle resting on its side, because of its vertical stance and narrowing base, is considered to be in a state of unstable equilibrium. The goal is to lower its center of mass to the support or base level to achieve a state of stable equilibrium.

There are numerous methods for cribbing and stabilizing vehicles, such as box cribbing, struts, step chocks, wedges, shims, ratchet lever jacks, stabilizer jacks, rope, chain, cable, winches, ratchet straps, and tow trucks. This chapter discusses how to stabilize common passenger vehicles in multiple resting positions following a crash incident.

SAFETY TIP

During stabilization, responders should always be aware of the potential for vehicles to shift.

To facilitate the learning comprehension of this chapter, review Chapter 3, *Tools and Equipment*, for the various stabilization tools working load limits (WWL) of stabilization devices, and cribbing configurations.

Cribbing

As discussed in Chapter 3, cribbing is the most basic physical tool used for vehicle stabilization. Cribbing is commonly available as wood or composite materials, with some products being made of steel. Several cribbing designs are used for extrication incidents, such as step chocks, wedges, shims, and the basic 4-in. × 4-in. (10-cm × 10-cm) sections of timber (commonly referred to as "four-by-fours") that are cut at various lengths, most commonly 18 to 20 in. (46 to 51 cm) and 3 to 6 ft (0.9 to 1.8 m) or longer.

Wood Characteristics

Understanding the basic characteristics of wood used for cribbing is essential to the technical rescuer, whether you are stabilizing a vehicle, shoring a structure, or supporting a load.

Wood is heterogeneous in nature, meaning that it is composed of a mixture of different materials or has a lack of uniformity. Wood is also considered anisotropic in that the properties of each wood species are different according to its growth ring placement and direction of the grain. These two facts are important because not all wood types are suitable for cribbing and/or shoring. Soft woods, such as southern yellow pine or Douglas fir, are commonly used for cribbing because they are well suited for compression-type loads. Hard wood, such as an oak species, is very strong but may split easily under certain stresses.

When considering wood species for cribbing, the primary concern is the measurement of applied stress (which is a unit of force), without failure, of that particular species of wood. The applied stress factors may be compression, tension, or shear. All of these stress factors, including the proportional strain of the wood, occur when a force is applied and a section of wood bends, which is considered the elastic performance of the wood.

Stress and strain are proportional, which means that any incremental increase in stress is proportional to an incremental increase of strain. The maximum stress and proportional strain on an object beyond its proportional limit will result in the failure of the material. Wood is considered elastic up to its proportional limit; beyond that limit, failure occurs.

The American Society for Testing and Materials (ASTM) International has adopted standardized testing guidelines for measuring the relative stress resistance or strength values of particular species of wood. The maximum stress a board can be subjected to without exceeding the elastic range or proportional limit is known as its fiber stress at proportional limit (FSPL) rating.

When the downward force of an object rests or applies pressure on the surface of a section of wood and it is perpendicular to the grain, such as when a section of cribbing is set up in a crosstie or box-crib configuration, the cribbing strength is determined using a formula.

The dimension of the surface area at the **contact point**, or weight-bearing section of cribbing, is multiplied by the FSPL rating of that particular species of wood. For example, the FSPL rating of the southern yellow pine and Douglas fir is 500 psi (3447 kPa), meaning 500 psi (3447 kPa) is the load capability in pounds for each contact point. Now, apply this formula to a 4-in. × 4-in. (10-cm × 10-cm) box crib. Multiply the surface area of contact of a 4-in. × 4-in. (10-cm × 10-cm) section, which is generally configured to be 3.5 × 3.5 in. (9 × 9 cm), or 12.25 in.^{2} (79 cm^2):

500 psi (3447 kPa) (FSPL rating) × 12.25 in.^{2} (79 cm^2) (surface area of contact) = 6125 lb (3.1 short tons) per area contact point

The load capacity is 6125 lb (3.1 short tons) per area of contact point. If you have a simple box-crib configuration with only four points of contact, then this setup will support a uniform load capacity of 24,500 lb (12.25 short tons):

6125 lb (3.1 short tons) × 4 points of contact = 24,500 lb (12.25 short tons)

Wood Box Cribbing

NFPA 1006, *Standard for Technical Rescue Personnel Professional Qualifications*, 6.2.12, lists five types of wood box-cribbing configurations with which the technical rescuer needs to be familiar (**FIGURE 8-3**):

- Two-piece layer crosstie
- Three-piece layer crosstie

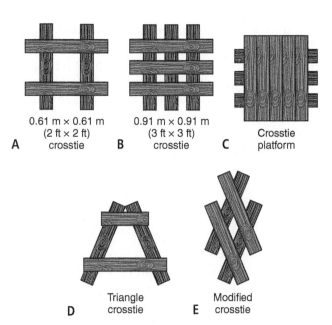

FIGURE 8-3 Five wood box-cribbing configurations. **A.** Two-piece layer crosstie. **B.** Three-piece layer crosstie. **C.** Crosstie platform. **D.** Triangle crosstie. **E.** Modified crosstie.

- Platform crosstie
- Triangle crosstie
- Modified crosstie

The two-piece layer crosstie, three-piece layer crosstie, and crosstie platform are the most commonly used wood box-crib configurations; these will be used to demonstrate a majority of the various cribbing scenarios discussed in this chapter. The triangle crosstie and modified crosstie are unique types of wood box-crib configurations that are specific to the type of stabilization incident presented; they are generally used for tight or odd-shaped spaces.

When you are setting up a basic two- or three-piece crosstie crib configuration, make sure that all the individual sections are uniform, with one on top of the other, providing a 1- to 1.5-in. (2.5- to 3.8-cm) gap from the ends. Most ends on a cut section of a four-by-four are cracked or splintered, creating a potential for failure. Avoid placing the contact point, or the weight-bearing section of cribbing, at the ends; you must ensure a safety margin if the load shifts and the crosstie moves (**FIGURE 8-4**). Remember that when using a four-by-four, either southern yellow pine or Douglas fir, each contact point has an estimated weight- or load-bearing capacity of 6000 lb (3 short tons).

> **LISTEN UP!**
> Take the necessary steps to ensure that all cribbing configurations are structured and uniform, with one on top of the other.

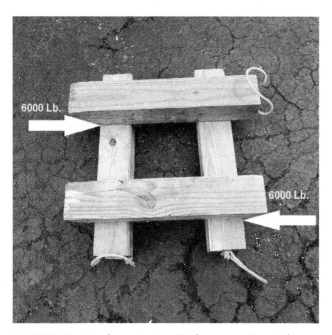

FIGURE 8-4 Each contact point has an estimated weight-bearing capacity of 6000 lb (3 short tons).
Courtesy of David Sweet.

Vehicle Positioning

NFPA 1006 Annex A is not a part of the NFPA requirements but is included for informational purposes. Annex A.8.2.3 lists five directional vehicle movements that the officer or technical rescuer in charge must consider during the process of vehicle stabilization of a common passenger vehicle:

1. **Horizontal movement**: Vehicle moves forward or rearward on its longitudinal axis or moves horizontally along its lateral axis.
2. **Vertical movement**: Vehicle moves up and down in relation to the ground while moving along its vertical axis.
3. **Roll movement**: Vehicle rocks side to side while rotating on its longitudinal axis and remaining horizontal in orientation.
4. **Pitch movement**: Vehicle moves up and down about its lateral axis, causing the vehicle's front and rear portions to move left or right in relation to their original position.
5. **Yaw movement**: Vehicle twists or turns about its vertical axis, causing the vehicle's front and rear portions to move left or right in relation to their original position.

Four post-collision vehicle positions are most commonly encountered at an accident scene:

- The vehicle may be in a regular or normal upright position resting on all four tires.
- The vehicle may be resting on its side.
- The vehicle may be resting on its roof.
- The vehicle may be on top of another vehicle, some other object, or an object may be on top of the vehicle.

The following sections will outline the stabilization process for these four post-collision vehicle positions that are most commonly encountered at an accident scene on a level plane. Keep in mind that there are numerous additional scenarios or complexities that can be presented with each of these positions, such as elevated or declining planes, bodies of water, snow, ice, mountainous terrain, or heavy brush. These scenarios will require additional stabilization techniques and/or equipment and resources.

The Vehicle in Its Normal Position

The main objective for stabilizing a vehicle in an upright position is to gain control of all vehicle movement by minimizing the vehicle's suspension system and creating a solid and safe base to work from (**FIGURE 8-5**). A vehicle's suspension system can cause

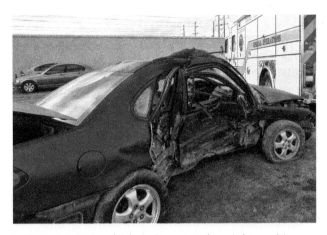

FIGURE 8-5 A vehicle in its normal upright position.
Courtesy of David Sweet.

the body of the vehicle to move up and down, potentially causing further injury to a victim. A victim with a suspected spinal injury needs to be properly immobilized immediately; any vehicle movement can exacerbate a spinal injury, potentially causing paralysis of the victim. The goal is to create a balanced platform to work from and minimize the movement of the vehicle's suspension system.

To better illustrate how to create this balanced platform and minimize the movement of the vehicle suspension system with cribbing, look at the shape of the underside of a common passenger vehicle that is completely stripped. If the vehicle's frame, undercarriage, underside, or platform is rectangular or square in design and all the vehicle's upper body components are removed, including side panels, parts, and wheels, you are left with a rectangular or square frame or platform. To balance out this object that is shaped like a rectangle or square, the best practice is to access four or more solid points or areas under the object and insert cribbing equally at these points to establish a balance, whether you build a wood box-crib configuration or insert a step chock. In a perfect world, you would always have access to all four sides of a vehicle, but the reality is that you may have access to only one or two sides of the vehicle. In such scenarios, use your best judgment, and crib the sides that you have access to. Properly cribbing just one side of the vehicle helps minimize movement of the vehicle. The overall objective for crib placement is to position cribbing in four or more solid areas spread out equally to create a balanced platform.

Also, you must consider placing cribbing at the front and rear tires to eliminate the potential for forward or backward movement of the vehicle. This is particularly a factor when the tires remain inflated. If the tires are deflated and the vehicle is resting firmly on cribbing, then the need for placing cribbing at the front and rear is not a high priority unless the vehicle is positioned on an elevation or decline. The decision to add more cribbing is up to the technical rescuer in charge of the operation.

When placing the cribbing, the need to choose areas that are solid cannot be stressed enough. Areas such as directly under the firewall/dash section or just in front of the rear tires are generally very solid points to work from. For example, if you were to change a flat tire, you would place the car jack under a solid area of the vehicle and avoid weaker areas, such as the fender sections behind the rear tire; these weaker sections can fold or collapse under weight or pressure. Also, avoid areas that can potentially block the extrication process or impede the normal swing of a door.

To eliminate potential problems, always think ahead before placing any cribbing sections. Ask yourself, "If cribbing is placed in this area, will it block my door from any movement or removal? Will the cribbing catch any section of metal when the door is manipulated?" When you are playing a game of billiards, each shot you take sets up your next series of actions; you strategize each shot and placement of the cue ball to set up each successive step in advance. This same strategy should be applied to cribbing placement—and to the extrication process as a whole. Each action the technical rescuer takes should set up the next step rather than impede it. Therefore, it is vital to know where and how to place cribbing strategically.

> **LISTEN UP!**
>
> The technical rescuer should always plan several steps ahead.

Determining the height distance from the ground to the bottom frame area will vary depending on the vehicle. For example, the amount of cribbing needed to stabilize a large sport utility vehicle (SUV) is significantly more than that needed to stabilize a small sports car. Step chocks will remove a lot of the guesswork because of the increased height adjustment on each successive step; also, consider the use of adjustable step cribbing or a scissor jack. When using cribbing, whether it is a basic four-by-four or a step chock, the goal is to make the contact area from the ground to the undercarriage tight, filling up any void spaces (**FIGURE 8-6**).

If a void space still exists after inserting a step chock, a wedge can be added under the step chock to build up the height and increase the contact area between the vehicle and the cribbing; tap the wedge

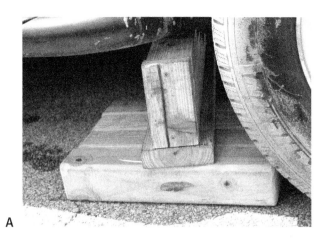

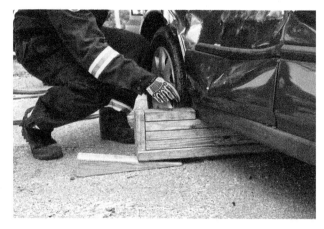

FIGURE 8-7 If a void space still exists after inserting step cribbing, a wedge can be added under the step chock to build up the height and increase the contact area between the vehicle and the cribbing.
Courtesy of Edward Monahan.

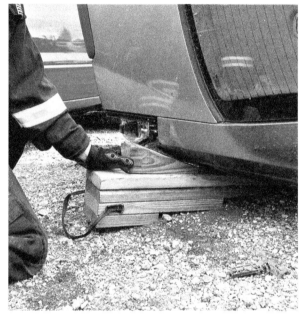

FIGURE 8-6 When using cribbing, whether it is a basic four-by-four or a step chock, the goal is to make the contact area from the ground to the undercarriage tight, filling up any void spaces.
Courtesy of Edward Monahan.

section in position using the butt end of a four-by-four, or use a rubber mallet (FIGURE 8-7). Also, if you are dealing with a vehicle that is high off the ground, such as an SUV, a crosstie platform–crib configuration can be set up with a step chock placed on top of it and then set into position.

One question that is continually asked is whether the vehicle's suspension can be lifted manually, just enough to insert the cribbing, and then let back down to rest on the cribbing that is now properly adjusted to the required height. This is a loaded question. If done correctly, then yes, this method can be attempted and is very effective. The proper technique includes positioning your back against the body of the vehicle near the front or rear wheel well, lifting with your legs and not your back, and lifting the suspension only and not the vehicle itself.

The problem comes from a poor lifting posture or from overexertion by an adrenalin-fueled rescuer who tries to lift the vehicle rather than just move the suspension; injuries will absolutely occur when the latter happens. Safe practice is always the main objective on any operation, so the decision to use or recommend this technique rests solely upon the officer in charge of the operation or should come from a directive outlined in a departmental policy, standard operating guideline (SOG), and/or approval of an agency's risk manager. Also, when determining whether to attempt this technique, consider the position of the vehicle, approximate estimated weight of the vehicle, and the physical condition of the rescuer or rescuers who will be performing the lift.

Tire Deflation

An often debated topic is whether the tires of the vehicle should be deflated after the cribbing has been inserted. One benefit of deflating the tires on a passenger vehicle is that it forces the vehicle to rest firmly on the cribbing, creating a solid base to work from. As sections of the vehicle are removed, such as the doors or roof, the vehicle becomes lighter. With a vehicle's tires still inflated and the vehicle becoming lighter, the suspension system causes the vehicle to rise and the cribbing to come loose. When the tires are deflated, the vehicle settles onto the cribbing with the suspension system virtually eliminated.

A drawback of tire deflation is that the stability of the vehicle may shift, or if there is an object or another vehicle positioned on top of the vehicle, then that object or vehicle can also shift. Other negative factors include design features that impede deflation, such as run-flat tires and steel tire valve stem assemblies as well as tire pressure monitor sensors that are built into the tire and attached to the stem valve. Determining whether to deflate the tires is purely a judgment call by the officer in charge and can be determined only at the time of the incident and by the type of situation being presented.

Some agencies do not advocate deflating tires because eliminating a means of measuring tire pressure can interfere with law enforcement's investigation. If your agency does not support tire deflation, then an alternative would be to insert a wedge section of cribbing under the crib configuration and strike the end of it with a mallet or the butt end of a four-by-four until the desired height or stability is achieved.

There are several tools that can be used to deflate a tire. Four types of tools to use for this objective are those that depress the valve core, those that remove the core from the valve stem, those that remove the entire valve assembly (a stem puller or a channel lock wrench), and a portable drill and step bit for puncturing the sidewall (**FIGURE 8-8**).

If the decision is to deflate a tire by removing the entire valve stem assembly, then a few criteria must be in place before proceeding with this procedure. If the stem is flexible and not a metal clamp-in type (which can be locked to the rim) and the valve is not recessed into the tire rim, a simple channel lock wrench can accomplish the task. When using a channel lock wrench, grab hold of the tire stem and rotate the tool so that the head of the wrench rests on the tire rim. Using the rim as a leverage point, move the tool downward, causing the stem to dislodge from its housing. One of the fastest techniques to deflate a tire with virtually no limitations is utilizing a battery-powered drill equipped with a step-bit attachment. Take the drill and place the tip of the step bit against the sidewall of the tire. Engaging the tool will quickly puncture the side wall, immediately deflating the tire as shown in Figure 8-8.

LISTEN UP!

Ensure that some form of stabilization is in place before deflating tires because the rapid release of air pressure can cause an unwanted shift in the vehicle's position.

Another option for tire deflation is to use the forked end of a Halligan bar. This technique also has limitations and can be applied only to the wheel rim with a flexible protruding valve stem, in addition to the hubcap being removed. Slide forward one side of the fork inside the tire rim just over the area where the stem protrudes from the wheel; the key is positioning the blade of the tool at the correct angle, which can take some practice to achieve. Sliding this tip section of the fork forward over that area cuts off the end of the rubber tire stem at the base where it protrudes from the rim (**FIGURE 8-9**). Remember that this technique works only on a wheel rim with a flexible protruding valve stem; any hubcaps need to be removed prior to attempting this technique. Also, never use the spiked end of a Halligan bar to puncture the tire. This is a very dangerous practice that can potentially cause injury if the tool rebounds off the tire. This approach is also very unprofessional; as technical rescuers, we strive to demonstrate skill through control, not through force.

Lastly, in addition to inserting cribbing for stabilization, the technical rescuer must always consider the basic or simple internal forms of stabilizing a vehicle. These steps include placing the vehicle in park, turning off the engine and securing the key, and applying the parking brake. These are steps that can easily be overlooked because the focus is on setting cribbing or step chocks into place quickly; yet these basic steps require very little effort to accomplish.

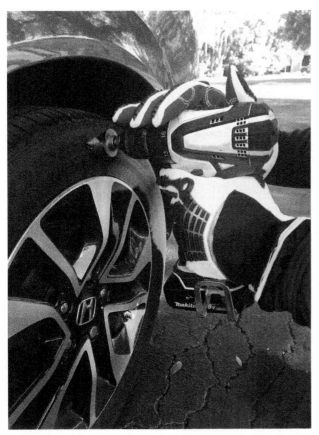

FIGURE 8-8 One of the fastest techniques to deflate a tire is utilizing a battery-powered drill equipped with a step-bit attachment.
Courtesy of David Sweet.

Voice of Experience

The fire and rescue services are in a time of rapid technological advancement, with rapid advances taking place every few months; in years past, huge leaps only occurred every five or ten years. There are more manufacturers, products, and vendors than ever before. While it may seem progressive to be early adopters and jump on board with new products and technology, rescuers should never lose those time-tested, fundamental skills.

Before taking a full-time position as a rescue instructor, I worked for a combination department in a small town served by three fire stations; two were career and one was all-volunteer. The career firefighters would check off all seven apparatus every morning, noting any new equipment that had been placed on any apparatus. Often training on the new gear would come later. That is exactly what happened one morning when I took note of four shiny yellow Rescue Jack RJ3's on the rescue. Back then, the concept of buttressing was new, and we had acquired one of the first buttress systems in our state. My indifference and lack of curiosity about our new rescue tools would come back and bite me a short while later.

The main highway in and out of town was two lanes and was often occupied with farm tractors with disks or combines and harvesters. Impatient drivers would often attempt to pass these farmers at high rates of speed, causing spectacular motor vehicle crashes.

We were dispatched to an MVA, a multiple car crash involving a farm tractor. Upon arrival, the tractor and disk were unharmed, but a driver had tried to pass, causing a head-on collision and secondary rear-end collision with the third vehicle. The scene was chaotic with a late-model sedan on its side, a truck with heavy front-end damage causing light entrapment, and a small SUV with heavy intrusion and moderate entrapment. We confirmed a fatality of an elderly man in the bottom of the sedan on its driver side. The assistant chief rode officer seat on Rescue 3. His first order was to stabilize the sedan with the buttresses. I felt like I looked like a deer in the headlights as I had never laid hands on them. I was determined to figure it out and not disappoint my assistant chief. I grabbed the jacks and fiddled with the height adjustments. I used the cam-buckle straps and married the base to the vehicle. Ultimately, I muddled my way through and put on a good show. My deployment of this tool was definitely sub-par and only marginally effective.

Our attention turned elsewhere as we had a classic brake pedal-foot entrapment in the vehicle resting on its side. The pedal relocation was in a very confined space. We worked top-down from the passenger doors, gaining access via the attic ladder. The buttress position obstructed our ability to remove the roof. Once we had the victim free, we passed him up through the doors and over the body of the car.

Lessons Learned:
- Do not risk placing new tools on any apparatus until all personnel have had the opportunity to train on them.
- When placing buttresses, have a plan for the extrication of the victim. It is easy to be lured into placing a strut in a position that prevents the roof from being flapped or removed. This forced us to struggle with extrication in the confined area and awkwardly hoist the body out of the car when the victim's foot was finally freed.
- Never forget the basics. In my panicked state, not knowing the Rescue Jacks, I forgot the *initial stabilization*. Step cribbing, wedges, and shims can be hugely instrumental in mitigating the "mouse-trap" hazard that the car on its side presents.

It was a close call on the buttressing, and this scene would teach me some valuable lessons that I would carry for the rest of my career.

Russell McCullar
Senior Instructor, Mississippi State Fire Academy
Jackson, Mississippi

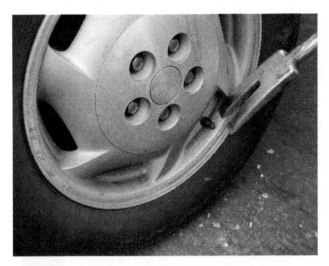

FIGURE 8-9 Sliding the flat section of the fork of a Halligan bar forward over the area of the rubber tire stem will cut off the end of the tire stem at the base where it protrudes from the rim.

To stabilize a common passenger vehicle in its normal upright position, follow the steps in **SKILL DRILL 8-1**.

The Vehicle Resting on Its Side

A vehicle resting on its side is a very dangerous scenario and requires the officer to develop an incident action plan (IAP) particular to this unique scenario. As was stated in Chapter 1, no two emergency incident responses are the same. Each response will require a different approach to developing a functional IAP. The officer must have the ability to adapt to the ever-changing dynamics an incident will present. (**FIGURE 8-10**). The IAP for a vehicle resting on its side should be developed using the following items:

Scene size-up: Is there a single car or multiple vehicles? Are the vehicles involved gasoline, diesel, or

SKILL DRILL 8-1
Stabilizing a Common Passenger Vehicle in Its Upright Normal Position
NFPA 1006 8.2.3

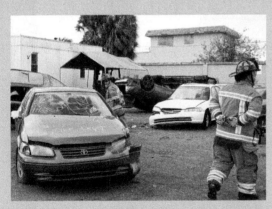

1 Don PPE. Enter the secure work area safely. Assess the scene for hazards, and complete the inner and outer scene surveys. Lay out a tarp at the edge of the secure work area for staging tools and equipment if indicated. Apply basic or simple internal forms of stabilization by placing the vehicle in park, turning off the engine, and/or applying the parking brake.

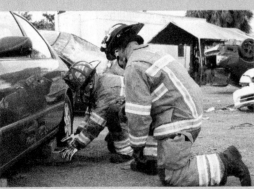

2 Insert a step chock, or build a wood box-crib/crosstie configuration under four solid points of the vehicle. If your agency supports tire deflation, deflate the tires by removing the tire valve stem assembly or puncturing the sidewall with a battery-operated drill equipped with a step-bit attachment. If your agency does not advocate tire deflation, use wedges to force the vehicle to rest firmly on the cribbing, and consider placing additional cribbing at the front and rear of the tires to prevent any unexpected forward or backward movement. Reassess to confirm stabilization. Perform all of these tasks in a safe manner. Notify command that the vehicle has been stabilized.

Courtesy of Davie Fire Rescue.

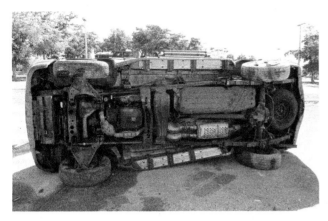

FIGURE 8-10 A vehicle resting on its side.
Courtesy of David Sweet.

hybrid vehicles? What is the ground condition (i.e., hard surface [asphalt] vs. soft [sand])? What is the terrain (i.e., level surface, embankment, or mountainous)? How many victims are involved?

Risk assessment: What type of hazards are present (e.g., fuel, electric lines, gas lines, terrain, inclement weather, or bodies of water)?

Resource availability and capability: What resources can you call to assist (i.e., large tow unit, high-angle rescue etc.)? Does your apparatus carry the correct type and supply of equipment to conduct the proper stabilization procedures?

Witness information: Are there possible ejections of victims from the vehicle? Did anyone leave the scene?

Reference materials: Check available references if needed (e.g., the *Alternative Fuel Vehicle Handbook* or *Emergency Response Guidebook*).

Remember that the company officer develops the IAP using the base procedures outlined in the organization's SOPs for an operations-level response to stabilizing a vehicle resting on its side. The company officer then builds off the SOPs, uses the information collected, and presents the IAP's Plan A (vehicle stabilization and entry plan including tactical assignment), Plan B (victim access and removal plan), and emergency plan (including immediate evacuation procedures for the team and victim[s]).

As with other scenarios, the vehicle resting on its side needs to be properly stabilized before any operations can be conducted. This section describes a technique using cribbing and tensioned buttress struts. Struts are structural supports used as a buttress to stabilize and reinforce an object. Because a technical rescuer must always be cognizant of time, the A-frame technique, described later, is designed for a very rapid and simplistic setup. When done correctly, this technique, including the inner and outer surveys, should take no longer than 5 minutes to complete. Keep the techniques basic unless you and your crew are well versed in multiple advanced stabilization scenarios; the time to attempt a new technique is not on the emergency scene.

There are many ways to stabilize a vehicle resting on its side, and the technical rescuer should research and train with the various manufacturers of stabilization equipment to become familiar with the wide array of tools that are offered. Taking this proactive initiative determines which tools are best suited to meet the needs of a particular organization.

One of the greatest advances in the rescue industry, with the exception of hydraulic tools, was the introduction of buttress stabilization struts with a tensioning attachment (**FIGURE 8-11**). These tools have simplified the stabilization process tremendously and make it much safer to conduct emergency operations on a vehicle.

SAFETY TIP

It is imperative that the team fully understand the stabilization technique before attempting it. Stabilization of a vehicle is a critical component of the extrication process; establishing a solid incident action plan will assist personnel in remaining on the same page to avoid potential breakdowns and/or harm or injury.

A vehicle resting on its side has a center of mass that is high and a comparatively narrow track or base, which can cause it to topple over very easily. The center of mass is the area of the object upon which all of the weight is centered; in this case, the center of mass is high because the vehicle is on its side. The goal is to lower the vehicle's center of mass by expanding the vehicle's **footprint**, or the area of the vehicle in contact with the ground. This can be accomplished with strategically placed struts, cribbing, and ratchet strapping. Ratchet straps are designed for tie-down purposes only and are not to be used for lifting. The main

LISTEN UP!

After the inner and outer surveys have been completed and all hazards cleared, the officer or technical rescuer in charge of the operation keeps his or her hands on the front or rear section of the vehicle to feel for any shifting or movement of the vehicle as the other crew members begin cribbing.

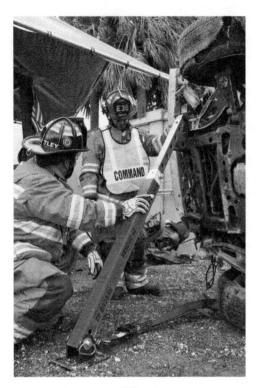

FIGURE 8-11 Buttress stabilization struts are structural supports that can be made of steel, aluminum, composite/Kevlar® wrap, and wood. They are used as a buttress to stabilize and reinforce an object, expanding a vehicle's base or footprint while also lowering its center of mass.
Courtesy of Edward Monahan.

objective is to position the struts to form an A-frame configuration. The A-frame configuration stabilizes the vehicle (just as the outriggers on an aerial apparatus are designed to work).

The first step that the technical rescuer takes is to examine whether the vehicle is leaning in a particular direction. If the vehicle is on its side on a level plane and with all of its tires/wheels intact, then the tendency is for the vehicle to roll toward the roof side; the roof side is considered the "hot side," or the most unstable, and will need to be the first side that is stabilized. To accomplish the scenario of stabilizing a vehicle resting on its side, the crew members should have a full complement of cribbing sections and struts to work with, such as wedges, shims, four-by-fours, and step chocks.

After the inner and outer surveys have been completed and all hazards cleared, the officer or technical rescuer in charge of the operation places his or her hand on the front or rear section of the vehicle (depending on where he or she best positions himself or herself) to feel for any shifting or movement of the vehicle as the other crew members begin cribbing. This safety technique allows the officer or rescuer in charge to warn crew members if the vehicle is going to roll or shift. Crew members who are inserting the cribbing are generally unable to determine vehicle movement

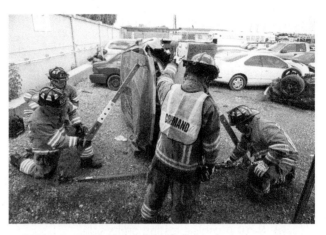

FIGURE 8-12 The position of the technical rescuer in charge of the operation should be at the front or rear of the vehicle; this provides full control of the operation by providing visibility to both sides of the vehicle.
Courtesy of Edward Monahan.

because their focus is at ground level where the cribbing is being placed. This safety technique gives the officer full control of the operation by providing visibility to both sides of the vehicle (**FIGURE 8-12**).

When operating at ground level around an unstable vehicle, such as inserting or positioning cribbing, the technical rescuer must always work from one knee in a semi-kneeling stance. This provides better mobility for moving quickly to avert any unexpected events as opposed to being planted with both knees on the ground. The scene safety officer or the technical rescuer in charge of the operation must keep a keen eye open for any improper techniques and remind personnel to always work safely.

LISTEN UP!

When operating at ground level around an unstable vehicle, such as when inserting or positioning cribbing, the technical rescuer must always work from one knee in a semi-kneeling stance.

To stabilize a vehicle resting on its side using buttress stabilization struts, follow the steps in **SKILL DRILL 8-2**.

Initial crib placement focuses on the most unstable area, or hot side, which in this particular scenario is the roof side of the vehicle. The objective here is to place some basic cribbing configurations initially on the hot side of the vehicle, thus enabling an A-frame strut setup using a tension buttress system. Placing cribbing under the front and rear sections of the vehicle leaves the roof area unobstructed and open to work on.

As an additional safety factor, another set of struts can be applied in the same manner to the rear section of the vehicle for extra stability, but generally one set of

SKILL DRILL 8-2
Stabilizing a Vehicle Resting on Its Side NFPA 1006 8.2.3

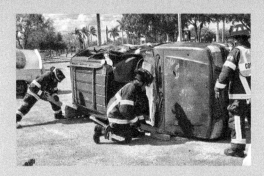

1 Don PPE. Enter the secure work area safely. Assess the scene for hazards, and complete the inner and outer scene surveys. Lay out a tarp at the edge of the secure work area for staging tools and equipment if indicated. Position an officer at the front or rear of the vehicle. The officer should position a free hand on the vehicle to feel and look for movement or shifting of the vehicle. Place cribbing under the hood and rear section of the vehicle using step chocks, wood cribbing, and wedges.

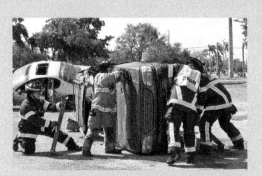

2 Place a tensioned buttress strut at a solid section of the undercarriage at the front of the vehicle. Adjust the strut height to maintain an angle of not less than 45 degrees to the vehicle and lock it into place. Move to the opposite (hood) side of the vehicle. Measure and then mark a purchase point location in the hood. Create a purchase point in the hood by using a battery-operated, cordless drill equipped with a step-bit attachment, or if a drill set is not available, use the spike end of a Halligan bar and striking tool to penetrate the hood section. Rotate the inserted Halligan bar 180 degrees and pry or pull down on the bar to create a lip on the top of the purchase point.

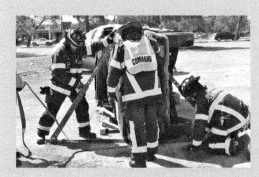

3 Place the tip of the strut into the purchase point, adjust the strut height, and lock it into place. Attach the hooks of the ratchet strap to the base of each strut with the ratcheting mechanism on the wheel side of the vehicle.

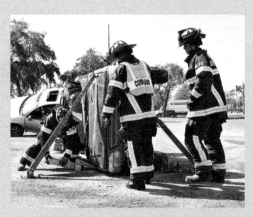

4 Double-check the placement of the struts before ratcheting. Tighten the ratchet strap, locking the struts into place. Reseat all cribbing to be sure the vehicle is stabilized.

Courtesy of Edward Monahan.

struts in the front section of the vehicle with the cribbing configurations at the front and rear is sufficient to accomplish the task. Also, if the grade level of the surface is sloping, depending on the position of the vehicle, additional cribbing or struts can be added to the front or rear to prevent any potential shifting. A basic operation should take the technical rescuer and crew no longer than 3 to 5 minutes to deploy and complete the stabilization of a vehicle resting on its side. The main advantage of using an A-frame technique is that the roof area is free of any cribbing, and an uncomplicated roof removal can be accomplished if called for by the officer in charge. Other techniques require cribbing to be inserted under the roof line in the area of the A-, B-, C-, or greater posts, which can impede a roof-removal operation.

The Vehicle Upside Down or Resting on Its Roof

When a vehicle is involved in a rollover, the roof posts can be compromised by the crash impact and subsequent weight of the vehicle now on the posts; this makes the vehicle unstable (**FIGURE 8-13**). Roof posts that have been compromised from a rollover impact are not guaranteed to support the weight of the vehicle; therefore, the roof needs a solid artificial support system before any operation can be conducted.

Federal Motor Vehicle Safety Standard (FMVSS) 216, *Roof Crush Resistance*, establishes a minimum requirement for roof strength. This standard, which has mandated full compliance since September 2015, states that a vehicle weighing 6000 lb (3 short tons) or less is required to have a roof that can withstand three times the weight of the vehicle when it is positioned on its roof. Some manufacturers impose even higher standards. This is an incredible safety feature for the consumer, but rescuers must not get lulled into a false sense of security by thinking that compromised roof posts are secure. The FMVSS test was not designed for post-crash roof supports. Always take the extra safety precaution and properly support the roof structure with struts and cribbing.

Stabilizing a vehicle on its roof on level ground involves using struts and applying cribbing, at a minimum, in a four-point configuration. Looking at the vehicle's position, the weight of the engine normally drives the hood or front area of the vehicle lower to the ground, with the trunk area presenting much higher. This scenario is based on the standard US automobile with a front-end engine compartment, where the roof area has not been completely flattened. With unobstructed access, there are usually three points of entry: the driver's side, the passenger's side, and the trunk area. Stabilization should always be set up to keep these potential entry points open and unobstructed.

Initial crib placement should focus on the most unstable area. In this particular scenario, the unstable area is the trunk side of the vehicle. The objective is to set up an A-frame configuration at the rear of the vehicle using struts by building up cribbing under the rear roof section and hood/dash areas of the vehicle. It is also possible to use crosstie box-cribbing configurations that are stacked on top of one another and placed under the trunk area on both sides. The rule of thumb is to never stack box cribbing any higher than two times its width. For example, a 20-in. (51-cm) wide box-crib formation should not exceed 40 in. (102 cm) in height (roughly 3.5 ft [1 m]).

Understand that by placing box cribbing under the trunk, you eliminate any possible trunk entry using a tunneling option. **Tunneling** is the process of gaining entry through the rear trunk area of a vehicle; this technique is more commonly used for a vehicle resting on its roof. Remember that it is always important to keep all options open to quickly compensate and change directions for any unexpected events.

To stabilize a vehicle resting on its roof, the crew members should have a full complement of cribbing sections and struts to work with, such as wedges, shims, four-by-fours, and step chocks.

To stabilize a vehicle resting on its roof on level ground, follow the steps in **SKILL DRILL 8-3**.

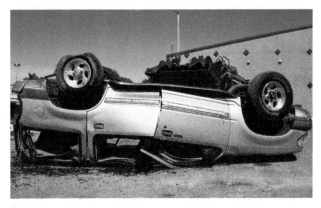

FIGURE 8-13 A vehicle upside down or resting on its roof.
Courtesy of Edward Monahan.

> **LISTEN UP!**
>
> Federal Motor Vehicle Safety Standards (FMVSS 216) establishes a minimum requirement for roof strength. This standard states that a vehicle weighing 6000 lb (3 short tons) or less is required to have a roof that withstands three times the weight of the vehicle when it is positioned on its roof. Some manufacturers impose even higher standards.

SKILL DRILL 8-3
Stabilizing a Vehicle Resting on Its Roof NFPA 1006 8.2.3

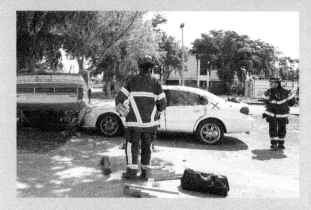

1. Don PPE. Enter the secure work area safely. Assess the scene for hazards, and complete the inner and outer scene surveys. Lay out a tarp at the edge of the secure work area for staging tools and equipment if indicated.

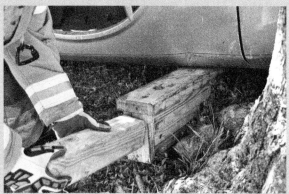

2. Place cribbing under the hood and rear section of the vehicle using step chocks, wood cribbing, and wedges. Set up buttress struts on both sides of the rear quarter panel/trunk area to form an A-frame configuration.

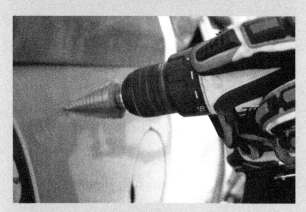

3. On both sides of the rear quarter panel, measure and mark an area for purchase points to place the tip of the struts. Other options can be used as long as the trunk seam is avoided (which keeps the option of tunneling through the trunk available if needed). Use a cordless drill with a step bit to penetrate the panel for the tip of the strut, or use a Halligan bar and flat-head axe combination.

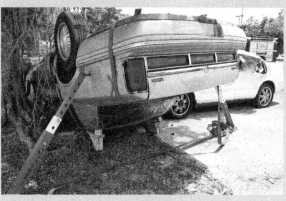

4. Connect the struts to each other by attaching the ratchet strap to the base of each strut. Pull up all the slack in the ratchet strap, and make it snug before ratcheting. Once completed, the remaining cribbing needs to be firmly reseated with the butt end of a four-by-four or rubber mallet.

Courtesy of Edward Monahan.

Vehicle on Vehicle or Multiple Concurrent Hazards

When the technical rescuer encounters a vehicle on top of another vehicle or an object on top of a vehicle, such as a large pole or concrete post, or where multiple concurrent hazards are present, he or she may be presented with two objects that are independently unstable (**FIGURE 8-14**). To stabilize both objects, they need to be married, or joined together, in their current position. **Marrying** vehicles eliminates any independent movement of the two objects. For the purpose of this discussion, we will use the example of a vehicle on top of another vehicle. Joining the two vehicles is best accomplished using industrial-grade ratchet strapping (**FIGURE 8-15**).

Because of the high degree of instability in this situation, it is extremely important to marry the two vehicles before operations are conducted. Stabilize the bottom vehicle first by inserting cribbing where there is access. Never crawl under the top vehicle because you may become trapped by a sudden collapse or shift; always work around the vehicle, remaining aware of and ready for any potential failure or collapse. If you need to pass a strap under a vehicle to the other side, hook the strap end to a long pike pole and safely pass it under the vehicle to the other side (**FIGURE 8-16**).

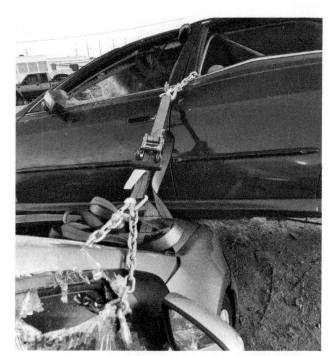

FIGURE 8-15 Industrial-grade ratchet strapping.
Courtesy of David Sweet.

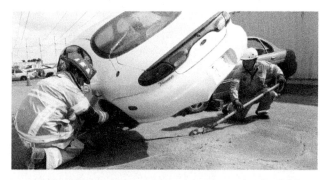

FIGURE 8-16 If you must pass a strap under a vehicle to the other side, hook the strap end to a long pike pole, and safely pass it under the vehicle to the other side.
© Jones & Bartlett Learning. Photographed by Glen E. Ellman.

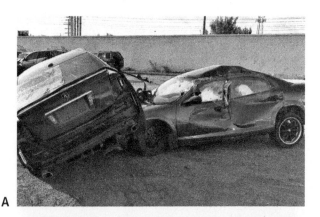

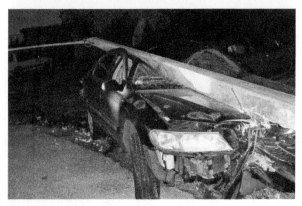

FIGURE 8-14 A. A vehicle on another vehicle.
B. Concrete pole on a vehicle.
Courtesy of David Sweet.

Other guidelines to remember about marrying vehicles using ratchet straps are:

- Always look at the top vehicle and determine where it wants to roll, shift, or move. Strap it in the opposite direction, pulling it in that direction and locking it into place.

LISTEN UP!

Use a long pike pole to pass straps under the vehicle to the other side.

- For more secure anchoring, wrap the ratchet strap around the object and hook it back into itself. If you must use the hook into the object, make certain that the object is strong material that will not tear and that the hook itself is the double-wire type.

Various factors will determine how the operation will be conducted. What are the positions of both vehicles? How is the top vehicle resting on the bottom vehicle? Is any section of the top vehicle touching the ground? Where are the victims in relation to the top vehicle? Are there any victims inside either vehicle? Where are the entry or access points to both vehicles? Will strapping or marrying the vehicles together block any access points? These are just a few questions that need to be addressed before any operation can be conducted, but additional questions will probably come up. This section reviews only one of the many possible vehicle-on-vehicle scenarios.

The objective is to stabilize the bottom vehicle and then marry the two vehicles together, eliminating any independent movement. To stabilize, or marry, a vehicle on top of another vehicle, follow the steps in **SKILL DRILL 8-4**.

SKILL DRILL 8-4
Stabilizing/Marrying a Vehicle on Top of Another Vehicle NFPA 1006 8.2.3

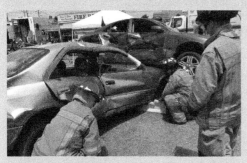

1 Don PPE. Enter the secure work area safely. Assess the scene for hazards. Complete the inner and outer scene surveys. Lay out a tarp at the edge of the secure work area for staging tools and equipment, if indicated. Stabilize the bottom vehicle. Cover the victim in the bottom vehicle with a blanket and manage the glass, utilizing the appropriate technique described in the text.

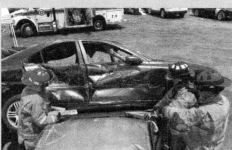

2 Fill the void spaces where the rocker panel of the top vehicle meets the hood section of the bottom vehicle.

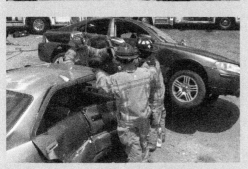

3 Anchor the ratcheting section of the ratchet strap to the lowest area of the passenger-side A-post of the bottom vehicle. Loop the loose end of the ratchet strap through the B-post of the top vehicle, and then loop the strap back through and secure it to itself. Tighten the ratchet strap, and lock or marry the top vehicle to the bottom vehicle.

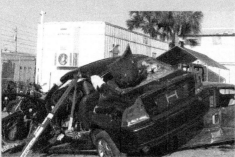

4 Once the top vehicle is secure, place cribbing or tension buttress stabilization struts to the lower section of the top vehicle and reseat all cribbing on the bottom vehicle. With both vehicles secured, a rescuer can be placed inside the bottom or top vehicle to treat and package the victim.

Courtesy of David Sweet.

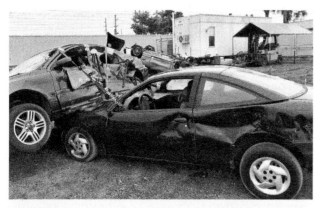

FIGURE 8-17 Marrying two vehicles using the technique in Skill Drill 8-4 allows for full access to the opposite side of the vehicle where unobstructed operations can be conducted and victim removal can occur.
Courtesy of David Sweet.

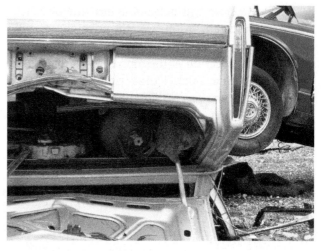

FIGURE 8-19 Hidden dangers such as this portable propane tank may be found in the trunk of a vehicle.
Courtesy of David Sweet.

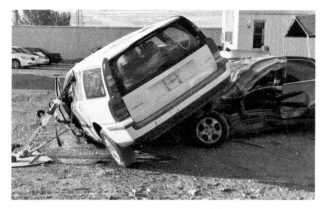

FIGURE 8-18 There are several additional cribbing options that can be added to the side of the vehicle on top to prevent any potential sliding as the bottom vehicle is being stabilized.
Courtesy of David Sweet.

This marrying configuration gives you access to the victim through the entire door and roof area (**FIGURE 8-17**). Keep in mind that there are several additional cribbing options that can be added to the side of the vehicle on top to prevent any potential sliding as the bottom vehicle is being stabilized (**FIGURE 8-18**).

Monitoring Stabilization

The stabilization of a vehicle(s) requires the continuous monitoring of stabilization devices by a designated safety officer or one member of the team. This requires the designated member to continuously walk around the vehicle(s) and lightly tap all cribbing with a rubber mallet to ensure that the cribbing has not shifted and is remaining tight and in place. In addition, shifting may occur after every major application of a tool, such as the use of a hydraulic tool to remove a door or roof. All stabilization devices should be reassessed after the application of a tool to confirm stabilization placement and position.

Hidden Dangers and Energy Sources

Although vehicle fires and downed power lines are visibly prominent and require immediate action and mitigation before the vehicle is stabilized, there are other potential hazards that may be hidden and cause havoc or injury to personnel on scene. For example, a portable propane cylinder could be found in a vehicle's trunk or back passenger compartment, or a short from a damaged electrical system could start a post-crash engine fire (**FIGURE 8-19**).

Once the vehicle has been stabilized, the proactive technical rescuer can mitigate hidden potential hazards by, for example, removing the portable propane tank and disabling the energy system of the vehicle. Again, the best practice is to stabilize the vehicle and establish a solid base or platform for the rescuer to work from in addition to minimizing vehicle movement, which can potentially exacerbate victims' injuries. Unless there is an immediate danger to life and health (IDLH) hazard that will affect the safety of the operation, stabilizing the vehicle should precede opening a hood or trunk of a vehicle to eliminate power. This practice is a guideline that should be applied only for conventional vehicles; alternative-fuel, hybrid, and fuel-cell vehicles require special procedures where disabling the electrical system is incorporated into stabilizing the vehicle and may have to be accomplished before cribbing is applied. The sequence of these actions is a judgment call that the officer in charge will have to make based on the type of incident presented.

Isolating or eliminating a vehicle's electrical system consists of disabling the vehicle's 12-volt DC battery and/or removing fuses from the fuse box. Removing any smart keys out of the range area is also recommended if the 12-volt DC battery cannot be disabled (**FIGURE 8-20**). A smart key is an electronic key that allows the driver to remotely start the vehicle from a general range of up to 20 ft (6 m) away, depending on the manufacturer. Before the electrical system is disabled, make sure any electrically controlled devices defined by NFPA 1006 as a beneficial system, such as vehicle seats, automatic steering wheel adjustments, or power windows, do not have to be used to gain access or create space for the victims. This needs to be coordinated between members of the rescue team and the incident commander (IC).

Another issue that can be encountered in some conventional vehicles is the possibility of multiple batteries or batteries that may be located in places other than the front hood area, such as in the rear trunk, under the front or rear seat, or under the right or left wheel well. Various vehicle manufacturers more commonly install 12-volt DC batteries in the trunk or under the rear seats (**FIGURE 8-21**). You must be aware of this possibility. Also, be aware that some manufacturers provide access only to the negative battery cable for purposes of disconnecting the electrical system.

Another method of isolating the energy system (which is recommended in various manufacturers' emergency response guides as well as the NFPA Emergency Response Guides) is to locate the fuse box and remove the fuses, which isolates all the electrical components and disables them. This alternative method can be time consuming and difficult to execute because the fuses are small and concealed and the 12-volt DC battery remains live. Supplemental restraint system air bag control units come equipped with an energy capacitor that can store power, keeping the air bag system active and live even when the power has been disconnected for a varied amount of time (varies among manufacturers). Supplemental restraint systems are discussed in detail in Chapter 6, *Supplemental Restraint Systems*.

To disable a conventional vehicle's electrical system and mitigate the potential electrical hazards at an MVA, follow the steps in **SKILL DRILL 8-5**.

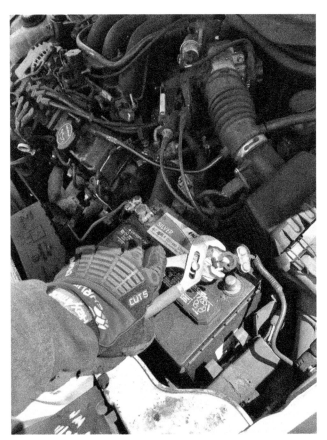

FIGURE 8-20 Isolating or eliminating a vehicle's electrical system consists of disabling the vehicle's 12-volt DC battery and/or removing fuses from the fuse box. Removing any smart keys out of the range area is also recommended if the 12-volt DC battery cannot be disabled.
Courtesy of David Sweet.

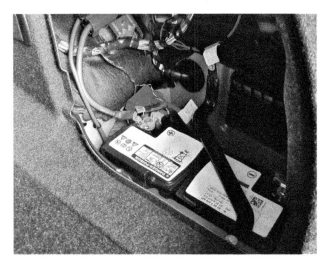

FIGURE 8-21 Vehicle manufacturers commonly install 12-volt DC batteries in the trunk or under the rear seat.
Courtesy of David Sweet.

SKILL DRILL 8-5
Mitigating Vehicle Electrical Hazards at an MVA NFPA 1006 8.2.3 and 8.2.4

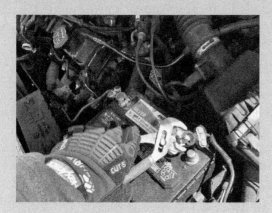

1. Don PPE. Stabilize the scene and the vehicle. Check the vehicle for a smart key, and move it out of range. Open the vehicle's hood. Locate the 12-volt DC battery system, and eliminate sources of ignition. The first option to disable the system is to remove the negative terminal connection first and then the positive terminal by loosening the cable connection from the terminal.

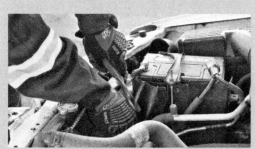

2. Alternatively, cut a section out of the negative battery cable first and then a section out of the positive battery cable. Prevent the cables from touching the terminals.

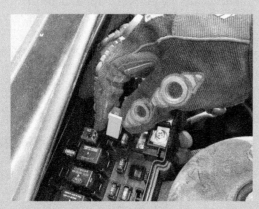

3. A third option to disable the vehicle's electrical system is to remove fuses from the fuse box.

Steps 1 and 3: Photos Courtesy of David Sweet; **Step 2:** Photo Courtesy of Edward Monahan.

After-Action REVIEW

IN SUMMARY

- Vehicle stabilization is a critical component of the extrication process.
- Proper vehicle stabilization provides a solid foundation to work from, which ensures safety for the emergency personnel as well as the victim and bystanders.
- Cribbing is the most basic physical tool used in vehicle stabilization.
- Soft woods are commonly used for cribbing because they are well suited for compression-type loads. Hard wood is very strong but may split easily under certain stresses.

- NFPA 1006 discusses five types of wood box-cribbing configurations: two-piece layer crosstie, three-piece layer crosstie, platform crosstie, triangle crosstie, and modified crosstie.
- There are five directional movements to consider during the process of vehicle stabilization: horizontal movement, vertical movement, roll movement, pitch movement, and yaw movement.
- There are four common post-collision vehicle positions that can be encountered at a collision scene:
  - The vehicle may be in a regular or normal upright position resting on all four tires.
  - The vehicle may be resting on its side.
  - The vehicle may be resting on its roof.
  - The vehicle may be on top of another vehicle or some other object, or an object may be on top of the vehicle.
- The basic or simple forms of internally stabilizing a vehicle include placing the vehicle in park, turning off the engine, and applying the parking brake.
- The main purpose for stabilizing a vehicle in its normal position is to gain control of all vehicle movement by minimizing the vehicle's suspension system and creating a solid and safe base to work from.
- When placing the cribbing, choose areas that are solid; areas such as the rocker panel just under the firewall/dash section or the area just in front of the rear tires are generally very solid points to work from.
- When using cribbing, the goal is to make the contact area from the ground to the undercarriage tight, filling up any void spaces.
- The purpose of deflating the tires is to have the frame of the vehicle settle down onto the cribbing, creating a balanced platform to work from and minimizing the suspension system.
- The goal of stabilizing a vehicle on its side is to lower its center of mass by expanding the vehicle's footprint, or base, such as seen with utilizing the outriggers on an aerial platform apparatus.
- When a vehicle is involved in a rollover, the roof posts will be compromised by the impact and weight of the vehicle, making the vehicle unstable. The objective is to set up an A-frame configuration at the rear of the vehicle using struts by building up cribbing under the rear roof rail section and hood/dash areas to maintain balance.
- When the technical rescuer encounters a vehicle on top of another vehicle or an object on top of a vehicle, he or she is presented with two objects that are independently unstable. These objects need to be joined together, or married, to eliminate any independent movement.
- Once the vehicle has been stabilized, the technical rescuer should mitigate any potential post-crash vehicle electrical hazards that can occur, which may require disabling the vehicle's electrical system.

KEY TERMS

Contact point When sections of cribbing are set on top of one another, the weight-bearing section of cribbing that crosses over the other. When using a 4-in. × 4-in. (10-cm × 10-cm) piece of timber, each contact point has an estimated weight-bearing capacity of 6000 lb (3 short tons).

Footprint A generic term used to describe an object's balance in relation to its center of mass as determined by how much of the object's base touches the surface and how much of the object spans the surface.

Horizontal movement One of five directional movements; the vehicle moves forward or rearward on its longitudinal axis or moves horizontally along its lateral axis.

Marrying The process of joining vehicles together to eliminate any independent movement.

Pitch movement One of five directional movements; the vehicle moves up and down about its lateral axis, causing the vehicle's front and rear portions to move left or right in relation to their original position.

Roll movement One of five directional movements; the vehicle rocks side to side while rotating about on its longitudinal axis and remaining horizontal in orientation.

Tunneling The process of gaining entry through the rear trunk area of a vehicle, a process more commonly used for a post-crash vehicle resting on its roof.

Vertical movement One of five directional movements; the vehicle moves up and down in relation to the ground while moving along its vertical axis.

Yaw movement One of five directional movements; the vehicle twists or turns about its vertical axis, causing the vehicle's front and rear portions to move left or right in relation to their original position.

On Scene

Your unit responds to a report of an MVA. Upon your arrival, you discover that multiple cars are involved. The IC assigns you the task of performing stabilization on vehicle number two.

As you perform your size-up of the vehicle, you note a late-model SUV that has come to rest on its roof. The vehicle has suffered major damage from an apparent rollover accident. There are victims trapped inside the vehicle who will require emergency medical care. You have access from all sides of the vehicle, and you do not see any secondary hazards, such as power lines or leaking fuel, as you and your crew complete the inner and outer surveys.

1. Stabilizing the vehicle will provide:
   A. tasks to keep the firefighters occupied.
   B. time for other resources to arrive.
   C. a stable foundation to work from.
   D. an alternative to rolling a vehicle back onto its wheels.

2. The most basic physical tool in vehicle stabilization is cribbing.
   A. True
   B. False

3. A vehicle resting on its side on level ground with all four wheels intact tends to roll toward its:
   A. trunk side.
   B. roof side.
   C. undercarriage side.
   D. The vehicle will not roll.

4. A vehicle that has been in a rollover and comes to rest on its roof is compromised because of the:
   A. engine block altering the center of gravity.
   B. potential for leaking fluids.
   C. potential for victims being underneath the vehicle.
   D. potential crash impact that compromised the integrity of the roof posts.

5. In this situation, struts and cribbing should be placed at a minimum of:
   A. one point.
   B. two points.
   C. three points.
   D. four points.

6. A vehicle that has come to rest on its roof provides a number of unique complications.
   A. True
   B. False

7. If no other routes of entry into the vehicle are available, such as when the sides are blocked, the victim can be reached through the rear via a method called:
   A. burrowing.
   B. tunneling.
   C. worm holing.
   D. belly crawling.

8. To stabilize the vehicle resting on its roof, the technical rescuer would likely use in addition to cribbing:
   A. electric winches.
   B. struts.
   C. chain hoists.
   D. come alongs.

9. The goal of the rescuer should be to create a strut configuration that is a(n):
   A. A-frame.
   B. lean-to.
   C. V-point.
   D. pivotless point.

10. Stabilization of a vehicle resting on its side should be focused on lowering the vehicle's:
    A. position.
    B. height.
    C. weight.
    D. center of mass.

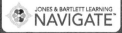 Access Navigate for more activities.

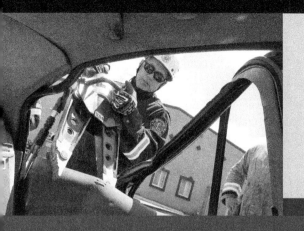

CHAPTER 9

Operations and Technician Levels

Victim Access and Management

KNOWLEDGE OBJECTIVES

After studying this chapter, you will be able to:
- Define the following terms and discuss their role in vehicle rescue incidents:
  - Glass management (pp. 224–226)
  - Expose and cut (p. 237–239)
- Detail the steps in victim access and removal. (**NFPA 1006: 8.2.5, 8.2.6, 8.2.7, 8.2.8, 8.3.6, 8.3.9**, pp. 222–224)
- Explain the differences between primary and secondary access. (**NFPA 1006: 8.2.5**, p. 223)
- Identify automotive window materials, and explain the challenges these materials pose to rescuers. (pp. 224–226, 227–231, 235)
- List dangers encountered in cutting vehicle components. (**NFPA 1006: 8.2.5**, pp. 233–234, 237–238, 249, 251–252, 255, 264, 266, 276)
- Describe the steps in roof removal. (pp. 235–237, 249–254)
- Compare and contrast the dash roll and the dash lift. (pp. 255–266)
- Describe the techniques available to rescuers for steering wheel relocation. (pp. 266–267)
- List the steps in addressing life-threatening injuries in vehicle crash victims. (pp. 271–276)
- Identify and use appropriate immobilization, packaging and transfer devices, and techniques to safely remove a victim from a vehicle. (**NFPA 1006: 8.2.7, 8.2.8, 8.3.9**, pp. 276–278)
- Identify signs and symptoms of compartment syndrome as a result of crush injuries (**NFPA 1006: 8.2.8**, p. 275)

SKILLS OBJECTIVES

After studying this chapter, you will be able to perform the following skills:
- Create access and egress openings for a common passenger vehicle that has come to rest on its wheels, roof, or side (**NFPA 1006: 8.2.6, 8.3.3, 8.3.4**, pp. 222–226).
- Ensure vehicle stabilization and entry/exit points are not compromised by vehicle movement, ensure stabilization points are structurally sound, tool placement, rescue activities, or equipment monitoring. (**NFPA 1006: 8.2.3, 8.3.2**, pp. 222–223)
- Perform an assisted backboard technique. (**NFPA 1006: 8.2.6, 8.2.7, 8.3.6, 8.3.9**, pp. 226–227)
- Break tempered glass using a spring-loaded center punch. (**NFPA 1006: 8.2.6, 8.2.7, 8.3.6, 8.3.9**, p. 229)
- Fracture tempered safety glass using a glass handsaw. (**NFPA 1006: 8.2.6, 8.2.7, 8.3.6, 8.3.9**, p. 230)
- Remove the windshield using a glass handsaw. (**NFPA 1006: 8.2.6, 8.2.7, 8.3.6, 8.3.9**, p. 232)
- Remove the windshield using a reciprocating saw. (**NFPA 1006: 8.2.6, 8.2.7, 8.3.6, 8.3.9**, p. 234)
- Remove windshield from a partially ejected victim. (**NFPA 1006: 8.2.6, 8.2.7, 8.3.6, 8.3.9**, p. 236)

- Expose air bag hazards by removing covering materials. (**NFPA 1006: 8.2.4, 8.2.6**, pp. 233, 234, 243, 246, 250, 251–252, 253, 255, 276)
- Execute the following vehicle extrication techniques using non-hydraulic tools:
  - Door removal (**NFPA 1006: 8.2.6, 8.2.7, 8.3.6, 8.3.9**, pp. 242–243)
  - Side-out (**NFPA 1006: 8.2.6, 8.2.7, 8.3.6, 8.3.9**, pp. 250–251)
  - Dash roll (**NFPA 1006: 8.2.6, 8.2.7, 8.3.6, 8.3.9**, pp. 258–259)
  - Dash lift (**NFPA 1006: 8.2.6, 8.2.7, 8.3.6, 8.3.9**, pp. 264–265)
  - Steering wheel relocation using a 2/4-ton rated come along and a First Responder Jack. (**NFPA 1006: 8.2.6, 8.2.7, 8.3.6, 8.3.9**, pp. 267–271)
- Execute the following vehicle extrication techniques using hydraulic tools:
  - Door removal (pp. 240–242)
  - Side-out (**NFPA 1006: 8.2.6, 8.2.7, 8.3.6, 8.3.9**, pp. 246–249)
  - Roof removal (**NFPA 1006: 8.2.6, 8.2.7, 8.3.6, 8.3.9**, pp. 253–254)
  - Dash roll (**NFPA 1006: 8.2.6, 8.2.7, 8.3.6, 8.3.9**, pp. 257–258)
  - Dash lift (**NFPA 1006: 8.2.6, 8.2.7, 8.3.6, 8.3.9**, pp. 261–263)
  - Wheel well crush technique (**NFPA 1006: 8.2.6, 8.2.7, 8.3.6, 8.3.9**, p. 244)
- Extricate a victim from a passenger car. (**NFPA 1006: 8.2.8, 8.3.9**, pp. 277–278)

You Are the Rescuer

You are on a vehicle rescue and extrication incident where a vehicle has impacted a concrete light pole, which has collapsed on the front end and hood of the vehicle, trapping the victim under the dash. The company officer orders your crew to perform a dash roll technique utilizing the hydraulic rams, but you know that this is not the proper technique for this type of entrapment.

1. As the technical rescuer on scene, what do you do?
2. Would you explain to the company officer that a dash roll technique will not work in this situation and that a dash lift is the correct technique?
3. Would you perform a dash lift technique to release the dash off the victim?

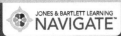 Access Navigate for more practice activities.

Introduction

Vehicle rescue and extrication is a step-by-step technical process consisting of three phases: stabilization of the scene, stabilization of the vehicle(s), and stabilization of the victim(s). This chapter discusses the third phase of the process, stabilizing the victim: victim access and management (**FIGURE 9-1**). With the scene and vehicle stabilized, it is time to access, manage, and transfer the victim. Managing the victim involves victim access, care, packaging, removal, and transport to the appropriate trauma-care facility. The main objective is not to remove the victim from the vehicle but to remove the vehicle from the victim by creating a large opening with systematic and precise techniques.

Access Points

After stabilizing a common passenger vehicle, the team must gain access into the passenger compartment to stabilize, protect, and disentangle victims. Plan A (the access plan, or initial entry plan) may be obtained in several ways. For example, simple and quick access may be obtained via an unobstructed and unlocked door adjacent to the victims, sliding in through an open or broken-out rear or side window, or an assisted backboard slide technique described in

CHAPTER 9 Victim Access and Management   **223**

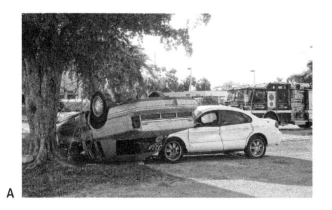

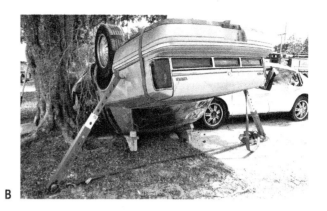

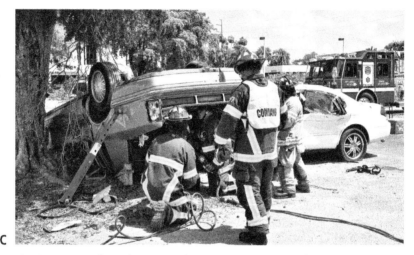

FIGURE 9-1 Vehicle extrication is a technical process that requires structured successive steps to produce favorable results. This chapter will discuss the third phase of this process "Stabilizing the victim: victim access and management." **A.** Phase 1: Stabilize the scene: site operations—dispatch, responding to the scene, scene size-up, scene safety zones, hazards, inner and outer surveys, incident action plan (IAP). **B.** Phase 2: Stabilize the vehicle: vehicle safety and stabilization—vehicle positioning; cribbing/struts; stabilization of vehicle in its normal position, on its side, or resting on its roof or on another object. **C.** Phase 3: Stabilize the victim: victim access and management—initial access points, using various rescue tools and equipment to gain access, providing initial medical care, packaging, and removal.
Courtesy of Edward Monahan.

the following text. The objective is to gain access to render immediate care. Options such as these may be referred to as primary vehicle access points, where no forceful techniques or special tools are required to gain entry. In the majority of vehicle accidents, access to victims may be gained simply by manually opening a door.

NFPA Glossary of Terms 2018 defines **primary access** as the existing openings of doors and/or windows that provide a pathway to the trapped and/or injured victim. NFPA Glossary of Terms 2018 defines **secondary access** as the openings created by rescuers that provide a pathway to remove/extricate trapped and/or injured victims, or Plan B (the removal plan and/or extrication plan). These two types of access are the basis for establishing Plan A and Plan B of the Incident Action Plan (IAP); if the team cannot gain entry through existing openings (the established Plan A), then Plan B is implemented to create and gain access.

Plan A and Plan B may be incorporated utilizing the same initial access area. For example, the initial access (Plan A) into the vehicle is through a rear door that is already opened from the damage of the impact. Once the victim is accessed and initially stabilized, Plan B (the removal plan) is to implement an all-door side-out technique using the primary access door as the starting point. If it is determined that more access is needed, then Plan B may evolve into a roof removal and dash displacement, depending on the level of entrapment. Incorporating additional techniques into the original Plan B may occur as the plan evolves; this takes coordination and acknowledgment from the officer to the entire team. The goal here is to create a large opening with a clear, unobstructed path for victim removal.

> **LISTEN UP!**
> The main objective is not to remove the victim from the vehicle but to remove the vehicle from the victim by creating a large opening with systematic and precise techniques.

It is also important to add that with Plan A and Plan B, an emergency escape plan must always be incorporated to address all unexpected emergencies that can happen at any moment. As discussed in detail in Chapter 7, the emergency escape plan is established immediately after the inner/outer survey is completed. The emergency escape plan is a designated area of temporary refuge that the team can immediately enter if an immediate danger to life and health is experienced, such as another vehicle entering the hot zone and crashing into an emergency apparatus.

Access Through Doors

One of the simplest ways to access a victim is to open a vehicle door (**FIGURE 9-2**). It is important to manually try all the doors before forceful methods are used; even if the doors appear to be badly damaged, sometimes, the latching mechanism still functions. An old adage and first rule of forcible entry is "Try before you pry." It is an embarrassing waste of time and energy to open a jammed door with heavy rescue equipment only to find that a door could have been opened easily without special equipment. Attempt to unlock and open the least damaged door first. Ensure that the locking mechanism is released prior to engaging the door handle. Then, try the outside and inside handles at the same time if possible. If the doors are locked, you might consider removing the glass from a window utilizing the techniques shown in this text and then attempt to manually release the locking mechanism to unlock the doors.

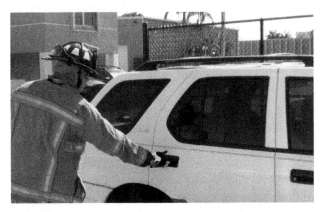

FIGURE 9-2 Manually attempt access into the vehicle through the doors first, if possible.
Courtesy of David Sweet.

> **LISTEN UP!**
> A fundamental rule of forcible entry is "Try before you pry."

Access Through Windows

If a victim's medical status is serious enough to require immediate care and entry cannot be made through a door of a common passenger vehicle in an upright position, consider removing the glass from a window and attempting to manually release the door's locking mechanism or conduct an assisted backboard slide technique (presented later in this chapter) to gain entry and render immediate aid. The side and rear windows can consist of tempered, laminated, or polycarbonate material. The rescuer must be prepared to take the appropriate action to manage the various window compositions encountered, which is explained in this chapter.

There are two basic ways to tell what type of glass you are dealing with. First, all vehicle glass contains small etched or embossed markings stating that it is "safety"/tempered glass and/or laminated glass (**FIGURE 9-3**). Internationally, the markings may appear in another language, such as German. *Verbund-Sicherheitsglas* (VSG) is translated in English to mean laminated safety glass; *EV-Verglasung* (ESG) means tempered glass glazing. These markings are generally very difficult to see, especially at night, because the manufacturers attempt to maintain the clear, unobstructed view and natural aesthetics of the glass. The second way to determine what type of glass you are dealing with requires the use of a center punch or other glass breaking tool. If the glass is laminated, then the center punch will not be able to penetrate the glass and will only partially fracture the outer glass section. This will be evident by a small spider-web ring around the point of impact. If the glass is made of a polycarbonate material, then again, the center punch will not be able to penetrate it; more than likely the tool will spring back.

Although it may not be a common procedure, entering through the windshield will require more aggressive steps utilizing hand and/or power tools, such as glass shears or a reciprocating saw, to gain entry. This method of entry may be required for a vehicle resting on its side. Remember that the front windshield on a common passenger vehicle is made of a laminated glass; it is generally sealed and held in place with a mastic-type adhesive that requires a cutting action of the glass itself to be properly removed.

Glass Management

There are multiple hazards that can be encountered at the scene of a motor vehicle accident, such as fuel

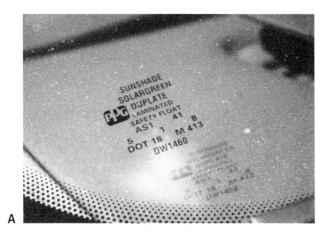

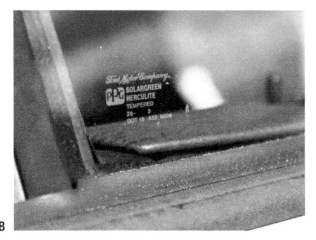

FIGURE 9-3 All glass contains small etched or embossed markings in one of the corners stating that it is "safety"/tempered glass and/or laminated glass. **A.** Laminated glass. **B.** Tempered glass.
Courtesy of Edward Monahan.

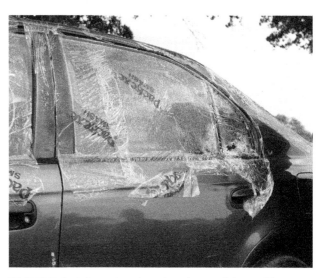

FIGURE 9-4 Securing the glass by applying a film product, such as Packexe SMASH®, prior to conducting the procedure allows for the decision either to leave the secured glass in place and proceed with the technique as normal or remove the glass section(s) entirely. Either decision gives the rescuer full control over the glass and prevents unexpected shattering from occurring.
Courtesy of Edward Monahan.

spills, electrical hazards, and biohazards, to mention a few. Some of these hazard types are a by-product of the accident itself and may exist based on factors such as the surrounding environment and the severity and type of impact of the vehicle and/or object as well as the damage that occurred. One hazard that remains constant and must be addressed in the IAP is vehicle glass. Vehicle glass can present a hazard to both the rescuer and the victims. Once broken, tempered glass produces small cube-like pieces of dull glass and fragment particles that can cover the victim and interior of the vehicle, where rescue personnel and, subsequently, their personal protective equipment (PPE) are exposed to it. When broken, laminated glass produces large shards as well as small, sharp particles that can also affect the rescuer and victim. **Glass management** is the process of identifying the need for controlling the removal of glass or maintaining the glass intact. With the implementation of Federal Motor Vehicle Safety Standard (FMVSS) 226, Ejection Mitigation, most vehicle manufacturers are moving toward utilizing laminated-type glass in the majority of the areas of the vehicle.

An excellent tool for managing glass is the application of self-adhesive film. Applying a self-adhesive film on the sides and rear sections of the vehicle glass strengthens and keeps the glass intact as well as controllable, whether the decision is to leave the glass in place or remove it. Securing the glass utilizing this type of product provides a safer working environment for the rescuer and victim by minimizing and/or eliminating all glass particles and shards (**FIGURE 9-4**). The process of removing a vehicle's roof requires all glass to be removed. This is a safety measure that must be performed to avoid glass unexpectedly shattering or falling on the victim when the roof is cut and removed. Securing a vehicle's windows with the self-adhesive film can quickly be accomplished, and then all the glass can be broken, with each section removed intact and placed in a designated debris area. The same procedure can be applied when a door is spread with a hydraulic tool; such rescue efforts will compress and twist the entire body of the vehicle, potentially causing an unsecured side or rear glass section that has not been removed to shatter. Applying a film to the glass prior to conducting the procedure allows for the decision either to leave the secured glass in place and proceed with the technique as normal or remove the glass section(s) entirely. Either decision gives the rescuer full control over the glass and prevents unexpected shattering from occurring.

When breaking unsecured glass, make certain that all personnel operating around the vehicle and the victim are aware that the vehicle's glass is going to be broken out. The statement "Breaking glass!" must be made before the action of breaking the glass begins. This safety practice ensures there are no surprises that can occur when someone haphazardly takes out glass without warning anyone. Ensure that the victim is fully aware of the action taking place and that the victim and the rescuer are covered before any glass is broken, unless all access to the victim is blocked. Attempt to break the glass beginning at the farthest point from the victim, and remember to clean out the tempered glass fragments from all the window frames using a hand tool or piece of 4-in. × 4-in. (10-cm × 10-cm) cribbing. Be extremely cautious when removing broken sections of laminated glass from the casing of the window with a gloved hand; even gloves are susceptible to a penetrating glass shard. All glass that has been removed, whether it is laminated windshield glass or secured tempered glass, should be placed in a debris pile in a safe area to avoid potential injuries.

The Backboard Slide Technique

The overall objective for using the backboard slide technique is to gain access to the victim as rapidly as possible to render care to a victim in a common passenger vehicle that is in the upright position. If the vehicle doors are locked, blocked, or not operable, initial access into the passenger compartment may be accomplished through a rear or side window utilizing an assisted backboard slide technique. Please be aware that the window openings may be extremely tight, with limited space to maneuver. The rescuer making entry may have to carefully slide headfirst, which requires the rescuer to be wearing the proper PPE and to be guarded when making entry to protect against any head or neck injuries. Also, ensure that the area of entry is clear of any harmful debris or biohazards.

To perform the assisted backboard slide technique through a rear window, follow the steps in **SKILL DRILL 9-1**.

LISTEN UP!

When breaking unsecured glass, begin at the farthest point from the victim. Remember to clean out the tempered glass fragments from all window frames using a hand tool or four-by-four cribbing.

SKILL DRILL 9-1
The Assisted Backboard Slide Technique NFPA 1006 8.2.6, 8.2.7, 8.3.6, 8.3.9

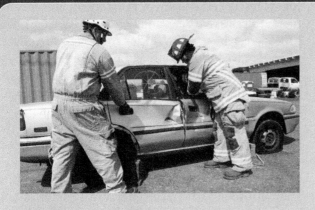

1 Don appropriate PPE, including mask and eye protection. Assess the scene for hazards, and complete the inner and outer surveys. Stabilize the vehicle that is in an upright position. Manually try to open all doors before beginning the technique to confirm they are locked or inoperable.

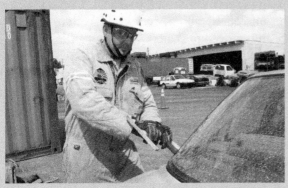

2 If there is no access, prepare to make entry through a window. Apply a safety film if available, and remove the rear window glass utilizing the appropriate techniques.

SKILL DRILL 9-1 Continued
The Assisted Backboard Slide Technique NFPA 1006 8.2.6, 8.2.7, 8.3.6, 8.3.9

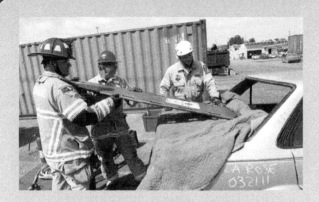

3 Place a tarp or blanket in the window frame to protect against any unsecured glass fragments. Ensure that the area of entry is clear of any harmful debris or biohazards. Place a long backboard up on the trunk area, with the front end just resting on the inside of the rear window frame.

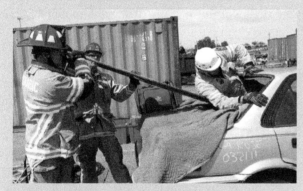

4 A technical rescuer will position himself or herself on the backboard, either headfirst or feetfirst depending on the type of vehicle, maneuverability, and the size of the opening. Two additional technical rescuers will grab hold of the board on opposite sides and raise the board to slide the technical rescuer on the board safely into the vehicle.

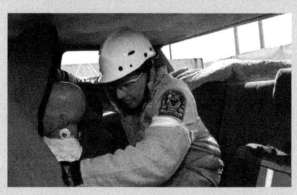

5 All appropriate medical gear is passed into the vehicle, and care is rendered to the victim.

© Jones & Bartlett Learning. Photographed by Glen E. Ellman.

Tempered Safety Glass

There are several tools designed for fracturing tempered glass. Some of them were discussed in Chapter 3, *Tools and Equipment*. The spring-loaded center punch is the most basic and common of all glass breaking tools (**FIGURE 9-5**).

When using a center punch to fracture tempered glass, the technical rescuer must follow several safety rules. First, wearing full PPE, including eye protection, position a gloved hand palm down against the lower corner of the window and frame area that is going to be broken (if this area is accessible). Your hand should be positioned with the thumb pointing upward, flush against the window and the window frame for support. With your free hand, rest the body of the center punch on the outer ridge of your palm, in the V of your hand, between the thumb and index finger. Place the tip of the tool at a 90-degree angle to and against the window. The positioning of your hand against the corner of the window and frame area

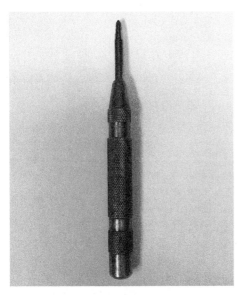

FIGURE 9-5 The spring-loaded center punch is the most basic and common of all glass breaking tools.
Courtesy of David Sweet.

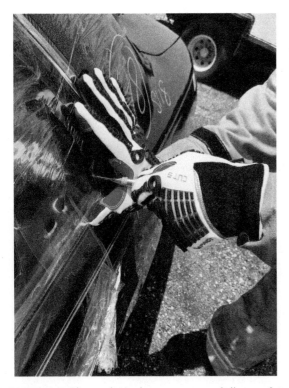

FIGURE 9-6 The technical rescuer must follow safety rules when utilizing a spring-loaded center punch to break tempered glass. This technique prevents the rescuer from accidentally putting a hand through the window as the glass is broken.
Courtesy of David Sweet.

will act as a safety stop, preventing you from accidentally putting your hand through the window when it fractures (**FIGURE 9-6**). Once you are ready, give the warning "Breaking glass!" and then commence plunging the tool into the window.

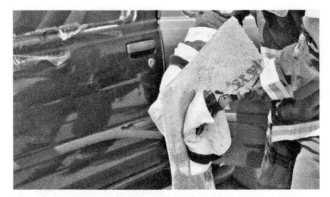

FIGURE 9-7 Tempered glass with tinting or safety film applied makes it easy to remove the entire section of glass when it is broken.
Courtesy of Edward Monahan.

If the tempered glass is unsecured, with no applied safety film or tinting film, use a hand tool or a four-by-four to clean out the window frame of any remaining fragments of glass. If the window is covered with safety film and/or tinting film, the glass will hold together even after it has been broken. Use the back section of the center punch, not your hand, and chip out a small section of glass in the corner of the window. Make the opening large enough to fit a gloved hand inside. Now, insert your gloved hand, and grab ahold of the glass. Pull the glass up and out, taking the entire section of glass out of the frame (**FIGURE 9-7**). With unsecured glass, if there is a large amount of accumulated glass fragments on the ground, use a broom or shovel to move them under the vehicle, or place the debris outside the hot zone in a designated debris pile.

Tempered safety glass goes through a process where the glass is heated and then quickly cooled; this process gives the glass its strength and resistance to impacts. When tempered glass is fractured, it is designed to break into small pieces, with no long shards. Tinting on tempered glass can be an added benefit for the technical rescuer because, when the glass is broken, the tinting normally holds all the small fragments together, making the glass easy to remove and dispose of. Adding a self-adhesive safety film to all the windows provides a stronger benefit similar to tinting where full control over glass management is maintained.

LISTEN UP!

Always use a hand tool, such as a Halligan bar or a four-by-four, to clean out the tempered glass fragments remaining in a window frame after the glass has been broken.

To break tempered glass using a spring-loaded center punch, follow the steps in **SKILL DRILL 9-2**.

SKILL DRILL 9-2
Breaking Tempered Glass Using a Spring-Loaded Center Punch NFPA 1006 8.2.6, 8.2.7, 8.3.6, 8.3.9

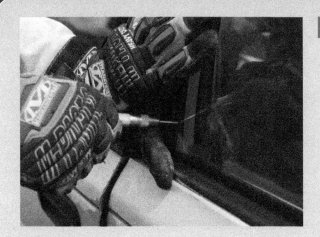

1 Don appropriate PPE, including mask and eye protection. Assess the scene for hazards, and complete the inner and outer surveys. Stabilize the vehicle and, if available, apply plastic safety film over all the glass. Ensure that the victim is properly protected from flying glass particles when breaking unsecured glass. Warn all personnel and victims that you will be breaking the glass with the verbal command "Breaking glass!" Beginning with the window farthest from the victim, place the palm of your hand against the lower corner of the window and frame, with your index finger and thumb facing upward. Rest the body of the tool in the ridge section of your palm (V of your hand) between your index finger and thumb.

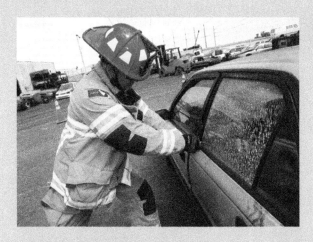

2 With the point of the center punch directly on the glass, apply forward pressure until the spring is activated and the glass breaks.

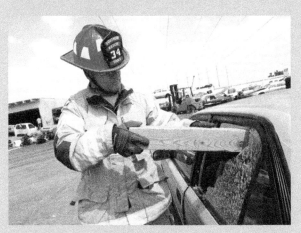

3 Once the glass breaks, remove all loose tempered glass fragments from around the window frame using a hand tool or a short section of a four-by-four. Follow this procedure until all glass has been removed from the frame.

© Jones & Bartlett Learning. Photographed by Glen E. Ellman.

The glass handsaw is a manually operated glass removal tool that has several unique features built into it, including a hand guard; a hollow slot for a center punch; and a notched section that fits over the top lip of the glass, which, when turned, causes the glass to fracture. The glass handsaw is capable of breaking tempered or cutting laminated glass.

When the glass saw is utilized to break tempered glass, a center punch is set inside the hollow slot located in the handle of the tool. The hand guard is then used as a bracing mechanism by placing it against the outer steel section of the window frame with the point of the center punch placed against the corner of the window. The tool is rolled forward, plunging the center punch into the glass. The glass handsaw can then be used to clean the remaining window frame of glass fragments.

To break tempered glass using a glass handsaw, follow the steps in **SKILL DRILL 9-3**.

A glass shearing tool is a device that is attached to a battery-powered drill or is a free-standing battery-powered tool that is designed to quickly cut out laminated glass. This tool gives the rescuer full directional control over the cut with minimal projected glass fragments, which are normally encountered when operating a glass handsaw or reciprocating saw (**FIGURE 9-8**). The glass shearing tool is designed for laminated glass only and requires a separate tool to make a purchase opening for insertion of the blade.

Laminated Safety Glass

Laminated safety glass is created by applying a layer of clear thermoplastic film or a binding agent between two layers of plate or sheet glass. This process holds the two pieces of glass together. Laminated glass is federally regulated for performance requirements under FMVSS 205, Glazing Materials, to use for windshields

SKILL DRILL 9-3
Fracturing Tempered Safety Glass Using a Glass Handsaw
NFPA 1006 8.2.6, 8.2.7, 8.3.6, 8.3.9

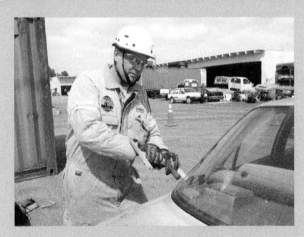

1 Don appropriate PPE, including mask and eye protection. Assess the scene for hazards, and complete the inner and outer surveys. Stabilize the vehicle, and apply plastic safety film over all outside vehicle glass if available. Ensure that the victim is properly protected from flying glass particles when breaking unsecured glass. Place a center punch inside the hollow slot located in the handle of the glass handsaw. Utilizing the hand guard as a bracing mechanism, place the guard against the outer steel section of the window frame using the window farthest from the victim.

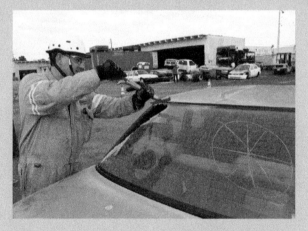

2 Warn all personnel and victims that you will be breaking the glass by announcing "Breaking glass!" With the point of the center punch placed against the corner of the window and the guard safety braced against the frame, roll the tool forward, plunging the center punch into the glass. Remove all loose tempered glass fragments from around the window frame using the glass handsaw.

© Jones & Bartlett Learning. Photographed by Glen E. Ellman.

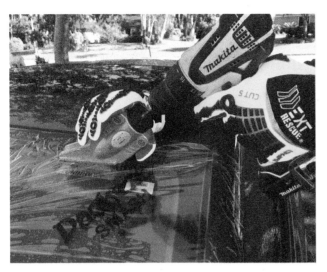

FIGURE 9-8 The glass shearing tool gives the rescuer full directional control over the cut with minimal projected glass fragments, which are normally encountered when operating a glass handsaw or reciprocating saw.
Courtesy of David Sweet.

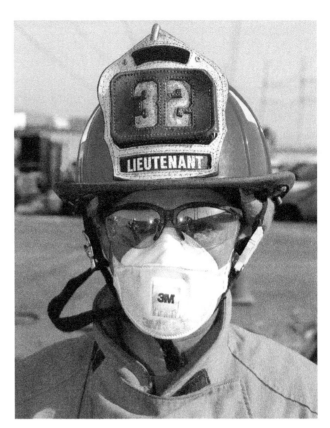

FIGURE 9-9 The technical rescuer must be wearing full PPE, including eye and respiratory protection, to protect against flying glass particles and dust.
© Jones & Bartlett Learning. Photographed by Glen E. Ellman.

but can also commonly be found in rear and side windows. When the window is fractured, the plastic film between the two layers of glass prevents big shards of glass from flying in on the occupant as well as keeping the occupants from being ejected from the vehicle through the laminated glass. Corning® Gorilla Glass® is another type of laminated glass that uses a three-layer fusion process to make this special, stronger laminated glass that is compatible for use in vehicles. Removal of this special type of laminated glass can be accomplished with any of the laminated glass removal techniques and tools.

As discussed, laminated glass found in a common passenger vehicle is generally sealed and held in place with a mastic adhesive that requires a cutting action of the glass itself to be properly removed. Attempting to scrape this adhesive seal out is difficult at best and extremely time consuming; doing so should be avoided.

Accessing a victim through a windshield is not a common procedure, but this approach could be performed with a vehicle resting on its side. The main purpose for removing the windshield glass is for safety. Utilizing a technique such as scoring the bottom of the windshield with an axe and removing part of the windshield is not an optimal technique, even though it is still utilized quite extensively throughout the world. This technique is not as effective or safe as completely removing the entire section of glass. It is highly recommended for safety purposes and consistency to remove the entire windshield by cutting it out with a battery-powered glass shears, glass handsaw, or reciprocating saw; it takes only seconds to complete the procedure.

The technique to remove the front laminated windshield is best accomplished using two technical rescuers positioned on opposite sides of the vehicle. It is recommended that, when sawing through laminated glass, respiratory protection, such as an N-95 filtered nose and mouth filter/respirator; eye protection; and protection of exposed areas around the face and neck should be utilized (FIGURE 9-9). The teeth of a glass handsaw blade are set at an inward angle, which will throw a large amount of glass particles back at the technical rescuer on each upward and dragging stroke. The glass particles stick to unprotected skin and irritate the respiratory tract of an unprotected rescuer who is in the immediate proximity or downwind. A filtered nose and mouth mask rated N-95 or higher is specially designed to block such fine particles. Consider applying plastic safety film over the laminated section to be cut, which will dramatically reduce glass particulates from the cutting action. Also, prior to cutting the windshield, attempt to cover the victim with a blanket that sufficiently protects against glass fragments and particles.

The proper technique for removing a windshield using a glass handsaw can be accomplished by following the steps in SKILL DRILL 9-4.

SKILL DRILL 9-4
Removing the Windshield Using a Glass Handsaw NFPA 1006 8.2.6, 8.2.7, 8.3.6, 8.3.9

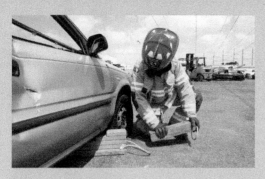

1 Don appropriate PPE, including mask and eye protection. Assess the scene for hazards, and complete the inner and outer surveys. Stabilize the vehicle and, if available, apply plastic safety film over the glass area to be cut to minimize the glass particles produced by the cutting action.

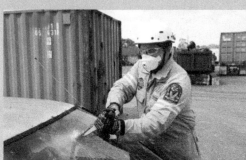

2 Ensure that the victim and the rescuer inside the vehicle are properly protected from unsecured flying glass particles. Remove the rearview mirror if it is still in place. If the mirror remains in place, the striking action of the spiked end of the glass tool (required to make an access point for the blade) onto the glass will generally dislodge the rearview mirror at a high velocity, potentially hitting the victim or the technical rescuer inside.

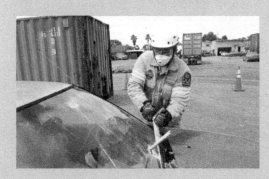

3 Using the spiked end of the glass handsaw, make a hole at the center top of the windshield, and then make a hole at the center bottom of the windshield.

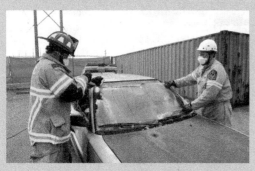

4 Insert the blade into the top hole, and begin a steady pulling/dragging of the blade rather than making short cuts. With one continuous cut and without removing the blade, cut a line all the way around the top of the roof line to just inside the A-post, working the tool to the bottom of the windshield. Try not to saw the glass or make short strokes because the continual downward insertion of the blade pushes glass fragments into the passenger compartment and onto the victim and rescuer. Pull the blade out, and insert it into the center bottom hole to finish the cut on the bottom section of the windshield glass. Because the windshield and dashboard meet at an acute angle, the blade of the glass handsaw must be turned sideways to prevent the blade from hitting the dash when cutting. Hand the tool to the technical rescuer on the opposite side of the vehicle so he or she can complete the cut on that side. Support the windshield section that you just cut to prevent it from falling in on the victim once the other side is cut. Push the loose windshield from inside the vehicle outward, toward the hood. Fold the glass in half on top of itself, and place it in a debris pile outside the hot zone.

© Jones & Bartlett Learning. Photographed by Glen E. Ellman.

Removing the Windshield Using a Reciprocating Saw

The high-speed reciprocating action of the blade of a reciprocating saw makes the process of cutting out laminated windshield glass very fast and leaves a straight edge on the glass. This occurs because the heat of the blade as it passes through the glass melts the laminate that is between the two layers of glass. The cutting process is very fast and different from using a glass handsaw; be prepared for the difference in speed, and ensure that everyone, including the victim and the rescuer inside the vehicle, is fully protected and aware of your action.

A reciprocating saw can be very effective for cutting through laminated glass when it is used correctly and a plan of action is followed. Always plan a few steps ahead. If the plan is to incorporate the removal of the roof and the windshield, then a reciprocating saw would be highly effective. The ideal situation would be to cut through both A-posts and cut out the windshield as opposed to using the reciprocating saw to cut out only the windshield. The technical rescuer must take into account the increased setup time to hook up an electric reciprocating saw versus using another glass tool, such as a battery-powered glass shear tool or glass handsaw, either of which requires no setup. Another option would be to use a battery-powered reciprocating saw, which minimizes the time of deployment to operation. The complexity of the incident and the number of skilled technicians on scene should determine the choice of action.

When using a reciprocating saw to cut into laminated glass, there are two schools of thought when choosing the teeth-per-inch (TPI) rating for the saw blade. (TPI measures the number of teeth on the blade per inch.) The first option is to use a bimetal blade with a high TPI, such as 14. This blade will produce a fine cut and minimize the chance of large particles of glass flying out. However, the high TPI rating will produce and throw a large amount of fine glass particles, mostly in a powdery cloud. The second option is to use a bimetal blade with a variable TPI of approximately 6 to 9. However, the larger size teeth will produce and throw large particles of glass everywhere. When utilizing a reciprocating saw to cut out laminated glass, regardless of the blade used, the saw will produce large amounts of glass fragments, particles, and dust comprising glass particulates. If it is available, apply plastic safety film over the glass area to be cut to minimize the glass particles produced by the cutting action. Proper respiratory, skin, and full eye protection is a must.

Another concern is the potential for an air bag cylinder to be located in the A-post (**FIGURE 9-10**).

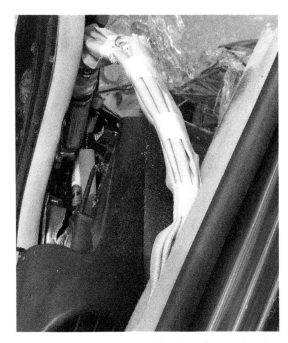

FIGURE 9-10 If an air bag cylinder is located, cut in an area that avoids that cylinder.
Courtesy of David Sweet.

Examine all areas prior to cutting; an air bag cylinder can be visualized by pulling back the plastic or fabric molding around the post with your gloved hand or prying it back with a large flat-head screwdriver or other type of small prying tool. If an air bag cylinder is located, cut in an area that avoids the cylinder (whether it is high or low). The actual nylon air bag that extends out of the cylinder and up around the roof rail can be cut. Avoid the cylinder and attached electrical components. Remember the saying "If an air bag cylinder is found, then cut around!" All personnel on scene must be made aware of the air bag's location. Once you are through the post, the rest of the windshield can be quickly cut, removed, and placed in a debris area outside the hot zone.

Remember that, before the windshield is cut, another technical rescuer with full PPE, including respiratory protection, must be placed in position to support the windshield from falling in on the victim when the cut is made. With the windshield removed, the technical rescuer will proceed to the other A-post and follow the same steps just described. Also, remember that, when you cut through any vehicle posts, there must be enough personnel to assist with supporting the roof to prevent it from collapsing on the victim. Although the B-posts are still intact, always yield to safety first. This may seem like an obvious statement, but this is a common occurrence because, often, all the focus is on the cut and removal of the roof and not on supporting the roof once it is cut. One factor you can count on to be present 100 percent of the time is gravity. Proper procedures for performing a roof removal utilizing a reciprocating saw are discussed in Chapter 10, *Alternative Extrication Techniques*.

The proper technique for removing a windshield using a reciprocating saw can be accomplished by following the steps in **SKILL DRILL 9-5**.

SKILL DRILL 9-5
Removing the Windshield Using a Reciprocating Saw
NFPA 1006 8.2.6, 8.2.7, 8.3.6, 8.3.9

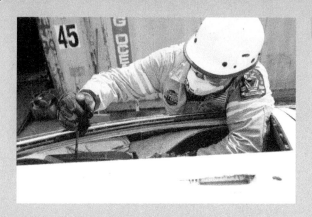

1. Don appropriate PPE, including mask and eye protection. Assess the scene for hazards, and complete the inner and outer surveys. Stabilize the vehicle, and if it is available, apply plastic safety film over the glass area to be cut to minimize the glass particles produced by the cutting action. Ensure that the victim and the rescuer inside the vehicle are properly protected from unsecured flying glass particles. If the A-posts will be incorporated into the cutting process, examine the posts for any air bag cylinders by removing or pulling back the moldings. If air bag cylinders are found, then cut around them.

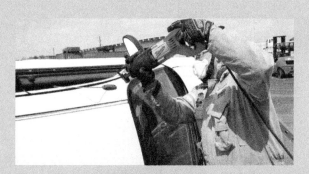

2. Utilize a reciprocating saw (battery or electric powered) to create a purchase point to start the cut. This can be accomplished by starting the cut at the top of the A-post or creating a hole in the glass with the spiked end of a Halligan tool or the spiked end of a glass handsaw.

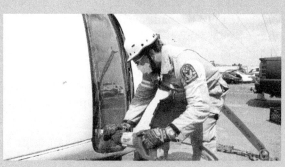

3. Begin at the top of one A-post, and make one continuous cut all the way through the post; continue into the top of the windshield and around the entire windshield frame, staying as close to the edge as possible.

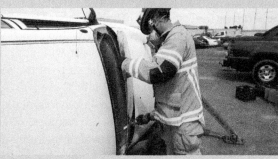

4. Another technical rescuer should be supporting the weight of the windshield. When all the glass has been cut, push the loose windshield from inside the vehicle outward, toward the hood. Fold the glass in half, and place the section in a debris pile outside the hot zone. Once the glass has been removed, the other A-post can be cut if a roof removal operation has been called for by the officer in charge.

© Jones & Bartlett Learning. Photographed by Glen E. Ellman.

Polycarbonate Windows and Ballistic-Rated Glass

Polycarbonate window material is a thermoplastic material that can used in vehicle window applications in lieu of traditional vehicle glass, whether tempered or laminated. Polycarbonate is a light and durable plastic that is up to 250 times stronger than glass; it is naturally designed to resist direct impacts by any striking tool carried on the apparatus (see Chapter 5, *Mechanical Energy and Vehicle Anatomy*).

When polycarbonate windows are encountered on a vehicle, the best technique to address this type of material is to treat it as a part of the vehicle body by removing the entire section as one piece, whether it is an entire roof or a door structure with the window. Another option is to utilize a prying tool or the hydraulic spreader to pry the polycarbonate window section out of its frame casing, which is held in place by a mastic or similar type of adhesive. If there happens to be an opening caused by a vehicle's crash deformity, you may be able to place the tips of a hydraulic spreader into the opening and release the section containing the polycarbonate material from its casing. Polycarbonate material that has a bend or some type of deformity caused by an impact may be loaded and can release from its casing, either on its own or from the force of a tool. It is designed to conform back to its original shape.

If removing a window section of polycarbonate is a must, then a purchase point can be made by crushing a section of the roof rail or accessible metal in which the seam of the window to be removed is seated. This action should cause an opening in the area just large enough to insert the tips of the hydraulic spreader and force the window out of its casing. The use of saws, such as a reciprocating saw, is not effective because the heat produced by the friction of the blade will melt the thermoplastic, and it will reseal itself in some areas as the cut is being made. Utilizing a powered rotary saw (K-12 saw) and reversing the carbide tip blade are effective for cutting this type of material, but this saw is impractical to use and time consuming to set up. Bullet-resistant glass utilizes multiple layers of tempered glass, laminated material, and polycarbonate thermoplastics, all sandwiched together to the desired thickness. The weight and thickness of the glass will increase depending on each increased level of protection, which can be as high as 3 in. (7.6 cm) or more, depending on the consumer's design request and the customization of the vehicle to fit and hold the weight of the glass. When ballistic glass is encountered on a vehicle, the best technique is to approach it just as you would polycarbonate material, by treating it as a part of the vehicle body and removing the entire section as one piece, whether it is an entire roof or a door structure.

> **LISTEN UP!**
>
> When polycarbonate windows are encountered on a vehicle, the best technique is to treat this material as a part of the vehicle body by removing the entire section as one piece, whether it is an entire roof or a door structure with the window.

Removing the Windshield from a Partially Ejected Victim

Occupants who are not properly restrained by a seat belt system can easily be ejected when a collision occurs. Remember the points brought up in Chapter 5 regarding the kinetics of energy and the law of motion. A body in motion will remain in motion until acted upon by anther force or object. If the vehicle is traveling at 50 mi/h (80.5 km/h) and abruptly stops because of a collision, the unrestrained occupant(s) will continue to travel at 50 mi/h (80.5 km/h) until they are stopped by an object or a force. In some incidents, the occupant is partially ejected with his or her head or torso breaching the front windshield, trapped in a constricting web of shattered glass and held in place by the laminate. The technical rescuers will be challenged in many ways to render immediate care and release the victim from the glass entrapment.

When encountering an occupant who has been partially ejected with his or her head protruding from the windshield, follow the steps in **SKILL DRILL 9-6**.

> **LISTEN UP!**
>
> When treating a victim who has been partially ejected through the windshield, slowly insert towels around the head and neck of the victim from the direction the windshield was impacted.

Using Hydraulic Rescue Tools to Gain Door and Roof Access

If technical rescuers cannot gain access by the previously mentioned techniques, the use of heavy extrication tools, whether they be hand-, electric-, or hydraulic-powered tools, to gain access to the victim is the next option. Hydraulic rescue tools for vehicle rescue and extrication have been around for several decades, originating from the auto racing industry

SKILL DRILL 9-6
Removing the Windshield from a Partially Ejected Victim
NFPA 1006 8.2.6, 8.2.7, 8.3.6, 8.3.9

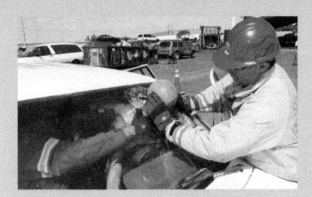

1 Don appropriate PPE, including mask and eye protection. Assess the scene for hazards, and complete the inner and outer surveys. Immediately support the victim's head from outside the vehicle. Stabilize the vehicle. Place a technical rescuer inside the vehicle to give additional support to the head and upper torso of the victim.

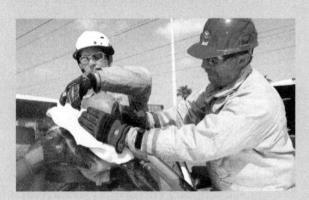

2 Carefully insert towels around the head and neck of the victim from the direction the windshield was impacted.

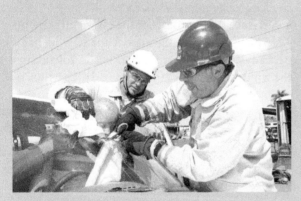

3 A technical rescuer positioned outside the vehicle will use trauma shears to slowly cut away sections of laminated glass that are entrapping the victim.

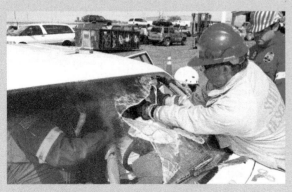

4 When enough space has been created to safely remove the victim's head, maintain cervical support, and properly immobilize and package the victim for removal from the vehicle.

© Jones & Bartlett Learning. Photographed by Glen E. Ellman.

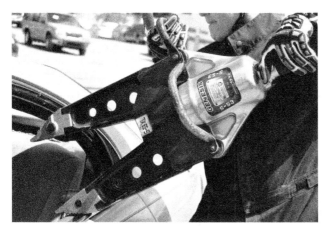

FIGURE 9-11 The use of a hydraulic spreader is a fast and efficient option for making a purchase point.
Courtesy of Edward Monahan.

and quickly becoming the staple for vehicle rescue and extrication across the world. As advances in technology continue to grow, new tools emerge that are faster and more powerful and designed to make vehicle rescue and extrication for the technical rescuer less complicated and cumbersome. Our knowledge in the use of these tools also needs to evolve and grow with new technology. Today's technical rescuer must shed the old style of spreading and tearing apart vehicles and look at the extrication process through the eyes of a surgeon to dissect and remove sections and fully understand the dynamics of moving metal. This section is about simplifying things, "working smarter," and accomplishing our goal of removing trapped victims in the safest, fastest, and most efficient way.

Making a purchase point is the process of gaining an access area to insert and better position a tool for operation. For example, a purchase point may be needed to expose the locking/latching mechanism or hinges of a door enough to insert a hydraulic cutter; this technique is known as expose and cut. The use of a hydraulic spreader is a fast and efficient option for making a purchase point (FIGURE 9-11).

Most hydraulic cutters today are rated to cut through hinges and locking/latching mechanisms located in vehicles; however, it is a good idea to check with the manufacturer to see whether the tool your organization uses is rated to do so. If the manufacturer does not recommend this procedure for the tool or your organization is absolutely against cutting into this type of material, then some alternative steps can be utilized, which are described in the next section.

Anyone can rip a door off a vehicle using a hydraulic spreader, but it is the mark of a true professional who understands how to properly apply that force and the movement of metal by removing a door with precise technique and total control. The goal is to increase the

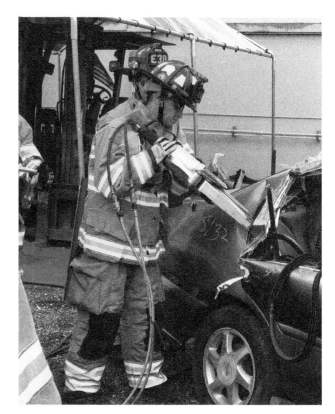

FIGURE 9-12 The goal is to increase the speed and efficiency of the operation through understanding how to properly approach spreading and removing a door using precise technique, maneuvering, and proper handling of hydraulic rescue tools.
Courtesy of David Sweet.

speed and efficiency of the operation through understanding how to properly approach spreading and removing a door using precise technique, maneuvering, and proper handling of these tools (FIGURE 9-12).

Door Access from the Latch Side: The Vertical Spread

Trying to release a door from its frame and/or latching mechanism can sometimes be a very difficult task. Depending on the level of intrusion as well as the integrity and type of the material that is being spread, this process can challenge even the best technical rescuer.

To gain access into a door, an older, traditional method that is still often taught would have two technical rescuers create a purchase point using a striking and prying tool to forcefully insert and bend the sheet metal at the edge or seam of the door near the latching/locking mechanism, just below the door handle. This is not good management of time and personnel because the technique requires multiple tools and personnel to accomplish a fairly simple task that can be accomplished with one person using one tool. Understanding how metal moves when force is applied is the

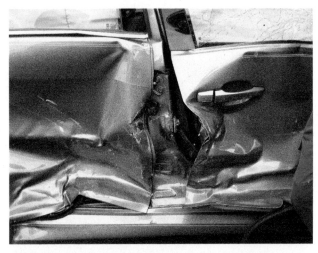

FIGURE 9-13 Tenting occurs when force applied causes the metal above and below the area of spreading to gradually collapse forming a tent around the arms or tips of the tool. This will limit the size of an opening, blocking the possibility of inserting a hydraulic cutter to cut the latching mechanism.
Courtesy of David Sweet.

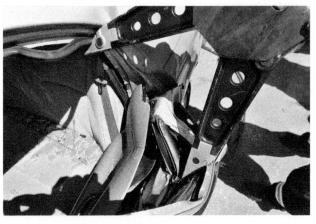

FIGURE 9-14 For hydraulic tool operations, the objective is to fully expose the door latching mechanism by utilizing a vertical spread technique, which forces the window frame and surrounding door structure down and outward.
Courtesy of Edward Monahan.

key to gaining access on every approach, whether the technical rescuer is utilizing a hydraulic spreader or hand tool such as a First Responder Jack (FRJ). When a spreading or jacking tool is inserted into an opening or positioned to create an opening, the force applied causes the metal above and below the area of spreading to gradually collapse and form a tent around the arms or tips of the tool. This action limits the opening by blocking the possibility of inserting a hydraulic cutter to cut the latching mechanism (**FIGURE 9-13**). This is an example of why a full understanding of how metal reacts and moves by the force of a tool is so important. Continuing to force the door in this direction will weaken the integrity and strength of the surrounding structure and no longer provide a vantage point to push from. The metal in this area becomes weakened and starts to tear and shred, much like an aluminum beverage can would, with the technical rescuer struggling and fighting the door, which causes physical exhaustion and frustration. The metal will eventually tear off the latch, but this process expends valuable time and effort, which could be avoided by simply reading the movement of the metal. Anyone can force a door off the latch or hinge with the sheer power of a hydraulic spreader or jacking tool, but only the skilled professional understands how metal reacts and moves by the force of a tool. Expose and cut!

For hydraulic tool operations, the objective is to fully expose the door latching mechanism utilizing a **vertical spread** technique, which forces the window frame and surrounding door structure down and outward (**FIGURE 9-14**). Correctly applying this technique creates a large, unobstructed opening to allow for the insertion of a hydraulic cutter to cut through the latching mechanism, thus releasing the door. If the hydraulic cutter is not rated for cutting the latching mechanism, then as an alternative, continue to work the spread vertically down and outward until the door can be rolled off the latch with controlled movements by working the tips of the spreader around the latch. There are heavier-gauge steel backer or reinforcement plates directly behind the latching mechanism, as well as the latching pin, which will prevent the metal from shredding; keep the tips of the spreader in this general vicinity (**FIGURE 9-15**). This technique is a faster and more efficient way of gaining access and requires the technical rescuer to expend less physical energy; it also limits the possibility of the door being violently released. Remember that you control the technique; the technique does not control you! When hydraulic tools are not available, hand tools, such as an FRJ, along with some powered tools, such as an air chisel or reciprocating saw, can also accomplish the same objective. The jacking device can be positioned in the door frame closest to the door handle with the tongue of the tool set on the door frame window sill and the base of the jack positioned just on and under the roof rail. A section of the window frame will have to be cut through using a cutting tool, which will allow the door to be pushed out untethered to the roof. As a safety measure, a strap or webbing can be fastened around the door and around the roof post, which is the most readily available vehicle section to control the door from releasing unexpectedly. Continued force applied to the jack will cause the door frame to move down and outward, causing it to separate

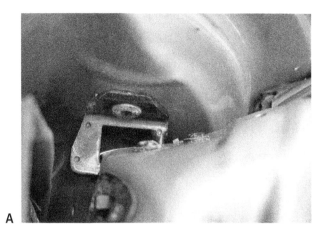

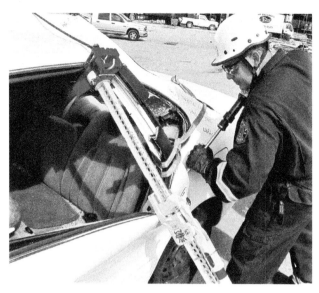

FIGURE 9-16 Force applied to the FRJ will cause the door frame to move down and outward and separate from the vehicle. It will eventually expose the latching mechanism, where an air chisel or other cutting tool can be applied to cut through the latching mechanism/pin.
Courtesy of Edward Monahan.

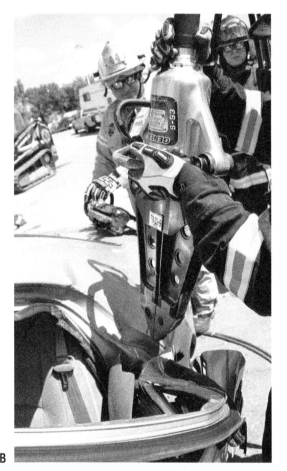

FIGURE 9-15 There are heavier-gauge steel backer or reinforcement plates directly behind the latching mechanism, as well as the latching pin, which will prevent the metal from shredding; keep the tips of the spreader in this general vicinity.
Courtesy of Edward Monahan.

LISTEN UP!

Remember that you control the technique; the technique doesn't control you! Understanding how metal reacts and moves by the force of a tool is critical to a successful outcome.

from the vehicle and eventually exposing the latching mechanism, where an air chisel or other cutting tool can be applied to cut through the latching mechanism/pin (**FIGURE 9-16**).

To release a door from its frame or perform the vertical spread, with and without hydraulics, follow the steps in **SKILL DRILL 9-7** and **SKILL DRILL 9-8**.

The importance of crew members working in tandem, understanding the technique that is being performed, and being prepared with the appropriate tools in hand and ready for action cannot be stressed enough. For trained technical rescuers, all of these techniques need to flow and transition seamlessly without needless interruptions, such as trying to locate or assemble a tool or waiting for the blades of a hydraulic cutter to be opened.

Door Access from the Hinge Side: Front Wheel Well Crush

Gaining entry into the interior of a vehicle by removing a door from the hinge side is not a common procedure because removing the door in this fashion goes against the natural swing of the door, which makes it very difficult to remove once the procedure progresses to the latch side. However, this technique may be needed for certain crash scenarios.

One such hypothetical crash scenario involves the front of a vehicle impacting a wall. The impact in this scenario crushes the front end of the vehicle and

SKILL DRILL 9-7
Releasing a Door from Its Frame or Performing the Vertical Spread (Hydraulic) NFPA 1006 8.2.6, 8.2.7, 8.3.6, 8.3.9

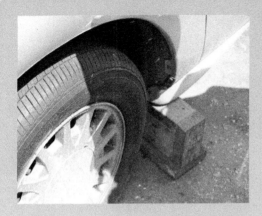

1 Don appropriate PPE, including mask and eye protection. Assess the scene for hazards, and complete the inner and outer surveys. Stabilize the vehicle. Ensure that the victim and the rescuer inside the vehicle are properly protected from unsecured glass particles. Secure all vehicle glass utilizing the appropriate glass management techniques demonstrated in this chapter.

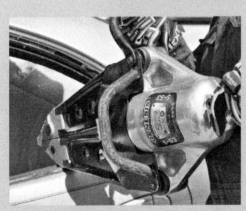

2 Place the hydraulic spreader with the arms positioned vertically in the door's window, close to where the door handle is normally located. Position the tips of the spreader with the bottom arm resting on the door's window sill and the top arm in position to catch the underside of the roof rail when the arm is fully opened. Push off of the roof rail; do not push off of the door's window frame. Pushing off of the window frame will only cause the window frame to tear off and thus compromise the technique. The tool operator should be positioned on the side of the tool opposite the door swing; this is a defensive position of safety in case the door is unexpectedly jarred open by the tool's force.

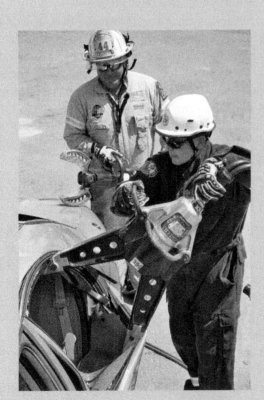

3 As the tool starts to open, adjust the positioning of the arms appropriately by lifting up on the back end of the spreader to maximize the spreading capacity of the tool. The vertical spreading of the door will cause the window frame just above the latch side to buckle and open up, thus providing an access point to reposition and insert the spreaders. Do not fail to make this adjustment; it could cause the tool to move forcefully inside the vehicle, which would negate any spreading ability and potentially cause further injury to a victim. The vertical spreading of the door will cause the window frame just above the latch side to buckle and open up, thus providing an access point to reposition and insert the spreaders.

SKILL DRILL 9-7 Continued
Releasing a Door from Its Frame or Performing the Vertical Spread (Hydraulic) NFPA 1006 8.2.6, 8.2.7, 8.3.6, 8.3.9

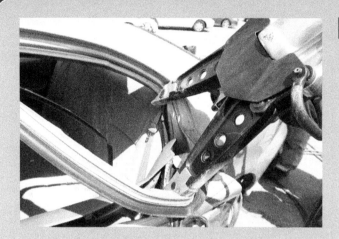

4 Position the tips of the spreader in this opening, and push the window frame out and downward, out of the way. The force of the spreader in this position will cause the window frame to pull the top section of the door out and down, thus exposing the latching mechanism.

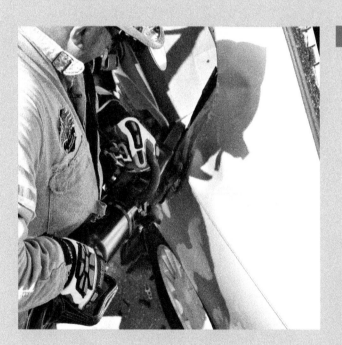

5 When the top corner of the door opens, reposition the spreader by dropping the tips of the tool down into this opening with the tool positioned almost vertically. The position of the tool at this point is critical for a successful outcome. Spread the metal outward, making the door start to fold out and down. At this point, the latching mechanism should be visible or fully accessible to position the hydraulic cutter to begin cutting. If the hydraulic cutter is not rated to cut this type of material, an alternative step would be to continue to work the spread vertically down and outward with controlled movements by working the tips of the spreader around the latch until the door can be rolled off of the latch. A second technical rescuer should stand with a hydraulic cutter in hand, powered up with the blades fully opened and ready to cut the latching pin, which encompasses the latching mechanism. Once the latching mechanism has been cut and the door released/opened, the technical rescue team can transition into the next operation, which will be determined by the company officer or incident commander (IC).

Courtesy of Edward Monahan.

SKILL DRILL 9-8
Releasing a Door from Its Frame or Performing the Vertical Spread (Non-Hydraulic) NFPA 1006 8.2.6, 8.2.7, 8.3.6, 8.3.9

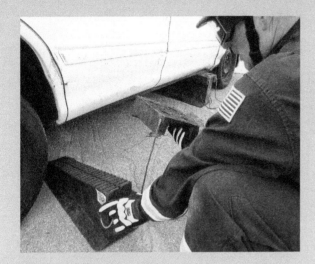

1 Don appropriate PPE, including mask and eye protection. Assess the scene for hazards, and complete the inner and outer surveys. Stabilize the vehicle. Ensure that the victim and the rescuer inside the vehicle are properly protected using a blanket to cover them from unsecured glass particles. Secure all vehicle glass utilizing the appropriate glass management techniques demonstrated in this chapter.

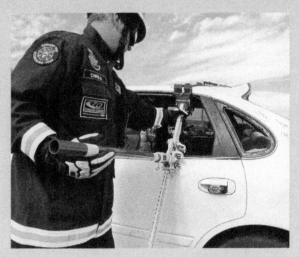

2 Position the FRJ with the base against the roof rail/window frame area closest to the door handle. The tongue of the tool will be positioned on the bottom of the window sill with the operating arm facing the rescuer.

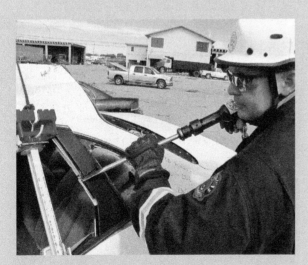

3 Cut through a section of the window frame with a cutting tool to release it, which allows the door to be pushed out untethered to the roof. As a safety measure, a strap or webbing can be fastened around the door and around the roof posts, which is the most readily available vehicle section to control the door from releasing unexpectedly.

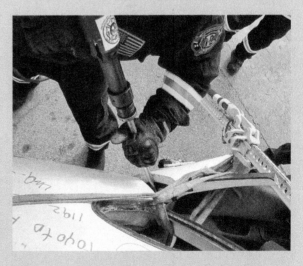

4 Operate the jacking device, and push the door frame down and outward, away from the latching mechanism. Once the latching mechanism has been exposed, an air chisel or other cutting tool can be applied to cut through the latching mechanism/pin.

SKILL DRILL 9-8 Continued
Releasing a Door from Its Frame or Performing the Vertical Spread (Non-Hydraulic) NFPA 1006 8.2.6, 8.2.7, 8.3.6, 8.3.9

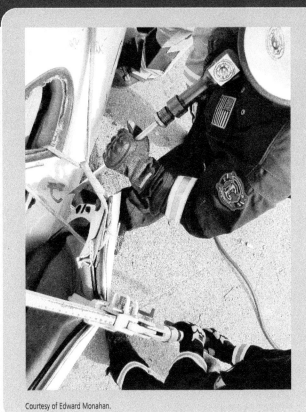

5 The latching mechanism is cut, and the door is released from its frame.

Courtesy of Edward Monahan.

compresses both doors, which will now require forcible entry. The vehicle is fully equipped with supplemental restraint devices and two front- and side-impact air bags located in both driver and passenger doors. The two front air bags deploy as designed, but the two side air bags remain live because there is no direct impact to any of the side-impact sensors. Any attempt at a door removal by the latch side could potentially trip the door sensors and activate the side air bag, deploying it on the occupants. One possible solution in this scenario is to enter the door from the hinge side, cut the hinges, and then pull the door back and away from the occupant and release it from the latch side (**FIGURE 9-17**). This is not a perfect science; an accidental air bag deployment may occur, but it provides the technical rescuer a viable option, including disconnecting the vehicle's 12-volt direct current (DC) battery. The best option would be to enter the vehicle

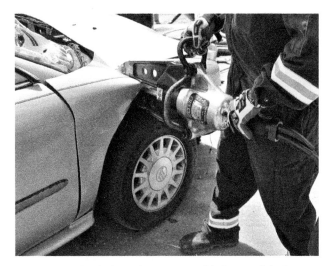

FIGURE 9-17 When door removal is impossible from the latch side due to air bag sensors, one possible solution is to enter the door from the hinge side.
Courtesy of Edward Monahan.

by removing the roof, but if the occupants are trapped under the dash, then the doors would have to come off anyway if a dash displacement technique is to be applied.

One of the more favorable techniques for gaining access to door hinges from the outside is a **wheel well crush technique**, which uses the hydraulic spreader and cutter. Using the hydraulic spreader to crush the wheel well creates a purchase point at the door's seam, which allows the hydraulic spreader space to get in and expose the hinges. The hydraulic cutter can then be inserted so the hinge can be cut.

To perform the wheel well crush technique, follow the steps in **SKILL DRILL 9-9**.

SKILL DRILL 9-9
The Wheel Well Crush Technique NFPA 1006 8.2.6, 8.2.7, 8.3.6, 8.3.9

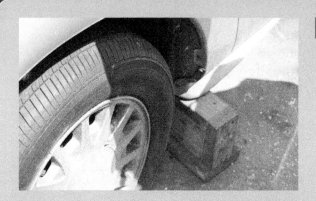

1 Don appropriate PPE, including mask and eye protection. Assess the scene for hazards, and complete the inner and outer surveys. Stabilize the vehicle. Ensure that the victim and the rescuer inside the vehicle are properly protected from unsecured glass particles. Secure all vehicle glass utilizing the appropriate glass management techniques demonstrated in this chapter.

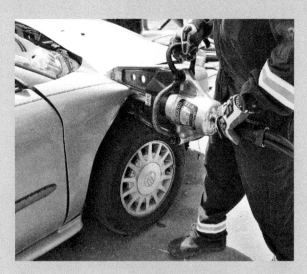

2 Locate and disconnect the vehicle's 12-volt DC battery if it is accessible. Prepare to crush the wheel well by locating an area just between the strut tower and the dash/firewall section. Open the arms of the spreader, and place the tip of the top arm on the hood or top section of the wheel well of the vehicle, making certain that the tip of the top arm is flush with the hood. It should not be positioned at an angle. As the bottom arm rises upward, ensure that it clears the tire and strut coil and falls into position under the wheel well. When this procedure is done correctly, it will seem like an optical illusion, where the bottom arm of the spreader appears to be the only arm moving with the top arm level and stationary.

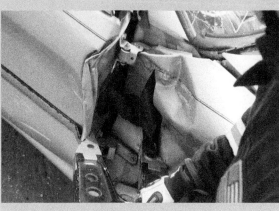

3 As the arms of the spreader lock onto the wheel well, prevent the tool from sliding off the angle and trying to conform with the slope of the wheel well. Hold the tool in position. The arms of the spreader will form a crease in the wheel well and upper rail area, causing the panel to buckle outward at the door seam where the panel and door meet and exposing the door's hinges. This creates a purchase point for the hydraulic spreader to create enough space around the door's hinges to insert a hydraulic cutter so the hinges can be cut.

Courtesy of Edward Monahan.

The Complete Side Removal Technique: The Side-Out

There are four basic types of impacts that a vehicle can sustain during a collision—a frontal impact, a side impact, a rear impact, or a rollover/roof impact. Side impacts have a higher rate of occurrence according to yearly statistics compiled by the Department of Transportation. The side-out technique is designed specifically for four-door vehicles involved in a side-impact collision. The technique allows technical rescuers to remove the front and rear doors as one unit on the same side of a four-door vehicle. This technique was first referenced in *Fire Engineering* magazine in November 1999, and it has made a tremendous difference for fire rescue agencies worldwide by dramatically reducing the time it takes to gain access through the doors of a four-door vehicle involved in a side-impact collision.

Understanding what occurs to the body structure of a vehicle after it has been involved in a side-impact collision is vital to comprehending the effectiveness of the side-out technique. The intrusion that occurs from a side-impact collision causes the entire door frame to fracture or partially fracture, which also causes the directional force of both doors at the B-post to move inward, toward occupants (**FIGURE 9-18**). If the technical rescuer attempts to spread the driver's-side door at the latching mechanism utilizing the hydraulic spreader, he or she will only cause the B-post, including both front and rear doors, to continue to move inward and collapse on the victim. This occurs because the directional force of the fracture caused by the impact is pushing inward, and it tends to continue in that direction. Because of the force applied to the metal, the metal will move and seek to find the path of least resistance—in this case moving inward.

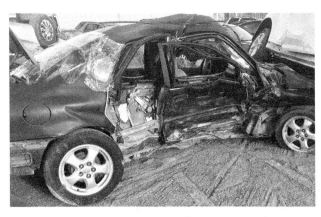

FIGURE 9-18 A side-impact collision causes the entire door frame to fracture or partially fracture, which also causes the directional force of both doors at the B-post to move inward, toward occupants.
Courtesy of David Sweet.

The correct action is to push the doors and B-post out and away from the victim. This technique utilizes the natural swing or directional movement of the doors and pushes or forces the doors and B-post outward, away from the occupant. This technique is best accomplished when two technical rescuers are working in tandem; one technical rescuer should carry out the hydraulic spreader assignment, and the other should carry out the hydraulic cutter assignment. The technique begins at the rear door and progresses forward.

If the door frames and B-post are pushed inward to a degree that any outside spreading application would cause further intrusion of the metal onto the victim, then this optional procedure can be attempted. As a first step, cut through the top of the B-post, and then place the spreader inside the vehicle, positioned at the best vantage point where one arm can push off of the rear floor transmission hump (additional cribbing may have to be used as floor reinforcement) and the other arm can push off of the interior B-post. This will relocate the framing off of the victim, close to its originally designed position. Once the B-post and door frame have been pushed back into position, then the technical rescuer can proceed with the all-door side-out technique as normal. This option is only one out of several options to address this type of intrusion scenario.

Other options include using a ram positioned with the base on the transmission hump and the tip positioned to push against the door or B-post, using a cross-ramming technique with a hydraulic ram pushing from B-post to B-post, or using an FRJ because there may be limited or no room to place a hydraulic spreader in the position previously described. Again, this procedure is about speed and efficiency, keeping in mind that adding or changing out tools will expend valuable time (**FIGURE 9-19**).

To perform the side removal/side-out technique on a vehicle resting on its side or its roof, follow the steps in **SKILL DRILL 9-10**.

SAFETY TIP

Never lean against a door that is being spread. The force of the hydraulic spreader can cause the door to violently release, driving it into the technical rescuer. Secure the door with webbing, and stand at a safe distance.

The side-out technique can be a very fast access technique when performed correctly. This technique, performed by skilled technical rescuers, has been accomplished in many scenarios in less than 5 minutes. The key is for the two technical rescuers operating the hydraulic spreader and cutter to thoroughly know the

246 Vehicle Rescue and Extrication: Principles and Practice

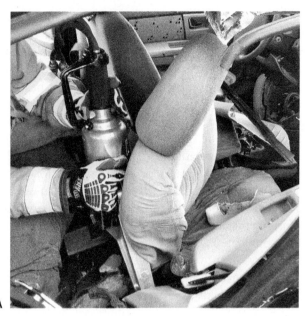
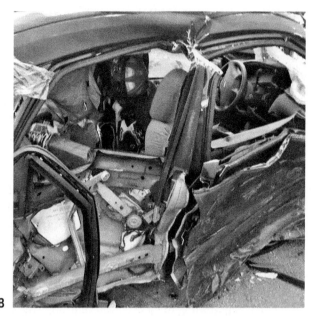

FIGURE 9-19 Utilize a hydraulic tool to push the B-post and doors off the victim and back to plane before attempting a door removal or side-out technique.
Courtesy of David Sweet.

SKILL DRILL 9-10
The Complete Side Removal/Side-Out Technique (Hydraulic)
NFPA 1006 8.2.6, 8.2.7, 8.3.6, 8.3.9

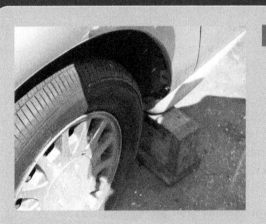

1 Don appropriate PPE, including mask and eye protection. Assess the scene for hazards, and complete the inner and outer surveys. Stabilize the vehicle. Ensure that the victim and the rescuer inside the vehicle are properly protected from unsecured glass particles. Secure all vehicle glass by utilizing the appropriate glass management techniques demonstrated in this chapter.

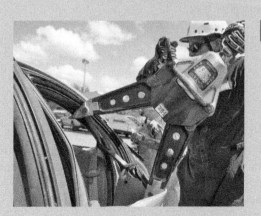

2 Disconnect the vehicle's 12-volt DC battery if the engine compartment is accessible. Cut the seat belt straps located on the B-post. Expose areas where potential air bag cylinders or seat belt pretensioning systems may be located to avoid cutting. Release the rear door from the latching mechanism, utilizing the vertical spread technique.

SKILL DRILL 9-10 Continued
The Complete Side Removal/Side-Out Technique (Hydraulic)
NFPA 1006 8.2.6, 8.2.7, 8.3.6, 8.3.9

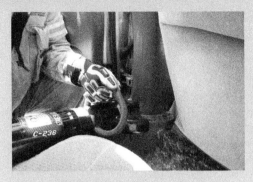

3 Open the door, and position the cutter at the bottom of the B-post, just above the area where the B-post meets the rocker panel. Make a small relief cut into the bottom of the post. Do not make a sectional, or pie, cut to get the cutter blades in deeper; it is not necessary and wastes valuable time. Also, do not make the mistake of positioning the blades incorrectly and accidentally cutting into the rocker panel; if the integrity of the area is compromised, the rocker panel and floor area will tear away instead of the B-post, posing a critical failure of the technique.

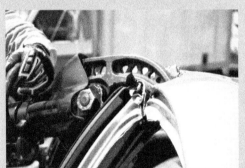

4 When the relief cut has been completed at the bottom of the B-post, move the cutter directly up toward the top of the B-post and roof rail area. Make an upward-angled cross-cut on both sides of the top section of the post and roof rail section. This cross-cut removes the jagged stump that would be left by just making one cut across the post. Do not make the mistake of leaving the top of the B-post uncut until the bottom of the B-post is detached. This action will disrupt the natural flow of the force and add more tension and resistance, which prevents the detachment of the bottom of the B-post.

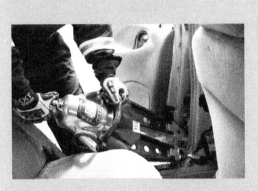

5 As the technical rescuer on the cutter is completing the cross-cut section on the opposite side of the B-post, the technical rescuer who is operating the hydraulic spreader should start to position the tool to spread the B-post off the rocker panel. The initial position of the hydraulic spreader is at the area where the relief cut was made at the bottom of the B-post. The objective is to angle the hydraulic spreader in a general 40- to 45-degree range, where the tip of the bottom arm is placed on the rocker panel and the tip of the top arm is angled near the bottom section of the rear door. This is only the starting point of the spread, as the tool will have to be repositioned once a better opening in the relief cut has been established.

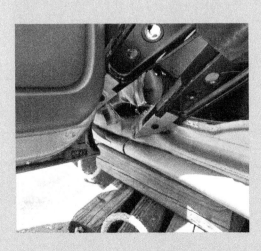

6 Once the spreader is in position (as described in Step 5) continue with that same initial angle; use cribbing to thoroughly shore up the area under the rocker panel where the bottom arm/tip of the hydraulic spreader rests. The cribbing must be inserted after the spreader has been positioned in place because the resting area of the bottom arm of the spreader will vary each time. The placement of the cribbing needs to be precise. It is very important that this area be fully shored because, once the hydraulic spreader is engaged, the tip of the tool can easily penetrate through the hollow rocker panel, tearing out the floor section. This will cause a critical failure of the technique.

(continues)

SKILL DRILL 9-10 Continued
The Complete Side Removal/Side-Out Technique (Hydraulic)
NFPA 1006 8.2.6, 8.2.7, 8.3.6, 8.3.9

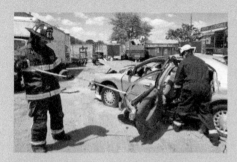

7 Before the spreader is engaged, as a safety measure, attach strapping, rope, or webbing to the rear door so a constant slight outward and upward pull can be applied to assist with the movement of the door from a safe distance.

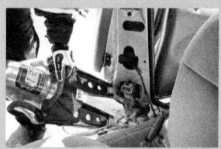

8 As the spreader is opened and the B-post starts to tear away from the panel, the position and angle of the spreader will have to be readjusted to gain better leverage to separate the lower B-post at the tear. If you do not reposition the spreader tips into the tear and continue to push off of the door and rocker panel, then the lower door hinge will violently separate. Remember that the goal is to separate the bottom B-post, not the door hinge. If the bottom of the B-post is spot welded to the rocker panel, it should tear off easily once force is applied by the opening of the spreader. If the B-post is molded as part of the rocker panel and force is applied, tearing can occur, separating the rocker panel in two sections. If this occurs, simply cut through the remaining small section of metal using the hydraulic cutter. The hydraulic cutter will have to be utilized as well if advanced high-strength steel (AHSS) is encountered and the post cannot be separated off the rocker panel with the spreader. With the addition of AHSS to the B-post framing, alternating between cutting and spreading may be required because the force of the spreader may not be enough to overcome and separate the AHSS.

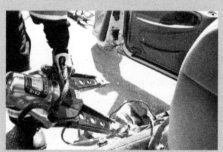

9 Once the B-post releases from the rocker panel, widen the front door opening or cut the front door hinges. The fastest and most efficient technique is to widen the door opening, eliminating the time spent on spreading or cutting hinges.

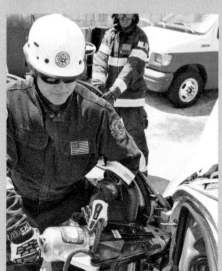

10 To widen the door, position the spreader in the front door's jamb around the midpoint area between the hinges. (If there is a door-limiting device, then position the tool just above that bar so it breaks away.) As the tool is engaged to open, the rescuer pulls back on the tool, using it as leverage, and slowly pushes backward against the door. This action bends the door back toward the front wheel, widening the door enough to provide equally sufficient access in half the time it would take to completely spread or cut the door off from the hinges.

SKILL DRILL 9-10 Continued
The Complete Side Removal/Side-Out Technique (Hydraulic)
NFPA 1006 8.2.6, 8.2.7, 8.3.6, 8.3.9

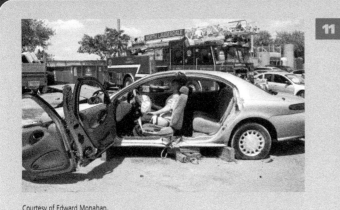

11 Cover any jagged metal that the procedure may have exposed at the bottom of the B-post. This procedure provides a large access point to safely remove the victim.

Courtesy of Edward Monahan.

technique and work in tandem by transitioning seamlessly between spreading and cutting. The perfect side-out technique will flow from the rear to the front of the vehicle, with each step performed one after the other without interruption. The all-door side-out technique can also be completed utilizing the combination of an FRJ and an air chisel and/or a reciprocating saw if hydraulic tools are not available.

To accomplish this without a hydraulic tool, follow the steps in **SKILL DRILL 9-11**.

Removing the Vehicle from the Victim

At times, the technical rescuer may encounter a situation where the intrusion of the B-post and doors is so severe that they have almost encapsulated the victim. The kinetics of the crash reveal that the force applied to the side doors and frame from the impact has caused the supporting metal to fracture and change its originally designed form. Any spreading of the doors in this situation, regardless of the location of the tool, will cause the metal to move inward and down onto the victim. This movement occurs because this is now the course of direction the metal tends to travel. The metal will follow the path of least resistance, which in this case, because of the impact, is inward and down. This is an important theory that the technical rescuer has to fully understand. In this extreme entrapment scenario, the objective is to first relocate the B-post and door frames to as close to their originally designed form as possible, thus creating enough room to place tools in the most advantageous position for a side removal technique to be applied. With the multitude of possible scenarios that can be presented, it is difficult to provide one technique that will be the most effective. Tool type and placement positions will vary with each entrapment. Several of these options and techniques for relocating the B-post and door frame from inside the vehicle are covered in Chapter 10 (**FIGURE 9-20**).

Roof Removal

One of the fastest ways to gain access and extricate a victim is by removing the roof. Victims are often needlessly manipulated by rescuers attempting to remove them through a door when removing the roof would provide better access and keep the victims in line without excessive manipulation as they are packaged and removed. Properly packaging victims by placing an immobilization device on them, along with keeping them in line as they are moved onto a backboard, provides the best victim care. Other benefits of removing the roof include better access to the victim with multiple rescuers in and around the vehicle and the ability to see the entrapment more clearly and to operate the tools with less obstruction and increased maneuverability for personnel.

The process of removing a roof can involve multiple tools, such as hydraulic tools, power tools, pneumatic tools, and hand tools. This section describes the process of removing a roof using only hydraulic tools (see Chapter 10 for a discussion of the use of other tools).

SKILL DRILL 9-11
The Complete Side Removal/Side-Out Technique (Non-Hydraulic)
NFPA 1006 8.2.6, 8.2.7, 8.3.6, 8.3.9

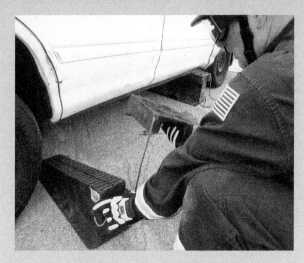

1 Don appropriate PPE, including mask and eye protection. Assess the scene for hazards, and complete the inner and outer surveys. Stabilize the vehicle. Ensure that the victim and the rescuer inside the vehicle are properly protected from unsecured glass particles. Secure all vehicle glass, utilizing the appropriate glass management techniques demonstrated in this chapter.

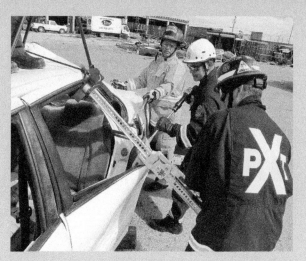

2 Locate and disconnect the vehicle's 12-volt DC battery if it is accessible. Cut the seat belt straps located on the B-post. Expose areas where potential air bag cylinders or seat belt pretensioning systems may be located to avoid cutting them. Release the rear door from the latching mechanism utilizing the vertical spread technique discussed earlier in the chapter.

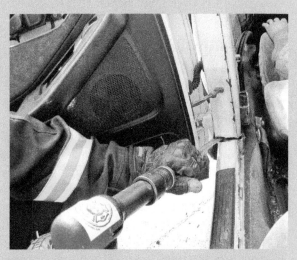

3 Open the door. Then, utilizing an air chisel or reciprocating saw, make a relief cut through the bottom of the B-post just above the area where the B-post meets the rocker panel. When the relief cut has been completed in the B-post, position an air chisel or a reciprocating saw toward the top of the B-post and roof rail area.

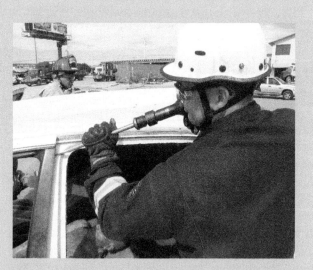

4 Make a cross-cut on both sides of the top section of the post and roof rail section ensuring that the entire post is cut through.

SKILL DRILL 9-11 Continued
The Complete Side Removal/Side-Out Technique (Non-Hydraulic)
NFPA 1006 8.2.6, 8.2.7, 8.3.6, 8.3.9

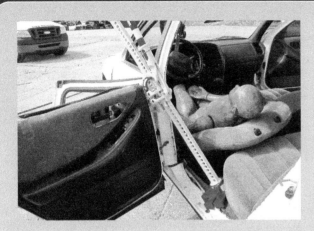

5 Position the FRJ with the base at the corner of the bottom section of the rear door and the tongue set inside the rear door at the area of the top hinge. As a safety measure, attach strapping, rope, or webbing to the rear door to apply a constant slight outward and upward pull to assist with the movement of the door from a safe distance.

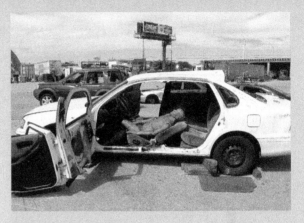

6 Engage the FRJ to separate the lower section of the B-post. The air chisel or reciprocating saw may have to be utilized as well if AHSS is encountered and cannot be separated with the force of the FRJ alone.

Courtesy of Edward Monahan.

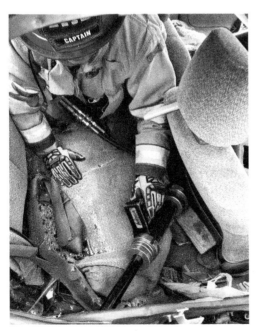

FIGURE 9-20 A telescoping ram is a versatile hydraulic tool. It is compact when closed and can be used in tight spaces to create a large opening when fully extended.
Courtesy of David Sweet.

When removing a roof, the technical rescuer must expose the interior of each post and the roof rail prior to cutting; this will reveal any problems that can potentially cause injury or halt or delay the process. Some of these problems may include air bag cylinders, boron rods or AHSS plates or blanks, seat belt harnesses, seat belt adjustment bars, or seat belt pretensioning systems. If any of these obstacles are encountered, the easiest solution is to avoid them by cutting above or below the object or area of concern. When cutting a roof post, the optimal position of the blade of the hydraulic cutter should be perpendicular to the object being cut. If the hydraulic cutter blades are not perpendicular to the object being cut, then the blades of the tool will start to bend sideways, potentially causing blade separation, failure of the blades, or multiple cutting attempts. It is recommended that the cuts be made as low as possible on the posts to keep the jagged post ends out of the way, but be aware that some manufacturers will put an air bag cylinder very low in the A-post, just at the level of or below the dash (**FIGURE 9-21**). Another option may be to cut where the least amount of metal is showing. In some

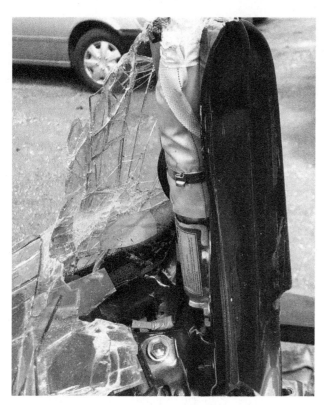

FIGURE 9-21 Be aware that some manufacturers will put an air bag cylinder very low in the A-post, at the level of or below the dash.
Courtesy of David Sweet.

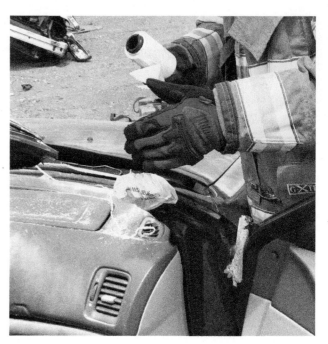

FIGURE 9-22 Cover cut jagged metal with a laminated sharps protection wrap, heavy blanket, or sections of precut hose sleeve.
Courtesy of David Sweet.

instances, it may be better to make a single cut high on a post rather than having to make several cuts at a lower section of the post because of the width or thickness of the post. Having to make multiple cuts will take valuable time away from the operation. If the post ends sharps are a concern, cover them with a laminated sharps protection wrap, heavy blanket, or sections of precut hose sleeve (**FIGURE 9-22**).

Another situation that commonly occurs when cutting a post is tool movement; when the tool is in the beginning stage of the cut, it can start to move forcefully inward toward the vehicle or outward away from the vehicle. This movement is caused by the blades of the tool trying to fracture and cut the metal where it finds the path of least resistance; the entire tool will move, and the blades will begin to make their own groove to cut into. To combat this problem and gain full control of the tool, be prepared to respond at the first instance of tool movement. As the tool closes around the post and movement is detected by the tool, the tool will want to forcefully shift away from you. Push or pull forcefully a few times in the direction opposite the tool's movement while continuing to engage the throttle and applying the cutting action of the blades. These two actions will force the blades of the hydraulic cutter to make a different groove in the metal, giving you full control of the cut and position of the tool.

When addressing the C-posts of a common passenger vehicle, there are several cutting options that the technical rescuer can utilize. Rear C-posts come in a variety of sizes and shapes. Wide C-posts may require several cuts using a hydraulic cutting tool because of the limited size of the opening created by the blades; a reciprocating saw would normally be the tool of choice for this situation. An option to minimize the number of cuts required on a wide C-post using a hydraulic cutter is to make a cut on one side of the post and then position the tips of the hydraulic spreader with one tip all the way through the cut section and the other tip on the uncut side section of the post with the tool set perpendicularly to the post. With the hydraulic spreader in place, close the tool on the cut; the tips of the spreader will tear through and crush the remaining section of metal. This will open up enough room to make one final cut in the center or on the uncut side of the post with the hydraulic cutter. To avoid a common error that can occur when attempting this technique, make certain that the tips of the spreader carry past the inside wall of the post and that the tool remains perpendicular to the post during the crush; doing so will prevent the tips from crushing only the outside wall and not the inside wall as well as preventing the entire tool from turning to the side. This technique, when carried out correctly, can eliminate multiple cuts that would otherwise have to be made utilizing a hydraulic cutter.

To remove the roof of an upright vehicle, follow the steps in **SKILL DRILL 9-12**.

CHAPTER 9 Victim Access and Management   253

SKILL DRILL 9-12
Removing the Roof of an Upright Vehicle NFPA 1006 8.2.6, 8.2.7, 8.3.6, 8.3.9

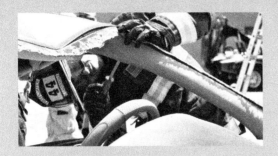

1 Don appropriate PPE, including mask and eye protection. Assess the scene for hazards, and complete the inner and outer surveys. Stabilize the vehicle. Ensure that the victim and the rescuer inside the vehicle are properly protected from unsecured glass particles. Secure all vehicle glass utilizing the appropriate glass management techniques demonstrated in this chapter. Locate and disconnect the vehicle's 12-volt DC battery if it is accessible. Expose the interior of each post and the roof rail prior to cutting to determine whether there are air bag cylinders, seat belt harnesses, seat belt adjustment bars, or seat belt pretensioning systems. Cut all seat belts that are attached high on the roof posts.

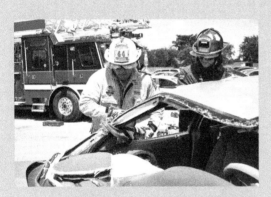

2 The proper order of cutting posts on a typical A-B-C-post roof structure will depend on the location of the victim. The last cut should be the post closest to the victim if this is an option. In this scenario, we will begin at the A-post. Position several rescuers on either side of the vehicle to assist in supporting the roof. With the hydraulic cutter perpendicular to the object being cut, start the cut on the A-post. The proper cutting angle of the hydraulic cutter should be perpendicular to the object being cut.

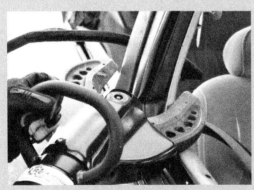

3 Work toward the B-post. Check again for any seat belt slide bars or reinforcement plates, and avoid cutting in this area, if possible. Before the cut is made, another rescuer must be positioned to support the roof when it is cut.

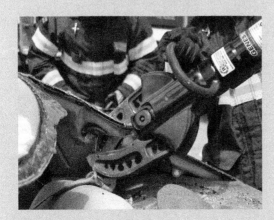

4 Once the B-post is cut, begin to cut the rear C-post. If the C-post is wide, make a cut on one side of the post, and utilize the hydraulic spreader to crush the remaining section.

(continues)

SKILL DRILL 9-12 Continued
Removing the Roof of an Upright Vehicle NFPA 1006 8.2.6, 8.2.7, 8.3.6, 8.3.9

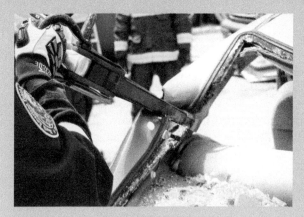

5 To avoid a common error that can occur when attempting this technique with a hydraulic spreader, make certain that the tips of the spreader carry past the inside wall of the post and the tool remains perpendicular to the post during the crush; doing so will prevent the tips from crushing just the outside wall, as well as preventing the entire tool from turning to the side. With the hydraulic spreader in place, close the tool on the cut. The tips of the spreader will tear through and crush the remaining section of metal, leaving one final cut to be made.

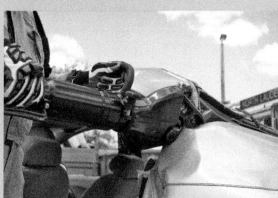

6 Cut the remaining section of metal on the C-post.

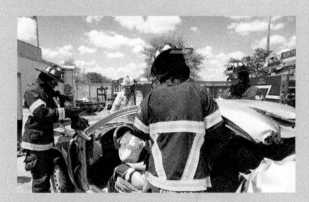

7 With crew members supporting the roof, move to the opposite side, and perform the same steps, cutting all remaining posts. Ensure that the roof is fully supported by personnel on both sides, preferably at all four posts, to prevent any accidental collapse.

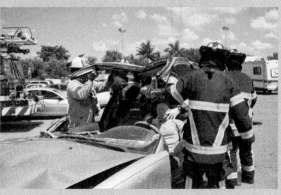

8 Walk the roof off the front or back of the vehicle, depending on where the victim is located. This step must be a coordinated effort between the crew members supporting the roof to prevent miscommunication and accidentally dropping the roof on the victim; it is best if one person takes the lead and directs the entire movement. Place the roof in an area outside the hot zone.

Courtesy of Edward Monahan.

> **LISTEN UP!**
>
> Expose the interior of each post and the roof rail prior to cutting to determine whether there are air bag cylinders, seat belt harnesses, seat belt adjustment bars, or seat belt pretensioning systems.

Relocating the Dash Section and/or Steering Wheel Assembly

Occupants can become trapped under the dash area of the vehicle following myriad crash scenarios. There are several techniques that are designed to move or lift the dash section that is entrapping the victim. Each of these techniques is designed to resolve a specific type of entrapment scenario that the technical rescuer may encounter. Utilizing the wrong technique for an entrapment that requires a specific application can potentially complicate the overall operation. Knowing when to use one technique over the others can greatly reduce the time it takes to safely release and remove the victim without causing further harm. Every entrapment scenario will present differently, and in some cases, combining techniques may improve the overall outcome. Problems can always occur, even after a technique has been initiated. A skilled technician will think outside the box, be able to apply multiple techniques using different tools, make adjustments, and overcome any issues that may arise.

The Dash Roll Technique

The traditional dash roll technique has been the standard technique for displacing the dash and steering wheel assembly for many years. The process involves pushing or rolling the entire front end of the vehicle, which encompasses the dash section and steering wheel assembly, off of the entrapped occupant utilizing hydraulic rams. The technique begins by removing the roof and gaining access to the front doors of both sides of the vehicle. Better maneuverability can be achieved if the doors are removed, but the technique can also be performed with the doors intact and in the opened position if rapid access and removal of the victim are needed. This technique can be performed with one ram positioned on the entrapment side or two hydraulic rams positioned on both sides of the vehicle for a more symmetrical push. The telescoping ram (about 20 to 60 in. [50.8 to 152.4 cm]) is the most effective type of hydraulic ram for this application because it eliminates the need to premeasure the opening.

When the dash roll technique is performed correctly, the vehicle's entire front end, including the dash, will lift up and forward, hinging from the relief cuts made on both sides. These relief cuts should tear slightly, giving the extra room needed to remove the victim. Another option is to insert cribbing wedges into the relief cuts once the push has been made with the dash lifted off the victim; this will assist in keeping the dash up and in place, or if one of the hydraulic rams is accidentally released or inadvertently moved, the cribbing wedges will prevent the dash from recollapsing onto the victim. Once the dash area is displaced, the victim should be properly packaged and removed toward the rear of the vehicle; the opened position of the hydraulic rams will prevent removal from the side.

If the vehicle is a two-door model, there is a product known as an L-bracket, which is made of steel and fits over the rocker panel and preferably up against the back of the door frame (the section that has the door latching pin attached to it). The welded steps on the L-bracket give the rescuer several sizing options for the ram to push from.

Another option to consider if the B-post has been removed is to stagger the height of the cribbing under the rocker panel so there is an incremental increase in steps and space. This formation will go from lower to higher, with the highest section of cribbing shored tightly under the rocker panel. Place the base of the hydraulic ram just over the lower section of cribbing where a gap has been purposely created, holding it in place until the ram is opened and the tip of the tool is placed into position. The tip of the hydraulic ram should be positioned at the bottom corner of the A-post where the dash and A-post join together.

Once the tip is in the correct position, push down on the base of the hydraulic ram as it is opened to resist the force of the tool kicking out. Applying pressure on the base of the hydraulic ram as the tool is opened will crush the hollow rocker panel down, causing it to conform to the gap created by the incremental cribbing formation, which in turn creates an artificial wall from which to push off. This technique takes a lot of practice to perfect, but it is very effective when performed correctly.

A less desirable option is to drive the spiked end of a Halligan bar into the rocker panel to create an artificial push point. The problem with this method is that it breaches the rocker panel, which weakens the area and can cause the Halligan bar to push back and tear open the hollow wall of the rocker panel when force is applied. If this occurs, there is a possibility of the Halligan bar dislodging forcefully, potentially causing injury.

Voice of Experience

Accurately evaluating all circumstances when arriving on an emergency scene that requires extrication is a critical component in prioritizing the necessary activities to safely remove trapped victims from vehicles. An initial scene size-up can help determine if there are any existing hazards, how many victims are involved, what additional resources are needed, and any other factors that may influence the success of an emergency operation. It is imperative to understand that every incident is unique and requires responders to conduct rapid assessments to determine the most appropriate method of accessing and treating victims. My personal experience with vehicle extrication has shown me that when doors are not an immediate option for victim removal because of damage, the window becomes a direct gateway to initiate patient care. This initial treatment may include basic things such as airway protection or cervical spine immobilization. The goal is to make contact with the victim as soon as possible.

Many years ago, as the captain of a truck company, we were dispatched to a motor vehicle accident (MVA) on a major highway with a report of people pinned. While en route to the incident, we received multiple updates about the situation, which were communicated to each member. This information allowed them to formulate their thoughts on what might be required of them upon arrival and provided a better situational awareness once on scene. We were the second unit to report on location and found a victim with agonal respirations, and her legs pinned beneath the dashboard. As I quickly assessed the situation, I determined the most important priority to be scene safety and requested the officer of the initial arriving company to shut down the highway.

As we approached the vehicle to begin extrication activities, an ambulance arrived on scene and immediately donned the required level of personal protective ensemble to operate within the hot zone. As they quickly approached, they suddenly noticed the condition of the trapped victim and determined that access to this victim was required immediately. I instructed one of our crew members to grant the medics access to the victim through the front window—away from the extrication activities. This action required the front windshield to be breached using a department-issued glass saw, which allowed patient care access without interfering with victim removal activities. From this opening, one of the attending medics was able to protect the airway, apply a cervical collar, and place the victim on oxygen before removing her from the vehicle. Victim access and management was critical to the life-saving efforts of the first responders and allowed essential functions to be conducted simultaneously.

The lesson learned from this incident is that victim access and management can be safely conducted while other activities occur. Had treatment been delayed in this situation, there may have been a different outcome. I believe that, when safety permits, victim assessment and treatment should be administered as quickly as possible to prevent the victim's condition from deteriorating. While this is the norm for our department, not all departments have the personnel or resources to conduct activities in the previously described manner and should prioritize their actions based on their current situation. Learn from the experiences of others and place that knowledge in your toolbox for situations that may require unconventional methods to be employed for the safe removal of a trapped victim.

Frank McKinley
Dallas Fire-Rescue Department
Dallas, Texas

CHAPTER 9 Victim Access and Management **257**

Another common practice that must be avoided is the use of the hydraulic spreader to push off from where the spreader is set in place to crush the rocker panel, leaving the spreader in the clamped position as a push point for the hydraulic ram. The hydraulic spreader was never designed for this type of maneuver or pressure, and this can damage the arms of the hydraulic spreader. There are many techniques that are far better and designed to use the tools for the right application.

To perform the dash roll technique (hydraulic and non-hydraulic), follow the steps in **SKILL DRILL 9-13** and **SKILL DRILL 9-14**.

SKILL DRILL 9-13
The Dash Roll Technique (Hydraulic) NFPA 1006 8.2.6, 8.2.7, 8.3.6, 8.3.9

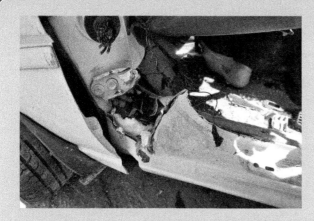

1 Don appropriate PPE, including mask and eye protection. Assess the scene for hazards, and complete the inner and outer surveys. Stabilize the vehicle. Ensure that the victim and the rescuer inside the vehicle are properly protected from unsecured glass particles. Secure all vehicle glass utilizing the appropriate glass management techniques demonstrated in this chapter. Locate and disconnect the vehicle's 12-volt DC battery if it is accessible. Scan the vehicle for supplemental restraint system (SRS) components (air bags). Release and open both front doors, utilizing the appropriate technique; the doors should be removed but can remain in place. Remove the roof of the vehicle, utilizing the appropriate technique. With both front doors in the opened position, use the hydraulic cutter to make an angled relief cut on each side of the vehicle, just under the bottom hinge where the firewall meets the rocker panel. A relief cut will need to be completed on each side of the vehicle.

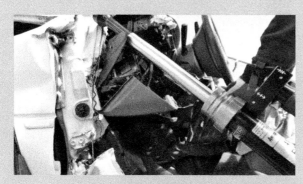

2 Premeasure for the appropriately sized hydraulic ram, or utilize a small to large telescopic model. Position the base of the ram at the bottom corner of the B-post and rocker panel, with the tip of the tool angled upward, extending out to reach the bottom corner of the A-post where the dash and A-post join.

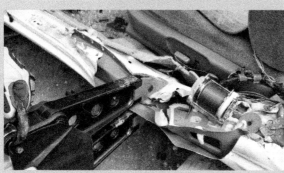

3 If the B-post has been removed, measure the proper distance of the ram as described in step 2, and then crimp the rocker panel in the area where the base of the ram rests using the hydraulic spreader. This creates a gap for the base of the ram to sit in and to push from.

(continues)

SKILL DRILL 9-13 Continued
The Dash Roll Technique (Hydraulic) NFPA 1006 8.2.6, 8.2.7, 8.3.6, 8.3.9

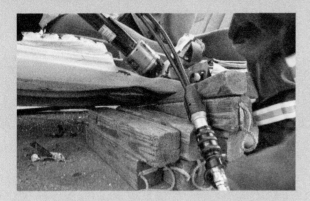

4. Insert and stagger the height of cribbing under the rocker panel beginning at the area where the gap was created so there is an incremental increase in steps and space. This formation will go from lower to higher, with the highest section of cribbing shored tightly under the rocker panel to prevent it from fully collapsing.

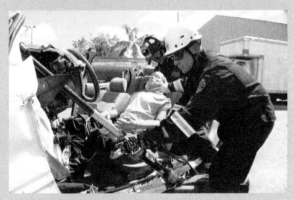

5. Position and open the ram. Once the tip is in the correct position, push down on the base of the hydraulic ram as it is opened to resist the force of the tool kicking out. Applying pressure as the tool is opened will force the rocker panel downward, causing it to conform to the gap and filling the space created by the incremental cribbing formation. This also creates an artificial wall to push off from. Operate the tool until enough room has been created to access and remove the victim. As the proper space is created, place cribbing/wedge sections in the opening to prevent the dash from falling back down on the victim. If more than one hydraulic ram is utilized, ensure that the procedure is coordinated and symmetrical.

Courtesy of Edward Monahan.

SKILL DRILL 9-14
The Dash Roll Technique (Non-Hydraulic) NFPA 1006 8.2.6, 8.2.7, 8.3.6, 8.3.9

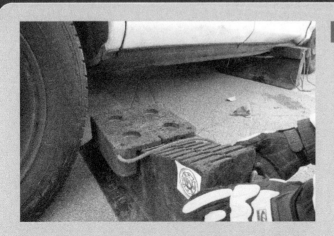

1. Don appropriate PPE, including mask and eye protection. Assess the scene for hazards, and complete the inner and outer surveys. Stabilize the vehicle. Ensure that the victim and the rescuer inside the vehicle are properly protected from unsecured glass particles. Secure all vehicle glass, utilizing the appropriate glass management techniques demonstrated in this chapter. Locate and disconnect the vehicle's 12-volt DC battery if it is accessible. Scan the vehicle for SRS components (air bags).

SKILL DRILL 9-14 Continued
The Dash Roll Technique (Non-Hydraulic) NFPA 1006 8.2.6, 8.2.7, 8.3.6, 8.3.9

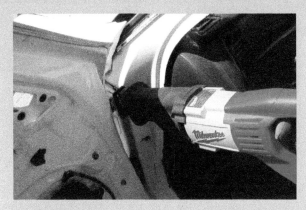

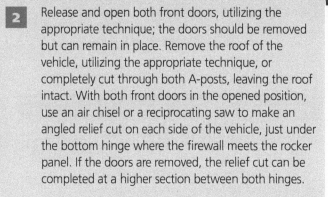

2 Release and open both front doors, utilizing the appropriate technique; the doors should be removed but can remain in place. Remove the roof of the vehicle, utilizing the appropriate technique, or completely cut through both A-posts, leaving the roof intact. With both front doors in the opened position, use an air chisel or a reciprocating saw to make an angled relief cut on each side of the vehicle, just under the bottom hinge where the firewall meets the rocker panel. If the doors are removed, the relief cut can be completed at a higher section between both hinges.

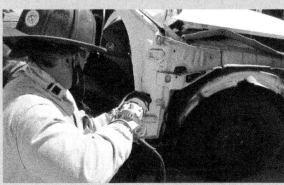

3 This relief cut will need to be completed on each side of the vehicle.

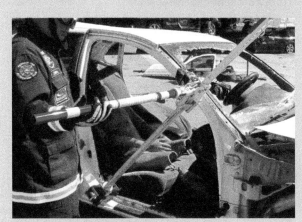

4 Place the FRJ at the bottom corner of the B-post and rocker panel, with the tongue of the tool angled upward, extending out to reach the bottom corner of the A-post. If the B-post is intact, then place cribbing under the B-post/rocker panel area, and push off from the corner of the B-post and rocker panel area. If the B-post has been removed, first crimp the rocker panel with the jack in the area where the base of the jack rests. This creates a gap for the base of the jack to sit in and to push from.

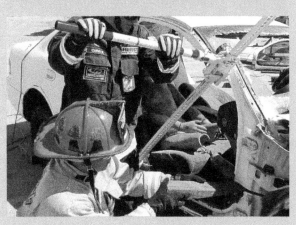

5 Insert and stagger the height of cribbing under the rocker panel beginning at the area where the gap was created so there is an incremental increase in steps and space. Position and open the jack. Once the tongue of the jack is in the correct position, have another rescuer push down forcefully on the base of the jack as it is opened to resist the force of the tool kicking out. Operate the tool until enough room has been created to access and remove the victim.

Courtesy of Edward Monahan.

> **LISTEN UP!**
> Do not use the hydraulic spreader to crush the rocker panel, leaving the spreader in the clamped position as a push point for the hydraulic ram. The hydraulic spreader was never designed for this type of maneuver or pressure, and this can damage the arms of the hydraulic spreader. There are many techniques that are far better and designed to use the tools in the right application.

> **LISTEN UP!**
> Every entrapment scenario will present differently, and in some cases, combining techniques may improve the overall outcome. Problems can always occur, even after a technique has been initiated. A skilled technician will think outside the box, be able to apply multiple techniques using different tools, make adjustments, and overcome any issues that may arise.

The Dash Lift Technique

Several vehicle accident scenarios may be encountered for which a dash roll technique will not be effective. Some of these incidents may include a vehicle impacting an object, such as a cement lamppost or large tree, which forces the vehicle's front end and dash onto the driver; a vehicle colliding with the rear end of a large commercial vehicle and causing an underride entrapment; or a vehicle ending up on the front end of another vehicle (**FIGURE 9-23**). A dash roll technique would not be effective in any of these situations. The weight and position of the objects or vehicles are locking and holding down the dash area. If the dash roll technique were used, the entire floorboard and rocker panel area, where the relief cuts would be made, would push up and create what is called a **tepee, or tenting, effect**. Rescuers would not be able to effectively release the dash area off of the victim.

> **LISTEN UP!**
> Use the right technique for the specific type of entrapment. Knowing when to use one technique over the other can greatly reduce the time it takes to safely release and remove the victims without causing them further harm.

Because the dash area needs to be released and lifted independently from the front end of the vehicle, the **dash lift technique**, rather than the dash roll technique, is the better option. Releasing a section of the dash from the front end of the vehicle requires a hinge point to be created at the upper rail section of the front end between the strut tower and the dash/firewall area. The strut tower, which is normally located above the center point area of the front wheel, is attached to the vehicle's upper rail frame. The goal is to release the strut tower from the dash/firewall section and create a hinge point for the dash to rise up and away from the trapped occupant.

To create this hinge effect, relief cuts are made in two areas. The first relief cut is made through the upper rail section as just described, and the second relief cut is made completely through the firewall area between the two hinges where the door was attached. When the technique is performed correctly, this section of the dash, including the steering wheel assembly, will lift straight up and off of the occupant, leaving the front end of the vehicle, including the front wheels, stationary. This is very important because the front section of the vehicle with the cement pole or tree imbedded or the other vehicle resting on top of it will not move when the dash section is lifted. This technique is designed to lift the dash on one side of the vehicle only; the steps will have to be repeated on the opposite side if that side of the dash needs to be lifted as well.

Prior to making any of the relief cuts, the hood area closest to the dash must be exposed and detached, with the hinge cut completely through, which releases it from the front end attachment. Once the hood is raised, the area can be examined for any possible hydraulic or gas-filled piston struts that are installed to assist in lifting the vehicle's hood (**FIGURE 9-24**). If a piston strut is installed in the area of operation, then it must be removed or disabled for safety purposes. To detach the hood hinge and verify whether there

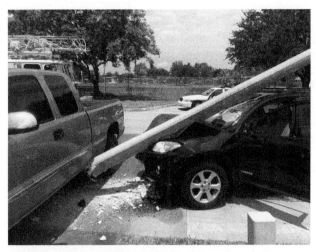

FIGURE 9-23 A dash roll technique would not be effective in this incident; the weight and position of the object or vehicles are locking and holding down the dash area, which prevents the forward movement of the dash.
Courtesy of Bill McGrath.

is a hydraulic or gas-filled piston, insert the tips of the hydraulic spreader under the top corner area of the hood where the dash and hood meet. Slowly open the spreader to lift up the corner of the hood just enough to get the hydraulic cutter in to cut the hinge attachment for the hood, releasing that side of the hood from the dash. If the hood is not cut from the dash at that particular hinge attachment, then the hood could impede the lifting of the dash. At the same time, examine the area for the presence of a hydraulic or gas-filled piston strut. If a piston is found, verify whether it is in the area of operation where the upper rail will be cut. If the piston strut is in the way, then it will need to be disabled and/or detached. To disable a hydraulic or gas-filled piston strut, with the spreader still in place supporting the hood with the hood's hinge cut, insert a hydraulic cutter and cut the section of the piston steel rod where it attaches to the vehicle (**FIGURE 9-25**). Do not cut into the piston cylinder body because there will be a rapid release of hydraulic fluid and/or a gas under pressure. Addressing these items can quickly clear the way to proceed with the remainder of the dash lift technique.

The dash lift technique is an advanced technique that first requires preparatory work to be completed and has multiple steps that must be carried out with strict discipline. Leaving out a step, which can happen in a high-stress environment, will almost always result in a critical failure; take the time to practice being proficient.

To perform the dash lift technique using hydraulics, follow the steps in **SKILL DRILL 9-15**.

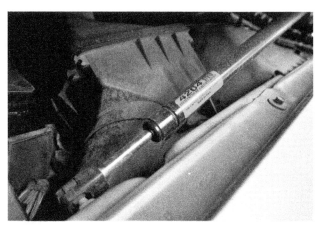

FIGURE 9-24 Piston struts assist in lifting the vehicle's hood.
Courtesy of Edward Monahan.

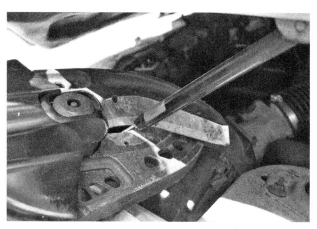

FIGURE 9-25 To disable a hydraulic or gas-filled piston strut, with the spreader holding open the hood and the hood's hinge cut, insert a hydraulic cutter, and cut the section of the piston where it attaches to the vehicle.
Courtesy of Edward Monahan.

SKILL DRILL 9-15
The Dash Lift Technique (Hydraulic) NFPA 1006 8.2.6, 8.2.7, 8.3.6, 8.3.9

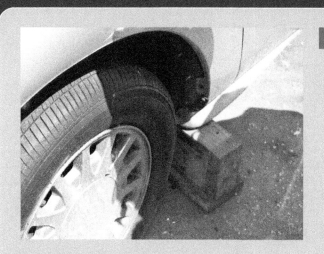

1 Don appropriate PPE, including mask and eye protection. Assess the scene for hazards, and complete the inner and outer surveys. Stabilize the vehicle. Ensure that the victim and the rescuer inside the vehicle are properly protected from unsecured glass particles. Secure all vehicle glass utilizing the appropriate glass management techniques demonstrated in this chapter.

(continues)

SKILL DRILL 9-15 Continued
The Dash Lift Technique (Hydraulic) NFPA 1006 8.2.6, 8.2.7, 8.3.6, 8.3.9

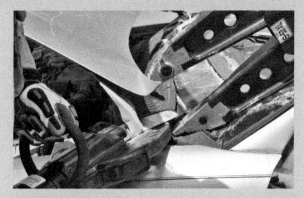

2 Locate and disconnect the vehicle's 12-volt DC battery if it is readily accessible. This technique can still be performed with the roof on; however, a section of the A-post connecting the dash area to be lifted must be removed. For best access to the victim, remove the roof. Remember to check the posts and roof rails for SRS components. Remove the vehicle's door on the side to be lifted. Lift and cut the vehicle's hood at the hinge attachment closest to the dash on the side to be lifted, and verify whether a hydraulic or gas-filled piston strut exists.

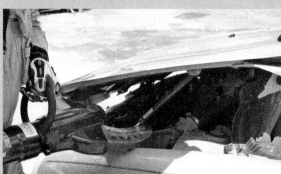

3 If a piston is found, then cut the steel rod (not the cylinder) and disable and detach the item as a safety measure.

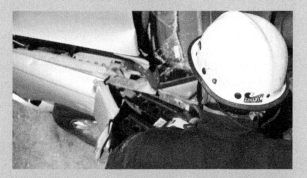

4 Remove the front wheel fender quarter panel.

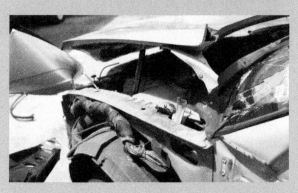

5 Expose the upper rail frame section of the engine compartment by removing the front wheel well fender panel cover by slowly and precisely spreading it off where it is attached. This is accomplished by inserting the tips of the spreader in the upper space between the firewall and the wheel well panel. Angle the spreader, and force the panel off the top front attachments leaving the bottom attachment by the rocker panel in place until the end. Slowly work the spreader across the inside top section of the wheel well panel, which will tear away from the upper rail if done correctly. If the bottom section of the wheel well panel releases (which is normally spot welded in) and tool leverage is lost, reposition the spreader. Clamp down on the panel where it is connected to the upper frame rail, and peel it back off of the area. This is thin sheet metal, and will tear easily. If it is a polycarbonate/plastic/fiberglass panel, then it will either break off or come off as one section.

SKILL DRILL 9-15 Continued
The Dash Lift Technique (Hydraulic) NFPA 1006 8.2.6, 8.2.7, 8.3.6, 8.3.9

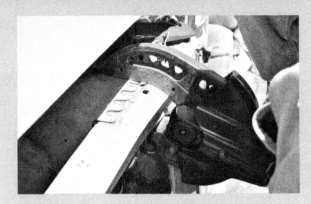 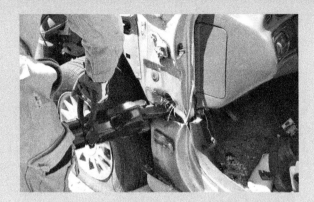

6 Once the wheel well panel is removed and the upper frame rail is fully exposed, a completed cut will be made through the upper rail at a section located between the strut tower and dash to ensure the proper release of the dash from the front end of the vehicle. As an option, the hydraulic spreader can be applied before the cut is made to pre-crush the upper rail section. This will assist in the cutting action of the blades, but remember that this adds a step, which can delay the operation. Insert a gloved hand, and feel the metal on the upper rail to assess the dimension, depth, and angle required for the cut, and then proceed with the cut. The number of cuts may vary depending on the type of vehicle construction or width of the area.

7 Once that cut has been made, reposition the hydraulic cutter, and make a complete cut through the entire firewall area directly between the top and bottom hinges. Again, the number of cuts may vary depending on the type of vehicle construction or width of the area. If a large firewall area is encountered or there is not enough room to get the cutter in, use the hydraulic spreader to crush the firewall. This is accomplished by making a smaller cut on one side of the firewall. Insert one tip of the hydraulic spreader into the cut side and one on the other side, compressing the metal enough to provide room for one final cut. As the final cut is made, there may be a slight visual release of the dash where the dash and steering wheel lift an inch (2.5 cm) or so. This is an indication that the cut has been made all the way through. If multiple cuts are required on the firewall, make the first cut away from the victim and close to the wheel well side to prevent the tool from rotating in on the victim.

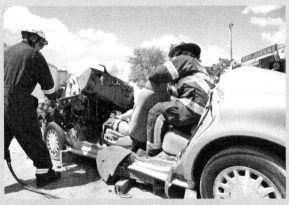

8 Insert cribbing under the rocker panel firewall area for support. Position the hydraulic spreader in line with the firewall (not off to the side), vertically set with one arm over the other, and insert the tips in the firewall that was cut. Slowly open the tool, using the top and bottom hinges (which are the strongest parts of that area) as guides and push points. As the arms open, carefully watch the tool for any signs of slippage or twisting. The spreader may have to be adjusted by repositioning and/or inserting deeper to get the proper angle. The goal is to have the top arm of the spreader eventually push/reach the dash cross/support bar that is hidden within the dash and normally extends from one side of the vehicle to the other. The dash will lift up and hinge at the section that was cut in the upper frame rail, taking the vehicle's front end completely out of the lift and supplying ample room for victim removal.

Courtesy of Edward Monahan.

Alternatively, to perform the dash lift technique without using hydraulics, follow the steps in **SKILL DRILL 9-16**.

One possible complication of the dash lift technique is the presence of metal brackets attached from the dash or dash cross bar to the floorboard. These metal brackets are located in the center console area where the radio, air conditioning unit, and other various components are located (see Chapter 5). The metal brackets are bolted or welded into the floorboard of the vehicle and designed to lock the dash in place to minimize any movement resulting from an impact.

SKILL DRILL 9-16
The Dash Lift Technique (Non-Hydraulic) NFPA 1006 8.2.6, 8.2.7, 8.3.6, 8.3.9

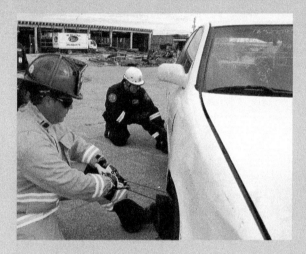

1 Don appropriate PPE, including mask and eye protection. Assess the scene for hazards, and complete the inner and outer surveys. Stabilize the vehicle. Ensure that the victim and the rescuer inside the vehicle are properly protected. Secure all vehicle glass utilizing the appropriate glass management techniques demonstrated in this chapter. Locate and disconnect the vehicle's 12-volt DC battery if it is accessible. Scan the vehicle for SRS components (air bags). Release the vehicle's door on the latch side using a combination of a pneumatic air chisel and an FRJ.

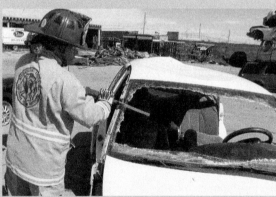

2 Remove the vehicle's roof. (This technique can still be performed with the roof on; a section of the A-post connecting the dash area to be lifted must be removed.) Perform this step using a reciprocating saw or pneumatic air chisel.

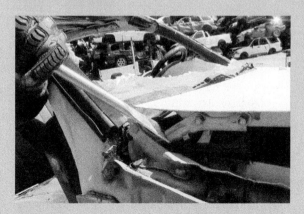

3 Remove the door on the hinge side. Remove all or part of the wheel well panel using a pneumatic air chisel. This will expose the upper rail frame section of the engine compartment. Expose the vehicle's engine compartment hood at the hinge attachment closest to the dash on the side to be lifted, and verify whether a hydraulic or gas-filled piston strut exists. If a piston is found, then disable and/or displace the item as a safety measure. Cut the hinge attachment connecting the hood to the dash.

SKILL DRILL 9-16 Continued
The Dash Lift Technique (Non-Hydraulic) NFPA 1006 8.2.6, 8.2.7, 8.3.6, 8.3.9

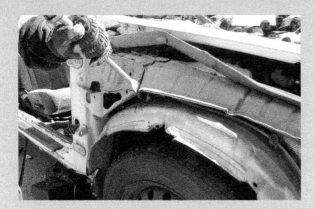

4. With the wheel well panel removed and the upper frame rail fully exposed, use the pneumatic air chisel or reciprocating saw to make a complete cut through the upper rail frame between the strut tower and dash. This will ensure the proper release of the dash from the front end of the vehicle.

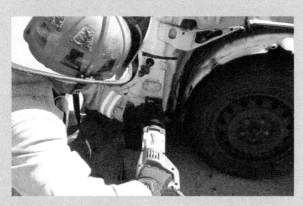

5. Using the pneumatic air chisel or reciprocating saw, make a complete cut through the entire firewall just above the area where the rocker panel meets the firewall. A larger section may have to be cut out to make room for the tongue of the FRJ.

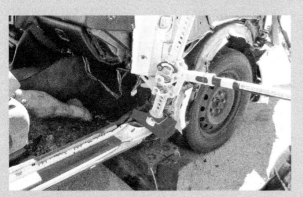

6. Insert cribbing under the rocker panel firewall area for support. Position the jack on the rocker panel, and insert the top lip of the tool in the firewall that was cut. As the tool arm is engaged for the lift, carefully watch the tool for any signs of slippage or twisting. If this occurs, insert cribbing to support the dash from coming back down on the victim, and readjust the tool.

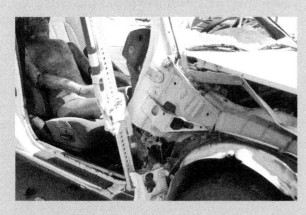

7. With the technique applied correctly, the dash will lift up and hinge at the section that was cut in the upper frame rail, taking the vehicle's front end completely out of the lift and supplying ample room for victim removal.

Courtesy of Edward Monahan.

Because of their inherent design and attachment points, these brackets can at times resist the upward movement of the dash lift technique, halting progress. If metal brackets are in place, the stopping of the dash's upward movement will occur almost immediately at the start of the lift, halting the force of the spreader or jack. It is extremely important for the technical rescuer to recognize the signs of this occurring. If the dash does not release and rise as the lift is being performed and/or the firewall area just starts to tear away and folds outward toward the technical rescuer with no vertical movement, there is the possibility that these brackets are not separating from the floorboard and are keeping the dash from releasing. The majority of the time, these brackets will break off and/or separate from the floorboard attachment when force is applied, but if they don't separate, then the two brackets may need to be cut before the dash will release. To accomplish this objective, the technical rescuer must gain access to the front passenger compartment opposite the entrapped victim and start to expose the brackets by removing the plastic molding surrounding the brackets. This plastic molding should break away and release with little effort (**FIGURE 9-26**).

Once the first bracket is exposed, use the hydraulic cutter or air chisel to cut through the bracket and then the remaining section to cut through the last side bracket next to the victim. The objective is to expose the metal brackets from the best vantage point of the rescuer that isn't impeded by victims. Once the brackets are cut, resume the dash lift technique and complete the lift.

If access is not possible to both sides because of an additional trapped occupant or objects, attempt another approach or angle, or consider another technique, such as a dash roll or steering assembly relocation, to gain access. Remember to always train on alternative techniques if Plan B has to change and evolve for these types of unexpected occurrences.

Steering Wheel Assembly Relocation

Relocating a steering wheel assembly utilizing a rated come along or an FRJ can be reliable options when other dash displacement techniques, such as a dash lift or dash roll technique, are not possible or a hydraulic tool fails. Techniques such as these come under a lot of scrutiny and will always be debated because of the fear of having the steering wheel and associated components come apart and break off under the extreme force applied from these tools, which can potentially send projectiles back into the victim. There is always an inherent danger in any technique applied in vehicle rescue and extrication; tools can fail, components can violently come apart unexpectedly, and poor application will almost always lead to problems as well. A risk versus reward assessment for the application of a technique or tool choice must be decided upon immediately and the action/technique executed. Overthinking, or "paralysis by analysis," is detrimental to the operation; make the decision and execute!

When the come along or FRJ and chain package have been properly applied, the technical rescuer has complete control over and feel of the entire movement. In addition, there is a safety feature for the handle component of the come along that is rated to fail by bending when a predetermined force is exerted. The properly rated come along for this technique is generally in the 2000- to 4000-lb (1- to 2-short tons) category; it has a rated handle and a complete chain package (see Chapter 3, *Tools and Equipment*). There is also a misconception about the amount of pull that is needed to release the steering column and free a trapped victim.

The proper operation of either tool does not require overexertion to be effective when the steering wheel is lifted and/or pulled through the dash; just a few inches of upward movement will create enough space to free the victim. If needed, more room may be created by cutting the section of the steering wheel ring that was impinging on the victim, but always make sure before attempting to cut a section of the steering wheel ring that it is not still impinging on the victim. The force and cutting action of the hydraulic tool as the ring is cut can drive a section of the steering wheel deeper into the victim before it releases. There is also a ratcheting cutting tool similar to a bolt cutter that is very effective in cutting steering wheel rings and is less aggressive than a hydraulic cutter. Again, it is best to relieve the pressure of the impinging steering wheel before attempting to cut the ring.

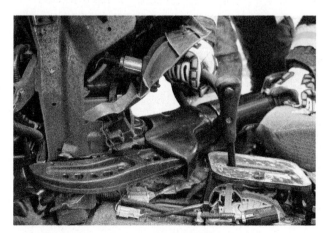

FIGURE 9-26 Remove the plastic molding to expose the dash brackets, and cut through both of them.
Courtesy of David Sweet.

CHAPTER 9 Victim Access and Management

One technique that is not recommended for relocating a steering wheel assembly is using hydraulic tools along with a rated chain package. This technique is very dangerous because the technical rescuer has no control over the amount of force that is applied; nor can the technical rescuer feel the force that is applied, as he or she can when using an FRJ or a rated come along.

When utilizing a come along, it is best practice to use two technical rescuers to complete the evolution, with both initial assignments being performed simultaneously.

To relocate the steering wheel assembly, follow the steps in **SKILL DRILL 9-17**.

To relocate the steering wheel assembly utilizing an FRJ, follow the steps in **SKILL DRILL 9-18**.

SKILL DRILL 9-17
Relocating the Steering Wheel Assembly Utilizing a 2/4-Ton–Rated Come Along NFPA 1006 8.2.6, 8.2.7, 8.3.6, 8.3.9

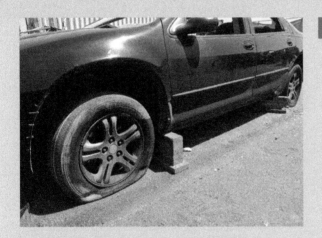

1 Don appropriate PPE, including mask and eye protection. Assess the scene for hazards, and complete the inner and outer surveys. Stabilize the vehicle. Ensure that the victim and the rescuer inside the vehicle are properly protected from unsecured glass particles. Secure all vehicle glass, utilizing the appropriate glass management techniques demonstrated in this chapter.

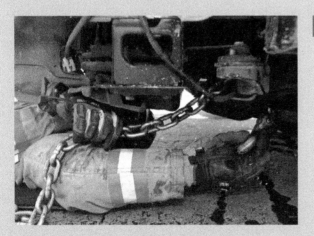

2 *Technical rescuer 1*: While positioned at the front of the vehicle, lay a section of **ladder cribbing** over the front hood/bumper area of the vehicle. Use a fastener to attach the ladder cribbing to the hood to temporarily hold the cribbing in place. Rest the support ring located at one side of the chain's end section on top of the ladder cribbing at the lower part of the hood (the come along will be attached to this). Using the other end of the chain, locate an area under the vehicle to secure it to. Loop the chain through, and take up the slack, utilizing the chain-shortener hook, which will lock in that loose section and secure the anchor point. To correctly position the come along, the operator should always place the flywheel (the operating wheel of the come along) in his or her right hand. Place the come along on top of the ladder cribbing, and secure it to the support ring of the chain.

(continues)

SKILL DRILL 9-17 Continued
Relocating the Steering Wheel Assembly Utilizing a 2/4-Ton–Rated Come Along NFPA 1006 8.2.6, 8.2.7, 8.3.6, 8.3.9

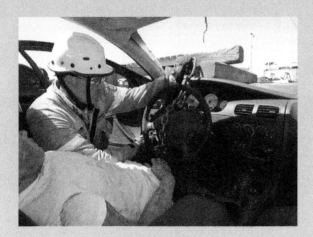

3 *Technical rescuer 2*: Use three four-by-fours to build a **slide cribbing** configuration on top of the dash directly in line with the steering wheel. Utilizing the second section of chain in the chain package, weave the support ring of the chain through the bottom section of the steering wheel ring starting from behind. Continue through the opening, and go around the front main base of the steering wheel, ending back through the top section of the steering wheel ring. Pull the support ring through, and lay it on the cross-section of the slide cribbing. Fasten one end of a bungee cord with hooks or another fastening device to the front hood and the other end to the support ring to hold it in place.

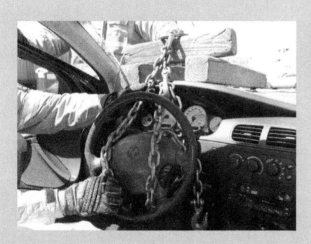

4 *Technical rescuer 2*: Wrap the other end of the chain clockwise around the steering wheel column twice, just behind the steering wheel ring. Pull it snug. Pull the end of the chain over, through, and around the steering wheel column. Once the chain has been tightly secured around the steering wheel column, with the end section of the chain mirroring the front section of chain, weave it through the bottom section of the steering wheel ring starting from behind. Continue through the opening, and go around the front main base of the steering wheel, ending back through the top section of the steering wheel ring. Pull up the slack in the chain, and secure the chain to the support ring utilizing the chain shortener.

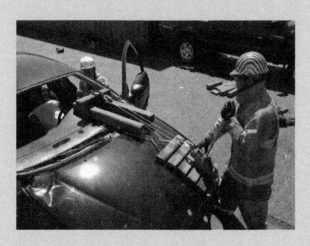

5 With both chain sections in place, technical rescuer 1 takes hold of the come along with the right hand on the flywheel and the left hand on the free spool lever located on the top left section of the device. Technical rescuer 2 takes hold of the hook-and-wire cable attachment of the come along and pulls out enough cable to attach it to the support ring located on top of the slide cribbing. Technical rescuer 1 releases the free spool lever and slowly lets out the wire cable by rotating the flywheel counterclockwise. Make certain that the release of the cable is controlled to prevent the cable from backlashing; this would be a critical error that makes it impossible to continue the technique.

SKILL DRILL 9-17 Continued
Relocating the Steering Wheel Assembly Utilizing a 2/4-Ton–Rated Come Along NFPA 1006 8.2.6, 8.2.7, 8.3.6, 8.3.9

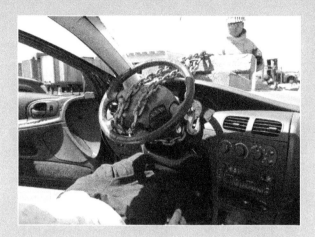

6 Once the wire cable has been attached and the slack has been taken up by turning the flywheel clockwise, complete a safety check of all connections, ensuring that the hooks are secure and facing upward and that the wire cable is not crossed on itself. Technical rescuer 1 now inserts the control handle into the come along and slowly pushes the handle forward and back, engaging the device's gear mechanism. As the tool is operated, technical rescuer 2 is positioned with the victim and verbally signals to technical rescuer 1 when enough clearance of the steering wheel has been established. When enough room has been created to free the victim, technical rescuer 1 removes the control handle of the come along and relocates it to the front of the device to ensure that the device is not accidentally engaged and released.

© Jones & Bartlett Learning. Photographed by Glen E. Ellman.

SKILL DRILL 9-18
Relocating the Steering Wheel Assembly Utilizing a First Responder Jack
NFPA 1006 8.2.6, 8.2.7, 8.3.6, 8.3.9

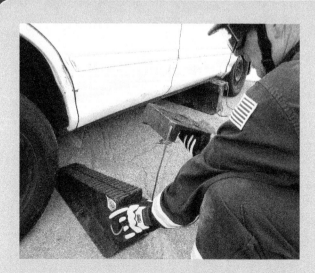

1 Don appropriate PPE, including mask and eye protection. Assess the scene for hazards, and complete the inner and outer surveys. Stabilize the vehicle. Ensure that the victim and the other rescuer inside the vehicle are properly protected using a blanket to cover them from unsecured glass particles. Secure all vehicle glass utilizing the appropriate glass management techniques demonstrated in this chapter.

(continues)

SKILL DRILL 9-18 Continued
Relocating the Steering Wheel Assembly Utilizing a First Responder Jack
NFPA 1006 8.2.6, 8.2.7, 8.3.6, 8.3.9

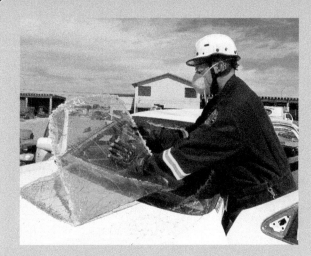

2 Remove the windshield, utilizing the techniques and tools described in this text.

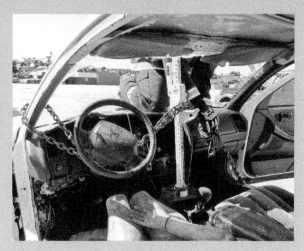

3 Place the FRJ inside the vehicle with the base resting on the center console area and the tongue of the tool facing the seats. Utilizing a rated chain package with a large J-hook, secure the chain to the A-post by wrapping it around the post.

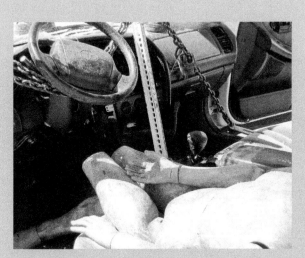

4 Continue wrapping the chain under the steering wheel and over the tongue of the FRJ, and then securely fasten it to the lower rocker panel on the opposite side, utilizing the J-hook.

Courtesy of Edward Monahan.

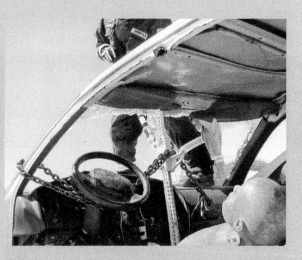

5 Operate the lever of the FRJ, which will tighten up the chains and thus lift the steering wheel assembly.

Providing Initial Medical Care

In vehicle rescue and extrication, an integral component to the IAP is obtaining an initial observation of the victim, managing threats to life, and quickly transporting the victim to the appropriate level of care. Any technique, procedures, and/or tools applied to gain access and extricate the victim are futile without a solid medical plan and a competent member or team that is preassigned to manage life-threatening injuries from trauma. Utilizing a similar concept adopted from the NASCAR and Formula One pit crew philosophy for cardiac resuscitation procedures, each member of the response team on the vehicle rescue and extrication incident has a position assignment with dedicated tasks that are carried out systematically without the direct intervention of the IC.

The medical position is a critical assignment. It requires medically trained personnel to utilize the critical thinking process to make the best medical decisions for victim care in a rapidly changing environment and chaotic conditions.

The medical position must rapidly evaluate the incident presented, develop a medical plan of action, integrate that plan into the overall IAP for the operation, initiate the plan, reassess the plan for effectiveness, and be prepared to adjust as the victim's condition and/or environment changes.

Upon the initial arrival of the emergency response team, the medical position will immediately engage in the operational process (standing by in a readiness state just outside the action zone) as the inner and outer survey crews complete the first phase of the scene stabilization process. With the basic trauma gear in hand, the medical position will move in the direction of the first victim who is identified by the survey team. The medical position can establish verbal contact with the victim but will not make physical contact with the vehicle or victim until an all-clear signal has been given by the survey team. Once either verbal or physical contact has been established, the victim now becomes the emergency medical services (EMS) care provider's victim (multiple victims will require rapid triage with the focus on the most critical based on available resources). Verbal communication with victim acknowledgment provides the EMS provider with immediate information on airway and basic neurological functions based on the response given as well as establishes a relationship with the victim. This relationship bond is important to establish early on to provide reassurance and trust.

The primary assessment can be conducted outside the vehicle if entry is delayed or cannot be made, but it is preferable to make access into the vehicle by self-entry or assistance to maximize the visual and hands-on examination process. Remember that your safety and that of your crew always precludes entering a vehicle that is unsafe, regardless of the incident that is presented, so ensure that an all-clear signal has been given by the survey team (**FIGURE 9-27**). While the EMS care provider makes entry into the vehicle, another rescuer positioned outside the vehicle can maintain manual temporary spinal immobilization of the victim and a neutral position of the victim's head to maintain the airway; it is best practice to protect the victim's cervical spine and keep the head in a supported neutral position at all times once initial contact has been established. The rescuer outside can continue maintaining this position if resources permit while the medical care provider inside the vehicle conducts the primary assessment.

The EMS care provider inside the vehicle should have all of the necessary medical gear inside the vehicle to render aid based on the level of medical service the jurisdiction provides.

As the primary survey is conducted in a rapid and logical order, the quick recognition of life-threatening injuries must be the priority of all EMS providers. The primary concern for life-threatening injuries in the assessment and management of the trauma victim

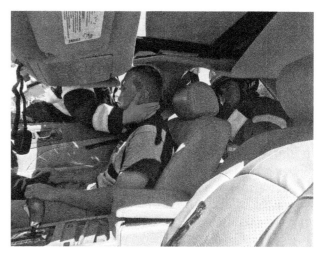

FIGURE 9-27 While the EMS care provider makes an entry into the vehicle, another rescuer positioned outside the vehicle can maintain manual temporary spinal immobilization of the victim and a neutral position of the victim's head to maintain the airway. It is the best practice to protect the victim's cervical spine and keep the head in a supported neutral position at all times once initial contact has been established.
Courtesy of David Sweet.

consists of the following components in the XABCDE mnemonic format:

eXsanguinating hemorrhage (severe, life-threatening bleeding)

A—Airway management

B—Breathing (ventilation)

C—Circulation

D—Disability

E—Exposure

The components of the primary survey are taught and displayed in a sequential manner but can be performed simultaneously. Any life-threatening conditions that are identified can immediately be addressed before completing the entire primary survey, such as applying a tourniquet to manage a severe hemorrhage or correcting an airway obstruction.

The goal of XABCDE is to prevent the onset of shock by maintaining the body's ability to deliver oxygen to the tissues via an intact circulatory system and to intake oxygen and expel waste products through the respiratory system.

Exsanguinating Hemorrhage

Hemorrhage must be immediately controlled to stop the onset of shock caused by the body's inability to sustain the proper volume to adequately perfuse the tissues and supply the needed oxygen for the production of energy. Hemorrhaging can occur either externally, internally, or both simultaneously from the traumatic injuries sustained. For external hemorrhaging, the course of action would be to apply direct pressure over the wound or use a tourniquet (**FIGURE 9-28**).

Quickly assess the victim's skin color and temperature. It is important to check the color of the victim's skin when you arrive at the scene so that you can monitor the victim's skin for color changes as time passes. Pale or ashen skin color is an indication of poor perfusion, which may be a sign of internal hemorrhaging.

Victims with deeply pigmented skin may show color changes in the fingernail beds, in the whites of the eyes, on the palm of the hand, or inside the mouth.

Airway

Immediately assess the victim for a patent airway, which again will be determined if the victim is exchanging clear verbal responses with the medical care provider. If on the initial exam it is found that the victim is not breathing where the airway is compromised and/or obstructed, attempt to access the vehicle safely

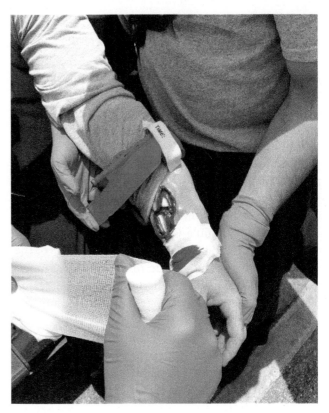

FIGURE 9-28 For external hemorrhaging, the best course of action would be to apply direct pressure over the wound or consider the use of a tourniquet.
Courtesy of David Sweet.

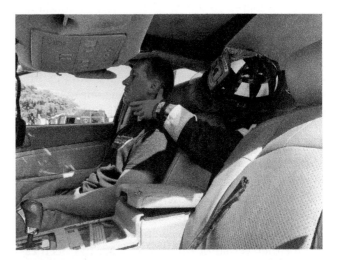

FIGURE 9-29 Use the jaw thrust maneuver if the victim is lying on the seat or floor and if there is any possibility that the collision could have caused a head or spinal injury.
Courtesy of David Sweet.

to apply the standard trauma jaw thrust maneuver/chin lift maneuver (**FIGURE 9-29**). Use the trauma jaw thrust maneuver if there is any possibility that the collision could have caused a head or spinal injury.

If the victim is in a sitting or semi-reclining position with an obstructed or compromised airway, grasp the victim's head with both hands, and put one hand under the victim's chin and the other hand on the back of the victim's head, just above the neck. Raise the head to a neutral position to open the airway.

Breathing

If the victim is conscious, assess the rate and quality of the victim's breathing. Does the chest rise and fall with each breath, or does the victim appear to be short of breath (**TABLE 9-1**)? If the victim is unconscious, check for breathing by placing the side of your face next to the victim's nose and mouth. You should be able to hear the sounds of breathing, see the chest rise and fall, and even feel the movement of air on your cheek. If the victim is having difficulty breathing or you hear unusual sounds, check for an object in the victim's mouth, such as food, vomitus, dentures, gum, chewing tobacco, or broken teeth, and remove it. However, do not put a finger inside the victim's mouth without the use of a bite block for protection.

If you cannot detect any movement of the chest and no sound of air is coming from the nose and mouth, then breathing is absent. Take immediate steps to open the victim's airway and perform rescue breathing. Because trauma is suspected after a motor vehicle collision, protect the cervical spine by keeping the victim's head in a neutral position and using the trauma jaw thrust/chin lift maneuver to open the airway. Maintain cervical stabilization until the head and neck are immobilized.

TABLE 9-1 Normal Vital Signs at Various Ages				
Age	Pulse Rate (beats/min)	Respirations (breaths/min)	Blood Pressure (mm Hg)	Temperature (°F)
Neonate (0 to 1 month)	Awake: 100 to 205 Asleep: 90 to 160	30 to 60	Systolic: 67 to 84 Diastolic: 35 to 53 Mean arterial pressure: 45 to 60	98 to 100 (37 to 38°C)
Infant (1 month to 1 year)	Awake: 100 to 180 Asleep: 90 to 160	30 to 53	Systolic: 72 to 104 Diastolic: 37 to 56 Mean arterial pressure: 50 to 62	96.8 to 99.6 (36 to 37.5°C)
Toddler (1 to 2 years)	Awake: 98 to 140 Asleep: 80 to 120	22 to 37	Systolic: 86 to 106 Diastolic: 42 to 63 Mean arterial pressure: 49 to 62	96.8 to 99.6 (36 to 37.5°C)
Preschooler (3 to 5 years)	Awake: 80 to 120 Asleep: 65 to 100	20 to 28	Systolic: 89 to 112 Diastolic: 46 to 72 Mean arterial pressure: 58 to 69	98.6 (37°C)
School-aged child (6 to 12 years)	Awake: 75 to 118 Asleep: 58 to 90	18 to 25	Systolic: 97 to 120 Diastolic: 57 to 80 Mean arterial pressure: 66 to 79	98.6 (37°C)
Adolescent (12 to 15 years)	Awake: 60 to 100 Asleep: 50 to 90	12 to 20	Systolic: 110 to 131 Diastolic: 64 to 83 Mean arterial pressure: 73 to 84	98.6 (37°C)
Early adult (18 to 40 years)	60 to 100	12 to 20	Systolic: 90 to 140	98.6 (37°C)
Middle adult (41 to 60 years)	60 to 100	12 to 20	Systolic: 90 to 140	98.6 (37°C)
Older adult (61 years and older)	60 to 100	12 to 20	Systolic: 90 to 140	98.6 (37°C)

Pediatric data from American Heart Association (AHA). Vital signs in children. Pediatric Advanced Life Support. Dallas, TX: AHA; 2015.

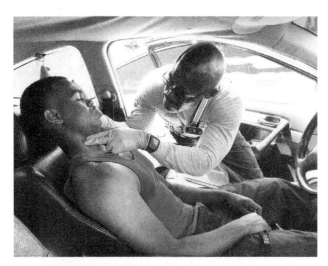

FIGURE 9-30 Check an unconscious victim's circulation by checking the carotid pulse.
Courtesy of David Sweet.

Circulation

Next, if the victim is unconscious, check the carotid pulse (**FIGURE 9-30**). Place your index and middle fingers together, and touch the larynx (Adam's apple) in the victim's neck. Then, slide your two fingers off the larynx toward the victim's ear until you feel a slight notch. Practice this maneuver until you are able to find a carotid pulse within 5 seconds of touching the victim's larynx (Table 9-1). If you cannot feel a pulse with your fingers in 5 to 10 seconds, begin CPR.

If the victim is conscious, assess the radial pulse rather than the carotid pulse (**FIGURE 9-31**). Place your index and middle fingers on the victim's wrist at the thumb side. You should practice taking the radial pulse often to develop this skill.

SAFETY TIP

Remember to wear the appropriate PPE to avoid contact with body fluids. Wearing medical gloves under the operational gloves can provide a protective barrier against these types of contaminants.

LISTEN UP!

Rescue operations are those activities directed at locating endangered persons at an emergency incident, removing those persons from danger, treating injured victims, and providing for transport to an appropriate trauma-care facility. *Recovery operations* are nonemergency activities undertaken by responders to retrieve property or remains of victims.

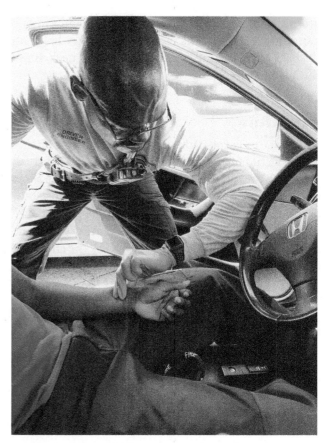

FIGURE 9-31 Take the radial pulse if the victim is conscious.
Courtesy of David Sweet.

Disability

Disability can be described as the cognitive reaction of the victim. Is the victim answering your questions with cohesive, complete sentences? Can the victim feel and move his or her extremities with minimal intervention? Medical care providers will utilize the Glasgow Coma Scale (GCS) score to determine the severity of traumatic brain injury by evaluating the victim's ability to respond based on three parameters.

Utilizing a weighted scale from 3 to 15, with 3 being the worst and 15 being normal, these three parameters measure the victim's best motor response, verbal response, and eye response. The GSC is a reliable way to measure the initial and subsequent level of consciousness throughout the operation, but factors such as alcohol and drug use as well as low blood sugar can alter the scoring.

Expose

To complete a thorough primary examination of the victim and rule out other potentially life-threatening injuries, the medical care provider will have to expose areas of the body that require the removal of clothing. Protecting the integrity of the victim as well as maintaining the body's temperature and preventing hypothermia by minimizing external exposure to inclement weather conditions is always a must when removing clothing. If the victim is conscious and alert, the medical care provider must explain every action taken and acknowledge consent prior to exposing the victim's body. This again stresses the importance of establishing a relationship and trust with the victim through compassion and understanding. Maintain a systematic approach when exposing areas of the body starting at the head and working down, checking for hemorrhaging, deformities, swelling and discoloration, hardness, firmness, warm, cold, diaphoresis, and pain from palpitation and/or manipulation.

Compartment Syndrome

Compartment syndrome occurs when compressive forces are applied to the body and blood is shunted away for a prolonged period of time from a tissue or organ. Compartment syndrome can occur from the crushing or traumatic injuries that are common in motor vehicle collisions. An example of a crush injury where compartment syndrome may be experienced is during the aftermath of a front-end collision where the dash area of the vehicle crushes down on the patient's lower torso and extremities. Immediate recognition and treatment of compartment syndrome is critical for patient survival. Signs and symptoms of compartment syndrome include severe pain, lack of a pulse in the extremity, obvious bone fractures, and loss of color to the extremity or area. The patient may be talking with you while still entrapped and then quickly decompensate when the crushing force is released from the body and the return of perfusion exposes the body to built-up waste products. This is why it is vital for the medical team to rapidly assess the patient before the patient is extricated. Compartment syndrome is an advanced life support emergency and intravenous fluids and medications may need to be administered to the patient before the patient is extricated from the vehicle.

Triage

Some incidents may involve multiple victims and may even be considered a mass casualty incident. Rapid and accurate triage will help bring order to the chaos of a scene with multiple victims and allow the most critical victims to be treated first for life-threatening injuries and then transported. Triage simply means to quickly sort victims based on the severity of their injuries with the premise of doing the greatest good for the greatest number of people.

There are four common triage categories. They can be remembered using the mnemonic IDME, which stands for immediate (red), delayed (yellow), minor or minimal (green; hold), and expectant (black; injuries incompatible with life or deceased) (**TABLE 9-2**).

It is important that each victim involved in the incident be given an initial color tag, which can simply be a plastic tear-off material that can be quickly tied and/or attached to the victim's extremity or body. Remember that this is a rapid initial assessment to sort out the most severe and critically injured victims. More detailed and thorough examinations will follow immediately after with the secondary survey once the critically injured have been identified. The color status of the victim can be changed upon further evaluation.

TABLE 9-2 Triage Priorities

Triage Category	Typical Injuries
Red tag: first priority (immediate)	Airway and breathing difficulties
Need immediate care and transport	Uncontrolled or severe bleeding
Treated first and transported as soon as possible	Severe medical problems
	Signs of shock (hypoperfusion)
	Severe burns
	Open chest or abdominal injuries
Yellow tag: second priority (delayed)	Burns without airway problems
Treatment and transport can be temporarily delayed	Major or multiple bone or joint injuries
	Back injuries with or without spinal cord damage
Green tag: third priority, minimal (walking wounded)	Minor fractures
	Minor soft tissue injuries
Require minimal or no treatment; transport can be delayed until last	
Black tag: fourth priority (expectant)	Obvious death
Already dead or have little chance for survival; salvageable victims treated before these victims	Obviously nonsurvivable injury, such as major open brain trauma
	Respiratory arrest (if limited resources)
	Cardiac arrest

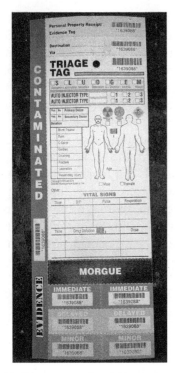

FIGURE 9-32 Triage tags should be color coded and clearly show the category of the victim. Triage tags will become part of the victim's medical record and should have a tear-off receipt with a number corresponding to the number on the tag.
Courtesy of David Sweet.

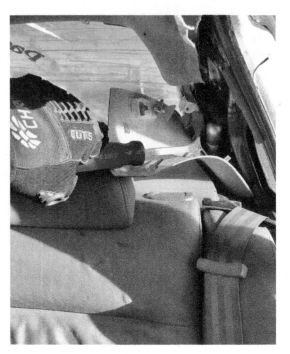

FIGURE 9-33 In addition to providing medical care, there are several other steps the rescuer inside the vehicle must carry out. Some of these tasks may include cutting all the seat belts to assist in roof removal, identifying any undetected air bag or SRS components, and relaying this information to the crew conducting the operation.
Courtesy of David Sweet.

On the secondary survey, a labeling triage tag system detailing the victim's condition should be attached to the victim. These detailed triage tags should be weatherproof and easy to read (**FIGURE 9-32**). They should be color coded and clearly show the category of the victim. Triage tags will become part of the victim's medical record. Most have a tear-off receipt with a number corresponding to the number on the tag, which assists in accountability and tracking a victim.

START triage is one of the easiest methods of triage. START stands for simple triage and rapid treatment. The staff members at Hoag Memorial Hospital in Newport Beach, California, developed this method of triage. It is easily mastered with practice and will enable you to rapidly categorize victims. START triage uses a limited assessment of the victim's ability to walk, respiratory status, hemodynamic status, and neurological status.

Lou Romig, MD, recognized that the START triage system does not take into account the physiological and developmental differences of pediatric victims. She therefore developed the JumpSTART triage system for pediatric victims. JumpSTART is intended for use in children younger than 8 years or who appear to weigh less than 100 lb (45 kg). Another system that is considered an all-hazard national triage guideline is called the SALT triage system, which stands for sort, assess, life-saving interventions, and treatment/transport.

In addition to providing medical care, there are several other steps the rescuer inside the vehicle must carry out. Some of these tasks may include cutting all the seat belts to assist in roof removal, identifying any undetected air bag or SRS components and relaying this information to the crew conducting the operation, attempting to see whether any of the seat adjustment mechanisms are operational (beneficial systems), and providing soft and hard protection for the victim and himself or herself against projectiles if tool operation will be in close proximity (**FIGURE 9-33**). It is important to note that the medical care provider is the eyes and ears of the crew operating outside the vehicle. Continuous communication has to be relayed back and forth from the medical care provider and the operational crew and officer/IC.

Victim Packaging and Removal

Maintaining alignment is one of the main objectives when removing a victim from a vehicle. Applying a victim immobilization tool, such as a Kendrick

Extrication Device (KED), can maintain alignment. The KED assists with managing and removing a victim by keeping the victim securely packaged to limit overmanipulation and free movement of the victim's body. If a KED is not available, consider utilizing a rolled blanket. A rolled blanket can be inserted around the upper torso and under the arms to create handles on both sides to grab and assist with the lift.

Regardless of the type of packaging tool or device utilized, several rescue personnel will have to be positioned inside the vehicle and around the victim to maximize and control the lift. The KED combined with a long backboard is one of the best complete package techniques to safely remove a victim (**FIGURE 9-34**). The following technique is one procedure that can be used to meet this objective.

To extricate a victim from a passenger car, follow the steps in **SKILL DRILL 9-19**.

Transport

Once the victim has been removed from the vehicle, transfer all pertinent medical information to the EMS personnel who will transport the victim to the appropriate trauma-care facility. Skilled verbal communication and written documentation will make it possible for you to effectively coordinate the transfer of care. Depending on the methods used in your jurisdiction, checklists, triage tags, or forms may be used to transfer the necessary information, including victim condition and history, to EMS. Documentation serves as an excellent record that the care delivered was appropriate, guarantees the proper transfer of responsibility, and ensures the continuity of victim care. The type of transport used to deliver the victim to the emergency department will vary depending on the severity of the victim's injuries and the distance to the medical facility.

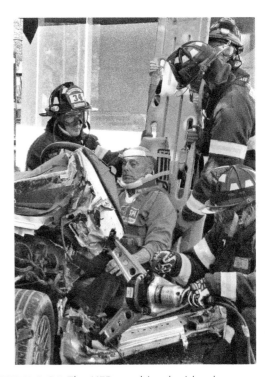

FIGURE 9-34 The KED combined with a long backboard is one of the best complete package techniques to safely remove a victim.
Courtesy of Edward Monahan.

SKILL DRILL 9-19
Extricating a Victim from a Passenger Car NFPA 1006 8.2.8, 8.3.9

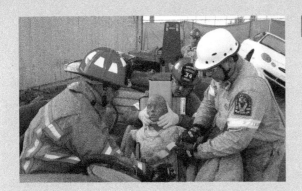

1 Don appropriate PPE, including mask and eye protection. Assess the scene for hazards, and complete the inner and outer surveys. Stabilize the vehicle. Ensure that the victim and the rescuer inside the vehicle are properly protected using a blanket to cover them from unsecured glass particles. Secure all vehicle glass, utilizing the appropriate glass management techniques demonstrated in this chapter. Locate and disconnect the vehicle's 12-volt DC battery if it is readily accessible. Access the victim using the appropriate method. Remove the vehicle's roof. Remember to check for SRS components. Remove work gloves, and replace with latex or similar medical gloves prior to touching the victim to prevent cross-contamination. Place an immobilization device on the victim.

(continues)

SKILL DRILL 9-19 Continued
Extricating a Victim from a Passenger Car NFPA 1006 8.2.8, 8.3.9

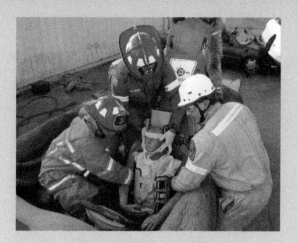

2 Insert a backboard behind the victim. Adjust the back of the seat in the down position if possible. If the seat adjustment is still operational (beneficial system) and can be reached, support the victim, and adjust the back of the seat in the down position if possible.

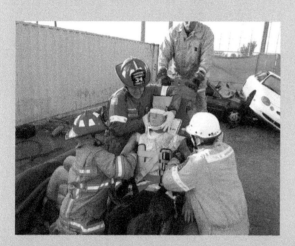

3 Position rescue personnel in a three-point position around the victim. The rescuer at the head of the victim will give the command to move the victim as a unit. Lift the backboard and the victim as a unit onto the trunk/rear dash area. Properly secure the victim to the backboard.

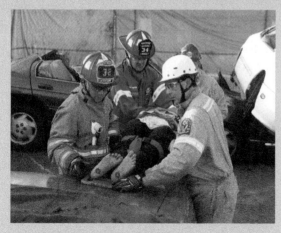

4 Once the victim has been properly packaged, use a four-point carry to transfer the victim to an awaiting stretcher. When performed correctly, this technique will maintain victim alignment with minimal manipulation required.

© Jones & Bartlett Learning. Photographed by Glen E. Ellman.

After-Action REVIEW

IN SUMMARY

- Victim management involves vehicle entry, victim packaging, and victim removal.
- The main objective is not to remove the victim from the vehicle but to remove the vehicle from the victim by creating a large opening with systematic and precise techniques.
- Primary access points are the existing openings into the vehicle, and secondary access points are openings created by rescuers.
- One of the simplest ways to access a victim is to open a vehicle door. It is important to manually try all the doors before other methods are used, even if the doors appear to be badly damaged.
- Polycarbonate glass is a light and durable thermoplastic that is up to 250 times stronger than glass; it is naturally designed to resist direct impacts by any striking tool carried on the apparatus.
- Making a purchase point/access opening is the process of gaining an access area to insert and better position a tool for operation. Once a purchase point has been established, the goal is to create a wide enough opening with the hydraulic spreader to expose the locking/latching mechanism or hinges and to insert a hydraulic cutter; this technique is known as expose and cut.
- For gaining door access, a vertical spread technique gives the technical rescuer the best vantage point from which to expose the latch and create enough room for the cutter blades to get in and cut the latching mechanism.
- A wheel well crush technique is utilized to gain access to door hinges from the outside, using the hydraulic spreader.
- The complete side removal technique (side-out) is a highly effective technique for four-door side-impact collisions; it pushes the door frame and B-post outward, separating them from the rocker panel, away from the occupant, utilizing the door's natural directional movement.
- When performing a roof removal, position rescuers on both sides of the vehicle to support the roof as the posts are cut.
- The dash roll technique involves pushing or rolling the entire front end of the vehicle, which encompasses the dashboard and steering wheel assembly, off of the entrapped occupant utilizing hydraulic rams.
- The dash lift technique involves lifting the dash upward with the hydraulic spreader by making precise relief cuts in the hood's upper rail and between the hinges of the firewall area, thus separating the dash section from the front end of the vehicle.
- Metal brackets attached to the dash can at times resist the upward movement of the dash lift technique, halting any progress.
- Relocating a steering wheel assembly, utilizing an FRJ or rated come along may be a reliable option when other dash displacement techniques, such as a dash lift or dash roll technique, are not an option or a hydraulic tool fails.
- Once inside the vehicle, the EMS care provider must assess the condition of the victim and render care, such as managing airway, breathing, and circulation.
- Because trauma is suspected after a motor vehicle collision, protect the cervical spine by keeping the victim's head in a neutral position and using the jaw thrust maneuver to open the airway. Maintain cervical stabilization until the head and neck are immobilized.
- Some incidents may involve multiple victims. Triage simply means to sort victims based on the severity of their injuries.
- There are four common triage categories. They can be remembered using the mnemonic IDME, which stands for immediate (red), delayed (yellow), minor or minimal (green; hold), and expectant (black; injuries incompatible with life or deceased).
- Once the victim has been removed from the vehicle, transfer all pertinent medical information to the EMS personnel who will transport the victim to the appropriate medical facility.
- Skilled verbal communication and written documentation will enable you to effectively coordinate the transfer of care.

KEY TERMS

Backboard slide technique An initial access technique that is used if the vehicle doors are locked, blocked, or inoperable; may be accomplished through a rear or side window.

Dash lift technique A technique used to lift and release a section of the dash from the front end of the vehicle using a powered tool, such as the hydraulic spreader, or a combination of hand tools and powered tools. It is performed by making precise relief cuts in the hood's upper rail and between the hinges of the firewall area, separating the dash section from the front end of the vehicle.

Dash roll technique The standard technique for many years for displacing the dashboard using a powered tool, such as the hydraulic ram, or a combination of hand tools and powered tools. The process involves the force of pushing or rolling the entire front end of the vehicle upward and forward, including the dashboard and steering wheel assembly, off of the entrapped occupant.

Expose and cut The process of creating a wide enough opening with the hydraulic spreader to expose the locking/latching mechanism or hinges and to insert a hydraulic cutter to cut.

Glass management The process of identifying the need for controlling the removal of glass or maintaining the glass intact.

Ladder cribbing Several 2-in. × 4-in. (5-cm × 10-cm) sections of wood attached together by a strip of webbing running along the sides.

Primary access The existing openings of doors and/or windows that provide a pathway to the trapped and/or injured victim.

Secondary access Openings created by rescuers using force that provide a pathway to trapped and/or injured victims.

Side-out technique A technique used to gain access to a four-door vehicle involved in a side-impact collision.

Slide cribbing Two sections of 4-in. × 4-in. (10-cm × 10-cm) cribbing positioned parallel to each other with a third section of cribbing on top traversing the two bottom sections.

Tepee, or tenting, effect A peak or tent shape that can result when using an ineffective dash roll technique; the floorboard and rocker panel area push up where the relief cuts are made when the dash area is locked down by an object or vehicle.

Vertical spread A door access procedure utilizing a hydraulic spreader; the tool is placed vertically in the window frame of the door and pushes off of the roof rail and window frame to create an access point to the door's latching mechanism.

Wheel well crush technique A technique utilized to gain access to door hinges from the outside.

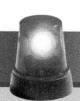

On Scene

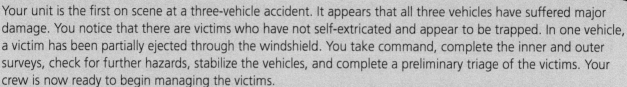

Your unit is the first on scene at a three-vehicle accident. It appears that all three vehicles have suffered major damage. You notice that there are victims who have not self-extricated and appear to be trapped. In one vehicle, a victim has been partially ejected through the windshield. You take command, complete the inner and outer surveys, check for further hazards, stabilize the vehicles, and complete a preliminary triage of the victims. Your crew is now ready to begin managing the victims.

1. The most desirable way for the rescuer to access the victim who has been partially ejected is to support the ejected head or torso from outside the vehicle and gain vehicle access:

   A. by removing the roof.
   B. through the rear window.
   C. through an open door.
   D. through the windshield.

2. Glass that breaks into small fragments is also known as:

   A. laminated glass.
   B. tempered glass.
   C. safety glass.
   D. polycarbonate glass.

On Scene Continued

3. The tool of choice to remove the windshield away from the partially ejected victim whose head or torso is protruding out of the windshield is a:
   A. reciprocating saw.
   B. glass saw.
   C. pair of trauma shears.
   D. pry axe.

4. To gain access to an area of metal on the vehicle to insert a tool, the rescuer should create a:
   A. position point.
   B. pivot point.
   C. pry point.
   D. purchase point/access opening.

5. The technique that refers to the removal of the front and rear door as one unit on the same side of a four-door vehicle is known as the:
   A. total-out technique.
   B. cutout technique.
   C. blowout technique.
   D. side-out technique.

6. The rescuer should lean against the door that is being spread to provide counter pressure.
   A. True
   B. False

7. When cutting posts with the hydraulic cutter, the blades should be positioned _____ to the posts to prevent the blades from twisting or separating.
   A. vertically
   B. horizontally
   C. perpendicularly
   D. tangentially

8. The weight of the dashboard can be pushed or rolled off of the victim using a technique known as:
   A. block-and-tackle snatch-and-pull technique.
   B. hydraulic ram dash roll.
   C. electric winch maneuver.
   D. bottle jack push procedure.

9. Exposing the interior of the post and the roof rail will reveal:
   A. air bag cylinders.
   B. cutting points.
   C. glass channels.
   D. crumple zones.

10. The rescuer's main objective should be to remove the victim from the vehicle.
    A. True
    B. False

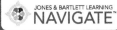 Access Navigate for more activities.

CHAPTER 10

Operations and Technician Levels

Alternative Extrication Techniques

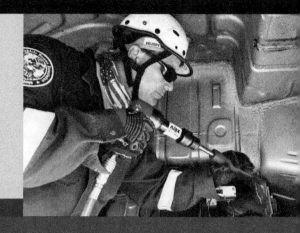

KNOWLEDGE OBJECTIVES

After studying this chapter, you will be able to:
- Describe the process of tunneling through a vehicle to gain access to victim(s). (pp. 283–286)
- Explain the dangers associated with tunneling and strategies to mitigate risks. (pp. 284–286)
- Identify when it is appropriate to remove front seats or seat-backs in alternative extrication operations. (pp. 287–290)
- Identify tools that can be utilized to replace or augment traditional extrication tools. (pp. 283–284, 293, 295–296, 298)
- Provide and explain alternate extrication strategies when traditional methods are inappropriate or unsuccessful. (pp. 283, 284, 287, 291–295, 297, 300, 308–313)

- Relocate the B-post or door frame with a hydraulic ram. (**NFPA 1006: 8.2.6, 8.2.7, 8.3.9**, pp. 291–292)
- Relocate the B-post or door frame with a First Responder Jack. (**NFPA 1006: 8.2.6, 8.2.7, 8.3.9**, pp. 293–294)
- Perform a cross-ramming operation using a hydraulic ram. (**NFPA 1006: 8.2.4, 8.2.6, 8.2.7, 8.3.9**, p. 297)
- Stabilize an impaled object. (**NFPA 1006: 8.2.4, 8.2.6, 8.2.7, 8.3.9**, pp. 299–300)
- Remove a roof using an air chisel. (**NFPA 1006: 8.2.4, 8.2.6, 8.2.7, 8.3.9**, pp. 302–303)
- Remove a roof from a vehicle using a reciprocating saw. (**NFPA 1006: 8.2.4, 8.2.6, 8.2.7, 8.3.9**, pp. 304–305)
- Remove a roof from a vehicle resting on its side. (**NFPA 1006: 8.2.4, 8.2.6, 8.2.7, 8.3.9**, pp. 306–307)
- Remove the vehicle door on the hinge side using an air chisel. (**NFPA 1006: 8.2.4, 8.2.6, 8.2.7, 8.3.9**, pp. 308–310)
- Perform a side removal on a vehicle upside down or resting on its roof. (**NFPA 1006: 8.2.6, 8.2.7, 8.3.9**, pp. 311–312)
- Relocate a pedal. (**NFPA 1006: 8.2.6, 8.2.7, 8.3.9**, p. 313)
- Removal of a victim under a vehicle using an FRJ. (**NFPA 1006: 8.2.3, 8.2.6, 8.2.7, 8.3.9**, p. 314)

SKILLS OBJECTIVES

After studying this chapter, you will be able to perform the following skills:
- Tunnel through the trunk. (**NFPA 1006: 8.2.4, 8.2.6, 8.2.7, 8.3.9**, pp. 284–286)
- Jacking the trunk. (**NFPA 1006: 8.2.6, 8.2.7, 8.3.9**, p. 288)
- Front seat-back removal. (**NFPA 1006: 8.2.4, 8.2.6, 8.2.7, 8.3.9**, p. 289)
- Front seat-back relocation. (**NFPA 1006: 8.2.6, 8.2.7, 8.3.9**, p. 290)

You Are the Rescuer

You arrive on scene of a motor vehicle collision where a common passenger vehicle is resting on its crushed roof. The inner and outer surveys reveal that one occupant is trapped in the rear passenger area and both doors are blocked and inaccessible because of positioning. There are no hazards, and the vehicle is not running.

1. What are some of the possible solutions to this scenario?
2. What steps are needed to stabilize the vehicle?
3. Will you perform a trunk-tunneling or jacking technique to gain access to the victim?

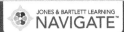
Access Navigate for more practice activities.

Introduction

Well-rounded technical rescuers have a diverse repertoire of alternative techniques that they are familiar with and can apply at any incident. This chapter will discuss several alternative methods that can be used on several incidents that may be encountered. Although some of these techniques may never be used, it is best to be prepared with as many options as possible to resolve an incident the moment a unique scenario is presented. The technical rescuer should be able to complete a technique utilizing various tools; seamlessly transitioning between hand tools, electric powered tools, and hydraulic tools to complete the task. An incident can demand this of the technical rescuer when tool failure occurs or when multiple operations occur simultaneously with limited tools available. A scenario involving limited access or a tight space may require the technical rescuer to transition to a different sized tool upon discovering that a hydraulic cutter cannot articulate an angle or fit, but a pneumatic air chisel may. The technical rescuer must be adaptable to changing situations, fully trained and prepared to apply the appropriate tools and/or an alternative technique to complete the task at hand despite complications or limited resources available.

Tunneling

As discussed briefly in Chapter 8, *Vehicle Stabilization*, **tunneling** is the process of gaining entry through the rear trunk area of a vehicle. The technique is more commonly performed for a vehicle that is resting on its roof, but it can be performed for a vehicle in any resting position following a multitude of crash scenarios, such as a vehicle underride where the impact has caused access to the doors and roof to be blocked

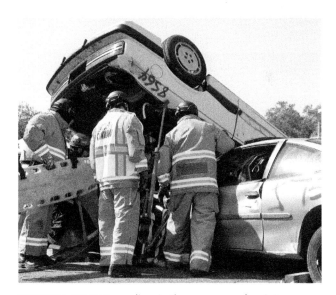
FIGURE 10-1 Tunneling is the process of gaining entry through the rear trunk area of a vehicle.
Courtesy of Edward Monahan.

off. At first glance, a tunneling scenario can be intimidating and can appear to be time consuming; however, with practice this technique can be accomplished fairly quickly and can enable in-line removal of the victim, thus minimizing the need for victim manipulation (**FIGURE 10-1**). A word of caution about attempting any tunneling operation involving hybrid, fuel-cell, and alternative-fuel vehicles: These vehicles may have high pressure fuel storage tanks and/or battery packs in the trunk area, so an alternative method of entry is recommended.

Let's consider a sample scenario. The vehicle on the left in **FIGURE 10-2** suffered a side-impact collision that flipped the vehicle over, blocking entry on both sides. The best option for this scenario is to tunnel through the back of the vehicle to gain access and extricate the victim. Using this scenario, start the technique by stabilizing the scene and the vehicle.

SAFETY TIP

The possible entrapment scenarios can be endless; this is when continual advanced training will assist in thinking outside of the box, preparing rescuers to overcome difficult incidents.

There are several tools that need to be set up and ready to use, such as an air chisel with several spare air bottles, an electric-powered reciprocating saw, and a hydraulic spreader/cutter. With the vehicle properly stabilized, the focus will be on removing the trunk to create a very large opening. The objective is to expose the latching mechanism using the hydraulic spreader and then cut the latching mechanism to release the trunk cover. In this scenario, gaining access to the latching mechanism will be demonstrated using a combination of the hydraulic spreader/cutter. This technique can also be accomplished using a reciprocating saw and/or air chisel. The decision for what tool or combination of tools to be used will depend on the type of vehicle, the body design, the presentation of the vehicle, and the skill level of the personnel and their familiarity with various tools.

Follow the steps in **SKILL DRILL 10-1** to tunnel through the trunk of a common passenger vehicle.

SAFETY TIP

Before opening the trunk of a vehicle on its roof, determine whether there are any hazardous or heavy storage items that may be in the trunk that can potentially come crashing down. Secure the trunk with a cargo strap to keep the trunk from opening when the latching mechanism is cut.

Jacking the Trunk

Jacking the trunk, or cracking the undercarriage and lifting the rear end of a vehicle, is an extreme technique that should be included in the technical rescue arsenal. A scenario may present where a tunneling operation through the trunk space of the vehicle is required but upon opening and examining the trunk area, it is found to contain a large fuel tank that

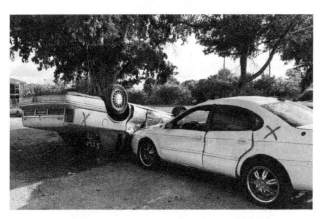

FIGURE 10-2 The vehicle on the left suffered a side-impact collision that flipped it over, blocking entry on both sides.
Courtesy of Edward Monahan.

SKILL DRILL 10-1
Tunneling Through the Trunk NFPA 1006 8.2.4, 8.2.6, 8.2.7, and 8.3.9

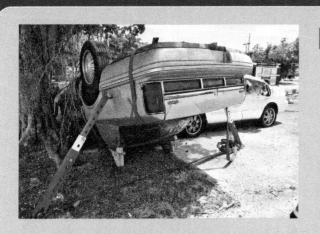

1. Don appropriate personal protective equipment (PPE), including mask and eye protection. Assess the scene for hazards, and complete the inner and outer surveys. Stabilize the vehicle. Ensure that the victim and the other rescuer inside the vehicle are properly protected. Secure all vehicle glass using the appropriate glass-management techniques. As a safety measure, secure the trunk with a cargo strap to keep the trunk from opening when the latching mechanism is cut.

SKILL DRILL 10-1 Continued
Tunneling Through the Trunk NFPA 1006 8.2.4, 8.2.6, 8.2.7, and 8.3.9

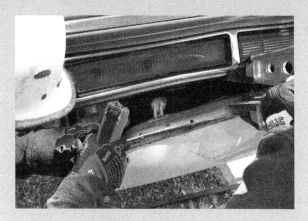

2 Locate the area where the trunk lip meets the rear bumper. Create a purchase point with the hydraulic spreader to squeeze/crush the area at the downward bend of the trunk cover. Use the hydraulic spreader to work the area around the latching mechanism to expose the latching mechanism. Do not try to force the trunk open by spreading it off its latch because this will cause the entire vehicle to shift and jeopardize the integrity of the stabilization struts and cribbing. Determine whether there are any hazardous or heavy storage items in the trunk.

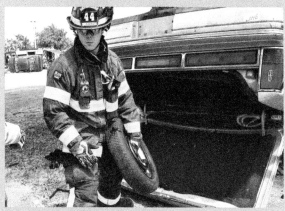

3 Insert the hydraulic cutter, and cut the latch area to release the trunk cover. With the trunk open, expose all metal within the trunk. Remove all interior lining, the spare tire, the vehicle tire jack, and any other items.

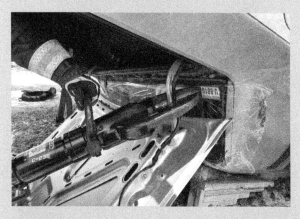

4 Use the hydraulic cutter to cut the arms that hinge the trunk cover open, and totally remove the trunk cover. Place the trunk cover in the debris pile.

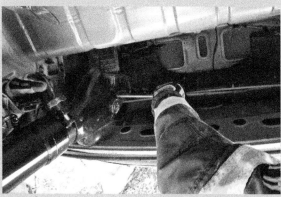

5 If the 12-volt direct current (DC) battery is located in the trunk area, disconnect the battery. If the trunk uses tension rods, maintain a safe position and cut and remove them using a hydraulic cutter. Carefully remove the rods by cutting them closest to the ends where they attach to the trunk hinge arms. The use of an air chisel or reciprocating saw will not work effectively in this situation because there is too much free movement of the rods for either tool to penetrate the metal.

(continues)

SKILL DRILL 10-1 Continued
Tunneling Through the Trunk NFPA 1006 8.2.4, 8.2.6, 8.2.7, and 8.3.9

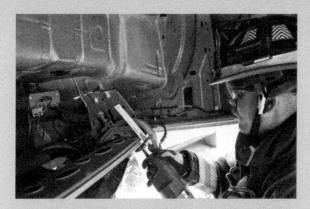

6 Remove the rear deck using a reciprocating saw, an air chisel, or a combination of both. In determining the best tool for this application, consider the amount of room or access that is presented to insert either tool.

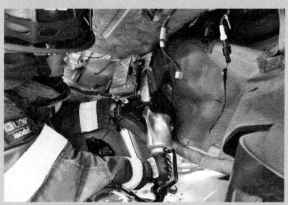

7 Remove the rear seats using the appropriate technique. Rear seats can be attached in multiple ways, so there is no single way to remove them that encompasses all techniques; it is best to access the attached areas and use the appropriate tool for removing the seats. Next, remove the front seat-backs if necessary. This is best accomplished by exposing the hinges on the seat-backs by cutting away the seat material with a knife or trauma shears.

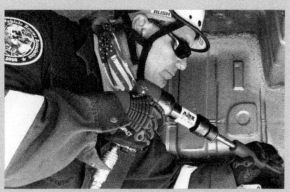

8 If the 12-volt DC battery has not been disconnected and/or cannot be accessed, scan the seats and roof structure for any indications of deployed supplemental restraint system (SRS) components (air bags) and/or seat belt pretensioning systems. Once the hinges on the seat-backs have been exposed, cut them using a pneumatic air chisel or hydraulic cutter.

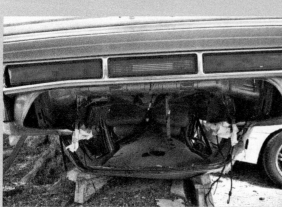

9 Once full access has been created to remove the victim, ensure that all jagged metal is covered with sharps wrap or blankets to prevent cut injuries when entering and exiting the vehicle.

Courtesy of Edward Monahan.

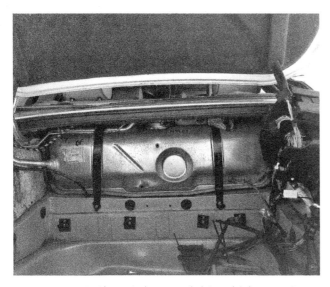

FIGURE 10-3 The trunk area of this vehicle contains a large fuel tank that will block any tunneling attempt at entry through this section.
Courtesy of David Sweet.

will block any attempt at entry through this section (**FIGURE 10-3**). Another incident may exist where the vehicle is a hybrid or electric system vehicle with the battery pack stored in the trunk, which creates too much of a hazard to attempt this approach. An alternative technique would be to crack the undercarriage and lift the rear end of the vehicle by following these steps. After stabilizing the vehicle using the procedures covered in Chapter 8, apply a powered tool, such as a hydraulic cutter or pneumatic air chisel, and make relief cuts at precise areas on opposite sides of the rocker panel/floorboard closet to the rear tires. The rear doors also must be released from the latch mechanisms to allow for the rear of the vehicle to separate and lift. Next, attach chains spanning from the front to rear of the vehicle, and position a First Responder Jack (FRJ) upright in the middle of the undercarriage. Next, lay the chain over the tongue of the FRJ, and engage the FRJ's lever until the chain is taut. As a safety measure, attach a come along to the front of the vehicle; extend the wire rope to the rear of the vehicle, and attach it to a secure area of the undercarriage. Engage the FRJ, which will tighten the chain and lift or jack up the rear of the vehicle, thus creating a large enough opening that will allow for access and removal of the victim while avoiding the fuel tank altogether.

A word of caution should be noted when considering this technique because the battery systems in some electric vehicles, such as the Tesla Model X, comprise the entire floor pan and thus negate the use of this technique. This technique again is considered extreme and very technical; every vehicle, regardless of the propulsion system, will have some differences in body structure, electrical components, and fuel system layout, so areas for relief cuts may vary. Follow **SKILL DRILL 10-2** to complete this task.

Seat Removal

Once a rescuer has tunneled inside the vehicle through the trunk, he or she may encounter a variety of victim-entrapment scenarios. If the opening is large enough, two rescuers should be positioned inside the passenger compartment. One rescuer will perform the victim disentanglement by gaining any additional access and removing sections of the vehicle that are entrapping the victim; the other rescuer will perform victim care as described in Chapter 9, *Victim Access and Management*. If the entrapment is heavy, evaluate what is impinging on the victim, and use the correct tool or tools to release the victim; it may take an air chisel or hydraulic cutter to remove the seats or a hydraulic ram to create more room.

Front Seat-Back Removal

Removal of a front seat can be difficult at times because of the various types of seat frames and advanced designs that may be encountered. Seats are attached to the floorboards of the vehicle in four or more places, with positional adjustments on slide tracks that are either fully automatic/motorized or manually operated. The floor attachments can be accessible in the simplest designs, or they may be fully enclosed and motorized with advanced designs. Seats will also contain hinges that allow the seat-backs to adjust forward or rearward either automatically/motorized or manually. The seat-back hinges are normally the best area of access for removing the seat-back from the seat frame. The material covering the seats may have to be removed using a knife or trauma shears to expose the area of attachment (hinges) where the seat-back is attached to the seat-bottom section. If removal is not an option, then consider (if access permits) making relief cuts on both sides of the lower seat-back. This will allow the seat-back to be folded down, which can provide access for a backboard to be placed behind the victim, keeping him or her in line for ease of removal.

To remove a front seat-back from a vehicle, follow the steps in **SKILL DRILL 10-3**.

SKILL DRILL 10-2
Jacking the Trunk NFPA 1006 8.2.6, 8.2.7, and 8.3.9

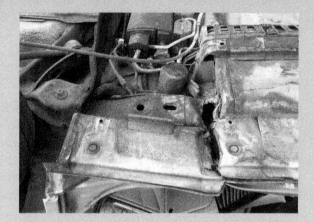

1 Don appropriate PPE, including mask and eye protection. Assess the scene for hazards, and complete the inner and outer surveys. Stabilize the vehicle. Ensure that the victim and the other rescuer inside the vehicle are properly protected. Secure all vehicle glass. Use a power tool, such as a hydraulic spreader, to release the rear doors from the latching mechanisms. This will allow for the rear of the vehicle to separate and lift. Use a power tool, such as a hydraulic cutter or pneumatic air chisel, and make a relief cut on opposite sides of the rocker panel/floorboard area just in front of the rear tires.

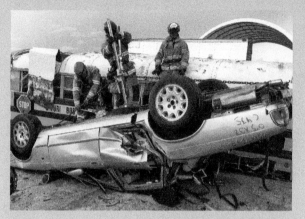

2 Attach chains spanning from the front to the rear of the vehicle, and position an FRJ upright in the middle of the undercarriage. Lay the chain over the tongue of the FRJ, and engage the FRJ's lever until the chain is taut. As a safety measure, attach a come along to the front of the vehicle; extend the wire rope to the rear of the vehicle, and attach it to a secure area of the undercarriage.

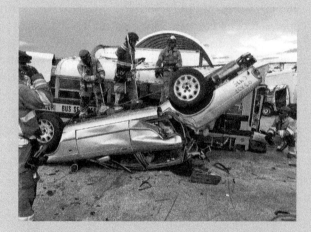

3 Engage the FRJ, and lift or jack up the rear of the vehicle, thus creating a large enough opening that will allow for access and removal of the victim.

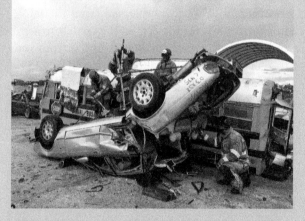

4 Once a large enough opening has been established to access the victim, evaluate the front and seat-backs to determine whether they require removal or they can be laid back. Ensure that all jagged metal is covered with sharps wrap or blankets to prevent cut injuries when entering and exiting the vehicle.

Courtesy of David Sweet.

SKILL DRILL 10-3
Front Seat-Back Removal NFPA 1006 8.2.4, 8.2.6, 8.2.7, and 8.3.9

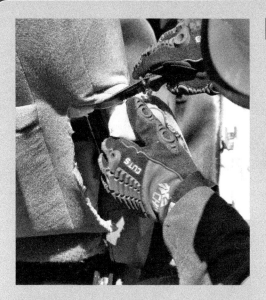

1 Don PPE. Assess the scene for hazards, and complete the inner and outer surveys. Stabilize the vehicle. Ensure that the victim is properly protected. Manage all vehicle glass using the appropriate technique. Check all seat-adjustment mechanisms if needed. Disconnect the 12-volt DC battery. Cut away the upholstery of the front seat to expose the metal frame of the seat.

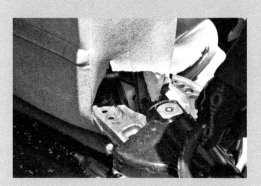

2 Assess the seat for any side air bag inflators that may be located in the seat-backs. Fully expose the inflator, and move any wires out of cutting areas. Remove the front seat by cutting the seat-back hinges, or make a relief cut on both sides of the lower seat-back. If accessible, the frame attachment of the seat at the floorboard can be cut using an air chisel or hydraulic cutter. This procedure may vary with each vehicle because of the differences in victim location, interior design, and frame structure of the seat. Ensure that the victim is fully supported before cutting the hinges or making a relief cut.

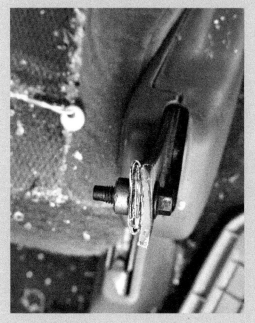

3 With the seat-back hinge cut on both sides, either remove this section or fold it down. Place a backboard behind the victim for removal.

Courtesy of Edward Monahan.

Front Seat-Back Relocation

Another option that can be used for managing seats to gain better access to the victim is to relocate the seat-back using an FRJ. This is a fast technique that can be applied to forcefully push the seat-back down, which allows a backboard to be placed behind the victim, keeping him or her in line for ease of removal.

To relocate a front seat-back in a vehicle, follow the steps in **SKILL DRILL 10-4**.

SKILL DRILL 10-4
Front Seat-Back Relocation NFPA 1006 8.2.6, 8.2.7, and 8.3.9

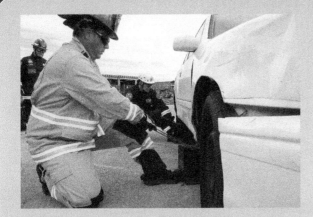

1 Don appropriate PPE, including mask and eye protection. Assess the scene for hazards, and complete the inner and outer surveys. Stabilize the vehicle. Ensure that the victim is covered with a blanket for protection from unsecured debris. Manage all vehicle glass using the appropriate technique. Manually check all seat-adjustment mechanisms for operability if needed. Disconnect the 12-volt DC battery.

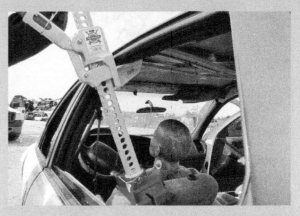

2 Place the FRJ with the base against the inside top of the seat-back. Adjust the tongue of the FRJ up against the inside of the roof rail and window frame. Ensure that the victim is properly supported at the head and body to prevent any shift from a sudden movement of the seat-back.

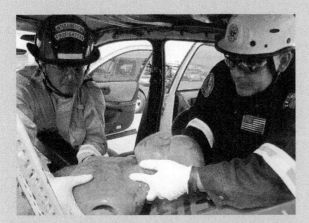

3 Engage the lever of the FRJ, which will forcefully collapse the seat-back downward. Once the seat-back has been relocated, place a backboard behind the victim.

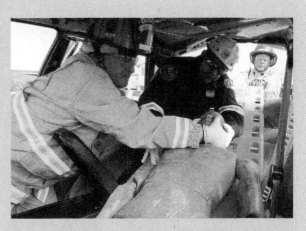

4 Package the victim appropriately for in-line removal.

Courtesy of Edward Monahan.

Impingement and Penetrating Objects

In a vehicle incident where the initial impact has caused the B-post to be pushed into the occupant compartment space and it is now impinging on and entrapping the victim, the B-post will have to be pushed back or relocated to its original position prior to attempting any other type of technique for victim access and removal. Just as discussed in Chapter 9 under the side-out technique, the force of the impact has now caused the metal to collapse or flow inward. Any force applied to remove the door will cause the B-post and surrounding structure to move further inward and crush down more on the victim (**FIGURE 10-4**). One possible solution to this situation is to push or relocate the B-post or door section off of the victim from the inside using a hydraulic ram, hydraulic spreader, or an FRJ. There are many factors that will influence the correct positioning and use for each tool; the main factor is accessibility, which again cannot be predicted. The key is to cut the top of the B-post completely away from the roof rail and then locate an effective base to push from inside the vehicle. The area inside the vehicle where the transmission hump is located is generally an effective base from which to work if it can be accessed.

Another area that can be used is the opposite-side B-post by applying a cross-ramming technique using a long, extending telescopic hydraulic ram, which is explained in the following paragraphs and in **SKILL DRILL 10-5**. If you have gained access to the

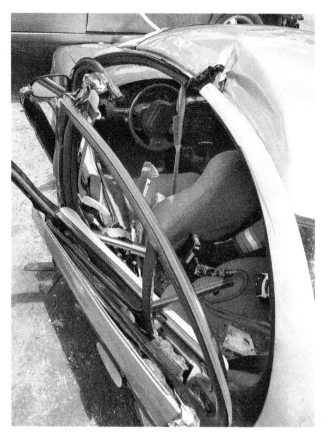

FIGURE 10-4 The initial impact on this vehicle has caused the B-post to be pushed into the occupant compartment space, and it is now impinging on and entrapping the victim. The B-post will have to be pushed back or relocated to its original position prior to attempting any other type of technique for victim access and removal.
Courtesy of David Sweet.

SKILL DRILL 10-5
Relocate the B-Post or Door Frame with a Hydraulic Ram NFPA 1006 8.2.6, 8.2.7, and 8.3.9

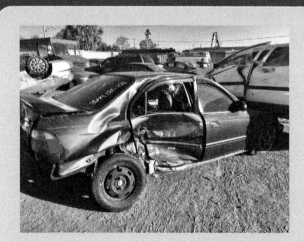

1. Don appropriate PPE. Assess the scene for hazards, and complete the inner and outer surveys. Stabilize the vehicle. Ensure that the victim is covered with a blanket for protection from unsecured debris. Manage all vehicle glass using the appropriate technique. If the 12-volt DC battery can be accessed, disconnect it. Scan the vehicle for all SRS components (air bags), including exposing all the roof posts and roof liner.

(continues)

SKILL DRILL 10-5 Continued
Relocate the B-Post or Door Frame with a Hydraulic Ram NFPA 1006 8.2.6, 8.2.7, and 8.3.9

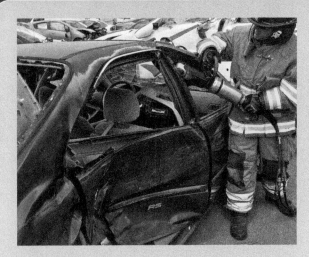

2 Make a cross cut on the top of the B-post.

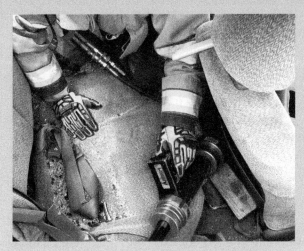

3 Place the hydraulic ram inside the vehicle. Place one or more 4-in. × 4-in. cribbing sections inside the vehicle against the transmission hump, and position the base of the ram against this cribbing and the tip angled upward against the inside of the B-post. The tip may have to be maneuvered in various positions or angles to accomplish this task.

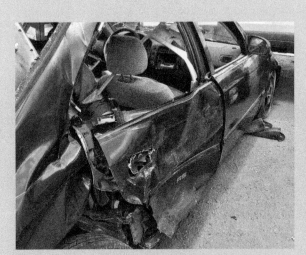

4 If an extremity is trapped between the seatback and B-post, incrementally insert cribbing sections above and below the crushed extremity as the B-post is pushed back into position. This will support the post from potentially collapsing back in if the hydraulic ram were to slip or be removed. Extend the ram just enough to release the impingement from the victim and to relocate the B-post back to its original plane prior to the impact.

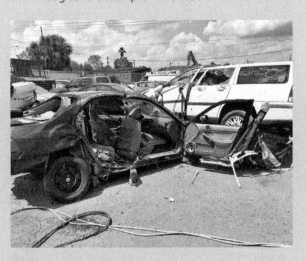

5 Once enough room has been established and the impingement is off the victim, the side-out or door-removal technique can be initiated.

Courtesy of David Sweet.

center transmission hump area, the next step will be to position the base of the ram or the arm of the spreader against the hump of the transmission to push from. When using the hydraulic ram, maneuver the tip of the tool to meet the area on the B-post that will best push the metal off of the victim; the tip may have to be maneuvered in various locations to accomplish this task. When using the hydraulic spreader, place one or more 4-in. × 4-in. (10-cm × 10-cm) cribbing sections inside the vehicle against the transmission hump, and position one arm of the spreader against this cribbing and the opposite arm angled upward against the inside of the B-post. The arms may have to be maneuvered in various positions or angles to accomplish this task. Once enough room has been established, the side-out or door-removal technique can be initiated. See Skill Drill 10-6 for further explanation of this technique. As an option, if hydraulic tools are not available or access or positioning inside the vehicle is not possible, then an FRJ and chain package can be applied, and the B-post can be pulled away from the victim to allow for another door-removal technique to be initiated.

To relocate the B-post or door frame using a hydraulic ram, follow the steps in Skill Drill 10-5.

To relocate the B-post or door frame using an FRJ, follow the steps in **SKILL DRILL 10-6**.

Impingement

The **cross-ramming technique** can be applied when limited access prevents positioning a hydraulic spreader or hydraulic ram against the rear floor panel

SKILL DRILL 10-6
Relocate the B-Post or Door Frame with a First Responder Jack
NFPA 1006 8.2.6, 8.2.7, and 8.3.9

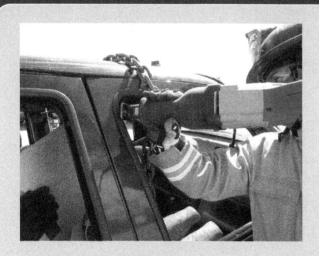

1 Don appropriate PPE. Assess the scene for hazards, and complete the inner and outer surveys. Stabilize the vehicle. Ensure that the victim is covered with a blanket for protection from unsecured debris. Manage all vehicle glass using the appropriate technique. If the 12-volt DC battery can be accessed, then disconnect it. Scan the vehicle for all SRS components (air bags), including exposing all the roof posts and roof liner. Use a power tool, such as a reciprocating saw or pneumatic air chisel, and cut completely through the top of the B-post.

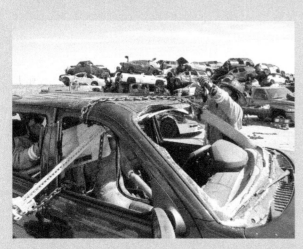

2 Take a long 15- to 20-ft (4.6- to 6-m) Grade 70 or higher rated chain, and wrap one end around the opposite-side A-post, locking it in with a chain-shortener hook. Place the running section of the chain over the top of the roof through the window opening where the victim is located. Wrap the remaining section of chain around the B-post, and leave a loop on the outside of the B-post.

(continues)

SKILL DRILL 10-6 Continued
Relocate the B-Post or Door Frame with a First Responder Jack
NFPA 1006 8.2.6, 8.2.7, and 8.3.9

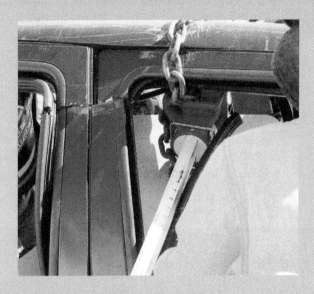

3 Place the base of the FRJ through the window and over the chain, inserting a chain link through the chain-lock device located at the base of the FRJ. Place the loop of the chain that is wrapped around the B-post over the tongue of the FRJ; engage the FRJ to tighten the entire chain section. Check all the chain connections and hooks to ensure that all sections are in the correct position and will not slip out when the jack is fully engaged.

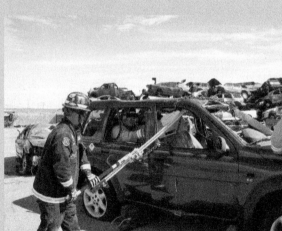

4 Engage the lever of the FRJ, and slowly pull the B-post off of the victim and back into its original position or plane.

Courtesy of Edward Monahan.

transmission hump. A large telescopic ram can be positioned to push off of the opposite side of the interior of the vehicle. A hydraulic telescoping ram provides the ability to maneuver the tool's arm to push out multiple areas, thus relieving the pressure of the impinging metal on the victim (**FIGURE 10-5**). The hydraulic ram can also be used to push up a crushed roof section, creating additional room and eliminating the potential for the roof to push down on the victim while it is being cut for removal. A crushed roof that is impinging on a victim needs to be raised off the victim prior to applying a cross-ramming technique. If the roof is not raised off of the victim prior to applying a technique, then the roof may be forced down onto the victim as that technique is applied. A hydraulic spreader, a hydraulic ram, or an FRJ can be used effectively to raise up the crushed roof section before any posts or sections are cut.

When performing a cross-ramming technique, have several 4-in. × 4-in. (102-mm × 102-mm) sections of cribbing (or "four-by-fours"), wedges, and shims to insert between the B-post and side of the seat-back once the impingement has been relieved by the hydraulic ram (**FIGURE 10-6**). The cribbing

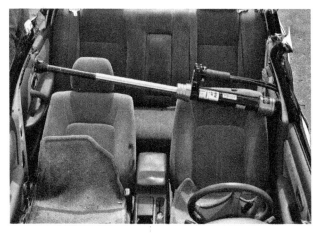

FIGURE 10-5 A hydraulic telescoping ram provides the ability to maneuver the tool's arm to push out multiple areas, thus relieving the pressure of the impinging metal on the victim.
Courtesy of Edward Monahan.

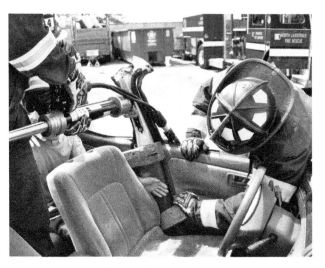

FIGURE 10-6 When performing a cross-ramming technique, have several four-by-four sections of cribbing, wedges, and shims to insert between the B-post and seat-back.
Courtesy of Edward Monahan.

sections will retain the space created by the ram, preventing any potential collapse of the metal back onto the victim if the ram is to be removed.

When applying a cross-ramming technique, be aware of the potential for tool slippage. This can occur when the hydraulic ram is extended under pressure and is forcing the B-post and door frame to spread beyond their vertical platform. The surface contact of the hydraulic ram tip is very small and can easily slip off, firing up or down under extreme force when a sloping angle is created by the B-post or door frame pushing outward. It is imperative that all personnel be made aware of this potential hazard. Slippage can be prevented by recognizing the signs and repositioning the tool. Adding a four-by-four between the B-post or door frame and the tip of the hydraulic ram may work in theory by increasing the footprint of the ram, but in reality, the four-by-four will normally roll, break, or kick out under extreme force; therefore, this is not a recommended practice. If the seat belt harness is positioned low enough on the B-post, then this would be a good place to position the tip of the hydraulic ram to push from. Remember from Chapter 5 that there is a steel reinforcement plate located inside the B-post directly behind the seat belt harness, giving this area added strength and support.

The following skill drill outlines a cross-ramming technique. In this scenario, an occupant traveling in the rear passenger area has an extremity trapped at the B-post area following a side-impact collision. Tools needed to perform a cross-ramming technique include a large hydraulic ram, preferably one that is telescopic and extends to 50 in. (1.3 m) or greater; assorted cribbing sections; and a backboard.

To perform a cross-ramming operation using a hydraulic telescoping ram, follow the steps in **SKILL DRILL 10-7**.

Roof Lift

At times, the roof may be crushed down to such a degree that it is now impinging on the victim. Before any technique or roof removal can be applied, the roof will need to be lifted off the victim. The forces that were applied during the crash caused a deflection of the roof into the passenger compartment. Any cutting action on any section of the roof can potentially continue that deflection, further crushing the victim. Lifting the roof up with a hydraulic spreader or ram or an FRJ changes the force direction of the metal to move upward away from the victim. Any technique or roof removal can now be applied without concern for the roof impinging back on the victim. To lift the roof using a hydraulic spreader, the placement of the tool will depend on the location of the victim, the area of the roof that requires lifting, and the amount of intrusion that is presenting. A simple lift would consist of placing the spreader in the rear window area using the rear deck as a base. This requires some four-by-fours to support the spreader from crushing down the rear deck when the force of the tool is applied. The bottom arm of the spreader would push off of the four-by-fours, and the top arm would aim for the roof line. Slowly work the tool upward until the top arm creates a tenting effect and the entire rear roof section lifts upward away from the victim.

If hydraulic tools are not available, then this same technique can be accomplished with an FRJ. Place two

Voice of Experience

The importance of being well versed in alternative extrication techniques is very important for everyday extrication incidents as well as having that backup plan in your toolbox should the need arise. Early in my career our station was dispatched for a car versus semi head-on, with entrapment of the driver of the car. Upon arrival, we found the driver of the semi walking around while the driver of the car was pinned with heavy front end and driver side impact damage.

I was assigned to the cutter by my officer with another person assigned to the spreader. While the rest of the crew made quick work on stablizing the vehicle, we readied our hydraulic tools. With stabilization complete, I started with the first operation which was cutting out the A-post of the vehicle due to its location in relation to the victim. As I started my first cut, the tool stopped mid-way through the cut. I tried to release the tool with no success. I called back to my crew to double check the connections, yet they found there to be no issues. My officer and my crew quickly realized we had equipment failure. My officer called to have another crew dispatched to bring hydraulic tools, while the rest of us went back to the apparatus to grab alternative tools. While not as originally planned, we were able to successfully extricate the victim using traditional tools: a reciprocating saw, a flat head axe, a halligan tool, an air chisel, high lift jacks, and a manual come along. By the time the mutual aid engine was on scene, the victim was free from the vehicle and on the way to the hospital.

This experience has forever changed my thoughts of how we mitigate vehicle entrapments. The problem ended up being a failure inside the hydraulic pump, causing no hydraulic flow. We now train as much on hydraulic tools as we do on alternative tools. Given this level of proficiency across all extrication techniques, we have found that nearly half of the extrication techniques used by our crews now are not utilizing hydraulic tools, but the traditional tools and techniques.

Brandon Sy
Valders Fire Department
Valders, Wisconsin

SKILL DRILL 10-7
Performing a Cross-Ramming Operation Using a Hydraulic Ram
NFPA 1006 8.2.4, 8.2.6, 8.2.7, and 8.3.9

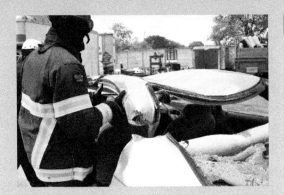

1 Don appropriate PPE. Assess the scene for hazards, and complete the inner and outer surveys. Stabilize the vehicle. Ensure that the victim is covered with a blanket for protection from unsecured debris. Manage all vehicle glass using the appropriate technique. If the 12-volt DC battery can be accessed, then disconnect it. Scan the vehicle for all SRS components (air bags), including exposing all the roof posts and roof liner. Remove the roof of the vehicle using the appropriate technique described in this chapter. The roof may need to be lifted first if it is impinging on the victim.

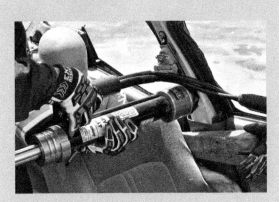

2 Position several rescuers inside and around the vehicle for support. The victim may require medical interventions depending on the injuries presented. Place the base of the hydraulic ram at the B-post. Extend the ram so the tip is aiming for the seat belt harness located on the opposite-side B-post. If an extremity is trapped between the seat-back and B-post, incrementally insert cribbing sections above and below the crushed extremity as the B-post is pushed back into position. This supports the post from potentially collapsing back in if the hydraulic ram under pressure were to slip or be removed.

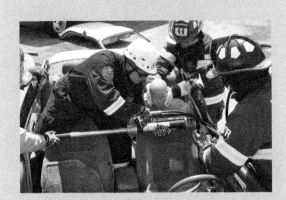

3 Extend the ram just enough to release the impingement off the victim and to relocate the B-post back to its original plane prior to the impact. Be careful not to overextend the post beyond the vertical position as this can cause the hydraulic ram to slip from its position.

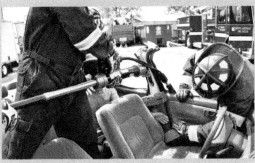

4 Once the victim has been released with sufficient access gained, then properly prepare the victim for removal using the techniques covered in this text.

Courtesy of Edward Monahan.

four-by-fours parallel on the rear deck of the vehicle. Place the base of the FRJ on the four-by-fours for support. Slide the tongue of the FRJ to sit just under the roof line, and engage the lever until a tenting effect occurs and the entire rear roof section lifts upward away from the victim. Lastly, a hydraulic ram can be inserted inside the vehicle and the roof systematically pushed upward away from the victim (**FIGURE 10-7**).

SAFETY TIP

A crushed roof with roof impingement on the victim needs to be raised off the victim prior to applying any access or cutting technique. If the roof is not raised off of the victim prior to applying a technique, then the potential for the metal to draw down on the victim as a technique is applied increases dramatically.

Penetrating Objects

Penetrating or impaled objects in victims can occur from sources outside the vehicle, such as road debris, vehicle components, or from vehicle cargo or objects inside the vehicle. When an object impales an occupant, the main objective is to stabilize the penetrating object at the entry and exit points if an exit point exists. Normally the penetrating object will need to be cut at the entry and exit areas so the victim can be properly extricated from the vehicle.

There are multiple impalement scenarios that can occur as well as multiple types of penetrating objects. This section will cover one such scenario involving cargo that came loose from a truck traveling at approximately 50 mi/h (80.5 km/h) and entered the vehicle traveling behind it. The cargo consisted of sections of 0.5-in. (13-mm) steel rebar and steel galvanized fencing post. One of these objects penetrated the vehicle from the front windshield and impaled the occupant in the front passenger seat at the area of the left shoulder, passing approximately 2 ft (61 cm) through the seat-back. Upon your arrival, the victim is in stable condition. The vehicle has not sustained any major damage, and no air bags have been deployed.

This is a very specific type of scenario that will encompass a majority of essential steps required for similar types of incidents that you may encounter. Obviously, some incidents will require additional steps or other interventions, but they are situational and can be determined only at the time the incident occurs. The cutting tools required for this scenario will be a metal-cutting circular saw with a carbide-tip blade or a pneumatic cut-off tool (whizzer tool) with a metal-cutting carbide blade and several spare air cylinders. A portable bandsaw is also very effective in these

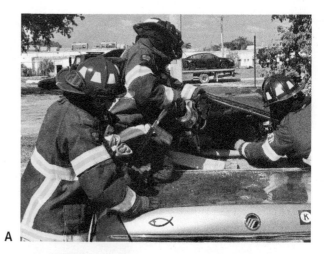
A

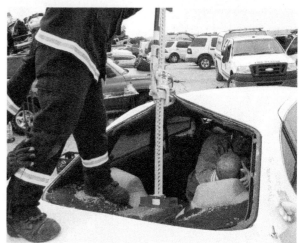
B

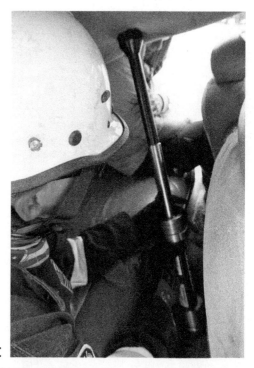
C

FIGURE 10-7 The three pictures shown here demonstrate raising a roof using three different tools. **A.** Hydraulic spreader. **B.** First Responder Jack (FRJ). **C.** Hydraulic ram.
Courtesy of Edward Monahan.

incidents. In addition, there should be a basic apparatus toolbox containing several types of hand tools, various cribbing sections, a water extinguisher, webbing material, towels, blankets, and pillows from a transport rescue. Using a hydraulic cutter, a reciprocating saw, or a handsaw for this scenario will cause too much movement or torqueing of the impaled object, possibly causing further injury and pain to the victim.

To stabilize an impaled object, follow the steps in **SKILL DRILL 10-8**.

SKILL DRILL 10-8
Stabilizing an Impaled Object NFPA 1006 8.2.4, 8.2.6, 8.2.7, and 8.3.9

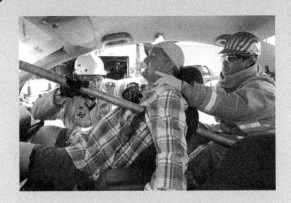

1 Don appropriate PPE. Assess the scene for hazards, and complete the inner and outer surveys. Stabilize the vehicle. Ensure that the victim is covered with a blanket for protection from unsecured debris. Manage all vehicle glass using the appropriate technique. If the 12-volt DC battery can be accessed, disconnect it. Scan the vehicle for all SRS components (air bags), including exposing all the roof posts and roof liner. Consider removal of the passenger-side door that provides direct access to the victim as well as the roof. Manually immobilize the victim and stabilize the impaled object. Determine necessary medical interventions.

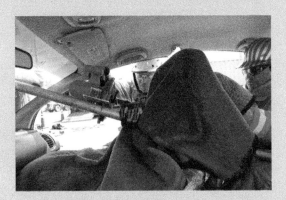

2 Ensure that the victim is still covered with a blanket for protection. Position a rescuer inside the vehicle with a water extinguisher to be applied if needed. The impaled metal object may need to be cooled as it is cut, depending on the tool used, or the rescuer may need to suppress any sparks that may occur. To suppress sparks, fan the tip of the water extinguisher with a gloved finger to mist the blade. Safely position the metal-cutting circular saw over the metal impaled object, pulling back the safety arm to release the blade. With two hands, cut off a section of the impaled object as close to the victim as possible.

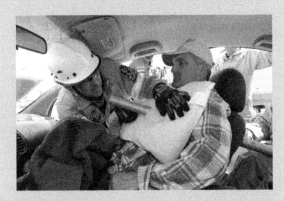

3 Place the impaled object in a debris pile. Cut the centers out of two or more pillows, and slip both pillows over the front end of the impaled object, and secure with tape. Cut the seat-back hinges using the steps outlined in this chapter. If the seat-back is light enough, it can be used as support for the object and held in place with tape.

(continues)

SKILL DRILL 10-8 Continued
Stabilizing an Impaled Object NFPA 1006 8.2.4, 8.2.6, 8.2.7, and 8.3.9

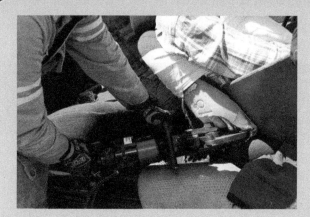

4 If the seat-back can be removed with minimal manipulation, then do so (this is a situational procedure that can be determined only at the time of the incident). If the seat-back is removed, the impaled object may require support from pillows.

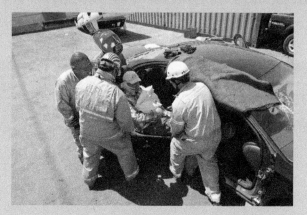

5 Remove the victim in a seated position and transfer to a stretcher.

© Jones & Bartlett Learning. Photographed by Glen E. Ellman.

Roof Removal

When cutting a roof with an air chisel or reciprocating saw, examine the roof damage for any tensioning or torsion deformities caused by the impact of the crash. Understanding this is very important because it will determine the proper angle to start the cut. Remember to remove all of the plastic molding on the posts and roof rail, and always keep half of the tip of the chisel blade showing through the entire cut, which will prevent the blade from getting stuck.

When a post is under tension or has a torsional bend to it, it is under a lot of pressure. Cutting such a post in the wrong location can cause the chisel blade or the blade of a reciprocating saw to pinch off and become stuck between the metal, stopping or jamming the tool. Always cut in an area away from the bend or torsion to minimize the chance of the chisel blade or reciprocating saw blade getting trapped by the metal collapsing around it from the pressure release. Take a moment and visualize how the post will react and where the metal will move when it is cut.

It is important to watch the reaction of the post throughout the entire cut; there may be a time when only half of the post can be cut at one angle and then another angle may be needed to complete the cut to avoid the tension releasing and trapping the chisel or reciprocating saw blade. An option that can assist the cutting action for either tool is using a steel wedging tool such as a large flat-head screwdriver or another flat-chisel blade, which can be inserted in the cut behind the tool and used as a block to prevent the tension of the cut roof metal from collapsing on the blade as it cuts through the rest of the roof area.

Some additional tips to remember when using an air chisel or reciprocating saw include the following:

- When cutting through a large or wide post, an inspection cut will have to be made to peel back the outer metal panel to reveal the inside panel so the cut can be completed. An air-chisel blade cannot cut through a wide two-piece roof post without completing this step first.

- When using a reciprocating saw, try to cut at a semi-downward angle to take advantage of the vehicle's center of mass and thereby limit tool vibration; to further limit vibrations, remember to keep the shoe of the tool firmly against the object being cut.

- As a post is being cut, if there seems to be an area that is very difficult to cut through where the penetration seems to halt, the probability of an impact or reinforcement bar located in the post is very high. Attempt the cut at a lower section of the post, preferably at the base.
- Remember that regardless of the tool used, hard protection should always be used to protect the victim and the rescuer inside the vehicle; if it is possible, try to angle or position all cuts away from the victim to eliminate any potential accidents.

Roof Removal Using the Air Chisel

As discussed in Chapter 3, *Tools and Equipment*, a high-pressure air chisel is a tool used for specific techniques requiring a well-trained technical rescuer to properly operate it. An air chisel requires continual repetitious training to keep skills at the optimum level needed to be effective on vehicle rescue and extrication incidents. When removing a roof for speed and efficiency, consider using a tool that provides a complete and thorough cutting action, such as a hydraulic cutter or reciprocating saw, prior to the use of an air chisel. Remember that a roof structure can have multiple layers of metal, support ribs, and hollow sections. An air chisel can go through only one section or layer of metal at a time, whereas a hydraulic cutter or reciprocating saw would require one cutting action to sever a post or roof section.

Multiple blades come with most air-chisel kits; the two most widely used blades are the panel-cutting blade, or T-blade, and the flat/curved blade (**FIGURE 10-8**). The two blades are different in use and appearance. The panel-cutting blade is used for cutting shallow, straighter cuts on small-gauge sheet metal, and the flat/curved blade is used for cutting through medium- to heavy-gauge steel.

Success with an air chisel is based on maintaining control throughout the entire operation. With this high-powered pneumatic system, it is very easy for an inexperienced operator to lose control of the blade while expending a bottle of compressed air within minutes and having very little progress to show from it.

To remove a roof using an air chisel, follow the steps in **SKILL DRILL 10-9**.

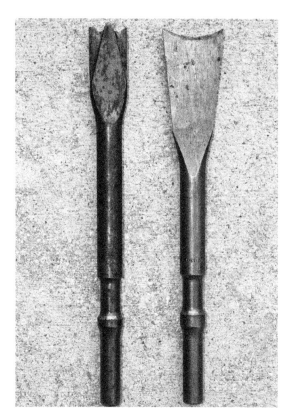

FIGURE 10-8 The two most widely used air-chisel blades. **A.** The standard/flat curved blade (right). **B.** The panel-cutter blade (left).
Courtesy of David Sweet.

Roof Removal Using the Reciprocating Saw

A reciprocating saw is an excellent tool for removing a vehicle's roof. It is fast and efficient, especially on vehicles with large C-posts. An electric reciprocating saw with a power output of around 11 to 15 amps will enable the operator to effectively cut through a wide range of grades and types of steel. Use a 9-in. (23-cm) bi-metal cutting blade with a teeth-per-inch (TPI) rating between 9 and 14. A lower rating, such as 5 TPI, will cause the tool to vibrate heavily, and the teeth will break off because of the inability of the blade to penetrate the metal effectively. A blade with a higher TPI rating, such as 18, is not aggressive enough and will dull quickly. Some reciprocating saws come equipped with a speed-setting dial or switch; this should be set at a moderate setting. To minimize blade overheating and warping, some manufacturers recommend starting the cut at a lower speed setting to establish the cut and then gradually building up to a higher setting as the cut progresses. It is also recommended to use a spray bottle with a soap-and-water mixture to reduce the high temperature of the blade, which

SKILL DRILL 10-9
Removing a Roof Using an Air Chisel NFPA 1006 8.2.4, 8.2.6, 8.2.7, and 8.3.9

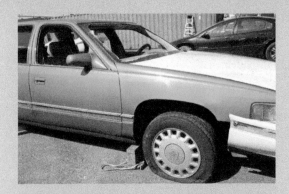

1 Don appropriate PPE. Assess the scene for hazards, and complete the inner and outer surveys. Stabilize the vehicle. Ensure that the victim is covered with a blanket for protection from unsecured debris. Manage all vehicle glass using the appropriate technique. Scan the vehicle for all/any SRS components (air bags), including exposing all the roof posts and roof liner.

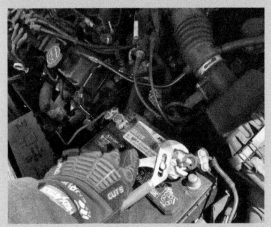

2 If the 12-volt DC battery can be accessed, disconnect it.

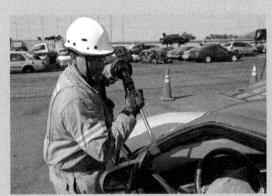

3 If possible, position a rescuer inside the vehicle to provide medical support and immobilization. Insert the long flat/curved blade into the air chisel. Hook up the regulator to the air cylinder; attach the hose to the regulator and the air chisel. Turn the air cylinder valve on with the blade and air chisel facing the ground to avoid an accidental discharge of the blade. Remove all plastic and molding around the posts and roof rail to identify any potential air bag cylinders. Avoid cutting into any plastic or rubber material as the air-chisel blade will bounce off rather than cut through it. Ensure that all seat belts have been cut. Check the roof for areas of damage causing metal tension and torsion. Cut around this area to avoid getting a blade pinched off by the metal under pressure when the pressure is suddenly relieved by the cut. Starting at the A-post, create a purchase point with the air chisel. Grip the blade in one hand, midshaft between the tip and collar to provide better control to maneuver the blade. Place one edge of the blade on the metal, and depress the trigger of the tool to make a purchase point. Once the blade has penetrated the metal, position the tip so at least half of the blade is always showing. It is extremely important to remember to keep half of the blade showing throughout the entire movement to avoid burying/trapping the blade. This is a common critical error made by inexperienced operators.

SKILL DRILL 10-9 Continued
Removing a Roof Using an Air Chisel NFPA 1006 8.2.4, 8.2.6, 8.2.7, and 8.3.9

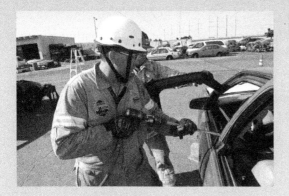

4 If there is a cut strip of glass attached to the A-post that was left from cutting out the windshield, ensure that most of the glass is removed prior to cutting the post. Apply sharps wrap around the post in the area to be cut to minimize glass fragmentation. If a boron rod or other advanced-strength steel-reinforced section is encountered, then reposition the cut higher or lower on the post to avoid the material. Work the tool around the A-post, mimicking the curvature of the post. Once a section of metal is loosened, pull or bend it out of the way to get to the inside of the post. A-posts are generally composed of rolled sheets of metal for reinforcement purposes; another layer may be revealed underneath the removal of the first layer. All layers must be removed as the rescuer works to avoid burying the blade. A hand light can be shone through the back side of the cut to verify if the post has been cut all the way through. Once the A-post is cut, move to the B-post. Avoid cutting into the seat belt bracket, which has a reinforced steel-backing plate. Choose an area at least 2 inches (51 mm) above or below the seat belt bracket. Another rescuer should be assigned to support the roof.

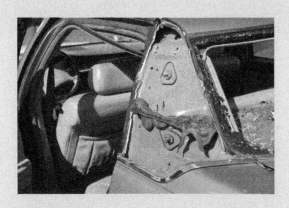

5 The technique used to cut the C-post will depend on the width of the post. A wide C-post is composed of two pieces of steel with a hollow center. It will require a sectional cut on the outside panel, exposing the inside panel so the cut can be completed through both sections. Once the cut has been made, the blade of the tool can be inserted to assist in peeling back the section cut. The inside panel may have holes that are used to pass wires or other materials through. These holes are beneficial because they mean less metal for the operator to cut.

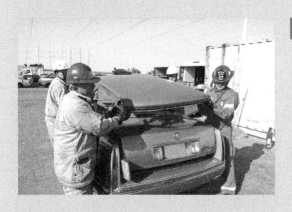

6 Move to the posts on the other side of the vehicle, and repeat the steps performed on the first side. Two rescuers must be assigned to support both sides of the roof as it is cut. Before the roof is removed, ensure that all attachments, such as plastic interior liners or wires, have been cut. Removal of the severed roof must be a coordinated and controlled movement, with one technical rescuer giving the order and direction of travel. Place the roof in a designated debris pile outside of the hot zone.

© Jones & Bartlett Learning. Photographed by Glen E. Ellman.

minimizes blade and teeth degradation and warping (**FIGURE 10-9**). To limit the possibility of tool failure or voiding the manufacturer's warranty, always check with the tool manufacturer for the proper tool operation and safety specifications.

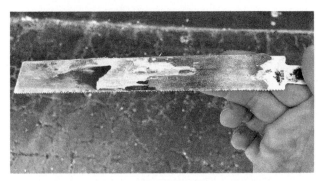

FIGURE 10-9 A reciprocating blade will degrade and warp from the high heat produced from the friction of a reciprocating saw operated consistently at a high speed.
Courtesy of David Sweet.

SAFETY TIP

Before the roof is removed, ensure that all the seat belts, wires, and cables have been cut.

To remove a roof using a reciprocating saw, follow the steps in **SKILL DRILL 10-10**.

Rapid Roof Removal: Vehicle on Its Side

There are multiple techniques to remove the roof of a vehicle that is resting on its side. One technique, designed for rapid entry, involves the use of a reciprocating saw and can be accomplished within minutes. Apply the methods described in Chapter 8 regarding stabilizing a vehicle on its side before initiating this process. To remove the roof of a vehicle on its side, follow the steps in **SKILL DRILL 10-11**.

SKILL DRILL 10-10
Removing a Roof Using a Reciprocating Saw NFPA 1006 8.2.4, 8.2.6, 8.2.7, and 8.3.9

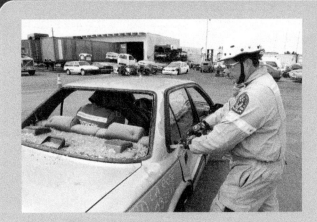

1 Don appropriate PPE, including mask and eye protection. Assess the scene for hazards, and complete the inner and outer surveys. Stabilize the vehicle. Ensure that the victim is covered with a blanket for protection from unsecured debris. Manage all vehicle glass using the appropriate technique. If the 12-volt DC battery can be accessed, disconnect it.

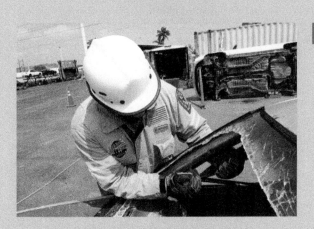

2 Remove all plastic and molding around the posts and roof rail to identify any potential air bag components. Ensure that all seat belts have been cut. Check the roof for areas of damage causing metal tension and torsion. Cut around this area.

SKILL DRILL 10-10 Continued
Removing a Roof Using a Reciprocating Saw NFPA 1006 8.2.4, 8.2.6, 8.2.7, and 8.3.9

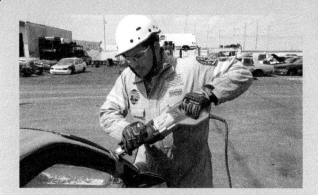

3 Begin at the A-post. Ensure that most of the glass near the area to be cut is removed prior to cutting the post. To minimize glass fragmentation, apply sharps wrap around the post in the area to be cut. If a boron rod or other advanced-strength steel-reinforced section is encountered, then reposition the cut higher or lower on the post to avoid the material.

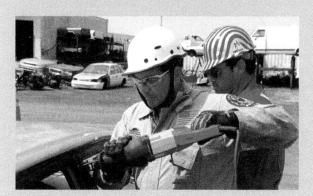

4 Once the A-post has been cut, move to the B-post. The technique for cutting the B-post will be the same as that used for cutting the A-post, but avoid cutting into the seat belt bracket, which has a reinforced steel-backing plate or adjustment bar. This area is heavy-gauge steel and will require time to cut through. Choose an area at least 2 in. (5 cm) above or below the seat belt bracket, or cut at the base of the post or roof line to avoid cutting through these stronger metals. Another rescuer should be assigned to support the roof.

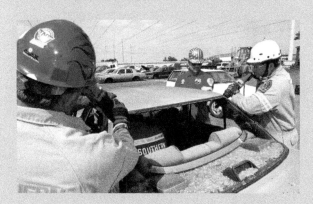

5 Once the B-post has been cut, move to the rear C-post. The reciprocating saw should rip through the metal C-post with ease, working best on a wider post. Keep the shoe of the reciprocating saw firmly against the metal, and cut on a semi-downward angle to take advantage of the vehicle's center of mass; this approach will minimize vibration and the potential for pinching off the blade.

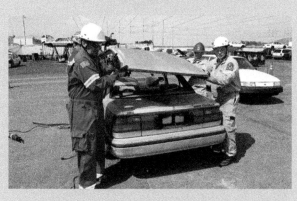

6 Move to the posts on the other side of the vehicle, and repeat the steps performed on the first side. Two or more rescuers must be assigned to support both sides of the roof as it is cut. Before the roof is removed, ensure that all attachments, such as plastic interior liners or wires, have been cut. Removal of the severed roof must be a coordinated and controlled movement, with one technical rescuer giving the order and direction of travel. Place the roof in a designated debris pile outside of the hot zone.

© Jones & Bartlett Learning. Photographed by Glen E. Ellman.

SKILL DRILL 10-11
Removing a Roof from a Vehicle Resting on Its Side NFPA 1006 8.2.4, 8.2.6, 8.2.7, and 8.3.9

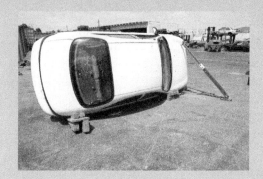

1 Don PPE. Assess the scene for hazards, and complete the inner and outer surveys. If the battery can be accessed, disconnect it. Stabilize the vehicle using the buttress-stabilization strut technique.

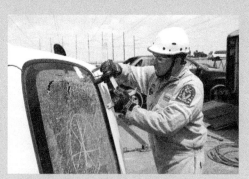

2 If possible, position a rescuer inside the vehicle to provide medical support and immobilization. Ensure that the victim inside the vehicle is covered with a blanket for protection from flying debris. Manage all vehicle glass using the appropriate technique.

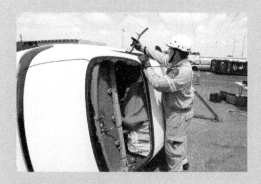

3 Remove all plastic and molding around the posts and roof rail to identify any potential air bag cylinders. This can be completed quickly with a large flat-head screwdriver or other small hand tool.

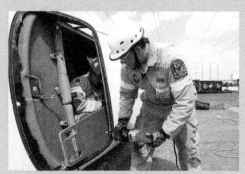

4 Ensure that all seat belts have been cut. Check the roof for areas of damage causing metal tension and torsion. Cut around these areas to avoid pinching off a blade from the metal when the pressure is suddenly relieved by the cut. Insert a long backboard lengthwise from the front or rear window of the vehicle; the rescuer inside the vehicle will use this as hard protection as the reciprocating saw blade passes through the roof. Insert a 6-in. (15-cm) bi-metal cutting blade with a TPI rating of 9 to 14 into a high-powered electric reciprocating saw. Rooftops are normally 2 to 3 in. (5 to 8 cm) thick, so a shorter blade is recommended to minimize the potential for hitting the victim or rescuer.

SKILL DRILL 10-11 Continued
Removing a Roof from a Vehicle Resting on Its Side NFPA 1006 8.2.4, 8.2.6, 8.2.7, and 8.3.9

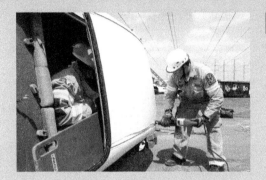

5 Make two lengthwise cuts to remove the inside section of the roof. Start at the lower section of the roof (closest to the ground). Make the initial cut just above the roof rail on the inside corner of the front A-post or at the rear post of the vehicle, which may be a C-post, D-post, or higher post depending on the type of vehicle. It is important to make the cut at the low end of the roof first; if the higher section were to be cut first, the bottom cut would be impossible to make because the roof would collapse onto itself, pinching off the blade of the saw. Follow a straight horizontal line, completing the cut through the roof to the opposite side. As the technical rescuer outside the vehicle makes the cut, the rescuer inside the vehicle will position the backboard to provide hard protection from the blade.

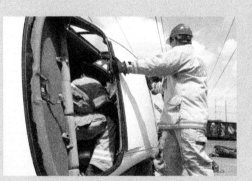

6 After the bottom cut has been made, cut the top section. Follow the same cutting pattern used on the bottom section. Position two personnel on either side of the roof to support it and prevent it from falling in on the victim and rescuer as the cut is completed. In a coordinated effort, place the roof section in a designated debris pile outside of the hot zone.

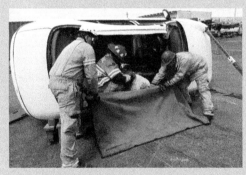

7 For added protection, place a tarp or large blanket over the bottom cut section of the roof to prevent any potential cut injuries.

© Jones & Bartlett Learning. Photographed by Glen E. Ellman.

To increase the speed of this technique, two reciprocating saws can be used. As the bottom line is cut midway through the roof, another technical rescuer can start cutting the top line with another reciprocating saw. This is a very aggressive technique that should be performed only by skilled technicians who have trained extensively on this type of procedure. Performing the technique in this fashion, through a coordinated and controlled effort, can lead to roof removal within 2 to 3 minutes. Because two operations are being conducted simultaneously, everyone involved in this technique has to be on the same page. The advantage of this technique, aside from the faster results, is that a section of the roof is actually removed; if the roof-flap technique is used, large sections of the roof with cut posts remain and may impede rescue efforts.

Door Removal on the Hinge Side

In Chapter 9, the technique of removing a door on the hinge side is described using a combination of a hydraulic spreader and hydraulic cutter; in this section, the same technique will be accomplished using an air chisel. Using an air chisel to cut through door hinges can be a challenging task, but with training, this is a very effective technique that can be quickly mastered.

To remove a door on the hinge side using an air chisel, follow the steps in **SKILL DRILL 10-12**.

SAFETY TIP

A technique that is commonly taught but that is not recommended here is dropping the floor pan just below the victim's feet where the brake and accelerator pedals are located. The reason this technique is not recommended is because of major safety concerns; fuel lines and high-powered electrical lines generally run in the area of the rocker panel/channel, and cutting into this area or tearing into this section can potentially rupture and/or sever one of these lines, causing additional problems or severe injury to the victim and crew.

SKILL DRILL 10-12
Removing a Door on the Hinge Side Using an Air Chisel NFPA 1006 8.2.4, 8.2.6, 8.2.7, and 8.3.9

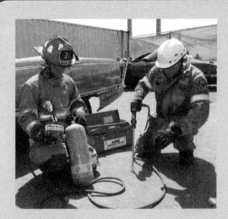

1. Don PPE. Assess the scene for hazards, and complete the inner and outer surveys. Stabilize the vehicle. If the 12-volt DC battery can be accessed, disconnect it. If possible, position a rescuer inside the vehicle to provide medical support and immobilization. Ensure that the victim inside the vehicle is covered with a blanket for protection from flying debris. Manage all vehicle glass using the appropriate technique. Ensure that all the seat belts have been cut. Examine the interior of the vehicle for air bags, including side-door air bags. Insert the long flat/curved blade into the air chisel. If a roof-removal technique will be performed, expose all of the posts and interior roof rail liners. Turn the air cylinder valve on with the blade and tool facing the ground to avoid an accidental discharge of the blade. Never fire the air chisel into the air to check the pressure; doing so can damage the tool. Check the pressure gauge by placing the blade against a solid surface and dialing up to the appropriate pressure in the general range of 200 psi (1379 kPa).

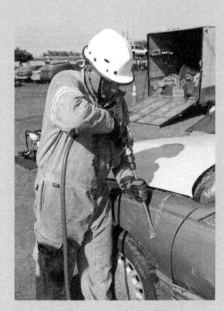

2. Cut away an opening in the top section of the quarter panel where the hood and quarter panel meet. The opening should be large enough to expose both hinges. Angle the blade downward, cutting toward the bottom of the panel around the wheel well.

SKILL DRILL 10-12 Continued
Removing a Door on the Hinge Side Using an Air Chisel NFPA 1006 8.2.4, 8.2.6, 8.2.7, and 8.3.9

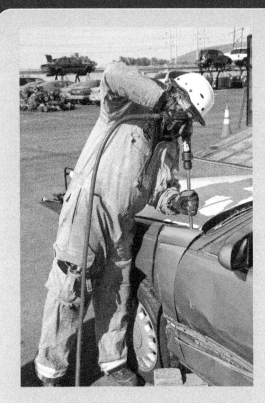

3 Bring the tool back to the top of the quarter panel, and prepare to make another vertical downward cut to the bottom end of the panel. The panel at that area bends at a 90-degree angle and attaches perpendicularly to the outside panel. Position the blade downward to cut on the inside of the panel directly on the angled 90-degree bend. As the blade moves down, bend the blade outward, manipulating the cut strip of metal away to maintain visibility of the cut.

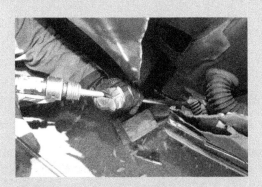

4 When the bottom is reached, cut the bottom section horizontally, and remove the entire section of the panel; the door hinges will now be exposed. Examine the door hinges to determine the design type and the approach that will need to be taken. Cut the bottom hinge first. Two types of hinges are commonly found: heavy-gauge, two-leaf overlay-type hinges with a center pin and spring (fairly common on larger vehicles) and lighter-gauge standard hinges (used on smaller compact vehicles). To cut through a heavy-gauge two-leaf overlay-type hinge with a center pin and spring, cut only one hinge leaf at a time. The hinge overlaps itself, and you will want to avoid cutting two sections of the hinge at the same time. Kneel on one knee, positioning the tip of the chisel on the area to be cut and bracing the back section of the air chisel against your chest. With one hand on the trigger and one hand on the shaft of the blade, lean into the gun; while depressing the trigger, apply a slight up-and-down rocking motion while pushing into the gun with the chest and shoulder. Maintain complete balance while applying pressure with the rocking motion. If there is a spring attachment on the hinge, beware of it flying off once the hinge is released.

(continues)

SKILL DRILL 10-12 Continued
Removing a Door on the Hinge Side Using an Air Chisel NFPA 1006 8.2.4, 8.2.6, 8.2.7, and 8.3.9

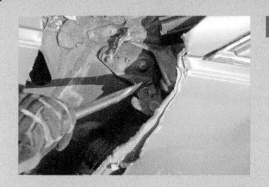

5. Once the bottom hinge is cut, move up to the top hinge, and follow the same technique. If the door comes equipped with a door-limiting device, the cut should be made with the blade angled on the bar section, closest to the door or firewall, not at the center. Attempting to cut through the center will cause the door-limiting device to bend from the pounding of the chisel. Remember that the air chisel works best by cutting through solid sections of metal with some type of backing.

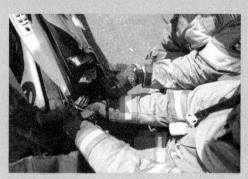

6. With the door hinges severed, pull back the door, and cut the wires that pass through the center to disconnect any air bags that may be present.

© Jones & Bartlett Learning. Photographed by Glen E. Ellman.

Side Removal: Vehicle Upside Down or Resting on Its Roof

Gaining entry through the side of a vehicle that has rolled over and is resting on its roof can require either a very basic procedure, such as forcing a door open, or a very involved process with multiple steps. The following skill drill will take you through the necessary procedures, starting with the basic steps and evolving to more advanced procedures. The scenario that will be used to explain the skill drill involves a four-door common passenger vehicle that has rolled over several times and come to rest on its crushed roof, trapping one victim upside down in the front-passenger compartment.

To perform side removal on a vehicle upside down or resting on its roof, follow the steps in **SKILL DRILL 10-13**.

Pedal Displacement and Removal

Acceleration and brake pedals are notorious for trapping or entangling occupants' foot extremities. Some instances occur where there is minor damage to the vehicle and the occupant happens to get a foot stuck under the brake pedal. Brake pedals can be designed with the standard hydraulic assistance and position, or they can be automatically height adjusted to a predetermined position that is programmed by the on-board computer system. Some manufacturers have designed a special air bag component that uses a piston rod and/or pillow-type bag that pushes the foot out of the way using the piston rod in conjunction with a rapidly inflating small air bag. This prevents the foot from getting trapped or injured from the impact.

Properly supporting a foot that is trapped under a pedal must be accomplished prior to any attempt

SKILL DRILL 10-13
Performing a Side Removal on a Vehicle Upside Down or Resting on Its Roof NFPA 1006 8.2.6, 8.2.7, and 8.3.9

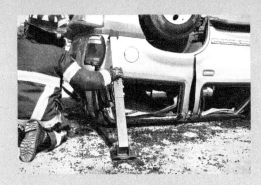

1 Don PPE. Assess the scene for hazards, and complete the inner and outer surveys. Stabilize the vehicle. Ensure that the victim inside the vehicle is covered with a blanket for protection from unsecured debris.

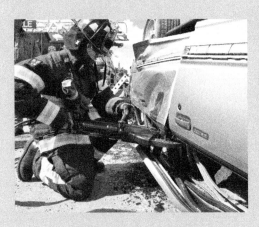

2 If accessible, use the hydraulic cutter to cut through the A-post and B-post at the bottom of the window frame. Remove the section of the window frame, and place it in the designated debris pile. This step releases the door from the ground. Using the hydraulic spreader, create a purchase point on the rear door to gain access to the latching mechanism. Pinch and partially collapse the area around the door seam and rocker panel. Be careful not to tear the metal and lose the integrity of the area to spread from. Work the door down and outward, exposing the latching mechanism. Cut the latching mechanism with a hydraulic cutter.

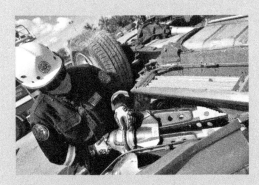

3 Once the rear door has been opened, perform a side-out technique by making a relief cut at the base of the B-post just above the rocker panel. Now, position the hydraulic spreader to separate the B-post from the rocker panel. The two doors attached together by the B-post should now be able to swing open using the natural movement of the front-door hinges. Remove the doors by cutting the hinges on the front door, and place them in the designated debris pile.

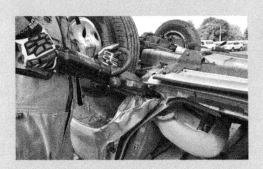

4 Using the hydraulic cutter, make a complete cut all the way through the firewall between the bottom and top hinges. Make an additional relief cut through the rear-wheel well/lower C-post just above the rocker panel. With the application of a hydraulic spreader and ram, these relief cuts will enlarge the side opening to provide greater access to the victim.

(continues)

SKILL DRILL 10-13 Continued
Performing a Side Removal on a Vehicle Upside Down or Resting on Its Roof NFPA 1006 8.2.6, 8.2.7, and 8.3.9

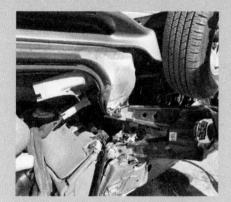

5 Secure cribbing under the dash area beneath the firewall section. Insert the tips of the hydraulic spreader into the opening in the firewall in a vertical position. This action will be the same as a dash-lift technique performed upside down.

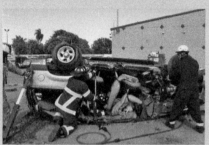

6 Simultaneously, with the hydraulic spreader in place, position a hydraulic ram with the base of the tool on the roof rail and the tip on the rocker panel closest to the C-post. The base of the ram must be positioned on the roof rail, not on the floor, or the vehicle will be lifted off the ground. Open both tools simultaneously, causing the floor of the vehicle to lift and separate at the relief cuts made in the B-post and firewall. The distance (lift) needed will be determined by the officer in charge of the operation. Both hydraulic tools must be maintained and controlled continuously throughout the entire operation to avoid any potential slippage of the two tools, and the stabilization struts will have to be adjusted to accommodate for the change in height. Immobilize and package the victim according to standard operating procedures.

Courtesy of Edward Monahan.

---

to move the pedal. Normally, the rescuer will find that the foot has been fractured or dislocated by the impact of the foot striking the floor panel and the repositioning of the pedal around the foot. The pedal arm can be cut and/or relocated using mechanical tools, such as a hydraulic cutter, reciprocating saw, air chisel, or pneumatic cut-off tool (whizzer saw); a come along and chain set; or a very simple tool such as a section of webbing or rope (**FIGURE 10-10**). What tool or combination of tools used will be determined at the time of the incident; there are many possible variables and presentations that will dictate which option is best. Some of the variables that may occur include the type of entrapment, the position of the foot, and the type of injury that was sustained to the foot as well as the overall condition of the victim, the involvement of air bags or other SRS components

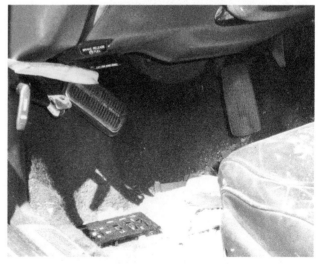

FIGURE 10-10 A pedal can be relocated using a section of webbing or rope.

in direct proximity to the pedal, other interventions or extrication procedures that have to be performed on the vehicle to release the occupant, and whether the pedals are standard-model or automatic height-adjustment pedals, which can be used prior to disabling the vehicle's 12-volt DC battery. These are only some of the variables that may occur that must be considered and planned for. As discussed, the process may require only a simple relocation of the pedal to free the foot.

The following skill drill describes relocating a standard pedal and does not involve any air bag or automatic height-adjustment components. The technique requires the swing of the driver's-side door to be operational. This technique can be applied to a door that has to be forced open; the only requirement is that the swing action using the hinges must remain operational.

To relocate a standard pedal void of any air bag or automatic height-adjustment components, follow the steps in **SKILL DRILL 10-14**.

Removal of a Victim Under a Vehicle Using an FRJ

Removing a person who has become trapped underneath a vehicle can be accomplished utilizing several tools, such as air-lift bags, hydraulic spreaders, or an

SKILL DRILL 10-14
Relocating a Pedal NFPA 1006 8.2.6, 8.2.7, and 8.3.9

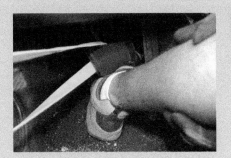

1 Don PPE. Assess the scene for hazards, and complete the inner and outer surveys. Stabilize the vehicle. Position a rescuer inside the vehicle to assess the condition of the victim and the entrapment of the extremity as well as support the foot throughout the operation. Ensure that the victim is properly protected from flying debris. Manage all vehicle glass using the appropriate technique. If a side-impact air bag is in the door or seat area, gain access to the engine compartment, and disconnect the 12-volt DC battery. Ensure that the swing of the driver's-side door is operational. Firmly attach a long section of webbing (no less than 15 ft or 5 m) to the pedal arm, stretching the webbing to the window frame on the driver's-side door.

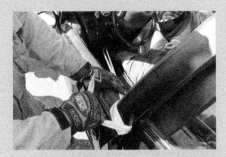

2 With the driver's-side door partially opened 1 in. (2.5 mm) or more, firmly secure the webbing to the window frame near the door's latching mechanism. There should be slight tension on the webbing from the door frame to the pedal.

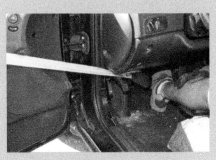

3 With the trapped foot extremity firmly supported by a rescuer, slowly open the driver's-side door to bend the pedal sideways and release the entrapment. This step must be a fully coordinated effort, as too much force can potentially cause further harm to the victim. Once the foot extremity has been released, take the appropriate steps to properly package and remove the victim from the vehicle. Place the victim onto an awaiting stretcher.

© Jones & Bartlett Learning. Photographed by Glen E. Ellman.

FRJ. One of the fastest tools to accomplish this task is an FRJ, based on minimal setup time, stability of the tool itself, and quick application. Regardless of the tool used, this procedure will require multiple personnel and cribbing support. The position of the victim, entrapment, and position of the vehicle (whether it is upright on wheels or on its roof or side) will affect tool placement and position assignment of personnel. Because there are so many possible scenarios for this type of entrapment, this section will focus on one basic entrapment scenario where a victim has become trapped under an upright vehicle with his or her upper torso exposed.

After the inner and outer surveys have been completed, the vehicle will require initial stabilization to prevent any movement from occurring, which includes securing the transmission and ignition and the chocking of all wheels. A minimum of five personnel are recommended to accomplish this task, with one positioned at the head of the victim, two on either side to insert cribbing as the lift is established, one to operate the FRJ, and one to monitor the opposite side for unwanted shifting or movement of the vehicle. Additional personnel can be added, such as a safety officer and overall incident officer.

Initial support cribbing has to be placed on the opposite side of the vehicle to maintain the lift and prevent any shifting of the vehicle. As the tongue of the FRJ is inserted under the rocker panel, personnel are in position on both sides of the victim and ready to insert cribbing as the vehicle is lifted. This is to support the lift should the FRJ fail or slip out. If there are suspected crushing injuries, then medical support should be initiated immediately prior to removal. Engage the FRJ until sufficient lift has been established to remove the victim.

To remove a victim trapped under a vehicle using an FRJ, follow the steps in **SKILL DRILL 10-15**.

SKILL DRILL 10-15
Removal of a Victim Under a Vehicle Using an FRJ NFPA 1006 8.2.3, 8.2.6, 8.2.7, and 8.3.9

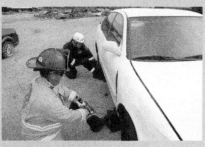

1 Don appropriate PPE. Assess the scene for hazards, and complete the inner and outer surveys. Stabilize the vehicle, which includes securing the transmission drive ignition and basic chocking of the wheels.

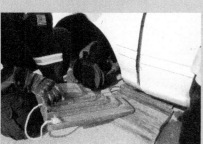

2 Position one rescuer at the head of the victim and two rescuers on either side to insert cribbing as the lift is established. One rescuer is needed to operate the FRJ while the other monitors the opposite side for unwanted shifting or movement of the vehicle. Place initial support cribbing on the opposite side of the vehicle to maintain the lift and prevent any shifting of the vehicle. If there are any crushing injuries to the victim, medical support should be initiated immediately prior to removal.

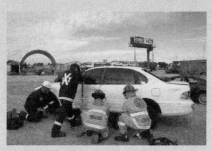

3 Personnel positioned on both sides of the victim should be ready to insert cribbing as the vehicle is lifted. This is to support the lift should the FRJ fail or slip out. Engage the jack until sufficient lift is established to safely remove the victim.

Courtesy of Edward Monahan.

CHAPTER 10 Alternative Extrication Techniques

After-Action REVIEW

IN SUMMARY

- Tunneling is the process of gaining entry through the rear trunk area of a vehicle. It is most commonly performed for a vehicle that is resting on its roof, but it can be performed for a vehicle in any resting position.
- Jacking the trunk, or cracking the undercarriage and lifting the rear end of a vehicle, is an extreme technique that should be included in the technical rescue arsenal. While attempting a tunneling operation, a scenario can present itself in which entry through the trunk area is blocked due to a large fuel tank or a battery pack stored in the trunk of a hybrid or electric system vehicle.
- There are multiple variations of the types of seat frames.
- Seats are attached to the floorboards of the vehicle in four or more places, with positional adjustments on slide tracks that are either fully automatic/motorized or manually operated.
- The material covering the seats may have to be removed using a knife or trauma shears to expose the area of attachment located on the floor or to expose the steel hinges where the seat-back is attached to the seat-bottom section.
- The cross-ramming technique is used when the impingement of metal on the victim requires a unique mechanism of movement.
- When an object impales a vehicle occupant, the main objective is to stabilize the penetrating object at the entry and exit points if an exit point exists.
- The pneumatic air chisel is a powerful tool with multiple blades. The two most widely used blades are the panel cutter, or T-blade, and the flat/curved blade. The panel cutter is used for cutting shallow, straight cuts on small-gauge sheet metal, and the flat/curved blade is used for cutting through medium- to heavy-gauge steel.
- A reciprocating saw is an excellent tool to use for removing a vehicle's roof, especially on vehicles with large C-posts.
- The technique of removing a door on the hinge side can be completed using a combination of a hydraulic spreader and hydraulic cutter, or it can be accomplished using an air chisel.
- Gaining entry through the side of a vehicle that has rolled over and is resting on its roof can require either a very basic procedure, such as forcing a door open, or it can be a very involved process requiring multiple steps.
- Acceleration and brake pedals are notorious for trapping or entangling occupants' foot extremities. The pedal arm can be cut and/or relocated using mechanical tools, such as a hydraulic cutter, reciprocating saw, air chisel, or pneumatic cut-off tool (whizzer saw); a come along and chain set; or a very simple tool such as a section of webbing or rope.
- Removing a person who is trapped underneath a vehicle can be accomplished using various tools: air-lift bags, hydraulic spreaders, or an FRJ. An FRJ is the fastest tool to accomplish this task, having minimal setup time, stability, and quick application.

KEY TERMS

Cross-ramming technique The use of a hydraulic ram to push off of the opposite door post, B-post, floor transmission hump, or inside rocker panel to move the interior of the vehicle away from the entrapped occupant.

Jacking the trunk (cracking the undercarriage and lifting the rear end of a vehicle) An extreme technique to be used when something such as a fuel tank or battery pack stored in the trunk blocks any attempt to enter the vehicle through tunneling.

Tunneling The process of gaining entry through the rear trunk area of a vehicle, a process more commonly used for a post-crash vehicle resting on its roof.

On Scene

You are dispatched for a motor vehicle collision in front of a large shopping center. You arrive to find two vehicles involved in the collision; one of the vehicles is on its roof and wedged between a parked vehicle on the driver's side and a concrete light pole on the passenger's side. There is no access on either side of the vehicle. There is also another passenger vehicle involved in the collision that is positioned upright. Both vehicles have sustained heavy damage. Your engine company is the first to arrive on scene.

1. Tunneling involves the process of making vehicle entry through:
   A. performing a side-out.
   B. the trunk of the vehicle.
   C. the roof of the vehicle.
   D. the front windshield of the vehicle.

2. Tunneling is more commonly used for vehicles:
   A. on their side.
   B. on their roof.
   C. down embankments.
   D. upright.

3. With the vehicle stabilized, victim protected, and glass removed, the first step of tunneling is to:
   A. remove the windshield.
   B. remove the dashboard.
   C. create an opening in the trunk.
   D. create an opening on the side of the vehicle.

4. The second step in tunneling before opening the trunk is to:
   A. determine whether there are any hazardous or heavy storage items in the trunk.
   B. create an opening in the side of the vehicle.
   C. expose the victim to fresh air.
   D. break all of the vehicle glass.

5. The optimal way to access the trunk would be to:
   A. expose and cut the latching mechanism of the trunk.
   B. crawl into the trunk area.
   C. remove the rear dashboard.
   D. remove the rear window frame.

6. The tool used to expose the latching mechanism of the trunk is the:
   A. hydraulic spreader.
   B. hydraulic cutter.
   C. screwdriver.
   D. come along.

7. To release the trunk cover, you will need to:
   A. use a come along to pull the trunk cover off.
   B. cut the latching mechanism using a hydraulic cutter.
   C. use a Halligan bar to pry the latching mechanism apart.
   D. use a circular saw to cut the latching mechanism.

8. The best tool for cutting tension rods located in the trunk of a passenger vehicle is a:
   A. pneumatic air chisel.
   B. hydraulic cutter.
   C. wire cutter.
   D. reciprocating saw.

9. You approach the upright vehicle and determine the roof will need to be removed. A tool that can be used to identify whether air cylinders are present in posts is:
   A. a large flat-head screwdriver.
   B. a hydraulic cutter.
   C. a hydraulic spreader.
   D. a pneumatic ram.

10. Seat belts should be cut prior to the roof being removed.
    A. True
    B. False

11. When using a reciprocating saw to remove the roof of a vehicle on its side:
    A. cut the higher section first.
    B. cut the lower section first.
    C. cut a vertical section.
    D. cut a horizontal section.

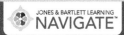

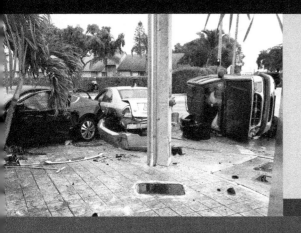

CHAPTER 11

Operations and Technician Levels

Terminating the Incident

KNOWLEDGE OBJECTIVES

After studying this chapter, you will be able to:

- Determine statutory requirements for responsible party notification. (**NFPA 1006: 8.2.9**, pp. 318–319)
- Record and document notification reporting methods based on statutory requirements. (**NFPA 1006: 8.2.9**, pp. 324–325)
- Determine and communicate potential or existing risks to responsible party. (**NFPA 1006: 8.2.9**, pp. 319–321)
- Recognize postincident stress indicators, and appropriately intervene or refer to protect emergency responders. (**NFPA 1006: 8.2.9**, pp. 321, 323)
- Identify information to include in a postincident analysis. (**NFPA 1006: 8.2.9**, p. 324)

SKILLS OBJECTIVES

After studying this chapter, you will be able to perform the following skills:

- Protect rescuers and bystanders during termination of a vehicle incident. (**NFPA 1006: 8.2.9**, pp. 318–319, 325–326)
- Terminate a vehicle rescue and extrication incident. (**NFPA 1006: 8.2.9**, pp. 325–326)
- Notify the party responsible for the operation, maintenance, or removal of the affected vehicle of modification, damage, and potential or existing hazards created by the extrication process. (**NFPA 1006: 8.2.9**, pp. 318–319, 325–326)
- Transfer scene control to a responsible party. (**NFPA 1006: 8.2.9**, pp. 318–319, 325–326)
- Decontaminate personnel and equipment. (**NFPA 1006: 8.2.9**, pp. 319–320, 325)
- Collect, document, and record required incident information per agency protocols and statutory requirements. (**NFPA 1006: 8.2.9**, pp. 324–325)
- Conduct a postincident analysis per agency protocols. (**NFPA 1006: 8.2.9**, p. 324)

You Are the Rescuer

After returning to the station from a mentally and physically difficult and traumatic vehicle rescue and extrication incident involving the fatalities of young children, you notice one of your crew members acting differently, somewhat quiet and withdrawn from the rest of the crew. When you approach him and ask if everything is alright, he responds firmly that he is fine and just wants to be left alone.

1. What actions can you take?
2. Should you encourage the crew member to talk and interact with the group rather than remaining isolated?
3. Does the agency support a department chaplain, peer counseling team coordinator, or critical incident stress management (CISM) team leader to assess the appropriate response needed?

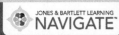

Access Navigate for more practice activities.

Introduction

With the victim extricated, properly packaged, and transported to the appropriate medical facility, the victim management phase of the incident is complete, but the incident is far from over. Getting the units back in service as quickly as possible is a priority for any organization, but personnel, equipment, and the scene must be secured before units are ready to respond to the next incident. This is a basic demobilization process. This chapter discusses the tasks that must be completed to terminate a vehicle rescue and extrication incident.

Terminating an incident includes securing the scene by removing the damaged vehicle and equipment from the scene, ensuring the scene is left in a safe condition, transferring the scene to a responsible party and notifying dispatch of the scene transfer, notifying dispatch that the units are in service, and completing documentation and reports, incident debriefing, and stress debriefing as appropriate. After you have secured the scene and packed your equipment, it is important to return to the station and fully inventory, clean, service, and maintain all the equipment (per the manufacturer's instructions) in preparation for the next call. Some items will inherently need repair, but most will need simple maintenance before they are placed back on the truck and considered in service.

Securing the Scene

Just because the victim has been removed from the wreckage and transported does not mean the scene can be abandoned. The proper transfer of a scene to a responsible party must be established; in the majority of incidents, if not all, this will be the law enforcement. Law enforcement will require the area to be secured so an investigation can be conducted to determine the cause of the crash or dispatch a specialty investigation unit and/or medical examiner if a fatality is involved. A potential crime scene shall be managed by law enforcement, who will preserve and secure any evidence and close off the scene or roadway. Once a scene has been released by law enforcement, vehicle removal is coordinated with a tow agency. In some cases, a vehicle may need to be turned right side up. Being proactive by standing by with a charged hose line is always a good practice during one of these procedures. There may be unique incidents where the roadway transit authority takes responsibility of a scene to ensure that the traffic flow has been restored or roadway debris is removed. A utility company may need to restore traffic signals, restore power to a damaged transformer, or remove power lines on a roadway. The utility company will take over once rescue and law enforcement have cleared the scene.

Prior to leaving a scene, ensure that all medical waste is accounted for and properly disposed of in approved biohazard waste containers, and any remaining body fluids, such as blood, vomit, and feces, must be neutralized with the appropriate solution (**FIGURE 11-1**).

Any fluid hazards that have spilled from the vehicle, such as gasoline, motor oil, transmission fluid, or radiator fluid, even if they were captured with absorbent or other products, are removed by the towing agency. Towing agencies must be licensed to transport and dispose of any hazardous substances;

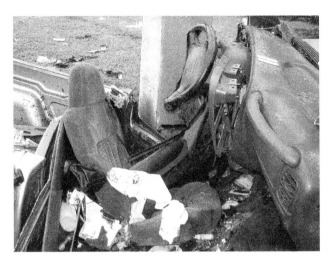

FIGURE 11-1 All agencies must properly secure a scene before clearing an incident. Properly disposing of used medical waste and biohazards is part of securing a scene.
Courtesy of David Sweet.

fire rescue agencies are typically not licensed to do so. To assist the towing agency, place any vehicle parts, such as doors, roofs, and fenders, back in a heavily damaged vehicle. Always ask the tow agency representative if he or she needs assistance before you start throwing items back into a vehicle. The tow agency may have procedures or a policy of their own for stowing and transporting loose objects. Being considerate of their preferences will help maintain a good working relationship with the tow agency for future endeavors, such as acquiring vehicles for use in a vehicle rescue and extrication class. It is also advisable to carry a contact list of various resources for any private and public organization or business that can offer a particular resource that can be used on the incident, such as public works/utilities, the Department of Transportation (DOT), or a heavy equipment company. Reestablishing the normal flow of traffic on major roadways is a priority for the jurisdiction's transit authority, so they will also have multiple resources that can be utilized as well.

LISTEN UP!

To assist the towing agency, place any vehicle parts, such as doors, roofs, and fenders, back in a heavily damaged vehicle, but first ask the tow agency representative if he or she needs assistance before you start throwing items back into a vehicle. The tow agency may have procedures or a policy of their own for stowing and transporting loose objects.

The exception to these procedures will be an incident involving a fatality or serious injury that may result in a fatality. Law enforcement acquires the scene immediately to conduct a fatality investigation. There are times when a victim of a fatality may be left in the vehicle, and your agency may be called back to the scene at a later time to extricate the body from the vehicle. This is often a very traumatic experience, and it is recommended that the crew that responded initially does not return to remove the body; dispatch another unit to complete this assignment.

Securing Equipment

Accountability and maintenance of equipment after the incident has concluded are critical components for properly terminating an incident (**FIGURE 11-2**). Crews are normally depleted both mentally and physically after the incident, and trying to gather all the equipment quickly to get back in service can lead to problems. There must be sufficient time allotted to gather the equipment properly; one person, normally the driver or engineer/chauffer of the apparatus, is in charge of inventory and overseeing that all on-scene equipment used is accounted for. The apparatus may need to be refueled, and the equipment must be properly placed back on the apparatus in a readiness status for the next incident.

Decontamination is also an important factor that cannot be overlooked. Any equipment or personal protective equipment (PPE) that is contaminated must

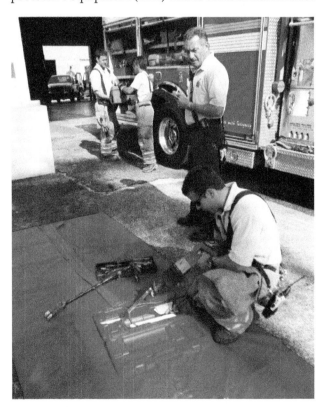

FIGURE 11-2 Accountability and maintenance of equipment after the incident has concluded are critical.
Courtesy of David Sweet.

be properly isolated and/or cleaned following your agency's decontamination procedures. Exposure to any biological or chemical contaminants must be reported immediately and followed up with the proper documentation, and any contaminated PPE must be initially deconned/washed down and placed in a secure containment system to prevent cross-contamination. There are many available programs on decontamination procedures. Some states, such as Florida's Division of the State Fire Marshal's office, offer grants for post-fire on-scene decontamination kits. The kits are designated to mitigate exposure to cancer-causing products of combustion after a fire incident, but can also be adapted for other types of contaminate exposures as well, such as biological, petroleum, and/or hydraulic fluid exposures. Always refer to your departmental procedures for handling the various types of exposures. In addition, there are excellent professional organization websites, such as the International Association of Fire Chiefs (IAFC) and the International Association of Fire Fighters (IAFF), that provide more information and research articles on exposures and denomination policies and procedures.

The following is an example of a postincident checklist that can be used for review after every incident as the equipment is placed back on the apparatus. This list is an example and should be modified to accommodate the agency's needs and type of equipment that is carried on the apparatus:

- Ensure that all gas-powered units are topped off with gasoline.
- Ensure that the hydraulic fluid levels for all power units are full and the correct hydraulic fluid is added if needed.
- Conduct a quick inspection of the hydraulic hoses for any damage as they are recoiled for storage.
- Check that the couplings are in good working condition and free of dirt or grime from the incident.
- Conduct an inspection of the hydraulic tools for any damage to the blades or arms.
- Engage the hydraulic spreader to fully close the tips, and then make a quarter turn in the open position to relieve the pressure before storing it away on the apparatus. Store the hydraulic cutter with the tips just touching each other.
- For all battery-powered tools, replace batteries with charged ones and recharge batteries used during the incident.
- Examine the teeth of the reciprocating saw blade, and replace the blade with a new one if significant wear is observed.
- Examine the electrical cord of the reciprocating saw for any damaged, flattened, or opened sections. Place out of service for any damage noted.
- Examine the air-chisel blade for any damage or chipping, and replace the blade if needed.
- Examine the regulator gauge for any damage.
- Lubricate pneumatic tools according to the manufacturer's recommendations.
- Change out any used air cylinders with topped-off bottles.
- Examine all wood cribbing for damage, such as cracks, splitting, or fastening screws that have become loose or backed out of their housing. Discard or recycle any damaged cribbing.
- Examine all strut stabilization systems and/or jacks for damage, and account for all securing pins and any other attachments that were included.
- Examine all cargo straps for tears or exposure to or absorption of any petroleum products that is deemed by the Authority Having Jurisdiction (AHJ) to be excessive and cannot be cleaned, which will eventually break down the material and potentially fail. Place out of service for any damage noted, such as that described.
- Examine chains and come along cables for any breaks in the strands or flattened sections. Place out of service for any damage noted, such as that described.
- Examine the handle of the come along for any bending or deformity. Place out of service for any damage noted, such as that described.
- Examine all air-lift bags, hoses, and regulators for any damage, such as leaks, dry cracking, and heat exposure causing warping or distortion. Place out of service for any damage noted, such as that described.

At first glance, this checklist may appear to be extreme or too time consuming; remember that it can be completed fairly quickly as the equipment is being loaded back onto the apparatus. Any heavy maintenance, such as washing, degreasing, and repairing, can be completed back at the station. There is no worse scenario than arriving at another accident, pulling off

LISTEN UP!

After you have secured the scene and packed your equipment, it is important to return to the station and fully inventory, clean, service, and maintain all the equipment (per the manufacturer's instructions) in preparation for the next call.

the equipment, and discovering that it has no fuel and/or has a drained battery, does not work, or is missing because it was not properly accounted for at the last incident. Take the time while still on scene to properly account for all the equipment before going back in service.

Securing Personnel

Stress is something that emergency response personnel experience every day. At one time, negative reactions to stressful incidents were suppressed or hidden, and it was a badge of honor to not show emotions. Great strides in research with immediate recognition and treatment protocols have greatly reduced the stigma and the negative side effects that cause debilitating emotional scars that can linger and impair normal everyday functions (**FIGURE 11-3**).

Programs in prevention and managing stress-related injuries are more prevalent today and are now considered a priority among fire rescue organizations across the globe. These programs are making a difference in extending the careers and post-careers of emergency personnel. One such program is the comprehensive Wellness/Fitness Initiative, which is a joint labor/management venture developed by the IAFC and IAFF. This program has multiple components within it, such as fitness, medical, injury rehab, and behavioral health, readily available to fire rescue organizations and can be awarded through grant funding provided by the Assistance to Firefighters Grant (AFG) program offered each year as appropriated by the U.S. Congress. One component of the wellness initiative focuses on physical fitness, which has been proven to be an effective measure in managing, reducing, and preventing both physical and behavioral stress-related injuries.

Stress

Stress is defined as a normal response to a stimulus, whether pleasant or unpleasant, that manifests itself in cognitive, physical, emotional, or behavioral signs. Stress is not necessarily a bad thing; it is our coping mechanism, or lack thereof, that determines how stress affects the body. There are several classifications of stress, two of which are eustress and distress. **Eustress** is stress that produces a positive response in the mind, body, and spirit, such as that experienced through physical exercise or a team sport. Eustress actually builds resistance to the negative aspects of stress. **Distress** is stress that produces a negative response, such as that experienced through the exposure to a critical incident. The continual exposure to critical incidents causes distress to accumulate, eventually leading to a breakdown of effectiveness and efficiency, including an erosion of concentration and self-confidence. Distress is the major contributor to most health issues. As stress builds over time, it can lead to burnout and become a major contributor of heart failure or other debilitating and/or fatal conditions.

Everyone reacts differently to a stressor, and a rescuer must be aware of common signs of distress. If left unresolved, distress can potentially disrupt a person's ability to properly function at the next emergency incident or heighten the risk for developing **post-traumatic stress disorder (PTSD)** or a depressive illness. PTSD is a delayed stress reaction to a prior incident. This delayed reaction is often the result of one or more unresolved issues concerning the incident.

Critical Incident Stress

Critical incident stress is a type of stress that emergency personnel are exposed to. The definition of a critical incident is an event that has the potential to create significant human distress that can overwhelm the body's normal coping mechanisms. This basically describes almost every emergency incident that a rescuer responds to. Remember that everyone reacts differently to a stressor; what may not affect you can drastically affect a co-worker. Also, reactions can occur immediately, several hours after the event, or several days later.

Rescuers who have been exposed to a traumatic or critical incident can exhibit negative stress reactions cognitively, behaviorally, emotionally, and physically.

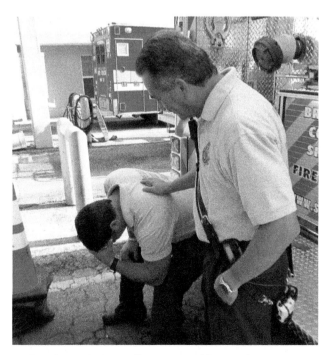

FIGURE 11-3 Immediate recognition and treatment of stress will greatly reduce the negative side effects and debilitating emotional scars that can linger and impair normal everyday functions.
Courtesy of David Sweet.

Voice of Experience

As a firefighter, the dispatch of a working fire or major accident with victims trapped creates a psychological and physical response unlike those of many other call types. During the response and operational phase of these incidents, firefighters use the knowledge, skills, and abilities that drove many of us into this occupation.

Extrications are often evaluated on the time it took from dispatch until that victim was successfully removed and transported to the appropriate medical facility. Many of these responses involve victims that are severely injured and involve multiple companies and agencies working in unison against the platinum 10 or that golden hour of survivability. A typical extrication call can involve such things as a hazardous material, a crime being committed, fire, electric vehicle hazards, or a mass casualty component. With the spread of a door or cut of a post, the victim is freed and often moments later the emergent part of the incident is under control.

The part that follows (though not as adrenaline draining) is as important or more important than the first stage. This involves documentation, incident stabilization, tailboard critique, the evaluation of equipment and personnel readiness, and releasing the scene. With documentation it is very important to gather as much information as possible prior to clearing the scene. Some camera phones, drones, and other devices can assist in properly documenting the incident. Always consider who is the target audience of your documentation. Depending on the type of call, have someone proofread your draft report and gather other responding unit's input prior to submitting your final report.

With incident stabilization, we always want to remove the hazards and return the scene as close as possible to pre-wreck status. Sometimes when clearing the accident scene, if you drive through the scene from a different direction you might see something you missed. The tailboard critique and evaluation of personnel/equipment go hand in hand. The driver engineer normally can give you a brief on apparatus and equipment status during this informal meeting as well as their thoughts on any other task that needs to be accomplished. As an officer, this also gives you a face-to-face with all your people. This time is critical for evaluating how the operation flowed, but more importantly it gives you an opportunity to evaluate your crews' post-incident behavior. Any behavior outside their normal interactions should be acted on immediately. Remember, if you as an officer think this was a tough incident, don't hesitate to act. Move it up the chain (take it out of your hands), as officers are affected also.

Finally, we hand this incident or scene off to law enforcement or another responsible agency. We should always remember that many extrication scenes go from "our scene" to crime scene. When we are in the rescue phase, patient care and removal top our priority list; however, crime scene preservation and processing may immediately become the next step.

In all responses, Life Safety, Property Conservation, and Incident Stabilization provide our magnetic North. Always remember, Life Safety includes responders, physically and mentally.

Everyone Goes Home…Well.

Rodney Smith
Cedar Hill Fire Department
Cedar Hill, Texas

Signs and symptoms of these four categories of reactions include the following:

- **Cognitive reactions**: attention deficit, nightmares, confusion, lack of concentration, decreased ability to problem solve, constant reliving of the event through flashbacks
- **Behavioral reactions**: withdrawing from others, emotional outbursts, extreme changes in normal behavior (such as silence or hyperactivity), repeated drunkenness, negative sexual reactions, insomnia, absenteeism
- **Emotional reactions**: depression, guilt, anger, fear, anxiety, feeling of doom, grief, perceived loss of control
- **Physical reactions**: headaches, muscle twitching/tremors, dry mouth, elevated blood pressure and/or heart rate, nausea, abnormally rapid breathing, profuse sweating, chest pains

A stress fracture left untreated causes continual pain or, eventually, a complete fracture of the bone. The same holds true for a negative stress reaction to a critical incident. Proper and immediate treatment is needed to alleviate further potential physical and psychological problems, and it should be available to the rescuer after any exposure to a critical incident.

Critical Incident Stress Management

Critical incident stress management (CISM) is another type of behavioral health mechanism for crisis intervention, specifically designed to help emergency personnel who have been exposed to a traumatic event process their response to the incident in a way that validates the normal stress reactions and stabilizes the potential negative results of the individual's response. It is geared toward enhancing natural coping mechanisms and facilitating a natural resiliency and recovery from the incident. Just as we provide emergency assistance to individuals in need of help, CISM is a kind of emergency psychological first aid for responders after an exposure to a traumatic incident. It is a resource that helps personnel deal with real-time issues from traumatic events that are momentarily suppressed or openly manifested.

A critical incident stress debriefing (CISD) is a structured and confidential group discussion among those who served at a traumatic incident to address emotional, psychological, and stressful issues related to the event (**FIGURE 11-4**). A CISD usually occurs within 12 to 72 hours of the incident. CISD is not an operational critique or a psychotherapy session. It is designed around three basic goals: (1) defuse the psychological impact of a traumatic event, (2) assist individuals in the normal recovery process, and (3) identify individuals who may need further help or require professional mental health assistance. The CISD lasts from 45 to 60 minutes in most cases.

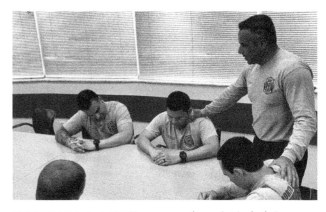

FIGURE 11-4 A CISD can greatly assist in helping personnel properly cope with an exposure to a traumatic incident.
Courtesy of David Sweet.

LISTEN UP!

CISM is geared toward enhancing natural coping mechanisms and facilitating natural resiliency and recovery from an incident.

Peer Support Groups

Emergency response personnel are subjected to an extreme amount of stress and trauma from the incidents and experiences that are encountered on the job. Anger, guilt, burnout, suicide, and divorce are some of the negative side effects that can manifest from these stressors when left untreated. Many fire rescue services form peer support groups to help alleviate these stressors. These groups employ trusted members of the organization who have had similar experiences to provide emotional support through nonclinical conversation and guidance. Peer support teams are designed to build trust and encourage communication among colleagues, which can open the door for reluctant or closed individuals to seek further professional counseling.

Fire rescue services also incorporate chaplain positions in staffing to provide nondenominational spiritual and personal counseling to emergency personnel, families, and staff members. Chaplains can also work well in coordinating peer counseling groups within the agency and providing liaison with other behavioral healthcare practitioners.

The IAFF established the IAFF Center of Excellence for Behavioral Health Treatment and Recovery, which is an inpatient residential facility provided to its members for the treatment of behavioral health injuries, such as post-traumatic stress and substance addiction recovery. Grant funding is also available for programs such as this through the annual AFG award.

Another therapy option which is recognized and recommended by the Department of Defense and the Veterans' Administration for PTSD treatment is EMDR, or Eye Movement Desensitization and Reprocessing. EMDR was developed by American psychologist Francine Shapiro. EMDR centers on teaching patients to reprocess traumatic information and to desensitize the emotions connected with the traumatic experience that occurred by initiating the neuro-mechanism of rapid eye movement or saccadic eye movements.

Postincident Analysis

A postincident analysis (PIA) is a review of the positive and negative aspects of an incident that identifies opportunities for improvement and addresses any necessary corrective actions that may be needed to improve the organization as a whole. There are two types of PIA: formal and informal. A formal PIA is a well-organized event with a structured agenda where all the critical information of the incident is gathered, reviewed, and discussed with all the personnel who responded to the incident. An informal PIA can be as simple as a discussion among the crews at the scene or a discussion back at the station either after the call or on the following shift (**FIGURE 11-5**).

An informal PIA allows the crew to have an open discussion about how the incident evolved. Talking in a no-pressure environment such as this allows everyone to determine ways to improve the response on the next call. Informal talks also build solid relationships and trust within the crew. The key is to be transparent and honest about the positives and negatives of the call. Being overly critical or demeaning is destructive and has no place in these types of meetings; to keep the discussion positive and proactive, all egos and tempers must be left at the door.

A PIA is a tool that is used to build on and improve, not break down; no one should be pointing fingers. If a deficiency is found, it needs to be addressed and corrected as a team. A PIA should be conducted after every incident, whether in a formal or an informal setting; the positive results and professional development gained are beneficial to both the personnel and organization as a whole.

Documentation and Record Management

As discussed in Chapter 2, *Vehicle Rescue Incident Awareness*, and Chapter 4, *Site Operations*, documentation, or record keeping, serves several important purposes, including tracking of equipment inventory, training, needs assessment, response times, and preincident planning. Adequate and accurate documentation also ensures the continuity of quality care; guarantees the proper transfer of responsibility; and fulfills the administrative needs of the department for local, state, and federal reporting requirements.

One form of documentation that is used after an incident has been terminated is an **after-action report (AAR)**. An AAR is a brief summary that analyzes the overall operations and effectiveness of the agency at a particular incident, measuring its capabilities through real-time on-scene evaluations. This summary goes hand in hand with the needs assessment planning discussed in Chapter 2. The AAR should be a formalized document that covers topics including:

- *Compliance to standard operating procedures (SOPs) and standard operating guidelines (SOGs)*: Were there any operational issues that were effective or not effective relating to the current SOPs/SOGs for the type of incident response? Is a policy change or recommendation(s) needed?
- *Medical protocols*: Were there any medical interventions that are outlined in the agency's medical protocols that need to be addressed through training or by the agency's medical director?
- *Staffing requirements*: Was the staffing on hand at the incident sufficient to accomplish the operation in a safe and efficient manner?
- *Mutual aid*: Was mutual aid requested? How did the integration of personnel, equipment, and procedures work to accomplish the scene objectives?

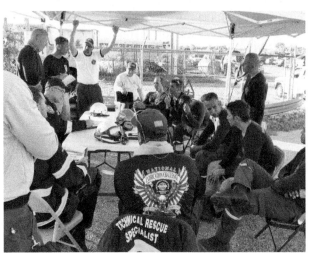

FIGURE 11-5 An informal postincident analysis can take place anywhere.
Courtesy of Carlos Eguiluz.

- *Equipment*: Were there any equipment issues? Was the equipment on hand effective in completing all tasks? Were there any deficiencies, or is there a need to upgrade the current equipment? Was there any equipment malfunction or breakage?
- *Training*: Are there any areas of improvement that can and should be addressed through training? Are there areas where subject experts need to be brought in to update or train personnel?

There may be other points that can be added to this list, but understand that this basic template gives the organization a clear idea of operational needs and performance by identifying strengths and shortfalls within the agency. The AHJ, fire chief, or chief of operations may request an AAR for significant incidents. The AAR should be revised after a PIA has been conducted.

In addition to the AAR, all state- and national-required reporting documents, such as those required by the National Fire Incident Reporting System (NFIRS) and the National EMS Information System (NEMSIS), should be filled out and submitted according to the required timeline set forth by the agency or the state of jurisdiction.

> **LISTEN UP!**
>
> The AAR, or documentation, should include specific details about an incident, such as compliance with SOPs/SOGs, staffing on the scene, mutual aid assistance, equipment used, and areas of training needed. The documentation helps the organization identify strengths and shortfalls.

> **LISTEN UP!**
>
> Documentation, or record keeping, serves several important purposes, including tracking of equipment, training, needs assessment, response times, and preincident planning. It also ensures the continuity of quality care; guarantees the proper transfer of responsibility; and fulfills the administrative needs of the department for local, state, and federal reporting requirements.

To terminate an extrication incident, follow the steps in **SKILL DRILL 11-1**.

SKILL DRILL 11-1
Terminating a Vehicle Rescue and Extrication Incident NFPA 1006 8.2.9

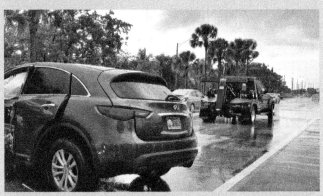

1 Secure the scene by returning it to its normal or pre-incident condition. This may involve preparing the vehicle for a towing company, containing hazardous fluids for removal, containment and disposal of medical waste, and notifying another resource such as the jurisdiction's public works division, power utility company, or excavation equipment company to remove debris and regain use of the roadway.

2 Secure the equipment and apparatus. Account for, maintain, and decontaminate all tools and equipment before placing them back on the apparatus for the next call. Transfer the scene to law enforcement so they can conduct their investigation of the accident. Notify dispatch of the scene transfer and when the units are back in service.

(continues)

SKILL DRILL 11-1 Continued
Terminating a Vehicle Rescue and Extrication Incident NFPA 1006 8.2.9

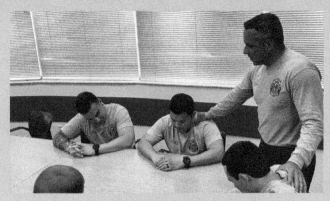

3 Secure personnel by initiating behavioral and physical health screening and/or appropriate rehab. The use of a department chaplain, CISM system, and/or peer counseling program may be needed if available. Conduct a formal or an informal PIA, and complete an AAR.

Steps 1 and 2: Courtesy of Edward Monahan; Step 3: Courtesy of David Sweet.

After-Action REVIEW

IN SUMMARY

- Before units are ready to respond to the next incident, personnel, equipment, and the scene must be secured and placed in a readiness state.
- A potential crime scene shall be managed by law enforcement to preserve and secure any evidence.
- Accountability and maintenance of the equipment after the incident has concluded are critical. There should be one person (normally the driver or engineer/chauffer of the apparatus) in charge of inventorying and overseeing that all the equipment that was used on scene is accounted for.
- A basic equipment checklist can be completed fairly quickly as the equipment is being loaded back onto the apparatus. Any heavy maintenance, such as washing, degreasing, and repairing, can be completed back at the station.
- Making sure that you and your personnel are physically, psychologically, and emotionally sound after the incident is vital not only to being able to properly function at the next incident but also to maintaining longevity in emergency services.
- Stress is something that a rescuer experiences every day. Great strides in research with immediate recognition and treatment protocols have greatly reduced the negative side effects and debilitating emotional scars that can linger and impair normal everyday functions.
- CISM is a type of behavioral health mechanism for crisis intervention specifically designed to help emergency personnel who have been exposed to a traumatic event process their response to the incident in a way that validates the normal stress reactions and stabilizes the potential negative results of the individual's response.
- Peer support groups are formed to help alleviate work-related stressors by using trusted members of the organization who have had similar experiences to provide emotional support through nonclinical conversation and guidance.
- A PIA is a review of the positive and negative aspects of an incident that identifies opportunities for improvement and any necessary corrective actions to improve the organization as a whole. An AAR may be completed following this analysis.
- Documentation, or record keeping, aids in keeping track of equipment inventory, training, needs assessment, response times, and preincident planning.

KEY TERMS

After-action report (AAR) A brief summary that analyzes the overall operations and effectiveness of the agency at a particular incident, measuring its capabilities through real-time on-scene evaluations.

Behavioral reactions Negative reactions that may present as withdrawal from others, emotional outbursts, extreme changes in normal behavior (such as silence or hyperactivity), repeated drunkenness, negative sexual reactions, insomnia, or absenteeism.

Cognitive reactions Negative reactions that may present as attention deficit disorder, nightmares, confusion, lack of concentration, decreased ability to problem solve, or constant reliving of the event through flashbacks.

Critical incident stress management (CISM) A type of behavioral health mechanism for crisis intervention specifically designed to help emergency personnel who have been exposed to a traumatic event process their response to the incident in a way that validates the normal stress reactions and stabilizes the potential negative results of the individual's response.

Distress Stress that generally produces a negative response, such as that experienced through the exposure to a critical incident.

Emotional reactions Negative reactions that may present as depression, guilt, anger, fear, anxiety, feeling of doom, grief, or perceived loss of control.

Eustress Stress that produces a positive response in the mind, body, and spirit, such as that experienced through physical exercise or a team sport. Eustress actually builds resistance to the negative aspects of stress.

Peer support groups A group to help alleviate the stress and trauma from the experiences encountered on the job. The group employs trusted members of the organization who have had similar experiences to provide emotional support through nonclinical conversation and guidance.

Physical reactions Negative reactions that may present as headaches, muscle twitching/tremors, dry mouth, elevated blood pressure and/or heart rate, nausea, hyperpnea, profuse sweating, or chest pains.

Post-traumatic stress disorder (PTSD) A delayed stress reaction to a prior incident. This delayed reaction is often the result of one or more unresolved issues concerning the incident.

Stress Any type of change, whether pleasant or unpleasant, that manifests itself in cognitive, physical, emotional, or behavioral signs.

On Scene

You and your crew have just completed your assignment at a difficult incident. The incident involved a fatality of a child. Your crew members all have children. After you arrive back at your station, your crew is noticeably more quiet than normal.

1. Securing the scene includes all of the following except:
   A. equipment.
   B. personnel.
   C. setting up a landing zone (LZ).
   D. scene/debris cleanup.

2. Due to the fatalities at this scene, _____ will acquire the scene.
   A. the morgue
   B. law enforcement
   C. an ALS crew
   D. a physician

3. A CISD usually occurs within _____ hours of the incident.
   A. 2 to 4
   B. 6 to 8
   C. 8 to 10
   D. 12 to 72

4. Peer support groups are made up of:
   A. members of the organization.
   B. medical professionals.
   C. chief officers.
   D. nurses.

(continues)

On Scene Continued

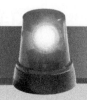

5. A delayed stress reaction to a previous incident is:
   A. distress.
   B. post-traumatic stress disorder.
   C. eustress.
   D. critical incident stress management.

6. An example of an emotional reaction is:
   A. elevated blood pressure.
   B. lack of concentration.
   C. confusion.
   D. grief.

7. Cognitive reactions include:
   A. attention deficit.
   B. withdrawing from others.
   C. depression.
   D. headaches.

8. _____ actually builds resistance to the negative aspects of stress.
   A. Anger
   B. Eustress
   C. CISM
   D. Distress

9. A physical reaction to a stress may be _____.
   A. confusion
   B. emotional outburst
   C. headache
   D. repeated drunkenness

10. A behavioral reaction to stress may include _____.
    A. confusion
    B. emotional outburst
    C. headache
    D. repeated drunkenness

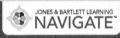 Access Navigate for more activities.

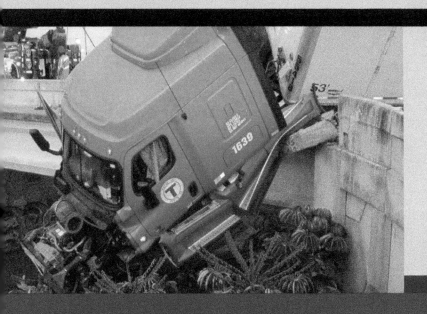

SECTION 3

Heavy Vehicle Incidents

CHAPTER **12** Commercial Vehicles

CHAPTER **13** School Buses

CHAPTER 12

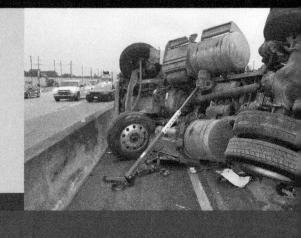

Heavy Vehicle Incidents

Commercial Vehicles

KNOWLEDGE OBJECTIVES

After studying this chapter, you will be able to:
- Define the following terms and explain their role in vehicle rescue incidents:
  - Commercial motor vehicle (CMV). (pp. 331, 347–348)
  - Semi-truck. (p. 333)
  - Semi-trailer. (pp. 333, 338–339, 343–345, 347–348)
- Identify the criteria for classifying a vehicle as a commercial vehicle. (pp. 332–333)
- Discuss the anatomy of a commercial vehicle. (pp. 333–343)
- Discuss the braking systems found in commercial vehicles. (pp. 341–342)
- Match the type of commercial vehicle with the hazardous materials it may be carrying. (pp. 343–346)
- Identify hazards present at commercial/heavy-vehicle extrication incidents. (pp. 343–346)
- Determine commercial/heavy-vehicle access and egress points. (pp. 348–349)
- Describe the role of placarding and shipping papers in heavy-vehicle extrication. (pp. 346–347)
- Cite types of commercial vehicles common in the AHJ response area. (pp. 332–333)
- Describe common commercial vehicle construction components. (pp. 333–343)

SKILLS OBJECTIVES

There are no skills objectives for this chapter.

You Are the Rescuer

As the officer on the engine, you and your crew pull up to an intersection where just moments prior a dump truck side-impacted a semi-tractor trailer with a MC-331 trailer. The trailer has broken at the kingpin and landed on its side.

1. What will be an important step to help you determine your actions at this incident?
2. What resources do you have that can be immediately dispatched or utilized?
3. What, if any, other agencies may need to be involved in the mitigation of this incident?

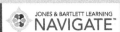 Access Navigate for more practice activities.

Introduction

This chapter covers material above and beyond the advanced technician level requirements as listed in Chapter 8 of NFPA 1006, *Standard for Technical Rescuer Professional Qualifications*.

The U.S. Department of Transportation (DOT) defines a **commercial motor vehicle (CMV)** as a motor vehicle or combination of motor vehicles used in commerce to transport passengers or property if the motor vehicle satisfies at least one of the following criteria:

- Has a **gross vehicle weight rating (GVWR)** of 26,001 lb (11,794 kg) or more inclusive of a towed unit(s) with a GVWR of more than 10,000 lb (4536 kg)
- Has a GVWR of 26,001 lb (11,794 kg) or more
- Is designed to transport 16 or more passengers, including the driver
- Is of any size and is used in the transportation of hazardous materials as defined in the regulation
- Vehicles designed or used to transport more than 8 passengers (including the driver) for compensation

The DOT established a vehicle classification scheme that is separated into categories depending on whether the vehicle carries passengers or commodities (see Chapter 3, *Tools and Equipment*). Non-passenger vehicles are further subdivided by number of axles and number of units, including both power and trailer units.

CMVs travel our roads, streets, and highways every day and are generally associated with the idea of carrying cargo. Many CMVs are utilized or designed for a special purpose, and the word "truck" is often combined with that vehicle's purpose, such as dump truck, fire truck, tow truck, or garbage

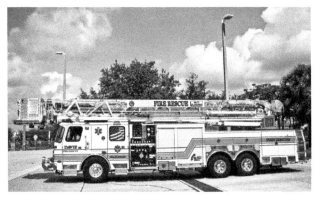

FIGURE 12-1 The tower ladder fire apparatus is one example of a CMV designed for a special purpose.

truck (**FIGURE 12-1**). CMVs also include box trucks, which utilize a single frame, and semi-tractor trailers, which use two or more separate frames that are equipped to haul machinery, chemicals, and a vast variety of commodities/supplies as well as livestock. Other specialized vehicles such as concrete mixers, vehicle transporters, buses, and cranes are also examples of CMVs that you may encounter when dealing with incidents requiring extrication. In England and some other European nations, a truck or CMV is referred to as a "lorry."

LISTEN UP!

GVWR consists of ratings established by manufacturers that take into account cargo, people, fuel, and the vehicle itself to determine the maximum total weight of the vehicle according to the manufacturer's specifications.

Commercial Trucks

Within the United States, the rules and regulations that are placed on CMVs are implemented through the DOT, which limits the amount of weight a CMV can transport, including the type of cargo being hauled with these vehicles. With literally thousands of CMVs traveling the streets and highways, the technical rescuer will in time encounter a collision involving one or more large commercial vehicles (**FIGURE 12-2**).

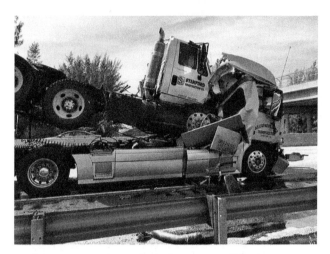

FIGURE 12-2 The technical rescuer will in time encounter a collision involving one or more large commercial vehicles.
Courtesy of Darren Wells.

Because of the overall design, which encompasses the heavier frame structure, size, weight, and cargo, CMVs that require extrication may involve special techniques, heavy equipment, and tools to complete the job. CMV rescue and extrication is a specialized field that is above the technician level in Chapter 8 of NFPA 1006. Qualified training for the proper management of a CMV rescue and extrication incident is an absolute requirement. Having qualified instructors and utilizing a standardized and validated training outline (with qualifying hands-on and written testing requirements) are the best practice model for an agency.

Commercial Truck Classifications

CMVs are classified into eight weight categories, which are based on a GVWR system and the work duty of the engine as it relates to emissions (light duty, medium duty, and heavy duty) (**TABLE 12-1**).

The lightest CMV carries a **class 1 commercial vehicle** rating, with a GVWR ranging from 0 to 6000 lb (0 to 2722 kg); a Ford Ranger is an example of a class 1 CMV. A class 2 commercial vehicle

TABLE 12-1 Weight Classifications for CMVs

Class	GVWR	Example	Work Duty
Class 1	0–6000 lb (0–2722 kg)	Ford Ranger pickup; Toyota Tacoma	Light duty
Class 2a	6001–8500 lb (2722–3856 kg)	Ford F-150; Dodge Dakota	Light duty
Class 2b	8501–10,000 lb (3856–4536 kg)	Ford F-250; Chevrolet Silverado 2500HD or GMC Sierra 2500HD	Light duty
Class 3	10,001–14,000 lb (4536–6350 kg)	Ford F-350; Chevrolet Silverado 3500HD or GMC Sierra 3500HD	Light duty
Class 4	14,001–16,000 lb (6351–7257 kg)	Ford F-450	Medium duty
Class 5	16,001–19,500 lb (7258–8845 kg)	Ford F-550; GMC C4500 and C5500	Medium duty
Class 6	19,501–26,000 lb (8846–11,793 kg)	Ford F-650; GMC C6500	Medium duty
Class 7	26,001–33,000 lb (11,794–14,969 kg)	Ford F-750; GMC C7500	Medium/heavy duty
Class 8	Above 33,000 lb (14,969 kg)	Tractor trailer; GMC C8500 or C8500-Tandem	Heavy duty

is subdivided into two categories (class 2a and 2b). A **class 2a commercial vehicle** is considered a light-duty vehicle, with a GVWR ranging from 6001 to 8500 lb (2722 to 3856 kg); a Ford F-150 is an example of a class 2a commercial vehicle. A **class 2b commercial vehicle** is still considered by many organizations as a light-duty truck, with a GVWR of 8501 to 10,000 lb (3856 to 4536 kg); a Ford F-250 is an example of a class 2b commercial vehicle. A **class 3 commercial vehicle** has a GVWR of 10,001 to 14,000 lb (4536 to 6350 kg); an example of a class 3 commercial vehicle is the Ford F-350. A **class 4 commercial vehicle** has a GVWR of 14,001 to 16,000 lb (6351 to 7257 kg); the Ford F-450 is an example of a class 4 commercial vehicle. A **class 5 commercial vehicle** has a GVWR of 16,001 to 19,500 lb (7258 to 8845 kg); the Ford F-550 is an example of a class 5 commercial vehicle. A **class 6 commercial vehicle** has a GVWR of 19,501 to 26,000 lb (8846 to 11,793 kg); the Ford F-650 is an example of a class 6 commercial vehicle. A **class 7 commercial vehicle** has a GVWR of 26,001 to 33,000 lb (11,794 to 14,969 kg); an example of a class 7 commercial vehicle is the Ford F-750. The heaviest commercial vehicle is a **class 8 commercial vehicle** with a GVWR of more than 33,000 lb (14,969 kg); a semi-tractor trailer is an example of a class 8 CMV. Class 7 and 8 CMVs have a GVWR that is greater than 26,000 lb (11,793 kg), which requires a minimum of a class B driver's license to operate in the United States. Other classifications that are utilized to determine weights are GAWR (gross *axle* weight rating), GCWR (gross *combined* weight rating), and GTWR (gross *trailer* weight rating).

Commercial Truck Anatomy

Vehicle rescue and extrication involving a commercial truck requires that the technical rescuer fully understand the general anatomy for these large vehicles. Almost all commercial trucks have similar construction features that are broken down into different sections, such as the cab, chassis, cargo area, and drive train. The **drive train (power train)** is a system that transfers rotational power from the engine to the wheels, which makes the vehicle move.

A **semi-truck**, or semi-tractor, is a commercial truck capable of towing a separate trailer that has wheels at only one end (semi-trailer) (**FIGURE 12-3**). When the semi-truck is combined with the trailer, it is known as a **semi-tractor trailer (semi-trailer)** (**FIGURE 12-4**). A semi-truck is normally designed with three axles, one in the front for steering purposes and two tandem axles in the rear.

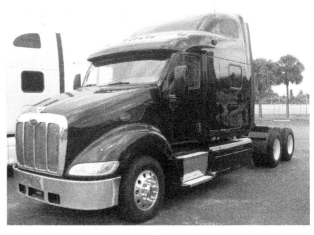

FIGURE 12-3 A semi-truck, or semi-tractor.

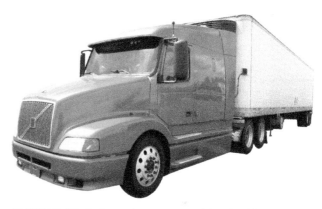

FIGURE 12-4 A semi-tractor combined with a semi-trailer is known as a semi-tractor trailer (semi-trailer).
© iStockphoto/Thinkstock.

Cab

The **cab** of a CMV is considered the enclosed space where the driver and passengers sit. The cab is usually made of a combination of steel, aluminum, and fiberglass (**FIGURE 12-5**).

There are three types of cabs found on commercial trucks:

- **Cab over engine (COE)** (often referred to as a tilt cab): This cab is lifted up over the engine to gain access to the engine itself. In a COE, the driver's seat is positioned over the engine and the front axle. This style of cab was developed to maximize truck cargo space where the overall truck lengths were federally regulated and limited. This body style was also designed to aid in the mobility of the vehicle itself (**FIGURE 12-6**).
- **Conventional cab**: In this design, the driver's seat is positioned behind the engine and front axle. The front end of the vehicle extends approximately 6 to 8 ft (1.8 to 2.4 m) from

Voice of Experience

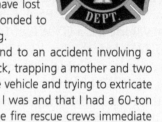

I have been working in the towing industry since 1990 and hold multiple certifications and levels in towing, recovery, and winching operations. I have lost count of the number of commercial vehicle accidents that I have responded to over the years, but one sticks out to me that was particularly frustrating.

I had been dispatched by the turnpike operations center to respond to an accident involving a tractor trailer and an SUV where the SUV impacted the rear of the truck, trapping a mother and two children. When I arrived, fire rescue crews were already working on the vehicle and trying to extricate the occupants. I walked up to the officer in charge and told him who I was and that I had a 60-ton rotator on scene that could lift the semi-truck off the SUV and provide fire rescue crews immediate access. The office told me to stand by, that his crews were working on it. It pained me to stand there and watch them struggle when we could have worked together and really made a difference.

That was several years ago, and since then I have been working with the local technical rescue teams in south Florida promoting joint training sessions which focuses on lifting large commercial vehicles off conventional vehicles. This training includes timed scenarios where fire rescue crews use the equipment off of their apparatus for one lifting scenario and then we conduct the same evolution with one of our 60-ton rotators. This proved to be a huge eye-opener for all of us, as it took fire rescue crews 45 minutes to accomplish what our large tow unit did in 5 minutes.

The towing industry is a huge resource that is under-utilized. These joint training sessions are an excellent way to share knowledge and learn to work cohesively together to accomplish the same goal of helping others.

Brett Holcombe
Owner, Westway Towing
Fort Lauderdale, Florida

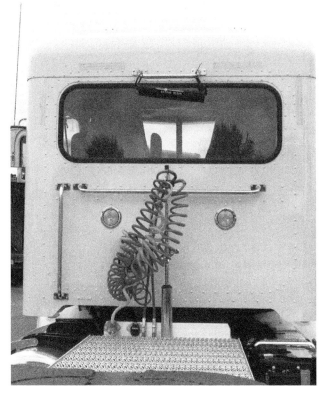

FIGURE 12-5 Rivet heads located on the outside panel of the cab or sleeper indicate the presence of heavy-steel or -aluminum framing directly underneath.

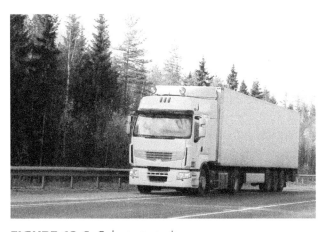

FIGURE 12-6 Cab over engine.
© Hemera/Thinkstock.

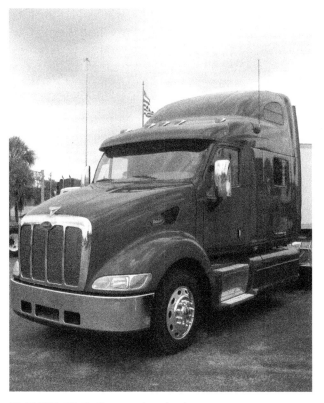

FIGURE 12-7 Conventional cab.

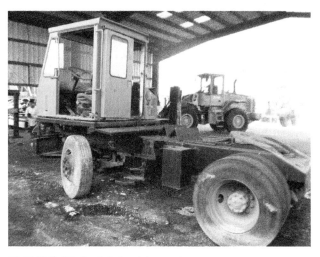

FIGURE 12-8 Cab beside engine.

the front windshield. Conventional cabs are more commonly found in the United States and Canada. To compensate for added wind resistance, a large wind/air deflector may be added to the top of the cab, which can add a lot more weight to the roof structure. The fuel tanks on these trucks also tend to be larger than those on COEs (**FIGURE 12-7**).

- **Cab beside engine (CBE):** In this design, the driver sits next to the engine. These trucks are mostly found in shipyards, freight yards, and baggage carriers within airports and seaports (**FIGURE 12-8**).

SAFETY TIP

Because of the tilt-cab design on a COE, for safety purposes, the cab may have to be secured to the frame of the vehicle prior to attempting any extrication procedures.

A cab may also have a **sleeper**, which is a compartment attached to the cab that allows the driver to rest while making stops during a long transport. Sleepers are most commonly found on a semi-truck. Sleepers can be factory installed to the rear of the cab with a separate access door on the side or at the center directly behind the cab or added on post factory. Like the cab, sleepers can also be made of aluminum, steel, or a combination of both. Generally, they are designed with steel or aluminum ribs or framing with an outer shell of fiberglass or a plastic injection molding. Between these layers are insulation and wires. Cutting into the cab and/or sleeper can require multiple tools, including hydraulic tools, reciprocating saws, and pneumatic air chisels.

> **SAFETY TIP**
>
> Always disconnect the battery system before conducting any entry operations.

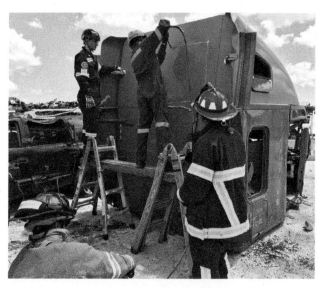

FIGURE 12-9 The height of the cab on a CMV requires that the technical rescuer build several platforms that surround the cab consisting of cross-tie box cribbing, backboards, and/or ladders or use a flatbed towing unit positioned against the cab to gain height and stability.
Courtesy of David Sweet.

The roof sections of the cab and sleeper can contain an air-conditioning unit as well as a wind deflector, which add a considerable amount of weight to the vehicle's roof; this weight increase must be compensated for when considering a roof removal procedure for a CMV that is upright. Also, the overall height of these cabs can range from 13.6 to 14.6 ft (4.2 to 14.5 m) from ground level. The height requires that the technical rescuer build several platforms that surround the cab consisting of cross-tie box cribbing, backboards, and/or ladders or use a flatbed towing unit positioned against the cab to gain height and stability (**FIGURE 12-9**). Working from a ground ladder placed against the cab is not the safest practice and requires multiple personnel to assist with stability.

> **LISTEN UP!**
>
> Reciprocating saws are one of the most effective tools for gaining entry into CMV cabs because of the large span of cutting that is required.

Glass

Windshield glass found in a CMV is composed of standard laminated safety glass and set in a rubber gasket similar to that found in a school bus. This type of rubber gasket setting can be removed with a prying tool, such as a large flat-head screwdriver. The glass can be removed without breaking or cutting it, although cutting the glass out with a battery-powered glass shear tool, glass handsaw, and/or reciprocating saw is also a fast and viable option. Some new models of CMVs use curved windshields that are set in place and sealed using a mastic adhesive; this setting requires that the glass be cut out for removal purposes. The side windows are composed of tempered safety glass, which can be much thicker than the glass found in conventional vehicles.

Chassis

The chassis makes up the main structural framework of the CMV and includes the braking, steering, and suspension systems (**FIGURE 12-10**). The frame structure, which is the strongest part of the CMV, is constructed of heavy-gauge steel to support the weight of the vehicle's cab, suspension system, engine, and cargo. It consists of two parallel boxed, tubular, or C-shaped rails or beams that are held together with crossbeams. These crossbeams, or crossmembers, are attached to the rails by welds or bolts.

Suspension. The suspension system for a CMV is designed to protect the cargo and frame system of the vehicle from damage and wear by absorbing the impacts of the tires as they drive over uneven terrain. Suspension systems can come in the form of large steel leaf springs, which can have an independent adjustment leaf spring system per axle, known as an independent suspension system (**FIGURE 12-11**), and/or spiral springs in addition to air bellows (bags), better known as an air ride system (**FIGURE 12-12**).

CHAPTER 12 Commercial Vehicles **337**

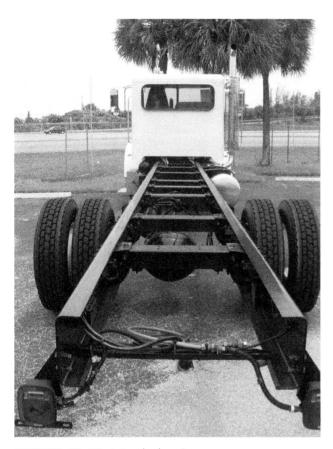

FIGURE 12-10 A truck chassis.

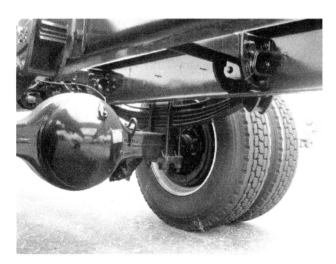

FIGURE 12-11 This suspension system has large steel leaf springs that may have an independent adjustment leaf spring system on each axle; this is known as an independent suspension system.

The **air ride system** is designed to inflate and deflate the suspension system through onboard air pressure tanks. The suspension system connects the axles, which include the wheels, to the vehicle. When the air brake (parking brake) is engaged, an air ride suspension system will release some air but remain stable. However, in some models, it can release air and drop

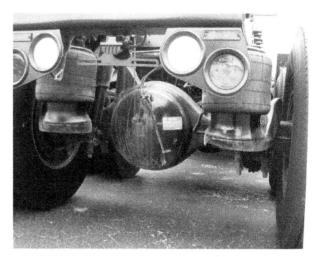

FIGURE 12-12 This suspension system has spiral springs in addition to air bellows (bags), better known as an air ride system.

several inches to accommodate the resting or parked position; this can exacerbate the crushing effect on a vehicle that it has collided with (underride) and is now trapped under the trailer (as further discussed later in this chapter). Also, if a bellows bag ruptures or leaks during an incident, it can cause the vehicle to settle or shift several inches. Most air ride bellows are interconnected per axle and will release air in all the bags sharing the same axle even if just one bag is damaged.

There are several tools, equipment, and techniques that can help the technical rescuer manage the stabilization of a CMV, but the weight of these vehicles will vary greatly, which must be calculated into any technique and/or procedure. The Federal Highway Administration's Office of Freight Management and Operations oversees state enforcement of heavy-truck and bus sizes and weight standards in the United States. The U.S. national weight standards that apply to CMV operations allow for a maximum of 80,000 lb (36,287 kg) for transport on the interstate highway system and does not require a permit. This maximum weight consists of the combined weight of the tractor, trailer, and cargo. Special permits can also be granted that exceed this gross weight. In addition, many states set their own CMV weight standards for CMVs that travel on roadways other than the interstate highway system.

The best piece of equipment to manage an unstable CMV is a large 50/60-ton rotating tow unit with an articulating boom, which can quickly apply two or more slings and a chain package to the CMV, thus stabilizing or lifting the unit to conduct safe operations and prevent shifting (**FIGURE 12-13**). Other options include placing tension stabilization struts with heavy lifting and weight management capabilities (check with the

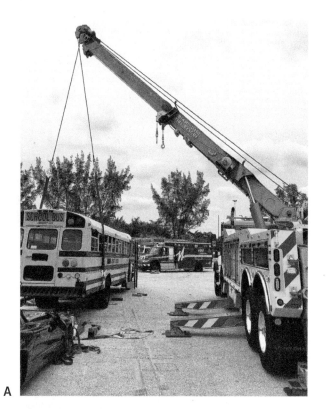

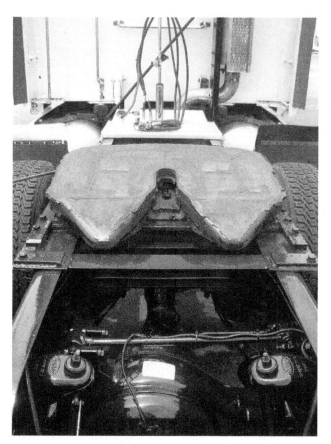

FIGURE 12-14 A fifth wheel.

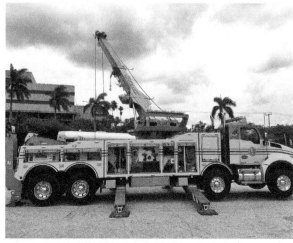

FIGURE 12-13 A large 50/60-ton rotating tow unit with an articulating boom can apply two or more slings and a chain package to the CMV, enough to conduct safe operations and prevent shifting.
Courtesy of Houston Holcombe.

manufacturer) around the CMV, locking the struts together with a heavy-cargo strap in the same fashion as stabilizing an upright school bus. This, in addition to utilizing First Responder Jacks (FRJs) and placing cribbing in front and back of each wheel to chock and prevent any rolling, can add support to maintain and/or raise (with the appropriate strut system) the CMV's suspension system and provide the stability to conduct safe operations.

Another tool that may be applied to certain types of cargo trailers for stabilizing and maintaining the trailer's suspension system is air-lift bags, which can be positioned between the frame and the top of the tires. Air-lift bags utilized in this manner must adhere to the safety rules discussed in Chapter 3. This technique can also be used in conjunction with a tension buttress stabilization strut system.

Cargo Area

The cargo area of a CMV can be attached to the same frame as the cab is attached to, as with a box truck, or there can be a separate frame from the tractor, as with the semi-tractor trailer. The vehicle manufacturer calculates the **gross combined weight rating (GCWR)** to determine the cargo capacity limitations.

The cargo trailer of a semi-tractor trailer, or semi-trailer, is connected to the tractor by a large locking pin called the **kingpin**. The kingpin sits in a flat, horseshoe-shaped quick-release coupling device called a **fifth wheel**, or a turntable hitch, mounted at the rear of the towing truck (**FIGURE 12-14**). The kingpin and fifth wheel allow for easy hookup and release. Fifth wheels are attached to the frame rails of the tractor, and the manual release of this device is located on the driver's side of the fifth wheel itself (**FIGURE 12-15**).

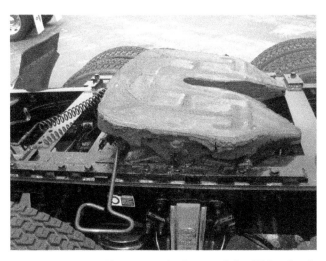

FIGURE 12-15 The manual release of the fifth wheel, which is on the driver's side of the fifth wheel itself.

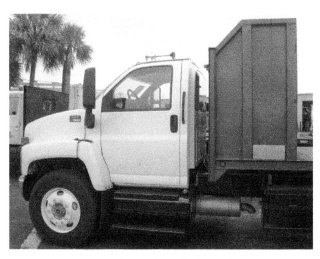

FIGURE 12-17 A dromedary deck or plate.

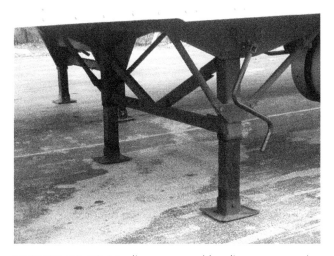

FIGURE 12-16 Landing gear and landing gear crank.

> **LISTEN UP!**
>
> The wide array of cargo transported in semi-tractor trailers or box trucks can add additional concerns for the technical rescuer when conducting rescue and extrication operations. The technical rescuer will need to be concerned not only with trapped victims, but also with cargo, which has the potential to wreak havoc and jeopardize safety on a scene. Cargo may include hazardous materials, livestock, or large amounts of debris. The officer and personnel must always maintain a situational awareness to the changing dynamics of the operation at hand; the potential for shifting cargo when stabilizing or lifting can be detrimental to the operation.

Cargo areas can contain all types of commodities and products and/or general goods (groceries, office supplies, and furniture), chemicals (liquid and solid), machinery, and other vehicles. Semi-trailers come equipped with a stabilizing device known as a **landing gear**. The landing gear is located at the front of the unit and can be lowered to stabilize the trailer when it is not attached to the tractor. This device is commonly operated manually by a hand crank (**FIGURE 12-16**). In addition to the traditional cargo area on a trailer, some CMVs can be equipped with a dromedary. A **dromedary (drom)** is a separate box, deck, or plate that is mounted behind the cab and in front of the fifth wheel on the frame of the tractor. A dromedary can be used to store products that should be kept away from the load in the cargo area, or it can be used to mount a power unit, such as a generator (**FIGURE 12-17**).

Axles

An **axle** is a shaft that is designed for wheel rotation (**FIGURE 12-18**). Axles are categorized as either live or dead. **Live axles** transmit propulsion or cause the wheels to turn. A **dead axle** is used for load support and is commonly set in the front section of a tractor where its function is for load support and steering; hence, it is also known as a steer axle. Another type of axle is the **lift axle**, which can be raised or lowered by an air suspension system to increase the weight-carrying capacity of the vehicle or to distribute the cargo weight more evenly across all the axles (**FIGURE 12-19**). As mentioned previously, tractors generally have three axles. One axle is set in the front of the vehicle and has one wheel on each side, and it controls the steering. The other two axles are under the rear of the tractor and have two wheels on each side; these axles can be set in tandem, with one or both used for propulsion.

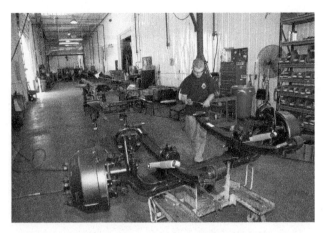

FIGURE 12-18 Axles are designed for wheel rotation.
© David R. Frazier/Science Source.

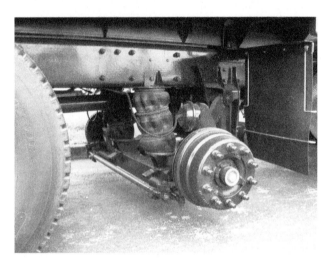

FIGURE 12-19 The lift axle.

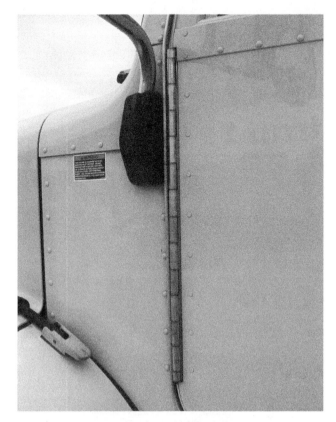

FIGURE 12-20 A piano-type hinge.

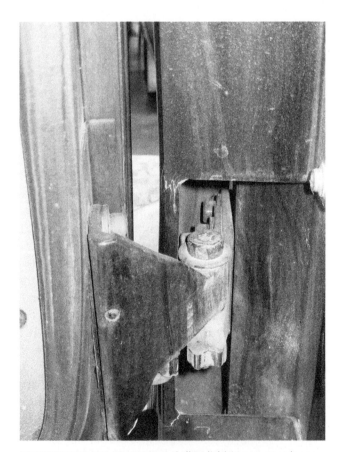

FIGURE 12-21 Two-piece full/solid hinges may be hidden on the inside of the door.

Doors

Doors on CMVs are very similar to doors found on conventional vehicles. They are, however, of a heavier construction from the increased amount of steel used. The door handle is usually located in the lower corner of the door, which makes access easier for vehicle occupants.

There may be a combination of hinges found on a CMV door, such as piano-type hinges (**FIGURE 12-20**); two-piece full/solid hinges, which can be hidden on the inside of the door (**FIGURE 12-21**) or fully exposed on the outside; and strap hinges, which attach on and extend to the outside of the door. The latching mechanism will usually consist of a latch pin and a latching device that grabs and locks the latch pin at two points rather than the standard latch that is found on a conventional vehicle. The latching mechanism and pin are normally located above the door handle, about midway on the frame.

Door removal techniques for CMVs apply the same philosophy as the door removal procedures in conventional vehicles, "expose and cut." Expose the latching mechanism and cut it. With hydraulic tools, create a purchase point with a vertical spread technique in the window frame, and start to spread the door down and away from the latch, creating a large enough opening to insert the hydraulic cutter and cut the latch mechanism. Gaining access through the hinge side of the door will be more complicated, depending on the type of hinge you encounter. Also, remember that you will be going against the natural swing of the door and will have to gain additional access to the latch system to release it. Exterior full/solid hinges can be cut with a high-pressure air chisel, or the area surrounding them can be spread enough with a hydraulic spreader to allow cutting with a hydraulic cutter. Piano-type hinges require a lot of work because they are attached in multiple areas along a vertical line. Interior hinges must be exposed and cut with either a hydraulic cutter or a high-pressure air chisel.

Braking Systems

The braking system on a CMV utilizes compressed air to actuate the system. There are three types of air brakes that make up the braking system on a CMV—the service brake, emergency brake, and parking brake. The service brake is the normal driving brake applied by the driver to slow and/or stop the vehicle during normal driving operations. The air brake (parking brake) is used when the vehicle is in a fully stopped position. An air-actuated release button or switch, which is engaged by the driver, bleeds out compressed air to hold back large springs located inside sealed chambers that release and lock the brakes in place (FIGURE 12-22 and FIGURE 12-23). The emergency brake utilizes a combination of the service and parking brakes to engage when a brake failure or air line break occurs. An added safety feature to the air brake system on all trucks, tractors, and trailers is an antilock braking system (ABS), which is federally mandated by Code of Federal Regulations, 49 CFR 393.55, *Antilock Brake Systems*, in addition to Federal Motor Vehicle Safety Standards (FMVSS) No. 121, *Air Brake Systems*. The power cables that carry ABS power to trailers are normally color coded with a lime-green color. Other power cables may be yellow, orange, and/or black.

Air is compressed by an onboard compressor that is run by the vehicle's engine. Air is stored in tank reservoirs that are located in various areas on the tractor as well as on the cargo trailer. The

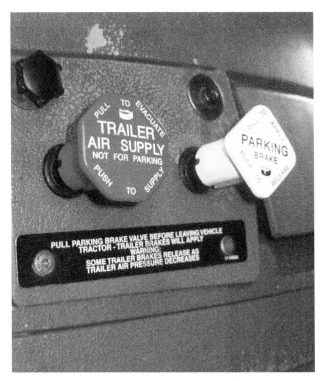

FIGURE 12-22 An air brake (parking brake).

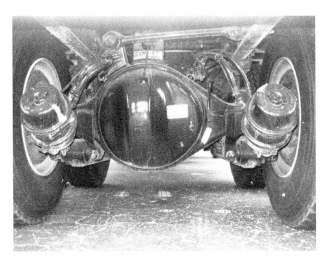

FIGURE 12-23 The parking brake bleeds out compressed air, holding back large springs located inside the sealed chambers (shown above) that release and lock the brakes in place.

compressor normally stores the compressed air at approximately 120 to 125 psi (827 to 862 kPa). When the pressure drops below 100 psi (689 kPa), the compressor will restart and fill the tanks to the appropriate pressure.

The air brake system on a tractor connects the trailer by a minimum of two air lines—the service air line, which is normally blue, and the emergency air line (supply line), which is normally red (FIGURE 12-24). The emergency line controls the air brake for the

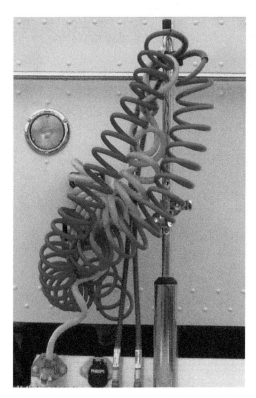

FIGURE 12-24 The air brake system consists of two air brake lines, usually red and blue in color, with an electrical line colored black; orange; or more commonly, lime-green (as shown in the picture).

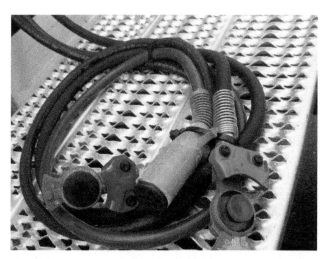

FIGURE 12-25 Glad hands are couplers that supply air to the braking system of the trailer.

trailer and is also utilized to fill the air reservoir tanks. The couplers that supply air to the braking system of the trailer are known as **glad hands** (**FIGURE 12-25**). In trailers that are designed to tow other trailers, there are shutoff valves at the rear of the towing trailer that control the service and emergency air lines and allow the closing of the air lines when not in use.

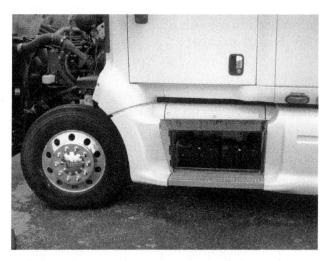

FIGURE 12-26 Battery trays are usually located underneath the step-up.

SAFETY TIP

Never attempt to engage the brakes by manually releasing the springs located in the sealed spring chamber.

Battery Systems

Battery systems for a CMV can consist of four or more 12-volt direct current (DC) batteries, which are hooked together in parallel, with all positive battery terminals wired together and all negative battery terminals wired together, thus increasing the energy storage capacity. Battery trays or storage areas can be located in several areas throughout the vehicle. In semi-tractor trailers, the battery trays are generally stored underneath the step-up to make entry into the vehicle easier, but this is not a standard feature (**FIGURE 12-26**). Battery trays can also be located behind the cab or in various other areas of the vehicle.

Fuel Tanks and Fuel Types

Fuel tanks for CMVs are usually constructed of aluminum but are also available in steel and range in size from 50 to 150 gal (189 to 568 L). There may be a single tank or two tanks positioned on either side of the tractor frame. These tanks may be referred to as "saddle tanks" because they saddle the sides of the vehicle (**FIGURE 12-27**). Fuel lines may lead from the top or the bottom of the tank depending on the manufacturer. These tanks are independently siphoned from the fuel pump; there is no crossover line or switch that

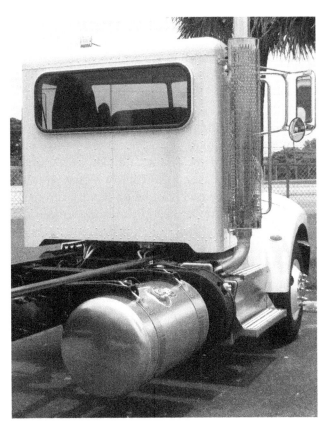

FIGURE 12-27 A saddle tank.

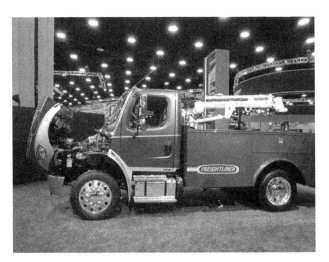

FIGURE 12-28 The HECMV utilizes either the internal combustion engine or an electric motor for propulsion.

connects each tank. The tanks also may be equipped with a shutoff valve on the tank itself or on the fuel line; the location of a shutoff valve varies among manufacturers. The fuel that is predominantly utilized in the trucking industry is diesel. Biodiesel is starting to gain some usage because it is less expensive than diesel.

Electric and hybrid CMVs are also beginning to be manufactured, and some are very similar in design to the systems in a conventional vehicle. The hybrid-electric commercial motor vehicle (HECMV) utilizes either the internal combustion engine or an electric motor for propulsion (FIGURE 12-28). Electric power is generated through an onboard battery pack with an ultracapacitor and/or through other means such as regenerative braking. The electric CMV has a propulsion system that relies completely on electric generated power. Tesla Corporation has introduced the Tesla Semi with a 500-mi (805-km) range, quick acceleration from 0 to 60 mi/h (0 to 97 km/h) in 20 seconds, and projected energy costs that are half the cost of diesel. Tesla is set to launch the Semi full electric CMV by 2021.

Hazardous Materials

One of the greatest concerns for the technical rescuer responding to a motor vehicle accident involving a CMV is the potential for the CMV to be transporting hazardous materials and for the cargo's or vessel's integrity to be compromised. According to the DOT's Pipeline and Hazardous Materials Safety Administration (PHMSA), there are more than 400,000 CMVs dedicated to the transportation of hazardous materials, with 18,000,000 shipments of gasoline and 125,000 shipments of explosives conducted each year by roadway travel.

The Federal Hazardous Materials Transportation Law (49 U.S.C. § 5101 et seq.) is a statute enacted to regulate hazardous materials transportation in the United States.

Section 5103 of the Federal Hazardous Materials Transportation Law (49 U.S.C. § 5103) defines a hazardous material as a substance or material including an explosive; radioactive material; infectious substance; flammable or combustible liquid, solid, or gas; toxic, oxidizing, or corrosive material; and compressed gas that the Secretary of Transportation has determined is capable of posing an unreasonable risk to health, safety, and property when transported in commerce and has been designated as hazardous under Section 5103. The term "hazardous material" includes hazardous substances, hazardous wastes, marine pollutants, materials with an elevated temperature, materials designated as hazardous in the Hazardous Materials Table (see 49 CFR 172.101), and materials that meet the defining criteria for hazard classes and divisions in part 173 of subchapter C—Hazardous Materials Regulations (HMR).

HMR refer to the regulations listed in 49 CFR, parts 171 through 180, and 49 CFR, parts 100 through 185. HMR apply to the transportation of hazardous materials in interstate, intrastate, and foreign commerce by aircraft, railcar, vessel, and motor vehicle. HMR are issued by the DOT's PHMSA, which governs the transportation of hazardous materials by highway, rail, vessel, and air. The PHMSA issues rules and develops and enforces regulations governing the safe transportation of hazardous materials.

Hazardous materials are divided into nine classifications with subdivisions as follows:

Class 1—Explosives

    Division 1.1—Explosives with a Mass Explosion Hazard

    Division 1.2—Explosives with a Projection Hazard

    Division 1.3—Explosives with Predominantly a Fire Hazard

    Division 1.4—Explosives with No Significant Blast Hazard

    Division 1.5—Very Insensitive Explosives with a Mass Explosion Hazard

    Division 1.6—Extremely Insensitive Articles

Class 2—Gases

    Division 2.1—Flammable Gases

    Division 2.2—Nonflammable, Nontoxic Gases

    Division 2.3—Toxic Gases

Class 3—Flammable Liquids

Class 4—Flammable Solids, Spontaneously Combustible Materials, and Dangerous-When-Wet Materials or Water-Reactive Substances

    Division 4.1—Flammable Solids

    Division 4.2—Spontaneously Combustible Materials

    Division 4.3—Water-Reactive Substances or Materials Dangerous When Wet

Class 5—Oxidizing Substances and Organic Peroxides

    Division 5.1—Oxidizing Substances

    Division 5.2—Organic Peroxides

Class 6—Toxic Substances and Infectious Substances

    Division 6.1—Toxic Substances

    Division 6.2—Infectious Substances

Class 7—Radioactive Materials

Class 8—Corrosive Substances

Class 9—Miscellaneous Hazardous Materials/Products, Substances, or Organisms

At any vehicle accident involving a CMV, the technical rescuer must anticipate, plan, and be prepared for the potential of the CMV to be transporting some type of hazardous material. Roadway transportation is the most common method of hazardous material transport. There are many different vehicle/vessel types that are used to transport hazardous cargo. According to 49 CFR 171.8(2) or local jurisdictional regulations (for example, Transport Canada), a cargo tank is considered bulk packaging that is permanently attached to or forms a part of a motor vehicle or is not permanently attached to any motor vehicle and that, because of its size, construction, or attachment to a motor vehicle, is loaded or unloaded without being removed from the motor vehicle. One clarification on cargo tanks is that the DOT does not view tube trailers (which consist of several individual cylinders banded together and affixed to a trailer) as cargo tanks. Some of the more common CMV cargo vessels are discussed next.

One of the most utilized and reliable transportation vessels is the MC-306/DOT 406 flammable liquid tanker (**FIGURE 12-29**). These cargo tanks frequently carry liquid food-grade products, gasoline, or other flammable and combustible liquids. The oval-shaped tank is pulled by a separate CMV tractor and can carry between 6000 and 10,000 gal (22,712 and 37,854 L) of product. The MC-306/DOT 406 is nonpressurized (with a working pressure between 2.65 and 4 psi [18.3 and 27.6 kPa]), is usually made of aluminum or stainless steel, and is off-loaded through valves at the bottom of the tank. These cargo tanks have several safety features, including full rollover protection and remote emergency shutoff valves (**FIGURE 12-30**).

A vehicle that is similar to the MC-306/DOT 406 is the MC-307/DOT 407 chemical hauler (**FIGURE 12-31**). This vessel is used to transport flammable liquids; it has a round or horseshoe-shaped tank and is capable of holding 6000 to 7000 gal (22,712 to 37,854 L) of liquid. The MC-307/DOT 407 also utilizes a separate CMV tractor to pull it. The MC-307/DOT 407 flammable liquid tanker typically hauls flammable and combustible liquids but can also carry mild corrosives

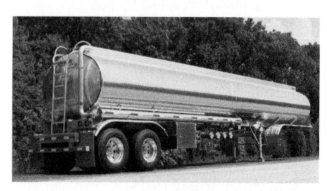

FIGURE 12-29 The MC-306/DOT 406 flammable liquid tanker typically hauls flammable and combustible liquids.
Courtesy of Polar Tank Trailer L.L.C.

CHAPTER 12 Commercial Vehicles 345

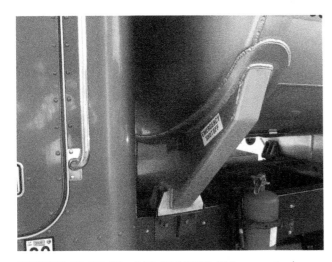

FIGURE 12-30 The MC-306/DOT 406 cargo tanker has a remote emergency shutoff valve as a safety feature.
Courtesy of Glen Rudner.

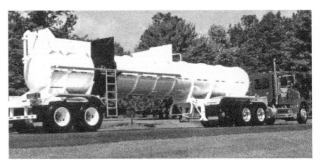

FIGURE 12-32 The MC-312/DOT 412 corrosives tanker is commonly used to carry corrosives such as concentrated sulfuric acid, phosphoric acid, and sodium hydroxide.
Courtesy of National Tank Truck Carriers Association.

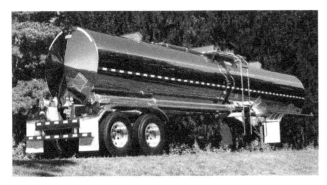

FIGURE 12-31 The MC-307/DOT 407 chemical hauler carries flammable liquids, mild corrosives, and poisons.
Courtesy of Polar Tank Trailer L.L.C.

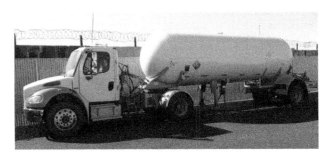

FIGURE 12-33 The MC-331 pressure cargo tanker carries materials such as ammonia, propane, Freon, and butane.
Courtesy of Rob Schnepp.

and poisons. This type of cargo tank may be insulated (horseshoe) or noninsulated (round) and may have a higher internal working pressure than the MC-306/DOT 406, in some cases up to 35 psi (241 kPa). Cargo tanks that transport corrosives may have a rubber lining to prevent corrosion of the tank structure.

The **MC-312/DOT 412 corrosives tanker** is commonly used to carry corrosives such as concentrated sulfuric acid, phosphoric acid, and sodium hydroxide (**FIGURE 12-32**). This cargo tank has a smaller diameter than the MC-306/DOT 406 or the MC-307/DOT 407 and is often identifiable by the presence of several heavy-duty reinforcing rings around the tank. The rings provide structural stability during transportation and in the event of a rollover. These cargo tanks have substantial rollover protection to reduce the potential for damage to the top-mounted valves. The MC-312/DOT 412 tanker operates at approximately 15 to 25 psi (103 to 172 kPa) and can hold up to approximately 6000 gal (22,712 L).

The **MC-331 pressure cargo tanker** is used to carry materials such as ammonia, propane, Freon, and butane (**FIGURE 12-33**). The liquid volume inside the tank varies from the 1000-gal (3785-L) delivery truck to the full-size 11,000-gal (41,640-L) cargo tank. The MC-331 cargo tank has rounded ends, typical of a pressurized vessel, and is commonly constructed of steel or stainless steel with a single-tank compartment. The MC-331 operates at approximately 300 psi (2068 kPa), with typical internal working pressures in the vicinity of 250 psi (1724 kPa). These cargo tanks are equipped with spring-loaded relief valves that traditionally operate at 110 percent of the designated working pressure. A significant explosion hazard arises if an MC-331 cargo tank is impinged on by fire, however. Because of the nature of most materials carried in MC-331 tanks, a threat of explosion exists because of the inability of the relief valve to keep up with the rapidly building internal pressure. Responders must use great care when dealing with this type of transportation emergency.

The **MC-338 cryogenic tanker** is designed to maintain high thermal protective qualities to transport materials such as liquid nitrogen and liquid oxygen (**FIGURE 12-34**). This low-pressure tanker relies on

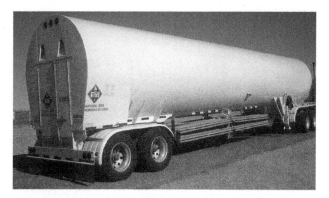

FIGURE 12-34 The MC-338 cryogenic tanker maintains the low temperatures required for the cryogens it carries.
Courtesy of Jack B. Kelly, Inc.

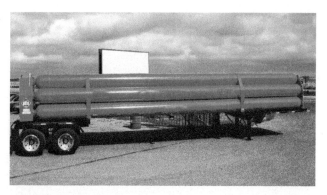

FIGURE 12-35 A tube trailer.
Courtesy of Jack B. Kelly, Inc.

tank insulation to maintain the low temperatures required for the cryogens it carries. A boxlike structure containing the tank control valves is typically attached to the rear of the tanker. Special training is required to operate valves on this and any other tanker. An untrained individual who attempts to operate the valves may disrupt the normal operation of the tank, thereby compromising its ability to keep the liquefied gas cold and creating a potential explosion hazard. Cryogenic tankers have a relief valve near the valve control box. From time to time, small puffs of white vapor will be vented from this valve. Responders should understand that this may not be an emergency, but just a normal occurrence; the valve is designed to maintain the proper internal pressure of the vessel.

Tube trailers carry compressed gases such as hydrogen, oxygen, helium, and methane (**FIGURE 12-35**). Essentially, they are high-volume transportation vehicles that are made up of several individual cylinders banded together and affixed to a trailer. These large-volume cylinders operate at working pressures of 3000 to 5000 psi (20,684 to 34,474 kPa). One trailer may carry several different gases in individual tubes. Typically, a valve control box is found toward the rear of the trailer with each cylinder having its own relief valve. These trailers can frequently be seen at construction sites or facilities that use large quantities of compressed gases.

Dry bulk cargo tanks carry dry bulk goods such as powders, pellets, fertilizers, or grain (**FIGURE 12-36**). These tanks are not pressurized but may use pressure to off-load the product. Dry bulk cargo tanks are generally V-shaped with rounded sides that funnel the contents to the bottom-mounted valves.

Placards

Hazard warning placards are a type of warning system that displays the hazardous classification type on

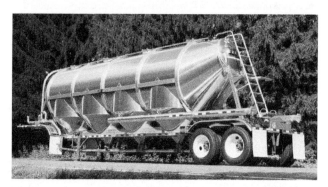

FIGURE 12-36 A dry bulk cargo tank carries dry goods such as powders, pellets, fertilizers, or grain.
Courtesy of Polar Tank Trailer L.L.C.

the sides of a vehicle using a diamond-shaped design. Federal law requires placards to be clearly displayed on each side and end of the vehicle.

The **gross weight** measurement of a product is the weight of the single item package plus its contents; so if there is one 55-gal (208-L) steel drum of chlorine that weighs 550 lb (249 kg), it is roughly 65 lb (29 kg) for the steel drum and 485 lb (220 kg) for the chlorine. The **aggregate weight** measurement combines all the packages to determine the total weight of the hazards. So if you have the same 55-gal (208-L) drum of chlorine weighing 550 lb (249 kg) and you are also transporting 1000 lb (454 kg) of ammonia, the aggregate weight of hazards is 1550 lb (703 kg).

A vehicle transporting hazardous materials is required to post warning placards when the gross weight of a single hazard or the aggregate weight of the combined hazards totals 1001 lb (454 kg) or more (**FIGURE 12-37**). Placards must be displayed for each product. Placards are also required for any explosives, poisonous gases, or radioactive materials, regardless of the weight. There is an exception to posting multiple placards when two or more classes of hazardous materials are loaded into the same vehicle and their aggregate weight is greater than 1001 lb (454 kg);

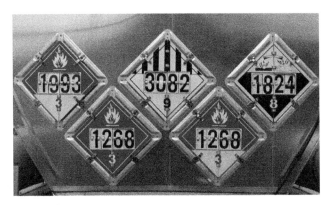

FIGURE 12-37 A placard is a large diamond-shaped indicator that is placed on all sides of transport vehicles that carry hazardous materials.
© Mark Winfrey/Shutterstock.

a placard displaying the word "DANGEROUS" can be used in lieu of separate placards to identify each hazard. The only exception to this is when 2205 lb (1000 kg) or more of a hazardous material consisting of a single hazard class is loaded on the vehicle; this requires a placard representing that hazard be displayed.

Hazardous materials classified as ORM-D materials (other regulated materials-domestic) can consist of a consumer commodity that is federally regulated but presents a limited hazard during transport and does not require hazard warning placards.

United Nations/North American Identification Numbers

United Nations/North American Hazardous Materials Code (UN/NA) identification numbers are another way to identify the hazardous material that is being transported. UN/NA identification numbers are given by the United Nations Committee of Experts on the Transport of Dangerous Goods.

When large quantities of a single hazardous material are transported by a vehicle or freight container in non-bulk packages, they must be marked on each side and each end with the UN/NA identification number specified for that hazardous material. The UN/NA number must be displayed on an orange label or on the placard itself. The following provisions and limitations must also apply:

- Each package is marked with the same proper shipping name and identification number.
- The aggregate gross weight of the hazardous material is 8820 lb (4000 kg) or more.
- All of the hazardous material is loaded at one loading facility.
- The transport vehicle or freight container contains no other material, hazardous, or otherwise.

Shipping Papers

Labels and placards may be helpful in identifying hazardous materials, but other sources of information are also available. Shipping papers are required by federal law to be carried on the transport vehicle when any hazardous materials are being transported. Shipping papers fully describe the content of the product(s) being transported. Several items must appear on all shipping papers, including:

- Identification of the shipper
- Identification of the receiver
- Hazard class or division
- UN/NA identification number
- Packing group number
- The total product quantity and weight with the exception of empty packages
- A 24-hour emergency contact number
- A certification statement certifying that the materials listed are the materials present
- The signature of the shipper and/or the shipper's agent verifying that all regulation requirements are met

Site Operations: Commercial Motor Vehicle

As stated earlier in this chapter, the greatest concern for the technical rescuer responding to a vehicle accident involving a CMV is hazardous materials. The cargo that the semi-tractor trailer or single frame box truck is transporting must be immediately identified before any physical approach or operation can commence. This one action, identifying a hazard, can mean the difference between a successful operation and a potential catastrophe.

Complete the following steps during the scene size-up involving a CMV:

- Survey the area and identify hazardous transport cargo through placard/UN number recognition.
- Dispatch additional resources—hazardous materials teams, a heavy tow unit (type C with an articulating boom), and other necessary resources.
- Locate the driver of the CMV if he or she is outside of the wreckage and is not injured, and confirm shipping cargo and location of shipping papers.
- Deploy at a minimum two 1.75-in. (44-mm) hose lines for protection, and consider an appropriate foam application for any significant fuel leaks.

- When it is deemed safe to enter, conduct the inner and outer surveys to clear all hazards within the operational area.
- Create hazard zones: hot, warm, and cold.
- Try to locate the shipping papers to confirm cargo before opening the cargo vessel/trailer.
- Stabilize all vehicles involved in the collision.
- Locate and disconnect the 12-volt DC battery system of the CMV and any other vehicle that may be involved.
- Disentangle and extricate the victim(s).

Victim Access: Commercial Motor Vehicle

One of the many challenges of a victim rescue and extrication involving a CMV is calculating the increased height of the cab because locating and accessing the victim requires the rescuer to be elevated by either stepping up onto the cab or utilizing another means of elevation. When conducting an inner survey upon arrival, the officer will have to make a complete 360-degree ground-level search around the CMV to clear all visual hazards and ensure the basic stability of the vehicle prior to stepping up onto the cab. Once the victim has been located and determined to be trapped or unable to self-extricate, the officer will call for additional resources and formulate the incident action plan (IAP), which will include the initial access/entry (Plan A), the removal/extrication (Plan B), and the emergency plan for unexpected contingencies that may occur. The officer will also need to set up hazard control zones (cold, warm, and hot), which can be enforced and maintained by utilizing the jurisdiction's law enforcement personnel. Next, the officer will determine the appropriate actions/procedures for stabilizing the vehicle. If the CMV is relatively stable, the entry (Plan A) can commence with one or two rescue personnel making entry into the vehicle to access the victim(s) and confirm the entrapment and procedure to carry out the removal/extrication (Plan B). Plan B may include removing doors, removing the roof, pushing the dash, and cutting into the rear cabin (**FIGURE 12-38**).

It is of vital importance that the IAP be communicated and acknowledged by all personnel to maintain safety, control, and continuity of the operation. All safety procedures must be strictly adhered to by all personnel and enforced by a designated safety officer or officers.

Several unique entrapment scenarios can occur, such as when a conventional vehicle rear impacts and underrides a semi-trailer. With this unique incident, there are safe and efficient techniques for lifting a semi-trailer off of the conventional vehicle

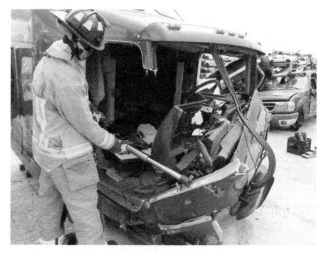

FIGURE 12-38 The removal/extrication (Plan B) may include removing doors, removing the roof, pushing the dash, and cutting into the rear cabin.
Courtesy of David Sweet.

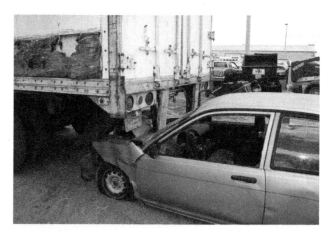

FIGURE 12-39 Conventional vehicles often underride semi-trailers.

(**FIGURE 12-39**). One of the fastest techniques to accomplish this task is to utilize a 50/60-ton tow truck with a rotating articulating boom. This tow unit can be used to lift the semi-trailer from the conventional vehicle utilizing two or more slings and a chain package, which are attached to the undercarriage of the trailer. This approach gives the tow operator full control of the trailer. The tow operator controls the boom's cable system with a remote controller box that he or she can operate at a safe distance in case anything should break and/or give way (**FIGURE 12-40**). A second, smaller tow truck or rated winching system should be positioned to pull the vehicle out from under the trailer to commence the rescue and extrication operations. The larger tow unit can also perform both functions by adding a snatch block and tackle. A snatch block consists of a single or multiple pulley system utilized to change cable direction (or limit line tension) toward the rear with a separate cable system, thus allowing removal of the vehicle simultaneously

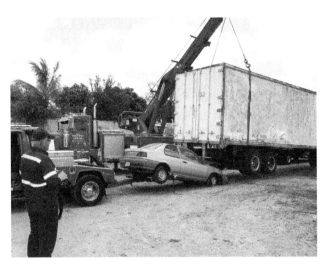

FIGURE 12-40 The tow operator operates the boom's cable system with a remote controller box that he or she can operate at a safe distance.

as the semi-trailer is raised. The larger 50/60-ton tow unit must be positioned at a specific angle for this to work, which may not be possible depending on how the wreckage presents. The technical rescuer must realize the importance of dispatching a tow unit immediately without delay.

Most states, as well as countries, have their own rating system to classify the size or towing/lifting capacity of a tow unit. There are also licensing standards and requirements that must be met to operate each type and size tow unit. The Towing and Recovery Association of America (TRAA) is a nonprofit organization for the towing industry that offers three levels of driver certification (Level III being the highest), depending on the type or classification of vehicle being driven.

LISTEN UP!

Tow units will be critical in some situations.
- Do you know how to contact this resource?
- What will be its response time?
- Have you trained with this resource?
- Do you have a backup plan?

After-Action REVIEW

IN SUMMARY

- The U.S. DOT defines a CMV as a motor vehicle or combination of motor vehicles used in commerce to transport passengers or property if the motor vehicle has a gross vehicle weight rating (GVWR) of 26,001 lb (11,794 kg) or more inclusive of a towed unit(s) with a GVWR of more than 10,000 lb (4536 kg); or a GVWR of 26,001 lb (11,794 kg) or more; or is designed to transport 16 or more passengers, including the driver; or is of any size and is used in the transportation of hazardous materials.
- CMVs also include box trucks, semi-tractor trailers, concrete mixers, vehicle transporters, buses, and cranes.
- Within the United States, the rules and regulations that are placed on CMVs are implemented through the DOT, which limits the amount of weight a CMV can transport, including the type of cargo being hauled with these vehicles.
- CMVs are classified into eight weight categories.
- One of the greatest concerns for the technical rescuer responding to a motor vehicle accident involving a CMV is the potential for that CMV to be transporting hazardous materials and for that cargo's or vessel's integrity to be compromised.
- Federal law requires placards to be clearly displayed on each side and end of the vehicle. UN/NA identification numbers are another way to identify the hazardous material that is being transported.
- There are five types or classifications of tow units to assist in a CMV extrication.

KEY TERMS

Aggregate weight A measurement combining all packages in a CMV to determine the total weight of all the hazards.

Air brake (parking brake) A brake used on some models of CMVs that causes the suspension system to release air and drop several inches to accommodate a resting or parked position.

Air ride system A system designed to inflate and deflate the suspension through onboard air pressure tanks to protect the cargo and the frame system of the vehicle.

Axle A structural component or shaft that is designed for wheel rotation.

Cab The enclosed space where the driver and passengers sit.

Cab beside engine (CBE) Design in which the driver sits next to the engine. These trucks are mostly found in shipyards and baggage carriers within airports and seaports.

Cab over engine (COE) (often referred to as a tilt cab) Design in which the cab is lifted over the engine to gain access to the engine itself. The driver's seat is positioned over the engine and the front axle.

Cargo tank Bulk packaging that is permanently attached to or forms a part of a motor vehicle or that is not permanently attached to any motor vehicle and that, because of its size, construction, or attachment to a motor vehicle, is loaded or unloaded without being removed from the motor vehicle.

Class 1 commercial vehicle A vehicle with a gross vehicle weight rating ranging from 0 to 6000 lb (0 to 2722 kg).

Class 2a commercial vehicle A vehicle with a gross vehicle weight rating ranging from 6001 to 8500 lb (2722 to 3856 kg); a light-duty vehicle.

Class 2b commercial vehicle A vehicle with a gross vehicle weight rating ranging from 8501 to 10,000 lb (3856 to 4536 kg); considered by many as a light-duty vehicle.

Class 3 commercial vehicle A vehicle with a gross vehicle weight rating ranging from 10,001 to 14,000 lb (4536 to 6350 kg).

Class 4 commercial vehicle A vehicle with a gross vehicle weight rating ranging from 14,001 to 16,000 lb (6351 to 7257 kg).

Class 5 commercial vehicle A vehicle with a gross vehicle weight rating ranging from 16,001 to 19,500 lb (7258 to 8845 kg).

Class 6 commercial vehicle A vehicle with a gross vehicle weight rating ranging from 19,501 to 26,000 lb (8846 to 11,793 kg).

Class 7 commercial vehicle A vehicle with a gross vehicle weight rating ranging from 26,001 to 33,000 lb (11,794 to 14,969 kg).

Class 8 commercial vehicle A vehicle with a gross vehicle weight rating of more than 33,000 lb (14,969 kg).

Commercial motor vehicle (CMV) Defined by the DOT as a motor vehicle or combination of motor vehicles used in commerce to transport passengers or property if the motor vehicle has a gross vehicle weight rating (GVWR) of 26,001 lb (11,794 kg) or more inclusive of a towed unit(s) with a GVWR of more than 10,000 lb (4536 kg); or has a GVWR of 26,001 lb (11,794 kg) or more; or is designed to transport 16 or more passengers, including the driver; or is of any size and is used in the transportation of hazardous materials.

Conventional cab Design in which the driver's seat is positioned behind the engine and front axle. The front end of the vehicle extends approximately 6 to 8 ft (1.8 to 2.4 m) from the front windshield.

Dead axle An axle used for load support more commonly set in the front section of a semi-truck; also functions for steering and is therefore also known as a steer axle.

Drive train (power train) A system that transfers rotational power from the engine to the wheels, which makes the vehicle move.

Dromedary (drom) A separate box, deck, or plate mounted behind the cab and in front of the fifth wheel on the frame of a semi-truck.

Dry bulk cargo tanks A tank designed to carry dry bulk goods such as powders, pellets, fertilizers, or grain. Such tanks are generally V-shaped with rounded sides that funnel toward the bottom of the tank.

Emergency air line (supply line) One of two air lines of an air brake system connecting a tractor to a trailer; the emergency air line is red.

Emergency brake A brake that utilizes a combination of both the service and parking brakes to engage when a brake failure or air line break occurs.

Fifth wheel A turntable hitch mounted at the rear of the towing truck or semi-truck.

Glad hands Couplers that are used to supply air to the braking system of the trailer.

Gross combined weight rating (GCWR) A rating set by the vehicle manufacturer that determines the vehicle's cargo capacity limitations.

Gross vehicle weight rating (GVWR) A rating set by the manufacturer; it shall not be less than the sum of the unloaded vehicle weight, rated cargo load, and 150 lb times the vehicle's designated seating capacity (49 CFR 567.4[g] [3]).

Gross weight The weight of the single item package plus its contents.

Hazardous material A substance or material including an explosive; radioactive material; infectious substance; flammable or combustible liquid, solid, or gas; toxic, oxidizing, or corrosive material; and compressed gas that the Secretary of Transportation has determined is capable of posing an unreasonable risk to health, safety, and property when transported in commerce and has been designated as hazardous under Section 5103.

Hybrid-electric commercial motor vehicle (HECMV) A CMV that utilizes either the internal combustion engine or an electric motor for propulsion.

Kingpin A large locking pin that connects the cargo trailer of a semi-tractor trailer or semi-trailer to the semi-truck or tractor.

Landing gear A stabilizing device that can be lowered to support a trailer when not attached to the tractor. This device is usually operated manually by a hand crank.

Lift axle An axle that can be raised or lowered by an air suspension system to increase the weight-carrying capacity of the vehicle or to distribute the cargo weight more evenly across all the axles.

Live axle An axle that transmits propulsion or causes the wheels to turn.

MC-306/DOT 406 flammable liquid tanker A tanker that typically carries between 6000 and 10,000 gal (22,712 and 37,854 L) of a product such as gasoline or other flammable and combustible materials. The tank is nonpressurized.

MC-307/DOT 407 chemical hauler A tanker with a rounded or horseshoe-shaped tank capable of holding 6000 to 7000 gal (22,712 to 37,854 L) of flammable liquid, mild corrosives, and poisons. The tank has a high internal working pressure.

MC-312/DOT 412 corrosives tanker A tanker that often carries aggressive (highly reactive) acids such as concentrated sulfuric and nitric acid. It is characterized by several heavy-duty reinforcing rings around the tank and holds approximately 6000 gal (22,712 L) of product.

MC-331 pressure cargo tanker A tanker that carries materials such as ammonia, propane, Freon, and butane. This type of tank is commonly constructed of steel and has rounded ends and a single open compartment inside. The liquid volume inside the tank varies from the 1000-gal (3785-L) delivery truck to the full-size 11,000-gal (41,640-L) cargo tank.

MC-338 cryogenic tanker A low-pressure tanker designed to maintain the low temperature required by the cryogens it carries. A boxlike structure containing the tank control valves is typically attached to the rear of the tanker.

Semi-tractor trailer (semi-trailer) A semi-truck, or semi-tractor, combined with a trailer; normally designed with three axles, one in the front for steering purposes and two tandem axles in the rear.

Semi-truck A commercial truck capable of towing a separate trailer, which has wheels at only one end (semi-trailer); may also be referred to as a tractor.

Service air line One of two air lines of an air brake system connecting a tractor to a trailer; the emergency air line is blue.

Service brake The usual driving brake that is applied by the driver to slow and/or stop the vehicle during normal driving operations.

Sleeper A compartment attached to the cab of a truck that allows the driver to rest while making stops during a long transport.

Tube trailers A high-volume transportation device made up of several individual compressed gas cylinders banded together and affixed to a trailer. Tube trailers carry compressed gases such as hydrogen, oxygen, helium, and methane. One trailer may carry several different gases in individual tubes.

On Scene

As the officer assigned to an engine company, you are dispatched to a commercial motor vehicle accident involving two trucks. On arrival you can see that a large semi-tractor trailer with a box trailer has side-impacted a MC-331 propane delivery truck. The delivery tank truck is lying on its side.

1. What is the greatest initial concern for this incident?
   - **A.** The number of victims
   - **B.** The number of personnel needed
   - **C.** The size of the semi-tractor trailer
   - **D.** Whether there are hazardous materials involved

2. Most wheels on a commercial motor vehicle can be flattened by cutting the air intake valve and releasing the air.
   - **A.** True
   - **B.** False

(continues)

On Scene Continued

3. Air brake lines are colored-coded red for the emergency brakes and blue assigned for the:
   A. electrical lines.
   B. water line.
   C. service brake.
   D. air release for the tanks.

4. An air ride system is designed to _____ through onboard air pressure tanks.
   A. protect the cargo and the frame system of the vehicle
   B. inflate and deflate the suspension
   C. inflate the passenger seats
   D. run at as little as 20 psi (138 kPa)

5. The cab of a traditional cab over engine (COE) design:
   A. can tilt forward to expose the engine.
   B. is secured to the frame and cannot tilt forward.
   C. has four doors.
   D. is known as a conventional design.

6. A fifth wheel located on a tractor:
   A. acts as a spare tire in case of a flat.
   B. can be dropped down in position to handle heavy loads.
   C. connects the trailer to the tractor by means of a kingpin located on the trailer.
   D. is the swivel used to turn the boom of a large tow truck.

7. In order to identify the contents of either truck, the rescuer may consult:
   A. shipping papers.
   B. placards on the vehicle(s).
   C. the shape of the container.
   D. All of these

8. The U.S. Department of Transportation defines a Commercial Motor Vehicle (CMV) as:
   A. semi-tractor trailers.
   B. box trucks.
   C. box trucks and concrete mixers.
   D. box trucks, semi-tractor trailers, concrete mixers, vehicle transporters, buses, and cranes.

9. Design in which the driver's seat is positioned behind the engine and front axle.
   A. Cab over engine
   B. Cab forward
   C. Conventional cab
   D. Short-nosed cab

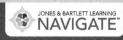 *Access Navigate for more activities.*

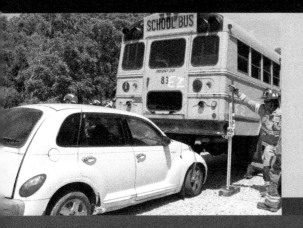

CHAPTER 13

Heavy Vehicle Incidents

School Buses

KNOWLEDGE OBJECTIVES

After studying this chapter, you will be able to:

- Define body-over-frame construction and explain its role in vehicle rescue incidents. (p. 357)
- Describe the four types of buses and four types of school buses and their subcategories. (pp. 356–357)
- Describe the anatomy and structure of a school bus. (pp. 357–360)
- List access points and emergency exits present in school buses. (pp. 357–360)
- Identify fire suppression and safety measures. (pp. 393–394, 394–395)
- Evaluate school bus stabilization needs. (pp. 363–367)
- Consider isolation methods and scene safety at school bus incidents. (pp. 360–361)
- Identify and document resource needs for future use. (pp. 360–363)
- Factor in time constraints for a school bus extrication incident. (pp. 360–363)
- Establish emergency escape routes for rescuers at school bus incidents. (pp. 360–363, 367–390)
- Enforce agency safety and emergency procedures in school bus incidents. (pp. 360–363)
- Identify the mechanisms of heavy vehicle movement and AHJ policies and procedures. (pp. 360–363)
- Identify the types of stabilization devices, stabilization points, and vehicle construction. (pp. 363–367)
- Manage commercial/heavy-vehicle systems and evaluate their beneficial use. (pp. 362, 366–368)
- Isolate and manage potential harmful energy sources. (pp. 393–394)
- Disentangle victims from a school bus. (pp. 367–390)
- Prevent victim injury. (pp. 360–363)

SKILLS OBJECTIVES

After studying this chapter, you will be able to perform the following skills:

- Create an incident action plan for a school bus incident. (pp. 360–363)
- Conduct initial and ongoing size-up for a school bus extrication. (pp. 360–363)
- Shut down a running commercial motor vehicle engine. (pp. 363, 365, 366, 370, 372, 374, 376, 378, 380, 383, 385, 388, 391, 393)
- Stabilize a school bus in upright, side, or inverted position. (pp. 363–367)
- Maintain heavy-vehicle stabilization during extrication. (pp. 363–369)
- Stabilize/marry a school bus on top of another vehicle. (pp. 368–369)

- Identify locations of victim(s). (pp. 367–390)
- Designate entry and exit points for victims, rescuers, and equipment. (pp. 367–368, 373–374, 376–382)
- Gain access into a school bus by removing the front windshield. (pp. 370–371)
- Remove a bench seat from a school bus. (pp. 372–373)
- Remove a section of the sidewall of a school bus. (pp. 374–375)
- Gain access through the roof of a school bus on its side. (pp. 376–377)
- Gain access through the rear door of a school bus in its normal position. (pp. 378–379)
- Gain access through the rear door of a school bus resting on its side. (pp. 380–381)
- Gain access through the front door of a school bus in its normal position. (pp. 383–384)
- Remove a victim from under a school bus resting on its side utilizing FRJs. (pp. 385–387)
- Remove a victim from under a school bus resting on its side utilizing air-lift bags. (pp. 388–389)
- Relocate a steering column in a school bus. (p. 390)
- Lift a school bus off an underride. (pp. 391–392)
- Disable the hybrid system on a type C or D school bus. (p. 395)

You Are the Rescuer

As the officer on the engine, you and your crew are first on the scene of a motor vehicle accident involving a dump truck that side-impacted a type C school bus, flipping the school bus onto its side. There are multiple adolescent students on the bus with injuries.

1. Does your agency have a pre-established emergency plan or mass casualty incident (MCI) protocols to manage this type of incident?
2. What resources do you have that can be immediately dispatched or utilized?
3. Have you trained for such an incident, and can you initiate a START (simple triage and rapid treatment) system utilizing the crew on hand?
4. What is your incident action plan (IAP)?

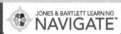

Access Navigate for more practice activities.

Introduction

This chapter covers material above the advanced technician level requirements in Chapter 8 of NFPA 1006, *Standard for Technical Rescuer Professional Qualifications*. This chapter presents bus anatomy and extrication operations utilizing a school bus. School buses are detailed in this chapter as an example of a commercial motor vehicle (CMV) and to help demonstrate the concepts of vehicle rescue and extrication for mass-casualty incidents (MCIs) involving CMVs (see Chapter 12, *Commercial Trucks*, for the definition of a CMV and a detailed description of the gross vehicle weight rating).

There is great diversity in the types of buses on the roadways today; accurately describing or classifying a bus can be difficult at best. The Federal Motor Carrier Safety Administration categorizes buses into carrier types or by function or purpose:

- **School bus:** Any public or private school or district, or contracted carrier operating on behalf of the entity, providing transportation for kindergarteners through grade 12 pupils (**FIGURE 13-1**).
- **Transit bus:** An entity providing passenger transportation over fixed, scheduled routes, within primarily urban geographic areas (**FIGURE 13-2**).
- **Intercity bus:** A company providing for-hire, long-distance passenger transportation between cities over fixed routes with regular schedules (**FIGURE 13-3**).

CHAPTER 13 School Buses **355**

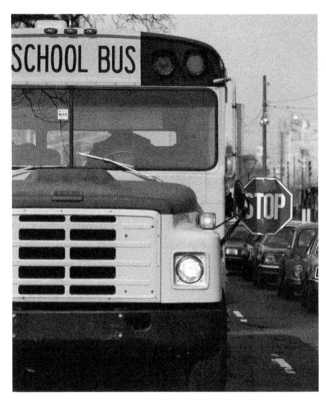

FIGURE 13-1 School bus.
© Photodisc/Getty Images.

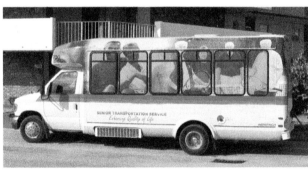

FIGURE 13-2 Transit bus.
Courtesy of David Sweet.

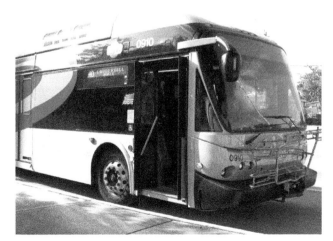

FIGURE 13-3 Intercity bus.
Courtesy of David Sweet.

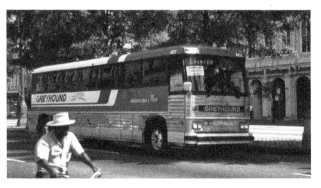

FIGURE 13-4 Charter or tour bus.
© Sylvia Pitcher Photolibrary/Alamy Stock Photo.

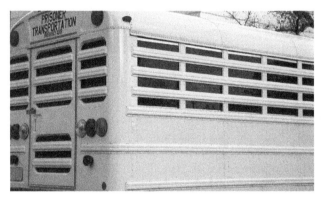

FIGURE 13-5 Other types of buses may include a department of corrections bus.
© Henryk Sadura/Alamy Stock Photo.

- **Charter/tour bus:** A company providing transportation on a for-hire basis, usually round-trip service for a tour group or outing. The transportation can be for a specific event or can be part of a regular tour (**FIGURE 13-4**).
- *Other:* All bus operations not included in the previous categories. Examples include private companies providing transportation to their own employees, nongovernmental organizations such as churches or nonprofit groups, noneducational units of government such as departments of corrections, and private individuals (**FIGURE 13-5**).

Classifying a particular bus type is further complicated because these buses can be interchanged and used for any of these purposes, depending on what country or region of the world you are in.

School Buses

On any given school day, there are multiple school buses crossing your path or traveling alongside of you. You may not even acknowledge their presence because they are just as common as any other vehicle on the road. The National Highway Traffic Safety

Administration (NHTSA) has reported that there are approximately 474,000 public school buses on the roads traveling approximately 4.3 billion miles annually to transport 23.5 million children and adolescents to and from school and school-related activities.

The NHTSA lists school bus travel as one of the safest forms of transportation, reporting approximately 0.001 accidents per every 100 million miles traveled. As an emergency responder, you may never come across a school bus accident, but it is vital to be prepared and know the makeup, structural components, and types of school buses that are on the roadways today.

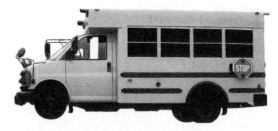

FIGURE 13-6 Type A school bus.
© Hemera/Thinkstock.

> **LISTEN UP!**
>
> The National Highway Traffic Safety Administration (NHTSA) has reported that there are approximately 474,000 public school buses traveling our roadways today.

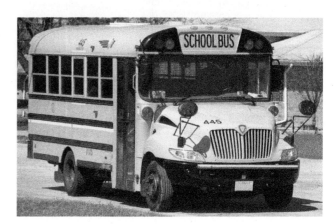

FIGURE 13-7 Type B school bus.
© Matt/Fotolia.

The U.S. Department of Transportation (DOT), through the NHTSA, issued statute 49 U.S.C. section 30125, which defines a "school bus" as any vehicle that is designed for carrying a driver and more than 10 passengers and that NHTSA decides is likely to be "used significantly" to transport "pre-primary, primary, and secondary" students to or from school or related events (including school-sponsored field trips and athletic events). The NHTSA has two classifications for school buses—small (gross vehicle weight rating [GVWR] of less than 10,000 lb [4536 kg]) and large (GVWR that is equal to or greater than 10,000 lb [4536 kg]). The school bus industry designates four classifications of school buses, with several subclassifications; be aware that these classifications can differ in various areas of the country or internationally. The occupant capacity for each type will also vary depending on different manufacturers' specifications. Regardless of the variations, all four types of school buses, including the subclassifications, must meet all Federal Motor Vehicle Safety Standards (FMVSS) for school buses:

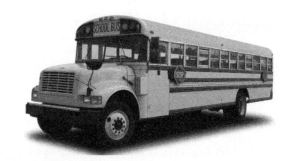

FIGURE 13-8 Type C school bus.
© Hemera/Thinkstock.

- **Type A school bus:** This type of school bus is a conversion type or bus constructed utilizing a cutaway front section vehicle with a left-side driver's door (**FIGURE 13-6**). This definition includes two subclassifications:
  - Type A-1, with a GVWR of 14,500 lb (6577 kg) or less
  - Type A-2, with a GVWR greater than 14,500 lb (6577 kg) and less than or equal to 21,500 lb (9752 kg)
- **Type B school bus:** This type of school bus is constructed utilizing a stripped chassis.

The entrance door is behind the front wheels (**FIGURE 13-7**). This definition includes two subclassifications:
  - Type B-1, with a GVWR of 10,000 lb (4536 kg) or less
  - Type B-2, with a GVWR greater than 10,000 lb (4536 kg)
- **Type C school bus:** This type of school bus, also known as a conventional school bus, is constructed utilizing a chassis with a hood and front fender assembly. The entrance door is behind the front wheels (**FIGURE 13-8**). These buses have a GVWR greater than 21,500 lb (9752 kg). Eighty-five to 90 percent of all school buses are type C or D.
- **Type D school bus:** This type of school bus, also known as a "transit-style" rear or front

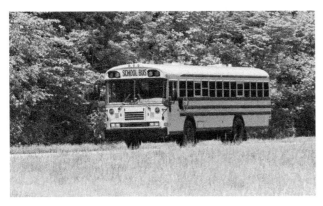

FIGURE 13-9 Type D school bus.
© iStockphoto/Thinkstock.

engine school bus, is constructed utilizing a stripped chassis where the outer body of the bus is mounted to the bare chassis. The entrance door is ahead of the front wheels, and the face or front section of the bus is flat (**FIGURE 13-9**). Type D buses have a passenger capacity of 80 to 90 people.

School Bus Anatomy

A school bus is designed with a body-over-frame construction. The body of the bus is composed of a full skeletal frame system consisting of steel trusses and studs, which are attached to and reinforced by steel crossmembers running the entire length of the bus. This body frame is encapsulated by inner and outer sheet metal panels. These inner and outer panels consist of 22- to 24-gauge steel and generally have fiberglass insulation inside that ranges from 1 to 1.5 in. (2.5 to 3.8 cm) thick for noise reduction and thermal protection.

The overall design features of the bus, such as metal thickness and spacing of channel beams, may vary among manufacturers, but all the features must meet the FMVSS for school buses. The standards include:

- Length of the bus shall not be greater than 45 ft (14 m).
- Width of the bus shall not be greater than 102 in. (2591 mm).
- Inside body height of the bus shall measure 72 in. (1829 mm) or more.
- Width of aisles will be at least 12 in. (305 mm), as measured from seat cushion to seat cushion with the top of the seat backs tapering inward, extending the spacing to a minimum of 15 in. (381 mm) in width.
- Aisle clearance for wheelchair accessibility will be at least 30 in. (762 mm) to the closest emergency door and/or lift area.
- School buses equipped with a power lift or a ramp shall have aisles a minimum of 30 in. (762 mm) wide leading from the wheelchair or other type of mobility device area to the emergency door, power lift, or ramp service entrance.

Chassis Frame

The chassis frame of the school bus consists of two long steel channel beams of 8- to 10-gauge steel that have steel crossmembers of 14-gauge steel. The crossmembers can vary in spacing but normally can be spaced up to 12 in. (305 mm) apart. Because of the extremely difficult work involved, the potential time expended, and the large amount of heavy-gauge steel located in this area, attempting to gain entry through the floor should not be attempted unless there are no other areas or alternative techniques to gain entry. Attached to the frame are components such as the engine, suspension system, fuel tank, wheels, and front and rear axles.

SAFETY TIP

Because of the extremely difficult work involved, the potential time expended, and the large amount of heavy-gauge steel located in this area, attempting to gain entry through the floor should not be attempted unless there are no other areas or alternative techniques to gain entry.

Floor Deck

The floor deck is composed of 14-gauge sheet metal panels, which are attached to the chassis frame. Plywood of 0.5- or 0.625-in (13- or 16-mm) thickness is fastened over the steel deck and covered with a thick corrugated rubber or vinyl matting. Because of the thickness of the floor, attempting any entry into the bus through the floor area is not recommended.

Bow Frame Trusses

The main body frame structure consists of steel sidewall **bow trusses** that run continuously from below the floor level on one side of the bus, vertically raising and bowing over to form the roof structure, and then extending over and down the other side of the bus, past the floor level. These structural members or ribs make up the support frame of the school bus and are normally composed of 12-gauge steel. Each roof pillar or side window frame makes up one of these structural members and has the crash and rub

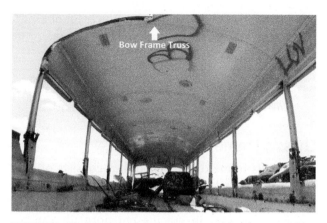

FIGURE 13-10 Bow frame trusses and stringers add structural support.
Courtesy of David Sweet.

rails attached to it along with exterior and interior sheet metal panels (**FIGURE 13-10**). The locations and spacing of these trusses are easy to determine because of the exterior rivets that attach the interior and exterior panels to the trusses. To give these bow frame truss members structural support at the roof level, steel longitudinal **stringers** are added that run continuously from the front of the school bus to the rear. Stringers consist of 16-gauge steel. There can be up to four stringers split, with two on each side of the roof emergency hatch.

Rub Rails

Rub rails, or guard rails, are visible exterior steel attachments that consist of 16-gauge corrugated metal. These steel members are 4 in. (102 mm) or more in width and are attached to the bow trusses. They run the entire length of the school bus, wrapping around to the rear of the vehicle. Rub rails are easily identifiable because they are usually painted black against the yellow background of the bus itself; from a distance, they look like black stripes running the length of the vehicle. These rub rails are strategically placed with the bottom rail positioned at the floor line and the middle rail positioned at the area of the seat cushion level. There can also be a top rail that ties into the bottom of the side and rear window frames.

Crash Rail

The **crash rail** is normally composed of 14-gauge steel and extends the entire length of the school bus just above the floor area between the floor and seat rub rail. As the name suggests, the crash rail is designed to protect the students from impact intrusions into the passenger compartment.

Entrance Door

The entrance door of the bus is designed in a two-section, split-type style and opens outward whereby the door folds to one side or the other. Other opening configurations may be encountered on older school buses, but they are less common than the outward-swinging type. The passenger door is located on the right side of the bus, opposite and in direct view of the driver. The opening can measure 24 in. (610 mm) in width and 68 in. (1727 mm) in height. On a type C bus, the front passenger door is located behind the front wheels, and on a type D bus, it is located in front of the wheels. The front door can be manually operated with a lever bar that the driver controls from his or her seat. The door may also be opened and closed with an air-actuated mechanism that pressurizes and releases air through a switch. This mechanism is also operated by the driver. In addition, an air-actuated door has a clearly marked emergency release valve that can be located on the upper right side or to the left or the right of the entryway; locations will vary among manufacturers. All entrance door glass is composed of tempered safety or laminated glass and is held in place by a gasket seal that can be manually removed, and the glass panels can be pushed in to release from the frame.

Emergency Exits

Rear doors are designed to swing outward from left to right, with the hinges being on the right side of the door (**FIGURE 13-11**). There are multiple types of hinge attachments that the technical rescuer might find on a rear or side door, such as piano-type hinges; three-bolt hinges; single-strap hinges; or nonexposed hinges, which may be on the inside of the school bus. The rear door on a school bus is a main access or egress point depending on the location of the victims and position of the bus itself.

Transit-style, or type D, school buses do not have a rear door because of the rear-mount engine design. This type of school bus will have an emergency escape window just above the engine access hatch; type D buses also have a side door, generally located in the middle section of the bus. There may also be special service entrance doors for repair technicians or wheelchair accessibility doors.

> **LISTEN UP!**
>
> The technical rescuer might encounter multiple types of hinge attachments on a rear or side door, such as piano-type hinges; three-bolt hinges; single-strap hinges; or nonexposed hinges, which may be on the inside of the school bus.

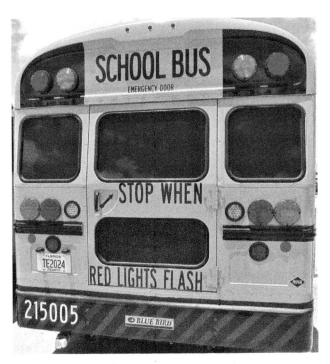

FIGURE 13-11 The rear emergency exit.
Courtesy of David Sweet.

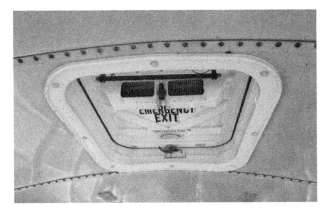

FIGURE 13-12 Emergency roof exits are operable from both inside and outside the vehicle.
© Jones & Bartlett Learning. Photographed by Glen E. Ellman.

Side Window Exits

Side windows can be composed of either tempered safety or laminated glass, depending on the manufacturer. Each side window has an opening of at least 9 in. (229 mm) in height but no more than 13 in. (330 mm) and at least 22 in. (559 mm) in width. The windows are designed to slide down to open. Some buses may also contain one window on each side of the bus that may be less than 22 in. (559 mm) wide. Side windows can easily be removed by cutting the attachment clips or bolts with a pneumatic air chisel and a prying tool (refer to Skill Drill 13-7 for an explanation of this).

The release mechanism of emergency windows follows FMVSS No. 217, *Bus Emergency Exits and Window Retention and Release*. Emergency windows are designed to release the entire frame, remaining hinged on only one side, which thus affords the escapee the full height and width of the opening. Removal of front windshield glass is discussed later in the chapter, including a skill drill technique for removal of the front windshield for gaining access into the vehicle.

Emergency Roof Hatches

Emergency roof exits are hinged on the front or forward side and are operable from both inside and outside the vehicle (**FIGURE 13-12**). The total opening is 16.5 in. (410 mm). The opening is large enough for a person self-escaping or entering the bus, but it is too narrow to allow a victim secured to a backboard to pass through.

Bench Seats

Standard bench seats are designed to have a 1-in. (25-mm) tubular steel frame and two outer leg posts attached to the floor by bolts or screws. The inside of the bench seat, which rests against the sidewall of the bus, is screwed or bolted to a lip that extends from the interior "skin" approximately 1 in. (25 mm). The one exception to this design are the seats located in the emergency egress way, whether it is a door or window; in this location, the seat section of the bench lifts up out of the way to make room for escapees.

Driver's Seat

The driver's seat is typically a single high-back chair with a fully integrated three-point seat belt harness. It is normally designed with an air-actuated suspension-type system (air ride), which is manually operated to the desired height of the driver.

Battery Compartment

The school bus batteries are secured on a pull-out sliding tray that is positioned inside the vehicle body and generally located near the front of the vehicle on the driver's side (**FIGURE 13-13**). There are normally two or more 12-volt direct current (DC) batteries connected in parallel configuration to increase the

LISTEN UP!

There are normally two or more 12-volt DC batteries positioned on a pull-out tray that are connected in parallel configuration to increase the amperage output.

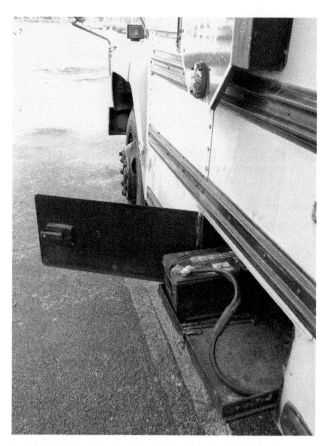

FIGURE 13-13 School bus batteries are secured on a pull-out sliding tray in the body and are generally located near the front of the vehicle on the driver's side.

amperage output. In type A and some type B buses, the batteries are normally located in the engine compartment similar to the battery's location in a conventional vehicle.

Exhaust After-Treatment Device

The Environmental Protection Agency (EPA) set emission control standards for all diesel-fueled engines built after January 2007. The standards called for a 90 percent reduction of particulate matter (soot and ash) and a 55 percent reduction of nitrogen oxide (NOx).

In compliance with the EPA standards, the school bus industry installed an **exhaust after-treatment device**, which replaced the standard muffler assembly. This device captures and converts soot to carbon dioxide and water through the combination of a diesel particulate filter (DPF) and a diesel oxidation catalyst (DOC). This conversion process is called regeneration, which entails three stages: passive, active, and manual. **Passive regeneration** occurs automatically when the particulate matter (soot) that is caught in the DPF is burned off naturally by the elevated temperatures of the exhaust system. When passive regeneration does not oxidize the soot sufficiently, the onboard computer system operates in an **active regeneration** mode. In this mode, fuel is injected into the system to burn and create higher temperatures, up to 1112°F (600°C). **Manual regeneration** occurs only when the parking brake is set and the engine is running. Manual regeneration is normally completed when the active regeneration fails to clear the system sufficiently. All three regeneration modes will engage automatically by the computer system independently of the driver's actions.

Site Operations: School Buses

One of the greatest concerns for the officer in charge at a school bus rescue and extrication incident is gaining and maintaining control of the incident through proper scene management and maintaining safety. Proper scene management is critical and can mean the difference between a successful, controlled operation and an operation where chaos and freelancing occur, jeopardizing the safety of victims and personnel. Any vehicle rescue and extrication incident with multiple victims (especially children) can be overwhelming to the first arriving officer. By applying the basic principles of incident management, breaking things down into manageable segments, and creating an IAP, the officer will gain control of the incident and gain confidence in his or her decision making. The jurisdiction's standard operating procedures (SOPs) on managing technical rescue incidents as well as all safety procedures must be adhered to and strictly enforced to avoid freelancing and stress-related actions. Ensure the proper planning for managing an incident such as that necessary for a large CMV such as a school bus. When agencies conduct preplanning for school bus accidents, local school authorities should be contacted and included in the planning. Many schools have a transportation emergency plan to ensure the accountability, safety, and security of the children. The first 10 to 15 minutes of the incident usually set the tone for how the operation goes. In these first minutes, everything is coming at the officer in charge at such a fast rate that the process of critical thinking can easily max out. The first rule for managing and gaining control of an incident is self-control. Think about what the priorities and objectives are for the incident:

- Size-up (scene safety)
- Scene stabilization (inner and outer surveys, hazard control zones, establishing the IAP)
- Resources available and needed (personnel, equipment, and apparatus), including the proper management of those resources

- Vehicle stabilization
- Victim access and management: START system (victim stabilization)
- Removal/extrication of victims
- Terminating the incident

Size-Up: Stabilize the Scene

Size-up begins with the initial dispatch of the incident. With a school bus incident, the officer should immediately ascertain from dispatch the number of occupants so the proper number of emergency response units can initially be dispatched; the number of response units can be adjusted and confirmed on arrival. Air rescue (if available to the jurisdiction) should also be placed on standby. Other factors must also be considered; time of day for traffic, weather, general geographic topography, and area can all play a factor in creating added contingencies.

Upon arrival, the officer must visually assess the scene for any notable hazards that will create obstacles for other incoming units or any immediate dangers to life and health that will halt all operations, such as electrical power lines involved in the incident. The officer may encounter a school bus on fire, which will require immediate suppression before any rescue operation can occur. As a safety measure, two hose lines should be laid out and charged at every school bus incident involving a rescue and extrication to prepare for any unexpected contingencies that may occur. The officer must also recognize the type of school bus involved, which can give an indication of the potential number of victims, as well as the position of the school bus (e.g., upright, on its side, etc.).

The initial report must also include the damage assessment of minor, moderate, or heavy, with additional resources requested or canceled based on this initial assessment. The inner and outer surveys are then initiated, with the company officer conducting the inner survey. Thorough inner and outer surveys will give the officer the proper information to identify and confirm known hazards as well as the number, general disposition, and general age of the victims to formulate the IAP. This identification of victims is not a medical triage but rather only a part of the information-gathering process to better request and/or allocate resources.

The IAP will include the initial access/entry (Plan A), the removal/extrication (Plan B), and the emergency plan for unexpected contingencies that may occur. Also, included with the IAP is setting up hazard control zones along with designated entry and exit areas for emergency personnel and victims. The entry and exit areas have to be separate because equipment and personnel can interfere with the removal and transfer of victims if these areas are combined.

The initial Plan A will include vehicle stabilization requirements before any entry is conducted. Plan A will also encompass the identification of the initial entry point for conducting the START system, which will quickly identify critical and noncritical victims. All noncritical, mobile victims will be removed, and trauma facilities will be notified of pending victims and triage findings. The incident commander (IC) will also have to initiate an incident clock through dispatch to monitor on-scene time, which is not only a critical component of victim care but also critical for monitoring the overall physical stress on emergency personnel operating on scene. Extended amount of work time on scene or within inclement weather will require crews to be rotated in a designated rehab area.

Plan B will encompass any procedures required to gain access and remove victims who are trapped and/or unable to self-extricate.

The emergency escape plan will vary based on each incident type and what is presented. It could be as simple as engaging the air horn on the closest apparatus three times at 30-second intervals, which will instruct all personnel to evacuate the hot zone immediately and meet at a designated area, preferably within the cold zone. All personnel must acknowledge and adhere to the emergency plan.

Stabilize the Vehicle

Once the scene has been determined to be safe, the overall stability of the vehicle shall be evaluated and the proper procedures enacted to ensure the vehicle is safe to operate on. Stabilizing a school bus or other CMV can be as simple as engaging the parking brake, turning off the engine, and chocking the wheels if the vehicle is upright with minimal structural damage. Stabilizing a school bus or other CMV, on the other hand, may be very complex and require heavy equipment and additional resources to accomplish a safe environment in which to work.

Stabilize the Victim(s)

Utilizing the existing front entry and side or rear exit to maintain the operational flow of personnel entering the vehicle and exiting with victims is the optimal setting. Physical interventions such as removing seats, sidewalls, and window frames or cutting an opening into a roof area to create an entry or exit point will require precise planning and coordination. Additionally, to conduct these type of procedures, personnel must be qualified.

Planning

Preplanning, or strategic planning, is the key to success for any organization. A needs assessment study covers a wide range of topics and basically answers the question of where the organization wants to be in relation to providing the necessary level of emergency services for the type of community it serves (see Chapter 2 for a discussion of the needs assessment). This model incorporates both long- and short-range goals for the organization.

A **SWOT analysis** (strengths, weaknesses, opportunities, and threats), which is mainly used in a corporate business environment, is a self-examination model that can be adjusted, adapted, and applied to any situation, incident, or project, large or small, that an organization is currently or will be involved in. Not many emergency organizations use this type of self-evaluation model, but it can be an invaluable resource tool for quickly addressing deficiencies and elevating an agency to the next level. If you were to apply a SWOT analysis to operating at a school bus rescue, you would consider questions such as the following:

- *Strengths*: What are the overall capabilities of the agency, including levels and types of training and pre-established response plans, to successfully operate at this type of incident with minimal to no hindrances?
- *Weaknesses*: What are the possible operational deficiencies that could cause the operation to fail? Is there a lack of adequate staffing, equipment, apparatus, or training?
- *Opportunities*: Are there any training opportunities, MCI drills, equipment needs, mutual aid agreements, or grant funding to help elevate the readiness stage and response capabilities of the organization?
- *Threats*: Are there any external elements such as inclement weather or time of season that would change the emergency plan or create additional challenges to overcome? Is it 98°F (36.7°C) with full sun exposure or 10°F (–12°C) in snow or ice?

Remember that this SWOT analysis of your organization is fully expandable, but to be effective, the analysis must be complete, honest, and objective.

Progressive agencies have preplanned and trained heavily for such an event and already have pre-established MCI protocols and/or emergency response plans that are in place. Depending on how your agency's MCI plan is set up, a level 3 MCI for your area may involve 50 or more victims, 10 transport units, and 8 fire apparatus automatically dispatched. Even the best plans fail if they are not properly carried out. As a technical rescuer or an officer in charge, you need to be prepared to properly manage this type of incident. If you do not have a pre-established plan, a suggestion would be to assign a resource, or staging officer with a separate response channel for all incoming units, keeping the operations, or tactical, channel free of unnecessary traffic. A lot of air traffic transpires during an incident of this type and scale; you will never be able to get one word of direction in on the radio if a separate response channel is not incorporated. There is absolutely nothing more frustrating to an IC who is fully engaged in the call than having to stop what he or she is doing to answer a routing request from an incoming unit that is lost. Consider two or more channels to make things more manageable and keep unnecessary conversation off the main operations channel. Some agencies also carry MCI kits on their apparatus, which can contain items such as a tactical worksheet or board that has preset benchmarks that the IC can reference and check off. Such items can help the IC determine what incident priorities need to be addressed. Also, some other items may include incident management system command vests, which visually establish position assignments for personnel, such as command, operations, safety, triage, and staging, and possibly some type of START system, which may include victim priority tags and flowcharts.

Scene Stabilization

With the dynamic nature of school bus rescue and extrication incidents, the need to maintain situational awareness should be a priority not only to the IC but also to every member of the team. Size-up of the incident begins the moment you are dispatched. Be proactive, and call for additional units and/or specialty units, such as a heavy-rescue team, a hazardous materials unit, or a tow agency (preferably a 50/60-ton rotating unit with an articulating boom), to respond. Put air rescue on standby as a prewarning. These units can always be canceled if the incident is found to be insignificant. In addition, preassignments should be directed to your crew while en route. When approaching a scene, a thorough visual scan of the entire area should be conducted prior to stepping off the apparatus. Easily recognized hazards, such as downed utility poles; variations in topography, such as embankments and slopes; or water hazards, such as canals, streams, and lakes, must be taken into consideration. Upon your arrival, give a clear and accurate account of what is presented, and conduct inner and outer surveys of the scene to formulate your IAP. Some basic initial considerations that need to be addressed include the following:

- What type of school bus are you dealing with (type C or D)?
- What is the damage level (minor, moderate, or heavy)?
- Is the school bus still running?
- What is its resting position (upright, side, roof, or override)?
- How many occupants are there (initial estimate)?
- What are additional resources needed (for example, apparatus, tow units, equipment, personnel, or command staff)?
- Do you have an established MCI plan that can be implemented?

Other considerations may need to be added here that pertain to your response area or jurisdictional requirements. This list is only a start; you should add to this list and customize it to your agency's needs and capabilities.

Stabilization: School Buses

As with most vehicles, there are basically four positions in which a school bus will present that the technical rescuer will have to stabilize—upright, on its side, on its roof, or on another vehicle. The main goal is to create a solid foundation from which to work, which includes lowering the bus's center of mass and preventing further unnecessary movement. The two more common suspension systems found on types C and D buses are either a metal leaf spring system or an air ride system with air bladders. The air ride suspension system is designed to protect the cargo and the frame system of the vehicle using air bladders. The bladders contain air under pressure ranging up to 120 psi (827 kPa). Stabilizing an upright school bus that utilizes an air bladder is extremely important because in the case of a bag rupture or leak, the bus will list or lean heavily to the side of the rupture.

To stabilize a school bus in its normal position, follow the steps in **SKILL DRILL 13-1**. Some steps may occur simultaneously.

SKILL DRILL 13-1
Stabilizing a School Bus in Its Normal Position

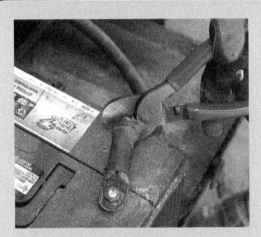

1. Don appropriate personal protective equipment (PPE). Assess the scene for hazards, and complete the inner and outer surveys. Activate the MCI protocols, depending on the number of victims. Call for additional resources, such as an appropriately sized tow truck unit, a technical rescue team (TRT) unit, or a hazardous materials unit. Set up the hazard control zones (hot, warm, and cold). Set up two 1.75-in. (44-mm) charged hose lines in defensive positions. Ensure that the vehicle is not running; if normal shutdown procedures (including disconnecting the battery system) cannot be accomplished, locate the air intake manifold in the engine compartment, and discharge a 10-lb (4.5-kg) minimum dry chemical extinguisher into the device to suffocate and shut down the engine. Locate and disable the battery system.

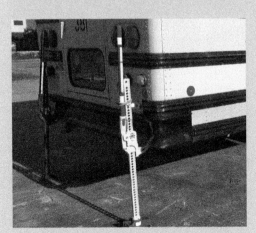

2. Place two First Responder Jacks (FRJs) at the rear of the school bus, lifting from the bumper.

(continues)

SKILL DRILL 13-1 Continued
Stabilizing a School Bus in Its Normal Position

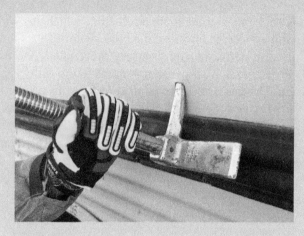

3 Position four tension buttress struts on the school bus with two at the front sides and two at the rear sides in an A-frame setup. Create purchase points for the tips of the struts to be set in place using a Halligan bar and flat-head axe or a pneumatic air chisel.

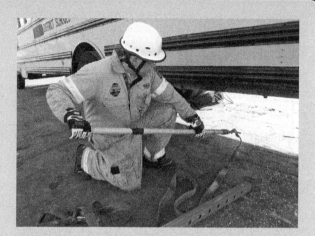

4 Pass the cargo straps under the school bus using a long pike pole to avoid going under the vehicle. Optional: Additional cross-tie box cribbing can be set in position under the frame at the rear of the school bus and at the front, under the bumper area. This will require a lot of cribbing, so ensure that the units on hand can support this task. The cribbing height for a cross-tie box crib should not exceed two times its width.

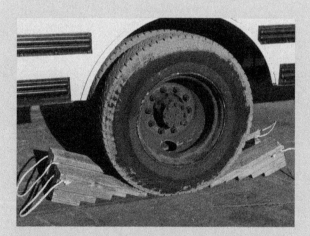

5 Prevent any forward or backward movement by positioning cribbing or step chocks upside down in a wedge-type setup in front of and behind each tire.

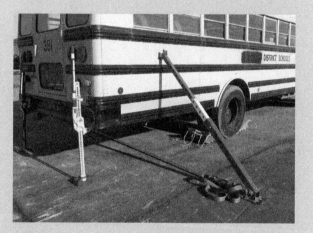

6 If access into the school bus can be established safely, then ensure that the air brake has been engaged if the driver has not already done so. Stabilize the school bus in its normal position.

© Jones & Bartlett Learning. Photographed by Glen E. Ellman.

To stabilize a school bus resting on its side, follow the steps in **SKILL DRILL 13-2**. Some steps may occur simultaneously.

Because of the shape and design of its semi-arched roof, a school bus will not normally come to rest on its roof after a collision or rollover incident. It will tend

SKILL DRILL 13-2
Stabilizing a School Bus Resting on Its Side

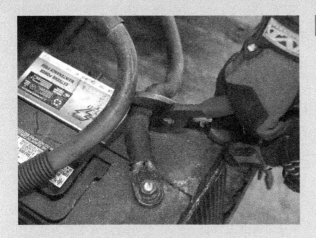

1. Don appropriate PPE. Assess the scene for hazards, and complete the inner and outer surveys. Ensure that there is no fuel leaking. Consider utilizing the appropriate foam for the type of fuel encountered. Activate MCI protocols, depending on the number of victims. Call for additional resources, such as an appropriately sized tow truck unit, TRT unit, or hazardous materials unit. Set up the hazard control zones (hot, warm, and cold). Set up two 1.75-in. (44-mm) charged hose lines in defensive positions. Depending on which side of the school bus is resting on the ground, locate and disable the battery system according to the procedures outlined in this chapter.

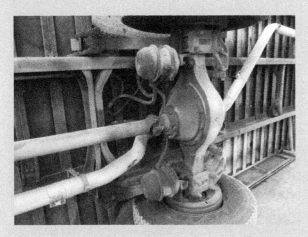

2. Ensure that the school bus is not running; if normal shutdown procedures (including disconnecting the battery system) cannot be accomplished, locate the air intake manifold in the engine compartment, and discharge a 10-lb (4.5-kg) minimum dry chemical extinguisher into the device to suffocate and shut down the engine. Secure the area around the muffler/regeneration device to ensure that this area is avoided because of burn potential from the heat of the device.

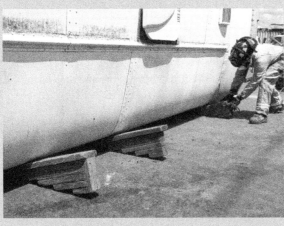

3. Stabilize the school bus. A school bus is relatively stable when positioned on its side on level ground; stabilization will generally require positioning wedge sections or step chocks upside down in a wedge-type setup under the roof line and the undercarriage or floor line of the school bus. Wedges set on top of a section of 4-in. × 4-in. (10-cm × 10-cm) cribbing (or four-by-four) can be utilized (see Chapter 8, *Vehicle Stabilization*, Skill Drill 8-2, for stabilizing a common passenger vehicle resting on its side).

© Jones & Bartlett Learning. Photographed by Glen E. Ellman.

366 Vehicle Rescue and Extrication: Principles and Practice

to remain upright or come to rest on its side. However, as rare as it may be, a school bus can come to rest on its roof.

To stabilize a school bus that is resting on its roof, follow the steps in **SKILL DRILL 13-3**. Some steps may occur simultaneously.

The elongated box shape of a school bus is designed to prevent overrides, in which the school bus comes to rest on top of another vehicle after a collision. The overall body design of a school bus is low to the ground, which allows it to bounce off an object rather than projecting upward on top of the object.

This design, however, was not effective in an accident that occurred when a type D school bus collided with a pickup truck and was then struck in the rear by another type D school bus. The force projected the first bus over the pickup truck and onto the cab of a semi-truck (**FIGURE 13-14**).

Such accidents involving a school bus are extremely rare and would challenge even the best prepared agency. However, once again, if the incident is broken down into manageable segments utilizing the incident management system, it can be handled and controlled with a high percentage of success. Multiple

SKILL DRILL 13-3
Stabilizing a School Bus Resting on Its Roof

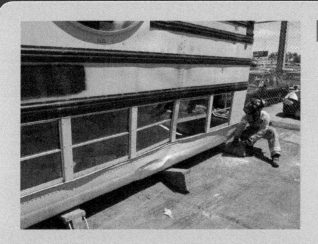

1 Don appropriate PPE. Assess the scene for hazards, and complete the inner and outer surveys. Ensure that there is no fuel leaking. Consider utilizing the appropriate foam for the type of fuel encountered. Activate MCI protocols, depending on the number of victims. Call for additional resources, such as an appropriately sized tow truck unit, TRT unit, or hazardous materials unit. Set up the hazard control zones (hot, warm, and cold). Set up two 1.75-in. (44-mm) charged hose lines in defensive positions. Locate and disable the battery system if it is accessible. Ensure that the school bus is not running; if normal shutdown procedures (including disconnecting the battery system) cannot be accomplished, locate the air intake manifold in the engine compartment, and discharge a 10-lb (4.5-kg) minimum dry chemical extinguisher into the device to suffocate and shut down the engine. Access may not be available with a front-mount engine found in type C buses. Secure an area around the muffler/regeneration device to ensure that this area is avoided because of the burn potential from heat retention of the device. Secure wedges and step chocks upside down in a wedge-type setup around the entire roof line to keep the school bus from rocking.

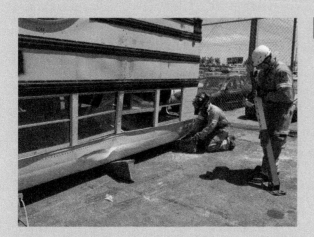

2 Position four tension buttress struts on the school bus with two at the front sides and two at the rear sides in an A-frame setup.

CHAPTER 13 School Buses **367**

SKILL DRILL 13-3 Continued
Stabilizing a School Bus Resting on Its Roof

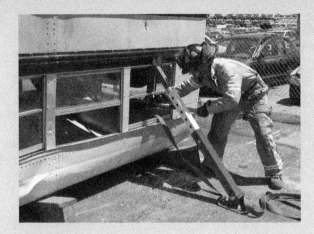

3 Create purchase points for the tips of the struts to be set in place using a battery-powered drill with a step bit attachment, a Halligan bar and a flat-head axe, or a pneumatic air chisel. The cargo straps used for tensioning of the struts can be passed through the windows to connect the struts together, or the strap can pass through a window around the truss bow and back through the adjoining window and be secured onto itself.

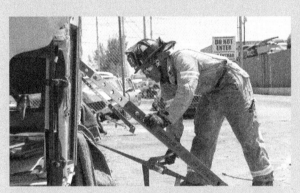

4 This image shows the stabilized school bus resting on its roof.

© Jones & Bartlett Learning. Photographed by Glen E. Ellman.

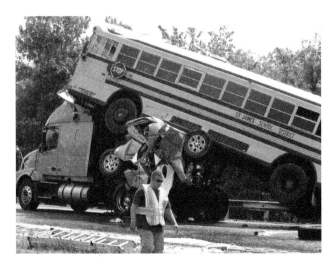

FIGURE 13-14 A type D school bus collided with a pickup truck and was then struck in the rear by another type D school bus.
© Jess Roberson/AP Photos.

stabilization tools and resources are required to properly stabilize a vehicle of this size in this type of resting position, some of which include a large tow unit, minimum 50/60-ton rotating unit with an articulating boom, large amounts of cribbing, ratchet/cargo straps, come alongs with chain packages, and tension buttress struts.

To stabilize or marry a school bus on top of another vehicle, follow the steps in **SKILL DRILL 13-4**. Some steps may occur simultaneously.

Victim Access: School Buses

Gaining or creating access into a school bus will depend on the vehicle's resting position. The goal is to create a main entry and exit area so the flow of rescuers and victim removal is consistent and controlled. The cage-like structure, with varying heavy-gauge

SKILL DRILL 13-4
Stabilizing/Marrying a School Bus on Top of Another Vehicle

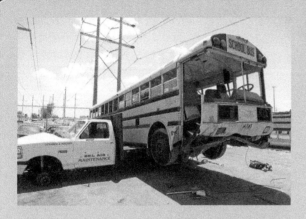

1 Don appropriate PPE. Assess the scene for hazards, and complete the inner and outer surveys. Ensure that there is no fuel leaking. Consider utilizing the appropriate foam for the type of fuel encountered.

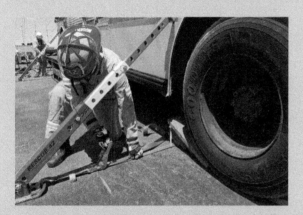

2 Activate MCI protocols, depending on the number of victims. Call for additional resources, such as an appropriately sized tow truck unit, TRT unit, or hazardous materials unit. Set up the hazard control zones (hot, warm, and cold). Set up two 1.75-in. (44-mm) charged hose lines in defensive positions. Locate and disable the battery system if it is accessible. Ensure the school bus is not running; if normal shutdown procedures (including disconnecting the battery system) cannot be accomplished, locate the air intake manifold in the engine compartment, and discharge a 10-lb (4.5-kg) minimum dry chemical extinguisher into the device to suffocate and shut down the engine. Position four tension buttress struts on the school bus with two at the front sides and two at the rear sides in an A-frame setup. Create purchase points for the tips of the struts to be set in place using a battery-powered drill with a step bit attachment, a Halligan bar and a flat-head axe, or a pneumatic air chisel. Pass the cargo straps under the school bus using a long pike pole to avoid going under the vehicle. This will lower the center of gravity on the bus and expand its overall footprint, thus preventing vehicle roll.

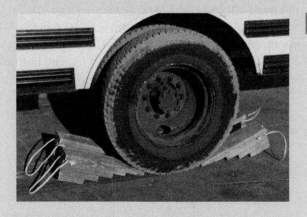

3 Position and engage two FRJs at each side of the rear bumper area. Optional cross-tie box cribbing can be set in position under the frame at the rear of the school bus and at the front under the bumper area. This will require a lot of cribbing; ensure that the units on hand can support this task. The cribbing height for a cross-tie box crib should not exceed two times its width. Prevent any forward or backward movement by positioning cribbing or step chocks upside down in a wedge-type setup in front of and behind each tire that is touching the ground.

SKILL DRILL 13-4 Continued
Stabilizing/Marrying a School Bus on Top of Another Vehicle

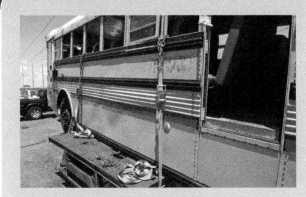

4 Marry the top vehicle to the bottom vehicle, utilizing cargo straps or come alongs with chain packages.

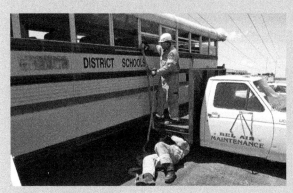

5 Attempt to marry the vehicles together in four or more areas for added stability.

© Jones & Bartlett Learning. Photographed by Glen E. Ellman.

---

steel throughout, is designed to provide occupant protection and safety. Thus, cutting into a school bus can be a difficult process that requires a lot of work and various specialized techniques. Again, the technique used will depend heavily on the bus's resting position. Because so many crash scenarios can occur, covering them all in detail would require a separate book. This chapter focuses on procedures that are the most commonly utilized; offer the highest percentage of success; and with practice, can be accomplished in the shortest amount of time. The tools used consist of but are not limited to a large assortment of cribbing sections; struts with tensioning straps; FRJs; hand tools, such as a battery-powered drill with a step bit attachment and a Halligan bar and a flat-head axe; electric-powered reciprocating saws with 20 to 30 spare blades; air chisels; hydraulic tools; air-lift bags; and an appropriately sized tow truck unit, preferably a 50/60-ton rotating unit with an articulating boom (**FIGURE 13-15**).

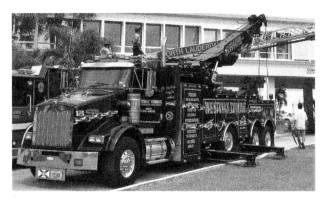

FIGURE 13-15 A 50/60-ton rotating unit with an articulating boom tow truck.
Courtesy of David Sweet.

Front Window Access

The front windows on a school bus are composed of laminated safety glass that, when removed from a bus on its side, can provide the rescuer a natural opening that is large enough to pass equipment through and remove victims on backboards with minimal restriction. There are two settings for installing the laminated glass in the vehicle—the gasket push-out type and the beaded mastic type.

The gasket push-out type uses a flat laminated glass and comes in several configurations. For example, the windshield may include one large panel of glass, two large panels of glass separated by a thin metal divider, or four sections of glass where the entire windshield extends outward with two large panels in the front and two small panels that square off the sides. These panels are held in place by a rubber gasket seal, which can be removed; once the seal has been removed, the glass can be pushed out from the inside of the vehicle or cut out with a battery-powered drill and glass shear attachment, an electric reciprocating saw, or a glass handsaw. It may be easier to use an electric reciprocating saw, which enables you to cut right through the metal glass divider while cutting the glass without having to stop. Utilizing a reciprocating saw to remove the windshield is the fastest procedure. Keep in mind that using the reciprocating saw will leave a glass edge. It is best to properly manage the glass by applying a self-adhesive film to secure the glass. The glass edge can also be pulled out along with the gasket, or a blanket can be placed over that section to protect people from being injured by the sharp edges if a film cannot be applied.

With the beaded mastic type of setting on a school bus windshield, the adhesive secures the laminated panel around the entire perimeter of the glass, which is similar to the mastic settings used on the front windshield of a standard conventional vehicle. The difference between the gasket setting and the mastic adhesive setting is that the laminated panel that is held in with the mastic adhesive is generally one section, or one panel, of glass, and it is curved instead of flat. This mastic setting requires that the windshield be cut out using a glass handsaw or an electric reciprocating saw.

To gain access into a school bus by removing the front windshield, follow the steps in **SKILL DRILL 13-5**. Some steps may occur simultaneously.

Seat Removal

Removing a bench seat can be a fairly easy process that can be accomplished quickly using a combination of a hydraulic spreader and a hydraulic cutter. Other tools such as a pneumatic air chisel or an electric reciprocating saw can also be utilized to accomplish the same task and may need to be used in some instances because of tight spaces, positioning, or precision cutting. For speed of operation, the combination of the hydraulic spreader and cutter is the best tool choice to accomplish the task.

To remove a bench seat from a school bus, follow the steps in **SKILL DRILL 13-6**. Some steps may occur simultaneously.

SKILL DRILL 13-5
Gaining Access into a School Bus by Removing the Front Windshield

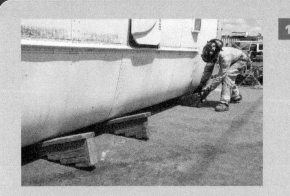

1 Don appropriate PPE. Assess the scene for hazards, and complete the inner and outer surveys. Ensure that there is no fuel leaking. Consider utilizing the appropriate foam for the type of fuel encountered. Activate MCI protocols, depending on the number of victims. Call for additional resources, such as an appropriately sized tow truck unit, TRT unit, or hazardous materials unit. Set up the hazard control zones (hot, warm, and cold). Set up two 1.75-in. (44-mm) charged hose lines in defensive positions. Locate and disable the battery system if it is accessible. Ensure the school bus is not running; if normal shutdown procedures (including disconnecting the battery system) cannot be accomplished, locate the air intake manifold in the engine compartment, and discharge a 10-lb (4.5-kg) minimum dry chemical extinguisher into the device to suffocate and shut down the engine. If the bus is resting on its side or roof, secure the area around the muffler/regeneration device to ensure that this area is avoided because of burn potential from the heat of the device. If the school bus is resting on its side, stabilization will generally require positioning wedge sections or step chocks upside down in a wedge-type setup under the roof line and the undercarriage or floor line of the school bus. Wedges set on top of a four-by-four can be utilized (see Chapter 8, Skill Drill 8-2, for stabilizing a common passenger vehicle resting on its side).

SKILL DRILL 13-5 Continued
Gaining Access into a School Bus by Removing the Front Windshield

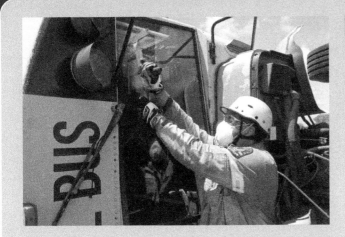

2 Use a large flat-head screwdriver or some type of prying tool to get a section of the gasket off of the glass, and then pull it off around the entire perimeter of the window. Use the prying tool to work a corner of the glass away from the frame, and then pull the entire glass toward you and out of the casing. This approach does not always work well as the gasket may have dry-rotted and/or become compromised by age; the glass may break, or the gasket may tear apart in sections. Use a Halligan bar or a glass handsaw to make a purchase opening at the top of the window.

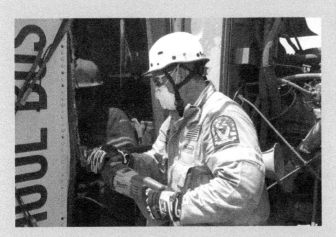

3 Use a reciprocating saw to cut out the two sections of glass, cutting through the center divider bar and working the blade around the inside perimeter of the windshield.

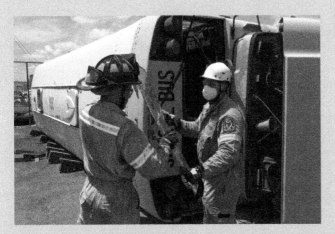

4 Remove the windshield, and place it in a designated debris pile outside of the hot zone.

© Jones & Bartlett Learning. Photographed by Glen E. Ellman.

SKILL DRILL 13-6
Removing a Bench Seat from a School Bus

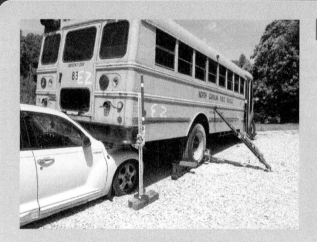

1 Don appropriate PPE. Assess the scene for hazards, and complete the inner and outer surveys. Ensure that there is no fuel leaking. Consider utilizing the appropriate foam for the type of fuel encountered. Activate MCI protocols, depending on the number of victims. Call for additional resources, such as an appropriately sized tow truck unit, TRT unit, or hazardous materials unit. Set up the hazard control zones (hot, warm, and cold). Set up two 1.75-in. (44-mm) charged hose lines in defensive positions. Locate and disable the battery system if it is accessible. Ensure the school bus is not running; if normal shutdown procedures (including disconnecting the battery system) cannot be accomplished, locate the air intake manifold in the engine compartment, and discharge a 10-lb (4.5-kg) minimum dry chemical extinguisher into the device to suffocate and shut down the engine. Stabilize the school bus from movement by utilizing the techniques outlined in this chapter.

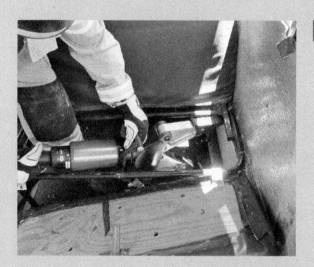

2 Position a hydraulic spreader with the arms vertical behind and under the bench frame closest to the lip that extends and attaches the seat to the sidewall. Slowly open the spreader, ensuring that the top arm catches the frame and detaches the seat from the sidewall lip attachment. This section of the seat must be removed first, or there will not be enough leverage for the spreader to operate effectively.

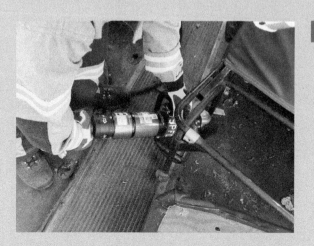

3 Use the hydraulic cutter to cut the seat frame where it is bolted to the floor next to the aisle. Attempting to take the bolts off by utilizing a pneumatic impact wrench will normally just spin the heads but will not remove them. Cutting the frame produces the most success even though a 0.5-in. (13-mm) section of cut frame protrudes from the floor.

SKILL DRILL 13-6 Continued
Removing a Bench Seat from a School Bus

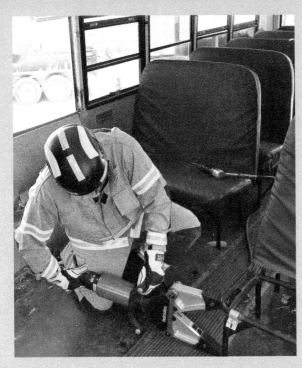

4 As an option, one leg can be spread off first, but the last leg must be cut.

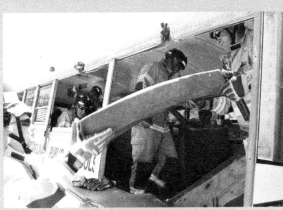

5 Remove the entire bench seat and place it in a debris pile outside the hot zone. It is best to hand off debris to someone outside of the bus because of the number of seats and material that may have to be removed.

Courtesy of David Sweet.

Sidewall Access

Removing a section of the sidewall can produce a large opening for victim removal. The technique involves removing two windows that are side by side; cross-cutting the roof bow truss that separates those two windows; removing two or more rows of bench seats; cutting down the sides of the sidewall, creating a relief cut on the bottom section of the center roof bow truss; and then pulling the entire section out and down. Multiple tools will be needed to accomplish this task, including but not limited to two electric reciprocating saws with multiple blades, a pneumatic air chisel, a hydraulic spreader, and a hydraulic cutter.

To remove a section of the sidewall of a school bus, follow the steps in **SKILL DRILL 13-7**. Some steps may occur simultaneously.

Roof Access

Gaining access into the roof of a school bus can be difficult because it requires cutting through multiple structural members composed of heavier-gauge steels.

SKILL DRILL 13-7
Removing a Section of the Sidewall of a School Bus

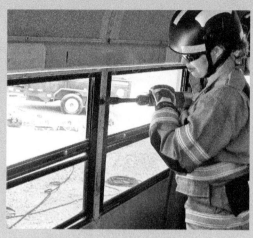

1. Don appropriate PPE. Assess the scene for hazards, and complete the inner and outer surveys. Ensure that there is no fuel leaking. Consider utilizing the appropriate foam for the type of fuel encountered. Activate MCI protocols, depending on the number of victims. Call for additional resources, such as an appropriately sized tow truck unit, TRT unit, or hazardous materials unit. Set up the hazard control zones (hot, warm, and cold). Set up two 1.75-in. (44-mm) charged hose lines in defensive positions. Locate and disable the battery system if it is accessible. Ensure the school bus is not running; if normal shutdown procedures (including disconnecting the battery system) cannot be accomplished, locate the air intake manifold in the engine compartment, and discharge a 10-lb (4.5-kg) minimum dry chemical extinguisher into the device to suffocate and shut down the engine. Stabilize the school bus from movement by utilizing the techniques outlined in this chapter. Enter the school bus. With a pneumatic air chisel, cut through the screw attachment, or cut off the attachments or screw heads that lock the windows to the school bus frame. This task can be accomplished without breaking any of the glass in the windows.

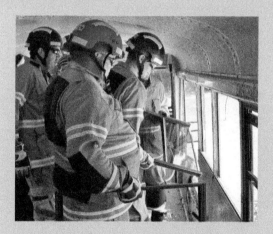

2. Once these attachments or screws are removed, the windows will pull right out of the frame casing.

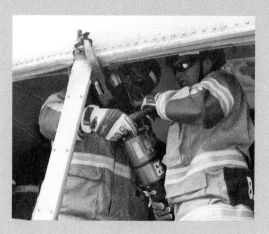

3. Remove two or more sets of seat benches utilizing the proper technique. Use the hydraulic cutter to cut the roof bow truss that divides the two windows. Utilize a cross-cut technique to keep the post stub from protruding downward. Another cut may have to be made at the top of the post to ensure it clears the frame when it is pushed forward.

SKILL DRILL 13-7 Continued
Removing a Section of the Sidewall of a School Bus

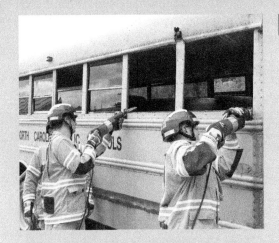

4 Position two technical rescuers outside of the bus with reciprocating saws. Simultaneously cut downward on two sections of the sidewall, beginning just inside the outer section of the window frame where two roof bow trusses form the outer frame of those two windows that were removed. Stay to the inside of the rivet heads that outline the position of a roof bow truss. Cut down past the first rub rail, which should be approximately at seat level; cutting any farther down will be difficult at best because you will encounter heavier-gauge steel with the crash rail, which will cause the reciprocating saw to slow down and the blade to melt or dull quickly.

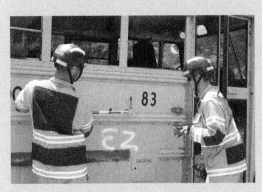

5 Using a Halligan bar and a flat-head axe, make two holes on both sides of the lower section of the center roof bow truss in the general area of the seat-level rub rail by driving the spiked end of the Halligan bar into the sidewall by striking it with the flat-head axe. The area in which the holes will be made is just below the first rub rail, near seat level; if you go any lower, you will encounter the crash rail area, which is composed of high-gauge steel and is extremely difficult to cut into.

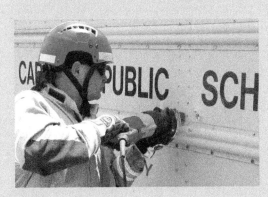

6 Insert the blade of a reciprocating saw into one of the holes just created, and cut through the roof bow truss; this will now act as a relief cut.

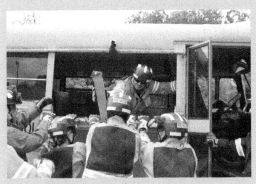

7 Grip the top center roof bow truss that was cut; pull out and downward, taking with it the entire sidewall that was just cut out. Move all the debris to the debris pile outside of the hot zone.

Courtesy of David Sweet.

LISTEN UP!

Avoid making the purchase-point holes in line with any row of rivets because there will be a structural member underneath the sheet metal that is held in place by the rivets.

To gain access through the roof of a school bus resting on its side, follow the steps in **SKILL DRILL 13-8**. Some steps may occur simultaneously.

Rear Door Access

There are several techniques that can be applied to gain entry into the rear emergency door of a school bus. The resting position of the bus will be a factor in deciding which technique to use. With the vehicle resting in the upright position, gaining access into the rear emergency door of a school bus requires removing the two safety glass panels located in the rear door prior to forcing entry. A vertical spread technique can

SKILL DRILL 13-8
Gaining Access Through the Roof of a School Bus on Its Side

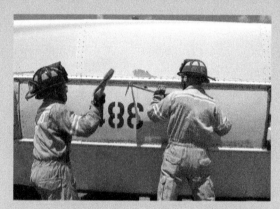

1 Don appropriate PPE. Assess the scene for hazards, and complete the inner and outer surveys. Ensure that there is no fuel leaking. Consider utilizing the appropriate foam for the type of fuel encountered. Activate MCI protocols, depending on the number of victims. Call for additional resources, such as an appropriately sized tow truck unit, TRT unit, or hazardous materials unit. Set up the hazard control zones (hot, warm, and cold). Set up two 1.75-in. (44-mm) charged hose lines in defensive positions. Locate and disable the battery system if it is accessible. Ensure the school bus is not running; if normal shutdown procedures (including disconnecting the battery system) cannot be accomplished, locate the air intake manifold in the engine compartment, and discharge a 10-lb (4.5-kg) minimum dry chemical extinguisher into the device to suffocate and shut down the engine. Secure the area around the muffler/regeneration device to ensure that this area is avoided because of burn potential from the heat of the device. Stabilize the school bus from movement by utilizing the techniques outlined in this chapter. Locate the area of the roof that will be designated as an exit/egress path. The height of this opening will vary depending on the structure and position of the bus as well as the overall height of the rescuer. Be aware that all school buses are not the same; some may have additional support members, such as roof stringers, that run perpendicular to the roof bow trusses. These stringers can be identified by the presence of rivets. A good rule of thumb is to count three roof bow trusses. Cut the outside dimensions of the opening just *inside* the two outer roof bow trusses; the center roof bow truss should be positioned directly in the middle of your opening. Use a battery-powered drill with a step bit attachment, a Halligan bar and a flat-head axe, or an appropriate striking tool to create four purchase-point holes just on the outside of the center roof bow truss at the top, which will mark the top dimension of your opening. The first two holes will be just on the outside of the center roof bow truss at the top, which will mark the top dimension of your opening.

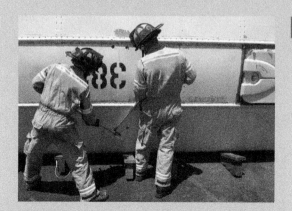

2 The second two holes will be at the bottom of that same center roof bow truss, which will mark the bottom dimension of your opening.

SKILL DRILL 13-8 Continued
Gaining Access Through the Roof of a School Bus on Its Side

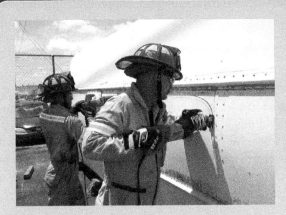

3. With the help of another responder, insert the blades of two electric reciprocating saws into the top purchase-point holes just created, and start the opening cuts; do not cut the top center roof bow truss until last to avoid excessive vibration or the blade becoming pinched and/or stuck in the metal. The two saws should move in opposite directions outward and then down, staying inside the rivets. You may have to cut through a roof stringer, which will slow your saw down because it is an approximately 16-gauge steel beam.

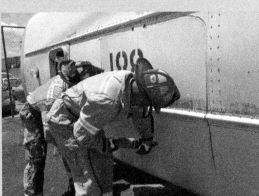

4. Once you have reached the bottom of the cut, two things can be done: The cut can continue back to the center roof bow truss with the intention of removing the entire section of metal, or the section can be pulled down or flapped. If the plan is to flap, then use one saw to cut the bottom center roof bow truss, inserting the blade into the purchase-point opening that was made and cutting completely through the roof bow truss.

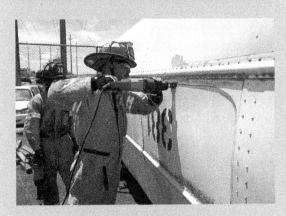

5. Make the same cut at the top section of the center roof bow truss in the same fashion; remember that this has to be cut last to avoid excessive vibration or the blade becoming pinched and/or stuck in the metal.

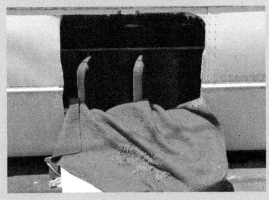

6. Pull downward the entire section of metal that was just cut. Place a tarp or covering over the flapped or cut section to avoid injury.

© Jones & Bartlett Learning. Photographed by Glen E. Ellman.

378 Vehicle Rescue and Extrication: Principles and Practice

> **LISTEN UP!**
>
> Be aware that all school buses are not the same and some may have additional support members, such as roof stringers, that run perpendicular to roof bow trusses; these can be identified by the presence of rivets.

be performed in one of the window frame openings of the door to create a purchase-point opening. The goal is to create a large opening near the latching mechanism, which will need to be cut and released with the hydraulic cutter. A standing platform utilizing two or more cross-tie box cribbing configurations and a backboard may need to be created to gain the proper height to operate the tools. The side emergency door that can be found on a type D bus will have only one glass panel.

Rear Door Access: School Bus in Its Normal Position. To gain access through the rear emergency door of a school bus in its normal position, follow the steps in **SKILL DRILL 13-9**. Some steps may occur simultaneously.

Rear Door Access: School Bus Resting on Its Side. The main goal of gaining access into a school bus is to create an adequate opening to rescue and remove victims as quickly as possible. Cutting out the entire rear section of a school bus is great practice for improving tool-handling skills, but doing so is not necessary and wastes valuable time. Opening the rear

SKILL DRILL 13-9
Gaining Access Through the Rear Door of a School Bus in Its Normal Position

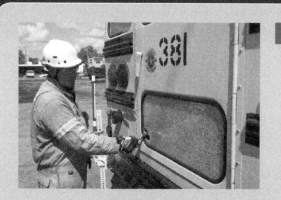

1 Don appropriate PPE. Assess the scene for hazards, and complete the inner and outer surveys. Ensure that there is no fuel leaking. Consider utilizing the appropriate foam for the type of fuel encountered. Activate MCI protocols, depending on the number of victims. Call for additional resources, such as an appropriately sized tow truck unit, TRT unit, or hazardous materials unit. Set up the hazard control zones (hot, warm, and cold). Set up two 1.75-in. (44-mm) charged hose lines in defensive positions. Locate and disable the battery system if it is accessible. Ensure the school bus is not running; if normal shutdown procedures (including disconnecting the battery system) cannot be accomplished, locate the air intake manifold in the engine compartment, and discharge a 10-lb (4.5-kg) minimum dry chemical extinguisher into the device to suffocate and shut down the engine. Stabilize the school bus from movement utilizing the techniques outlined in this chapter. Try to open the rear door manually. If the door won't open, remove the two safety glass panels located within the rear door frame. This can be accomplished by breaking the glass with a glass tool if it is tempered glass or by using a battery-powered glass shear tool or glass handsaw to cut it out if it is laminated glass. You may attempt to pull the gasket out to release the glass, but it may become a very time-consuming task if the gasket starts to tear apart from weathering.

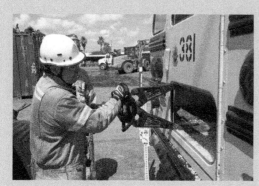

2 Place the hydraulic spreader with the arms vertical in the lower window frame opening, and perform a vertical spread technique.

SKILL DRILL 13-9 Continued
Gaining Access Through the Rear Door of a School Bus in Its Normal Position

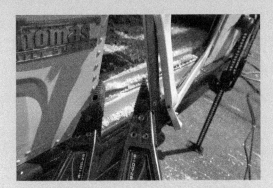

3 Once a purchase-point opening has been established, place the tips of the hydraulic spreader in the door frame, and create a larger opening; work the tool upward toward the latching mechanism.

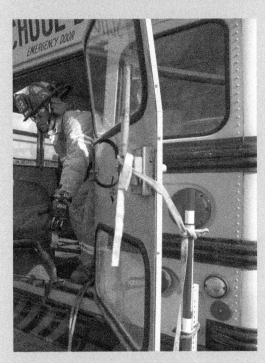

4 Once a large enough opening has been created around the latching mechanism, use the hydraulic cutter to cut the latch, releasing the door. Tie the door back in the open position utilizing rope or webbing.

© Jones & Bartlett Learning. Photographed by Glen E. Ellman.

door will create a large enough opening to safely remove occupants and save valuable time.

To gain access through the rear emergency door of a school bus resting on its side, follow the steps in **SKILL DRILL 13-10**. Some steps may occur simultaneously.

Front Door Access

Entry through the front door of a school bus will depend on the operability of the door itself. Always try to open the door manually. Otherwise, it may only require removing one of the glass panels in the door and inserting a pike pole into the bus to grip the lever bar that releases the door. This is a very fast technique that requires the least amount of forcible entry tactics and tool usage (**FIGURE 13-16**).

Gaining access through the door can also require cutting it out completely, utilizing hydraulic tools or a combination of hydraulic tools and reciprocating saws.

To gain access through the front entry door of a school bus in its normal position, follow the

SKILL DRILL 13-10
Gaining Access Through the Rear Door of a School Bus Resting on Its Side

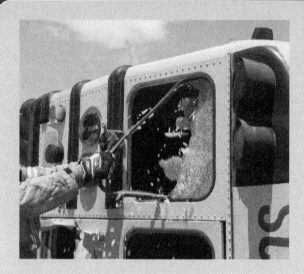

1. Don appropriate PPE. Assess the scene for hazards, and complete the inner and outer surveys. Ensure that there is no fuel leaking. Consider utilizing the appropriate foam for the type of fuel encountered. Activate MCI protocols, depending on the number of victims. Call for additional resources, such as an appropriately sized tow truck unit, TRT unit, or hazardous materials unit. Set up the hazard control zones (hot, warm, and cold). Set up two 1.75-in. (44-mm) charged hose lines in defensive positions. Locate and disable the battery system if it is accessible. Ensure the school bus is not running; if normal shutdown procedures (including disconnecting the battery system) cannot be accomplished, locate the air intake manifold in the engine compartment and discharge a 10-lb (4.5-kg) minimum dry chemical extinguisher into the device to suffocate and shut down the engine. Secure the area around the muffler/regeneration device to ensure that this area is avoided because of burn potential from the heat of the device. Stabilize the school bus from movement utilizing the techniques outlined in this chapter. Build a standing platform to work from so the tools are not elevated and operated over your head. This can be accomplished with two or more cross-tie box cribbing configurations and a large backboard or by other means. If the door will not open manually, remove all the safety glass from the rear using the appropriate technique.

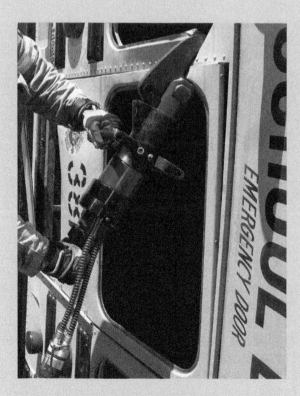

2. Use the hydraulic cutter to cut through the top section of the door frame; this is the post that connects the door to the adjacent upper window frame.

SKILL DRILL 13-10 Continued
Gaining Access Through the Rear Door of a School Bus Resting on Its Side

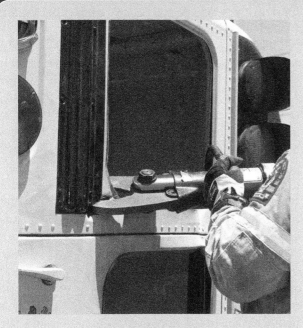

3 Cut diagonally into the bottom corner section of the top window where the door latch and the top window frame meet. The cut line should be directed downward toward the corner of the bottom window frame of the door.

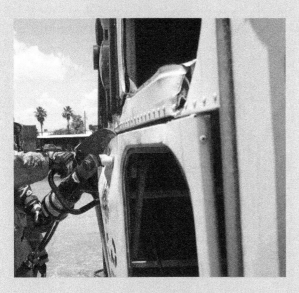

4 Cut diagonally upward toward the upper corner of the bottom door window frame, attempting to meet the first cut that was made.

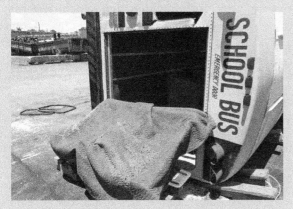

5 If the two cuts do not meet, then take a reciprocating saw and complete the cut or attempt to work the hydraulic cutter upward, cutting away the last remaining section. The goal is to cut around the latching mechanism, which will release the door without having to spread the latch away with the hydraulic spreader.

© Jones & Bartlett Learning. Photographed by Glen E. Ellman.

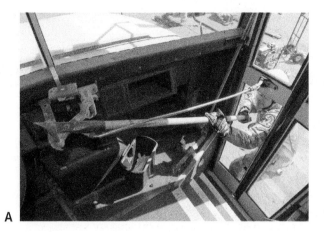

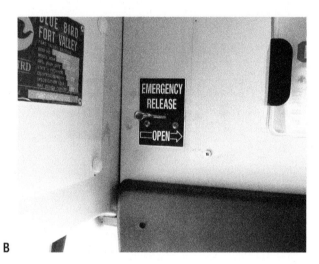

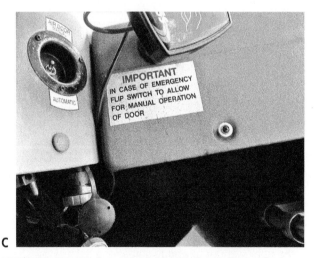

FIGURE 13-16 Entry through the front door of a school bus may only require removing one of the glass panels in the door and inserting a pike pole into the bus to grip the lever bar that releases the door or move the emergency air release switch to the open position.

A: © Jones & Bartlett Learning. Photographed by Glen E. Ellman; **B** and **C:** Courtesy of David Sweet.

steps in **SKILL DRILL 13-11**. Some steps may occur simultaneously.

Lifting Operations

On any given school bus rescue, an occupant can be ejected or partially ejected and trapped under the bus itself. There are multiple tools that can be used to safely and effectively lift and extricate a victim who has become trapped under a school bus. Ideal tools to accomplish the rescue include an appropriately sized tow truck unit (preferably a 50/60-ton rotating unit with an articulating boom), two FRJs, two heavy-lifting struts, or rescue air-lift bags (the high-pressure or the low-pressure high-lift type). Again, preplanning and training for incidents such as this cannot be stressed enough. There is not a tow agency out there that would not be willing to train with fire rescue agencies in sharing resources. Some fire rescue agencies in Europe, where tow agencies are incorporated in the response protocols for emergency services, are automatically dispatched on incidents such as this in their jurisdiction. They are well prepared because many have worked and trained together, and they have response protocols pre-established.

There are several tools and techniques that can be applied to lift a school bus off of a partially or fully entrapped victim. The action of moving or lifting a school bus, regardless of the tools or techniques utilized, must be a well-coordinated procedure, requiring precision from every emergency responder involved in the operation.

Occupant ejections can occur when any vehicle in motion is overturned with the vehicle potentially landing and entrapping the ejected victim. The following skill drills will describe two of the same scenario incidents utilizing two different methods and different tools to access and release a victim who is partially entrapped by an overturned school bus. The first technique explained is the use of two FRJs. This application is the fastest to set up, but this technique requires strict coordination and synchronization of the movement of both jack levers. These jacks have a working load limit (WWL) of 5000 lb (2268 kg), but remember that only a section of the bus will need to be partially lifted or tilted; the bus is not being fully uprighted.

To perform a jacking operation to access and release a person who has been ejected and trapped under a school bus that is resting on its side, please follow the steps outlined in the following **SKILL DRILL 13-12**. Some steps will occur simultaneously.

SKILL DRILL 13-11
Gaining Access Through the Front Door of a School Bus in Its Normal Position

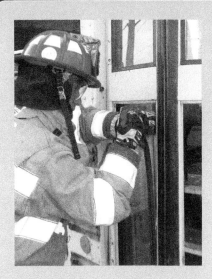

1 Don appropriate PPE. Assess the scene for hazards, and complete the inner and outer surveys. Ensure that there is no fuel leaking. Consider utilizing the appropriate foam for the type of fuel encountered. Activate MCI protocols, depending on the number of victims. Call for additional resources, such as an appropriately sized tow truck unit, TRT unit, or hazardous materials unit. Set up the hazard control zones (hot, warm, and cold). Set up two 1.75-in. (44-mm) charged hose lines in defensive positions. Locate and disable the battery system if it is accessible. Ensure the school bus is not running; if normal shutdown procedures (including disconnecting the battery system) cannot be accomplished, locate the air intake manifold in the engine compartment, and discharge a 10-lb (4.5-kg) minimum dry chemical extinguisher into the device to suffocate and shut down the engine. If the door will not open manually, remove all the safety glass from the front entry door by removing the gasket and pushing the panels inward or breaking and/or cutting the glass out using the appropriate techniques outlined in this chapter.

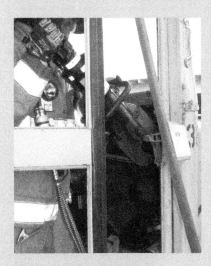

2 After you remove one side of the door and can make an entry into the bus, if the lever arm used to control the opening and closing of the door is inoperable, cut it loose using a hydraulic cutter.

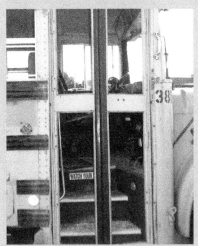

3 The door is composed of two sections that release outward. With the glass removed, the appearance of the door frame will resemble a cross, which is the frame section that will be cut out.

(continues)

SKILL DRILL 13-11 Continued
Gaining Access Through the Front Door of a School Bus in Its Normal Position

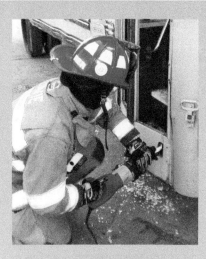

4 Cut the frame of both sections beginning at the bottom closest to the hinged section of the frame; do not attempt to remove the piano-type hinge of the door sections. Work your way to the top section of the door. Starting at the bottom first minimizes the vibration effect that can occur when using a reciprocating saw (a hydraulic cutter can also be utilized).

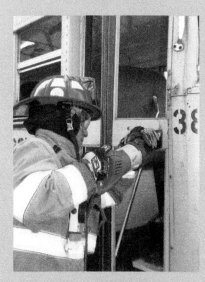

5 Moving upward, cut the middle section and finally the top section. The A-post and side/front windshield can also be incorporated in the removal process if needed to gain additional access.

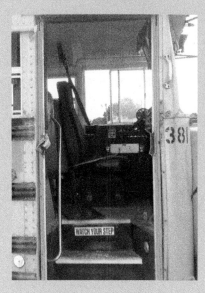

6 With the two sections of the door removed, place them in a designated debris pile outside the hot zone.

SKILL DRILL 13-12
Removing a Victim from Under a School Bus Resting on Its Side Utilizing FRJs

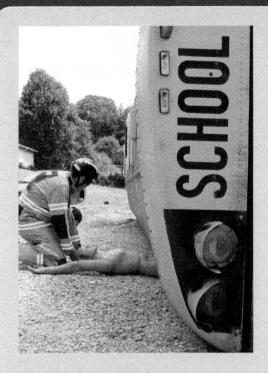

1 Don appropriate PPE, including mask and eye protection. Assess the scene for hazards, and complete the inner and outer surveys. Activate MCI protocols if they are pre-established and/or if needed based on the number of victims. Call for additional resources, such as an appropriately sized tow truck unit (preferably a 50/60-ton rotating unit with an articulating boom), TRT unit, or hazardous materials unit. Set up the hazard control zones (hot, warm, and cold). Set up two 1.75-in. (44-mm) charged hose lines in defensive positions. Depending on the resting position of the school bus, locate and disable the battery system according to the procedures outlined in this chapter. Ensure that the school bus is not running; if normal shutdown procedures (including disconnecting the battery system) cannot be accomplished, then locate the air intake manifold in the engine compartment, and discharge a 10-lb (4.5-kg) minimum dry chemical extinguisher into the device, which should suffocate and shut down the engine.

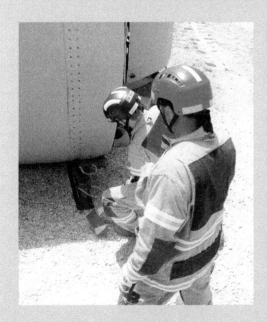

2 Assess the victim who is trapped under the bus, and maintain contact throughout the entire operation. Secure the area around the muffler/regeneration device to ensure that this area is avoided because of the burn potential from the heat of the device. Because a school bus is relatively stable when positioned on its side on level ground, the stabilization will generally require positioning wedge sections or step chocks upside down in a wedge-type setup under the roof line and the undercarriage or floor line of the school bus. Wedges set on top of a four-by-four can be utilized (see Chapter 8, Skill Drill 8-2).

(continues)

SKILL DRILL 13-12 Continued
Removing a Victim from Under a School Bus Resting on Its Side Utilizing FRJs

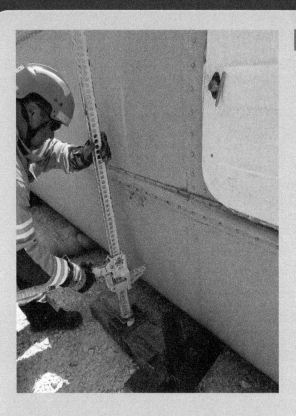

3 To properly and safely conduct a lifting operation, a minimum of six personnel are required: one tending to the victim, two on each side of the victim inserting cribbing as the bus is elevated, two managing the FRJs, and one overseeing and directing the operation. Medical rescue personnel with advanced life support training will need to immediately treat the victim when he or she is released. Some medical protocols recommend treating crushing injuries immediately before the victim is released. This will be a decision made by the authority having jurisdiction based on departmental medical protocols and medical direction. Position two FRJs spaced equally apart on opposite sides of the victim. If the ground is unstable, place four-by-four cribbing sections under the jacks for support and to expand their footprint.

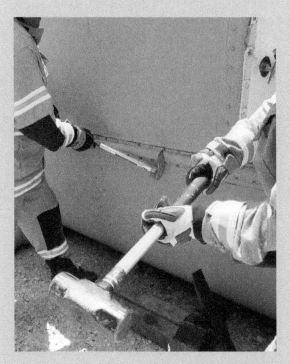

4 Make two large purchase-point openings just under the lower stringer rail that runs the length of the bus. If the stringer is not extruded, look for a series of rivets running the length of the bus, and make the purchase openings 2 to 3 in. (5 to 8 cm) below the rivets. The purchase-point openings should be large enough to allow the tongue of the FRJs to be inserted. This purchase-point opening can be made with a Halligan bar and a flat-head axe or a pneumatic air chisel. Once a large opening has been made, insert the FRJ, and engage the lever until the tongue is firmly seated just under the lower stringer rail.

SKILL DRILL 13-12 Continued
Removing a Victim from Under a School Bus Resting on Its Side Utilizing FRJs

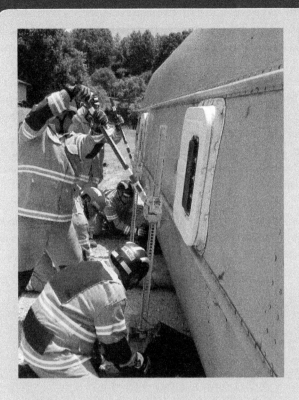

5 Each technical rescuer on cribbing assignment must be prepared with various sizes and types of cribbing by his or her side. Always remember to use a longer section of cribbing to push any box crib in position under the school bus; never put your body or extremities in a position where they can become trapped. As the order is given to engage and lift each jack, it is critical that the jacks be engaged and lifted in unison with each other. The officer can give the commands "Up on the jack!" or "Down on the jack!" to keep the rescuers in sync with each other. As the lift occurs, simultaneously insert the appropriately sized cribbing on both sides of the victim to support the lift and maintain an even lift. As the lift is increased by engaging the jacks, the cribbing will also need to increase in height.

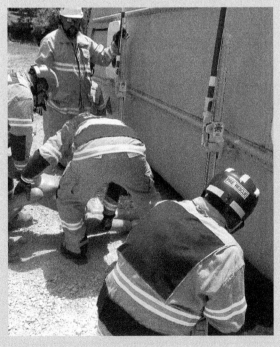

6 Once the proper height has been achieved with full support on both sides of the victim, insert a backboard under the victim. Place two or more personnel at each side of the victim and one personnel at the head to maintain spinal immobilization; simultaneously slide the victim in position onto the backboard. Once the victim is clear of the entrapment, secure the victim to the backboard and transfer to a medical team.

Courtesy of David Sweet.

Air-Lift Bag Operation

An air-lift bag operation for a person who has been ejected and become trapped under a school bus that is now resting on its side is very similar to an operation for a person who has become trapped under a conventional vehicle. This operation is actually less complicated because there is a much larger surface area to work from on a school bus. The key is to always lift evenly and from areas with structural support, such as roof bow trusses. The "lift an inch, crib an inch" expression applies; there should be ample amounts of cribbing on hand.

One issue that can hamper an air-lift bag operation is unstable terrain, such as muck or loose sand, termed "sugar sand," which can sink a bag when inflated. A solution is to place a large, flat, solid object, such as the steel or aluminum ground pads that are placed under aerial outriggers, under the bottom bag. Doing so expands the bag's footprint and equally distributes the lift point of the bag across the entire dimension of the plate. Remember, the larger the surface area covered, the greater the resistance to sinking. When dealing with unstable terrain, it is best practice to have some digging tools on hand, such as shovels and picks, because you may have to remove sand or dirt to gain a position to insert the bag(s). You may get only one bag in position initially, but once you lift the school bus a few inches and properly secure cribbing on both sides, you will be able to deflate the one bag and gain enough room to insert a second to help perform the full lift.

As a safety precaution, review the air-lift bag information detailed in Chapter 3, *Tools and Equipment*, before performing this skill drill.

To perform an air-lift bag operation for a person who has been ejected and is trapped under a school bus resting on its side, follow the steps in **SKILL DRILL 13-13**. Some steps may occur simultaneously.

SKILL DRILL 13-13
Removing a Victim from Under a School Bus Resting on Its Side Utilizing Air-Lift Bags

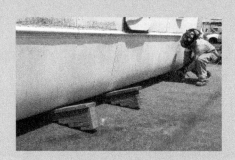

1 Don appropriate PPE. Assess the scene for hazards, and complete the inner and outer surveys. Ensure that there is no fuel leaking. Consider utilizing the appropriate foam for the type of fuel encountered. Activate MCI protocols, depending on the number of victims. Call for additional resources, such as an appropriately sized tow truck unit, TRT unit, or hazardous materials unit. Set up the hazard control zones (hot, warm, and cold). Set up two 1.75-in. (44-mm) charged hose lines in defensive positions. Locate and disable the battery system if it is accessible. Ensure the school bus is not running; if normal shutdown procedures (including disconnecting the battery system) cannot be accomplished, locate the air intake manifold in the engine compartment, and discharge a 10-lb (4.5-kg) minimum dry chemical extinguisher into the device to suffocate and shut down the engine. Secure the area around the muffler/regeneration device to ensure that this area is avoided because of the burn potential from the heat of the device. Stabilize the school bus from movement utilizing the techniques outlined in this chapter.

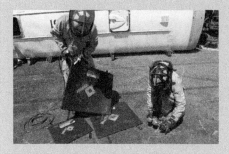

2 Determine the placement and number of air-lift bags needed to produce an even lift based upon where the victim is trapped and how the victim is presenting. Two bags may be sufficient, with the two placed on one side of the victim in conjunction with cribbing, or four bags may be needed, with two bags positioned on both sides of the victim in conjunction with cribbing. Position five rescuers around the victim: one personnel to tend to the victim, two personnel on each side of the victim inserting cribbing, one personnel managing the air-lift bag controls, and one personnel overseeing and directing the operation. Medical rescue personnel with advanced life-saving training will also be needed to immediately treat the victim when he or she is released. Medical protocols for treating crushing injuries will be decided by the authority having jurisdiction.

SKILL DRILL 13-13 Continued
Removing a Victim from Under a School Bus Resting on Its Side Utilizing Air-Lift Bags

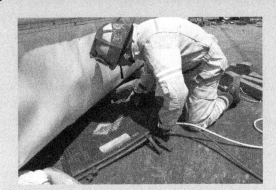

3. Position two air-lift bags, one on top of the other with the largest bag on the bottom, under the structural support of the school bus close to the victim. Remember, bag placement should be under a structural support, such as a roof bow truss. Otherwise, the roof section will cave in when the bags are inflated.

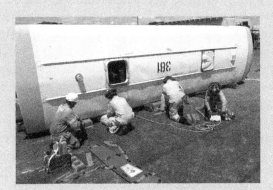

4. Each technical rescuer on cribbing assignment who is positioned on both sides of the victim must be prepared with a full complement of various sizes and types of cribbing by his or her side. Prebuilding a cross-tie box crib configuration can assist in preventing delays. Use a longer section of cribbing to push the box crib in position under the school bus; never put your body or extremities in a position where they can become trapped.

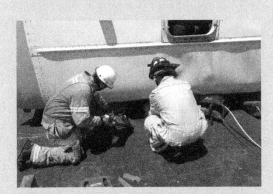

5. As the order is given to inflate the first (lowest) bag, simultaneously insert the appropriately sized cribbing on both sides of the victim to support the lift and to maintain an even lift. As the lift is increased by the inflation of the second bag, the cribbing will also need to increase in height.

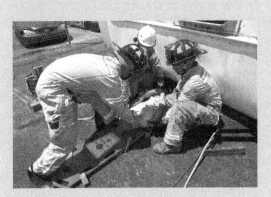

6. Once the proper height has been achieved with full support on both sides of the victim, insert a backboard under the victim. Place two or more personnel at each side of the victim and one personnel at the head to maintain spinal immobilization and simultaneously slide the victim in position onto the backboard. Once the victim is clear of the entrapment, secure the victim to the backboard and transfer to a medical team.

© Jones & Bartlett Learning. Photographed by Glen E. Ellman.

> **SAFETY TIP**
>
> To properly and safely conduct an air-lift bag operation, a minimum of five personnel are needed: one personnel tending to the victim, two personnel on each side of the victim inserting cribbing, one personnel managing the air-lift bag controls, and one personnel overseeing and directing the operation.

Steering Wheel Assembly

Relocating a steering wheel assembly off of a driver who has become trapped from a collision can be quickly and safely accomplished using a small tow truck unit that is equipped with a stationary boom. Personnel can back the tow unit to the front of the school bus, extend its lower brace bar to brace up against the front of the bus, pull the wire rope from on top of the boom, and wrap the rope securely around the steering wheel ring and column. The bracing bar is normally utilized to slide under the undercarriage and tires of a conventional vehicle to lift and haul a vehicle away. The stationary boom provides a height leverage advantage that, when operated, can easily relocate a steering column off of an entrapped occupant in minutes. Other techniques can be utilized, such as using a come along and a chain package (the same technique that is used for relocating the steering wheel assembly of a conventional vehicle, demonstrated in Chapter 9, *Victim Access and Management*, Skill Drill 9-14). This technique can be applied only to a type C bus or a bus with an extended front hood/engine compartment so the equipment can be properly set in place. A transit-style type D school bus will require the use of a tow unit as just described. There are other techniques that may be used, but the tow unit is the safest and fastest way to accomplish the objective.

Lifting a School Bus Off of an Underride

A vehicle that has impacted the rear of a school bus and has projected far under the rear chassis, entrapping the passengers, presents unique challenges to the rescuers. Depending on the number of victims within both the school bus and vehicle, this scenario will require multiple operations to be conducted simultaneously. Once all the victims in both vehicles are accounted for and properly triaged, determine whether the occupants within the vehicle underride are trapped and require extrication to be accessed and removed. The goal is to properly stabilize the school bus utilizing the technique described in this chapter and to determine if the vehicle underride is accessible to conduct rescue and extrication operations while still wedged under the school bus.

If access is blocked, the main objective will be to lift the school bus and pull the vehicle out from under it, far enough to allow for full access to conduct the proper technique to remove the entrapped victims. If access to a large-capacity tow unit is available, such as a 50/60-ton rotating unit with an articulating boom, then the operation of lifting the school bus and removing the vehicle underride will be fairly routine for a skilled and properly certified tow operator. The operator attaches a strapping and chain system under the bus, and the tow unit lifts with its boom extended. At the same time, a separate winch off of the same tow unit or another smaller tow unit positioned at the rear of the underride attaches to the rear of the vehicle and slowly pulls it out from under the bus.

When a tow unit is not available, the operation will instead focus on alternative options for lifting and removing the underride vehicle. One option is utilizing two FRJs, heavy-lifting struts, and additional equipment with multiple personnel in a highly coordinated evolution. Estimating the weight of the school bus is based on ranges within each class; additional factors such as number of passengers, fuel, cargo, etc. will make it very difficult to come up with exact numbers. When lifting occurs in the particular scenario presented, the rear section of the bus that is lifted accounts for one-quarter to one-half of the estimated overall weight. This estimated weight to be lifted has to be matched up with the WWL of the jacks and lifting struts applied.

A type C school bus is estimated to weigh between 21,500 and 30,000 lb (9752 and 13,508 kg). A basic calculation of one-half of the weight at 15,000 lb (6804 kg) and applying two FRJs at 5000 lb (2268 kg) WWL per jack and two lifting struts (such as Res-Q-Jack® Super X-Struts®) at 6000 lb (2722 kg) WWL per strut will yield a maximum lifting capacity of 22,000 lb (9979 kg). This will allow for adequate capacity to lift the rear of the school bus enough to remove the vehicle that is trapped underneath the chassis.

With the amount of weight and load that is placed on the jacks and struts, any shift from a noncoordinated and/or uneven jacking, tool failure, or heavy winds can potentially cause catastrophic consequences to occur. Because of the inherent risks associated with this advanced lifting scenario, the strictest discipline must be adhered to with all personnel, and extreme caution must be taken when applying this technique. This procedure requires two or more safety officers positioned on both sides of the school bus and a commanding officer who has full control of every action and direction of all personnel.

To perform this lifting operation, follow the steps in **SKILL DRILL 13-14**. Some steps will occur simultaneously.

SKILL DRILL 13-14
Lifting a School Bus Off of an Underride

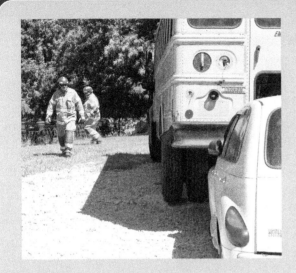

1. Don appropriate PPE. Assess the scene for hazards, and complete the inner and outer surveys. Activate MCI protocols, depending on the number of victims. Call for additional resources, such as an appropriately sized tow truck unit, a TRT unit, or a hazardous materials unit. Set up the hazard control zones (hot, warm, and cold). Set up two 1.75-in. (44-mm) charged hose lines in defensive positions. Ensure that the vehicle is not running; if normal shutdown procedures (including disconnecting the battery system) cannot be accomplished, locate the air intake manifold in the engine compartment, and discharge a 10-lb (4.5-kg) minimum dry chemical extinguisher into the device to suffocate and shut down the engine. Locate and disable the battery system.

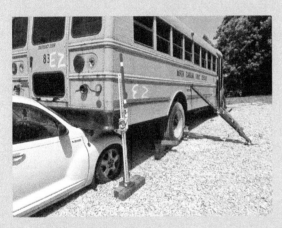

2. Place two FRJs at the rear of the school bus, lifting from the bumper. Position four tension buttress struts on the school bus, with two at the front sides and two at the rear sides in an A-frame setup. Create purchase points for the tips of the struts to be set in place; use a battery-powered drill with a step bit attachment, a Halligan bar and a flat-head axe, or a pneumatic air chisel. Pass the cargo straps under the school bus using a long pike pole to avoid going under the vehicle. Optionally, additional cross-tie box cribbing can be set in position under the frame at the rear of the school bus and at the front, under the bumper area. This will require a lot of cribbing; ensure that the units on hand can support this task. The cribbing height for a cross-tie box crib should not exceed two times its width. Prevent any forward or backward movement by positioning cribbing or step chocks upside down in a wedge-type setup in front of and behind each tire.

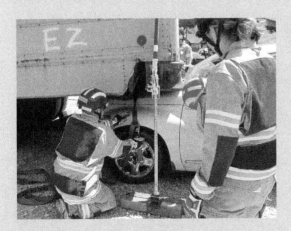

3. If access into the school bus can be established safely, ensure that the air brake has been engaged. Stabilize the school bus in its normal position. The vehicle that has driven under the rear of the bus must be assessed for risk–benefit analysis of removing versus remaining static, size and type of vehicle involved (common passenger/commercial vehicle, hybrid vehicle, sport utility vehicle, etc.), number of known or potential victims inside the vehicle and the possibility of ejections, identification of witnesses/bystanders, overall stability of the vehicle, and primary access into the vehicle. Attempt to lower and secure the front end of the vehicle by attaching a cargo strap over the front hood section of the vehicle and locking down the suspension system.

(continues)

SKILL DRILL 13-14 Continued
Lifting a School Bus Off of an Underride

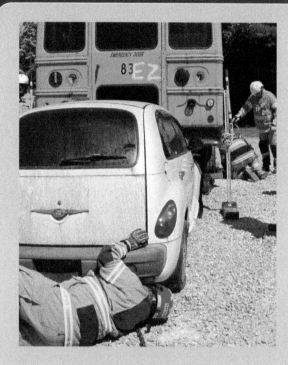

4 Position several personnel at each point of lifting. Assign a safety officer on both sides at the rear of the bus to oversee the direction of the lift and maintain the coordination of the crews. The IC should be positioned at the rear of the bus and direct commands to the two safety officers only. Attach a winch from an apparatus or small tow unit to the rear of the vehicle underride.

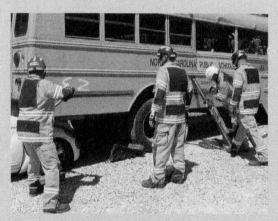

5 Prepare to pull the vehicle out from under the bus as space is created from the bus being lifted. The IC will order the jacks to be lifted simultaneously to avoid unwanted shifting or rocking from uncoordinated lifting while the struts are being adjusted to match the lift of the jacks.

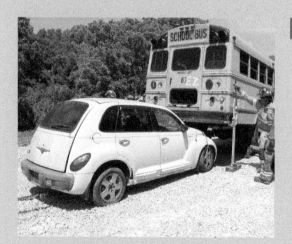

6 Continue the lift in the same fashion until enough room has been created to pull the vehicle out from the entrapment of the bus. Once the vehicle has been pulled out, stabilize the vehicle, and then perform the appropriate access procedure and remove the victim(s).

Courtesy of David Sweet.

Alternative-Fuel Buses

The majority of school buses on the road today utilize conventional diesel as their fuel source, with a smaller proportion of buses utilizing regular unleaded gasoline. However, just like the auto industry, school bus manufacturers are designing buses to operate on alternative fuels as well as advanced propulsion systems, such as hybrid and fuel-cell technology. Alternative fuels such as propane, biodiesel, liquefied natural gas, and compressed natural gas are starting to become more prevalent. Other systems such as bi-fuel or dual-fuel engines are designed to run on two different types of fuels by switching from one tank to another. There are also newer and cleaner types of petroleum-based fuels such as clean diesel, or reformulated gasoline, also known as oxygenated gasoline, or the E85 flex fuel.

Propane is one of the more prevalent alternative fuels used in school buses. Propane by itself has no scent, but a chemical odorant, ethyl mercaptan, has been added to alert of a leak or gas in the air.

The correct mixture of propane in air must contain 2.2 percent to 9.6 percent propane vapor for ignition to occur as well as an ignition temperature of 940°F (504°C). Fire suppression efforts include copious amounts of water to cool down the tanks below the ignition temperature or disperse the vapor. Propane tanks are constructed of carbon steel and are 20 times more puncture resistant than most diesel or gasoline tanks. They also are equipped with a pressure release device that automatically releases product when overpressing of the tank occurs (**FIGURE 13-17**). Propane gas has a heavier-than-air chemical property and a propensity to seek lower ground when released in the atmosphere. For this reason, propane tanks are positioned lower to the ground on the frame of the vehicle. In contrast, compressed natural gas has a lighter-than-air chemical property, and tanks are positioned higher on the frame and body of the vehicle. (Refer to Chapter 7, *Advanced Vehicle Technology: Alternative-Fuel Vehicles*, for more information on the chemical properties of these fuels as well as the general and emergency shutdown procedures.)

Hybrid technology for school buses utilizes the same design concept as conventional vehicles, where parallel (more common) or series propulsion systems are combined with a diesel- or gasoline-powered internal combustion engine (ICE). The industry standard orange-colored high-voltage wire is also used. A parallel system is more commonly used in types C and D school buses and is designed to work in tandem with a diesel-powered ICE. The propulsion of the bus can be operated either from the onboard electric generator

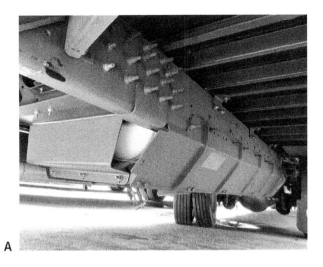

A

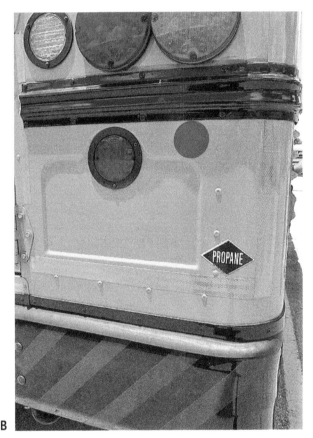

B

FIGURE 13-17 Propane tanks are constructed of carbon steel and are 20 times more puncture resistant than most diesel or gasoline tanks. They also are equipped with a pressure release device that automatically releases product when overpressing of the tank occurs.
Courtesy of David Sweet.

or through the diesel-powered ICE. In this particular parallel design, the hybrid system is placed behind the transmission, which allows the bus to operate solely on the battery system or the ICE. To engage the hybrid system, the driver must flip an operational switch located on a separate hybrid driver interface panel mounted on the dashboard. A hybrid school bus, regardless of the propulsion system, uses two or more 12-volt DC batteries located on a slide-out tray, normally positioned outside at the front of the bus on the driver's side area. These batteries function in the same fashion as those in a conventional school bus—that is, they start the bus, power the air conditioner, power basic electrical components, and so on.

> **LISTEN UP!**
>
> A hybrid school bus, regardless of the propulsion system, uses two or more 12-volt DC batteries located on a slide-out tray, normally positioned outside at the front of the bus on the driver's side area.

> **LISTEN UP!**
>
> Two types of parallel hybrid systems are in use for types C and D school buses:
> - *Charge-depleting hybrid system*: Utilizes a sealed lithium-ion (Li-Ion) battery pack comprising twenty-eight 12-volt DC batteries set in series and yielding 336 DC volts and requiring 4 to 8 hours of charging time depending on whether a 120- or 220-volt charge base system is used. The system is designed to utilize the battery system for up to 44 mi (71 km), depending on the terrain, and then must be recharged.
> - *Charge-sustaining hybrid system*: Utilizes nickel metal hydride (NiMh) batteries in 7.2-volt modules operating at a nominal 288 DC volts. Battery recharge is controlled by a continuous supply of power through regenerative braking.

Two types of parallel hybrid systems are in use for types C and D school buses; they consist of the **charge-depleting hybrid system**, which is a plug-in hybrid electric vehicle (PHEV), and the **charge-sustaining hybrid system**, which is a standard hybrid that operates on regenerative properties to charge its batteries. The battery pack for both systems is placed in a sealed unit, which comes in two designs. One is a single battery pack that weighs up to 1500 lb (680 kg) and is set in the undercarriage on the driver's side. Because of the weight load of this single battery pack, a counterbalance on the opposite side of the vehicle is used that weighs up to 1000 lb (454 kg). The other battery system design splits the battery pack into two battery packs that are set opposite each other on both sides of the undercarriage of the bus, thus eliminating the need for any counterbalancing weight. The battery packs also have a service disconnect switch that is designed to cut off voltage from the packs. This switch is easily recognizable and attainable, being mounted on the outside of the pack and in clear view.

A **series-operated propulsion system**, which is not as commonly found, is a system design that utilizes the electric motor by itself to propel the school bus, and the combustion engine is used only to regenerate the battery pack. These systems may be found on a type A school bus.

Emergency Procedures for the Hybrid Bus

The emergency procedures for disabling the hybrid system on a type C or D bus are directed at the current parallel system described in the preceding section; newer hybrid propulsion drive designs are in the developmental stages and will likely have different emergency procedures for disabling. It is the responsibility of the technical rescuer to stay current with the latest technology and research development in new types of hybrid propulsion system designs.

The following skill drill assumes that the vehicle has been in a collision and is upright; it will include additional appropriate steps for addressing this type of incident.

To properly disable the hybrid system on a type C or D school bus, follow **SKILL DRILL 13-15**. Some steps may occur simultaneously. Please note that there are no photos for this skill drill.

SKILL DRILL 13-15
Disabling the Hybrid System on a Type C or D School Bus

1. Don appropriate PPE. Assess the scene for hazards, and complete the inner and outer surveys. Avoid standing at the front or rear of the vehicle to protect against any sudden forward or backward movement of the vehicle. Activate MCI protocols if they are pre-established and/or if they are needed based on the number of victims. Call for additional resources, such as an appropriately sized tow truck unit, TRT unit, or hazardous materials unit. Set up the control zones (hot, warm, and cold). Set up two 1.75-in. (44-mm) charged hose lines in defensive positions. Ensure that the vehicle is not running.

2. Gain entry into the school bus, and disable the hybrid system. Turn off the operational switch located on the hybrid driver interface panel mounted on the dashboard. Turn off and remove the vehicle ignition key. Set the vehicle's parking brake.

3. Exit the bus, and turn off the battery pack service disconnect switch located on the outside of the battery pack. Locate and disable the conventional 12-volt DC battery system (not the hybrid battery pack) according to the procedures outlined in this chapter.

4. Place two FRJs at the rear of the school bus, lifting from the bumper. Position four tension buttress struts on the school bus, two at the front sides and two at the rear sides in an A-frame setup. Create purchase points for the tips of the struts to be set in place using a battery-powered drill with a step bit attachment, a Halligan bar and a flat-head axe, or a pneumatic air chisel. Pass the cargo straps under the school bus using a long pike pole to avoid going under the vehicle.

5. Additional cross-tie box cribbing can be set in position under the frame at the rear of the school bus and at the front under the bumper area. This will require a lot of cribbing; ensure that the units on hand can support this task. The cribbing height for a cross-tie box crib should not exceed two times its width. Prevent any forward or backward movement by positioning cribbing or step chocks upside down in a wedge-type setup in front of and behind each tire.

After-Action REVIEW

IN SUMMARY

- The Federal Motor Carrier Safety Administration categorizes buses into carrier types or by function or purpose, such as school bus, transit bus, intercity bus, and charter/tour bus.
- As an emergency responder, you may never come across a school bus accident, but it is vital to be prepared and know the makeup, structural components, and different types of school buses that are on the roadways today.
- The school bus industry has designated four categories of school buses: types A, B, C, and D.
- The overall design features of the bus, such as metal thickness and spacing of channel beams, may vary among manufacturers, but all must meet the FMVSS for school buses.
- Many of the design features of a school bus integrate safety.
- The greatest concern for the officer in charge at a school bus extrication incident is gaining and maintaining control of the incident through proper scene management.
- Progressive agencies have preplanned and trained heavily for such an event and have pre-established MCI protocols and/or an emergency response plan in place.

- Upon your arrival at the scene of a school bus extrication, give a clear and accurate account of what is presented, and conduct inner and outer surveys of the scene to formulate your IAP.
- As with most vehicles, there are basically four positions in which a school bus will present that the technical rescuer will have to stabilize: upright, on its side, on its roof, or on another vehicle.

KEY TERMS

Active regeneration The second of three stages of regeneration in which fuel is injected into the system to burn and create higher temperatures of up to 1112°F (600°C).

Bow trusses Structural steel members that run continuously from below the floor level on one side of a bus, vertically raising and bowing over to form the roof structure, and then extending over and down the other side of the bus, past the floor level.

Charge-depleting hybrid system A plug-in hybrid electric vehicle (PHEV).

Charge-sustaining hybrid system A standard hybrid that operates on regenerative properties to charge its batteries.

Charter/tour bus A company providing transportation on a for-hire basis, usually round-trip service for a tour group or outing. The transportation can be for a specific event or can be part of a regular tour.

Crash rail A rail designed to protect students from impact intrusions into the passenger compartment of a school bus; normally composed of 14-gauge steel and extending the entire length of the school bus just above the floor area between the floor and the seat rub rail.

Exhaust after-treatment device A device that replaced the standard muffler assembly. It captures and converts soot to carbon dioxide and water through the combination of a diesel particulate filter (DPF) and a diesel oxidation catalyst (DOC).

Intercity bus A company providing for-hire, long-distance passenger transportation between cities over fixed routes with regular schedules.

Manual regeneration The last of three stages of regeneration that occurs only when the parking brake is set and the engine is running. It is normally completed when the active regeneration fails to clear the system sufficiently.

Passive regeneration The first of three stages of regeneration that occurs automatically when the particulate matter (soot) that is caught in the DPF is burned off naturally by the elevated temperatures of the exhaust system.

Rub rails Visible exterior steel attachments that consist of 16-gauge corrugated metal. These steel members are 4 in. (102 mm) or more in width and are attached to the bow trusses. They run the entire length of the school bus, wrapping around to the rear of the vehicle.

School bus Any public or private school or district or contracted carrier operating on behalf of the entity, providing transportation for kindergarteners through grade 12 pupils.

Series-operated propulsion system A system that utilizes the electric motor by itself to propel a school bus, and the internal combustion engine is used only to regenerate the battery pack. These systems may be found on type A school buses.

Stringers Steel longitudinal structural members that give the bow frame truss members structural support at the roof level; they run continuously from the front to the rear of a school bus.

SWOT analysis A self-examination model that can be adjusted, adapted, and applied to any situation, incident, or project, large or small, that an organization is currently or will be involved in.

Transit bus An entity providing passenger transportation over fixed, scheduled routes, within primarily urban geographic areas.

Type A school bus A conversion-type bus constructed utilizing a cutaway front section vehicle with a left-side driver's door. This definition includes two subclassifications: type A-1, with a GVWR of 14,500 lb (6577 kg) or less, and type A-2, with a GVWR greater than 14,500 lb (6577 kg) and less than or equal to 21,500 lb (9752 kg).

Type B school bus A school bus that is constructed utilizing a stripped chassis. The entrance door is behind the front wheels. This definition includes two subclassifications: type B-1, with a GVWR of 10,000 lb (4536 kg) or less, and type B-2, with a GVWR greater than 10,000 lb (4536 kg).

Type C school bus (also known as a conventional school bus) A school bus that is constructed utilizing a chassis with a hood and front fender assembly. The entrance door is behind the front wheels. This type of school bus has a GVWR greater than 21,500 lb (9752 kg). Eighty-five to 90 percent of all school buses are type C or D.

Type D school bus (also known as a transit-style rear or front engine school bus) A school bus that is constructed utilizing a stripped chassis where the outer body of the bus is mounted to the bare chassis. The entrance door is ahead of the front wheels, and the face, or front section, of the bus is flat. Type D buses have a passenger capacity of 80 to 90 people.

REFERENCE

Blower, Daniel, Paul E. Green, and Anne Matteson. 2008. "Bus Operator Types and Driver Factors in Fatal Bus Crashes: Results from the Buses Involved in Fatal Accidents Survey." University of Michigan Transportation Research Institute for the Federal Motor Carrier Safety Administration. https://deepblue.lib.umich.edu/bitstream/handle/2027.42/61823/102176.pdf?sequence=1&isAllowed=y.

On Scene

You are the officer assigned to an engine company that has been dispatched to a motor vehicle accident involving a school bus. On your arrival you note that a type C school bus is lying on its side on the side of the road. It appears the right tires slipped off the edge of the road and caused the bus to roll right. You have occupants trapped inside.

1. What is the greatest initial concern for this incident?
   A. The number of victims
   B. The number of personnel needed
   C. The media
   D. Whether there are hazardous materials involved

2. A type C school bus is also known as:
   A. a traditional bus.
   B. the largest of all school bus types.
   C. a conventional bus.
   D. a transit-type bus.

3. Bow frame trusses on a bus run from floor level on one side of the bus to the:
   A. roof level.
   B. window sill level on the opposite side of the bus.
   C. floor level on the opposite side of the bus.
   D. rub rail on the opposite side of the bus.

4. What do exterior rivet heads on the outer panel of the school bus indicate?
   A. The panels are connected to the body.
   B. There is a structural member underneath the panel.
   C. Rivet heads are decorative only.
   D. The design is weak, and the rivet head will shear off.

5. Rub rails are strategically placed with the middle rail positioned at the area of the seat cushion level and the bottom rail positioned:
   A. at the floor line.
   B. at the window line.
   C. There is no set position for this rub rail.
   D. Newer buses no longer use rub rails.

6. The greatest concern for the officer in charge at a school bus extrication incident is:
   A. handling the media.
   B. gaining and maintaining control of the incident through proper scene management.
   C. having the proper equipment available to perform the rescue.
   D. making sure to document your Incident Management System.

(continues)

On Scene Continued

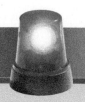

7. A rail designed to protect students from impact intrusions into the passenger compartment of a school bus, normally composed of 14-gauge steel extending just above the floor area between the floor and the seat rub rail, extending the entire length of the school bus is known as a:

   A. rub rail.
   B. stringer.
   C. side-impact rail.
   D. crash rail.

8. A school bus that is constructed utilizing a stripped chassis with the entrance door behind the front wheels is a:

   A. type A school bus.
   B. type B school bus.
   C. type C school bus.
   D. type D school bus.

9. This type of school bus is also known as a "transit-style" rear or front engine school bus.

   A. Type A school bus
   B. Type B school bus
   C. Type C school bus
   D. Type D school bus

10. As an emergency responder, it is vital to be prepared and know the makeup, structural components, and different types of school buses that are on the roadways today as you:

    A. may never come across a school bus accident.
    B. may respond to these incidents regularly.
    C. may respond to one or two of these incidents each month.
    D. may respond to these incidents frequently.

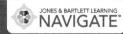 *Access Navigate for more activities.*

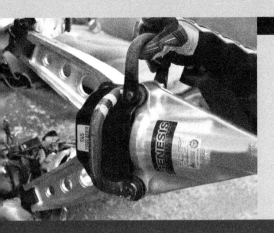

Appendix
NFPA 1006 Correlation Guide

NFPA 1006 Standard for Technical Rescue Personnel Professional Qualifications, 2021 Edition Correlation Guide

Awareness	Chapter(s)	Page(s)
8.1	1, 2, 3	3–93
8.1.1	2	42–43
8.1.1 (A)	2	42–43
8.1.1 (B)	2, 3	42–43, 50–57
8.1.2	1	6–7, 12
8.1.2 (A)	1, 2	6–7, 28–29, 42–43
8.1.2 (B)	2	25–26
8.1.3	2	35–36, 38, 40–42
8.1.3 (A)	2	23–24
8.1.3 (B)	2, 3	42–43, 50–57
8.1.4	2	21–22, 24, 32, 33–34, 36–45
8.1.4 (A)	2	21–22, 24, 32, 33–34, 36–45
8.1.4 (B)	2	42–43
8.1.5	2	21–22, 24, 26–32, 33–34, 36–45
8.1.5 (A)	3	50–57
8.1.5 (B)	2	26–32

Operations	Chapter(s)	Page(s)
8.2	4, 5, 6, 7, 8, 9, 10, 11	101–325
8.2.1	4, 5, 7	103, 111–115, 126–130, 132–136, 138–140, 169–170
8.2.1 (A)	4, 5, 7	103, 111–115, 126–130, 132–136, 138–140, 169–170
8.2.1 (B)	4, 7	108–109, 170–171
8.2.2	4	103, 111–113
8.2.2 (A)	4	103, 111–113
8.2.2 (B)	5, 7	112, 170–171
8.2.3	8	201–206, 208–212
8.2.3 (A)	8	201–206, 208–212
8.2.3 (B)	7, 8, 9, 10	170–171, 201–206, 208–216, 222–223, 314
8.2.4	5, 6, 7	123–124, 144, 161–164, 169–172, 175, 176, 178, 182, 186
8.2.4 (A)	5, 6, 7	123–124, 144, 161–164, 169–172, 175, 176, 178, 182, 186
8.2.4 (B)	6, 7, 8, 9, 10	161–162, 170-171, 173, 175–183, 186–188, 191–192, 193–194, 218, 233, 234, 243, 246, 250, 251–252, 253, 255, 276, 284–286, 297, 299–300, 302–310
8.2.5	4, 5, 8, 9	105–107, 130–131, 212, 222–224, 233–234, 237–238, 249, 251–252, 264, 267, 276
8.2.5 (A)	4, 5, 8, 9	105–107, 130–131, 212, 223
8.2.5 (B)	4	103, 105–108
8.2.6	5, 9	130–131, 222–224
8.2.6 (A)	5, 9	130–131, 222–224
8.2.6 (B)	4, 7, 9, 10	103, 105–108, 109–113, 201–206, 208–216, 222–227, 229, 230, 232–234, 236, 242–244, 246–249, 250, 251–252, 253–254, 255, 257–259, 261–263, 264–265, 267–271, 276, 284–286, 288, 289, 290–294, 297, 299–300, 302–314
8.2.7	9	222–224, 276–278
8.2.7 (A)	9	222–224, 276–278

Operations	Chapter(s)	Page(s)
8.2.7 (B)	9, 10	226–227, 229, 230, 232, 234, 236, 242–244, 246–249, 250–251, 253–254, 257–259, 261–263, 264–265, 267–271, 284–286, 288, 289, 290–294, 297, 299–300, 302–314
8.2.8	9	222–224, 276–278
8.2.8 (A)	9	275–278
8.2.8 (B)	4, 9	108–109, 277–278
8.2.9	11	318–321, 323, 324–325
8.2.9 (A)	11	318–321, 323, 324–325
8.2.9 (B)	11	318–320, 324–326

Technician	Chapter(s)	Page(s)
8.3	4, 5, 6, 7, 8, 9, 10	101–325
8.3.1	5, 7	126–130, 132–136, 138–140, 188–193
8.3.1 (A)	5, 7	126–130, 132–136, 138–140, 188–193
8.3.1 (B)	4	108–109
8.3.2	8	201–203
8.3.2 (A)	8	201–203
8.3.2 (B)	9	222–223
8.3.3	5	130–131
8.3.3 (A)	5	130–131
8.3.3 (B)	4, 9	105–108, 222–226
8.3.4	4, 5, 8	111–115, 126–130, 132–136, 138–140, 208–209
8.3.4 (A)	4, 5, 8	111–115, 126–130, 132–136, 138–140, 208–209
8.3.4 (B)	4, 9	108–109, 222–226
8.3.5	8	203–206, 208–212
8.3.5 (A)	8	203–206, 208–212
8.3.5 (B)	8	201–206, 208–216

Technician	Chapter(s)	Page(s)
8.3.6	5, 9	130–131, 222–224
8.3.6 (A)	5, 9	130–131, 222–224
8.3.6 (B)	4, 9	105–109, 226–227, 229, 230, 232, 234, 236, 242–244, 246–249, 250–251, 253–254, 257–259, 261–263, 264–265, 267–271
8.3.7	5, 8	126–130, 132–136, 138–140, 200, 203–205
8.3.7 (A)	5, 8	126–130, 132–136, 138–140, 200, 203–205
8.3.7 (B)	4	108–109
8.3.8	8	203–206, 208–212
8.3.8 (A)	8	203–206, 208–212
8.3.8 (B)	8	201–206, 208–216
8.3.9	9	222–224, 276–278
8.3.9 (A)	9	222–224, 276–278
8.3.9 (B)	9, 10	226–227, 229, 230, 232, 234, 236, 242–244, 246–249, 250–251, 253–254, 257–259, 261–263, 264–265, 267–271, 284–286, 288, 289, 290–294, 297, 299–300, 302–314

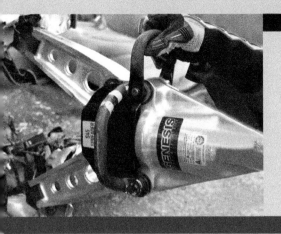

Glossary

A

Absorbed glass matt (AGM) A type of battery in which a glass mat is used to absorb and hold the electrolyte, preventing it from moving within the battery.

Accelerometer A sensor that detects a crash.

Active regeneration The second of three stages of regeneration in which fuel is injected into the system to burn and create higher temperatures of up to 1112°F (600°C).

Active restraint device A device that the occupant must activate; for example, a seat belt is an active device because the occupant has to engage the seat belt mechanism into the anchor unit.

Active risk–benefit analysis An analysis that entails an on-scene assessment of the risk to personnel and/or victims compared to the benefits that might result from the rescue.

Adapters Devices used to convert a battery-powered tool to a general-current tool.

Advanced high-strength steel (AHSS) Steel with a minimum tensile strength of 63 to 145 ksi (434 to 1000 MPa).

After-action report (AAR) A brief summary that analyzes the overall operations and effectiveness of the agency at a particular incident, measuring its capabilities through real-time on-scene evaluations.

Aggregate weight A measurement combining all packages in a CMV to determine the total weight of all the hazards.

Air bag An inflatable bag that inflates automatically to cushion passengers in the event of a collision. The air bag itself typically consists of a strong, durable nylon or blended material that is folded in a certain manner to facilitate inflation.

Air bag control unit (ACU) See *electronic control unit (ECU)*.

Air brake (parking brake) A brake used on some models of CMVs that causes the suspension system to release air and drop several inches to accommodate a resting or parked position.

Air compressors Equipment used to provide power to pneumatic tools or to provide breathing air.

Air impact wrench A pneumatic tool used to remove bolts/nuts of various sizes.

Air-lift bags Inflatable devices used to lift an object or spread one or more objects away from each other to assist in freeing a victim. They come in various sizes and types, such as low-pressure bags, medium-pressure bags, high-pressure bags, high-pressure flat bags, and multi-cell bags.

Air ride system A system designed to inflate and deflate the suspension through onboard air pressure tanks to protect the cargo and the frame system of the vehicle.

Air shores Shores extended by the use of compressed air; shores are used where the vertical distances are too great to use cribbing or the load must be supported horizontally.

Alloyed Created by combining two or more elements.

Alloyed steels Materials composed of steel and a mixture of various metals and elements. They are classified by both their strength range in megapascals and by their metallurgical type designation.

Alternative-fuel vehicle A motorized vehicle propelled by anything other than gasoline or diesel.

Aluminum alloyed metal A composition of various metals, including pure aluminum; its main design is to strengthen and lighten the vehicle.

A-posts/pillars Vertical support members located closest to the front windshield of a vehicle.

Authority having jurisdiction (AHJ) An organization, office, or individual responsible for enforcing the requirements of a code or standard or for approving equipment, materials, an installation, or a procedure. (NFPA 1006)

Automatic seat belt system A seat belt system that uses a shoulder harness that automatically slides on a steel or aluminum track system on the door window frame. When the door is closed, the shoulder harness automatically slides into place. The lap section of the harness has to be manually engaged.

Awareness level (1) This level represents the minimum capability of individuals who provide response to technical search and rescue incidents. (NFPA 1006) (2) This level represents the minimum capability of organizations that provide response to technical search and rescue incidents. (NFPA 1670)

Axle A structural component or shaft that is designed for wheel rotation.

B

Backboard slide technique An initial access technique that is used if the vehicle doors are locked, blocked, or inoperable; may be accomplished through a rear or side window.

Ballistic glass Glass that uses multiple layers of tempered glass, laminate material, and polycarbonate thermoplastics, all sandwiched together to the desired thickness. The weight and thickness of the glass increase depending on each increased level of protection, which can be as high as 3 in. (76 mm).

Behavioral reactions Negative reactions that may present as withdrawal from others, emotional outbursts, extreme changes in normal behavior (such as silence or hyperactivity), repeated drunkenness, negative sexual reactions, insomnia, or absenteeism.

Beneficial systems Auxiliary-powered equipment in motor vehicles or machines that can enhance or facilitate rescues such as electric, pneumatic, or hydraulic seat positioners, door locks, window operating mechanisms, suspension systems, tilt steering wheels, convertible tops, or other devices or systems to facilitate the movement (extension, retraction, raising, lowering, conveyor control) of equipment or machinery. (NFPA 1006)

Biodiesel A safe, nontoxic, biodegradable fuel used solely for diesel engines that is processed from domestic renewable resources, such as plant oils; grease; animal fats; used cooking oil; and, more recently, algae. Biodiesel can be used by itself as a diesel fuel or blended with petroleum diesel at varying percentages.

Body-over-frame construction Vehicle design in which the body of the vehicle is placed onto a frame skeleton and the frame acts as the foundation for the vehicle. The design consists of two large beams tied together by cross-member beams.

Boiling liquid expanding vapor explosion (BLEVE) An event that occurs when the temperature of the liquid and vapor (flammable or nonflammable) within a confining tank or vessel is raised by an exposure fire to the point where the increasing internal pressures can no longer be contained and the vessel ruptures and explodes.

Bow trusses Structural steel members that run continuously from below the floor level on one side of a bus, vertically raising and bowing over to form the roof structure, and then extending over and down the other side of the bus, past the floor level.

B-posts Vertical support members located between the front and rear doors of a vehicle.

Branches The organizational level having functional, geographic, or jurisdictional responsibility for major aspects of incident operations. (NFPA 1026)

Bumper system Front and rear vehicle frame attachment system designed to reduce the damage effect of a vehicle involved in low-speed collisions.

C

Cab The enclosed space where the driver and passengers sit.

Cab beside engine Design in which the driver sits next to the engine. These trucks are mostly found in shipyards and baggage carriers within airports and seaports.

Cab over engine (COE) (often referred to as a tilt cab) Design in which the cab is lifted over the engine to gain access to the engine itself. The driver's seat is positioned over the engine and the front axle.

Carbon One of the most abundant elements in the universe, classified as a nonmetallic element. It has the unique ability to bond with multiple elements.

Carbon fiber reinforced polymer (CFRP) An extremely strong and light fiber-reinforced plastic that contains carbon fibers.

Cargo tank Bulk packaging that is permanently attached to or forms a part of a motor vehicle or that is not permanently attached to any motor vehicle and that, because of its size, construction, or attachment to a motor vehicle, is loaded or unloaded without being removed from the motor vehicle.

Chain saw Gasoline-powered saws capable of cutting wood, concrete, and even light-gauge steel. Standard steel chains are used to cut wood, carbide-tipped chains can cut wood and light-gauge metal, and diamond chains are used for cutting concrete.

Charge-depleting hybrid system A plug-in hybrid electric vehicle (PHEV).

Charge-sustaining hybrid system A standard hybrid that operates on regenerative properties to charge its batteries.

Charter/tour bus A company providing transportation on a for-hire basis, usually round-trip service for a tour group or outing. The transportation can be for a specific event or can be part of a regular tour.

Chassis The basic operating motor vehicle including the engine, frame, and other essential structural and mechanical parts but exclusive of the body and all appurtenances for the accommodation of driver, property, passengers, appliances, or equipment related to other than control. Common usage might, but need not, include a cab (or cowl). (NFPA 1911)

Circular saw An electric- or battery-powered saw that moves in a circular motion; these saws come in a variety of sizes and are used primarily for cutting wood, although special blades are available that will cut metal or masonry.

Class 1 commercial vehicle A vehicle with a gross vehicle weight rating ranging from 0 to 6000 lb (0 to 2722 kg).

Class 2a commercial vehicle A vehicle with a gross vehicle weight rating ranging from 6001 to 8500 lb (2722 to 3856 kg); a light-duty vehicle.

Class 2b commercial vehicle A vehicle with a gross vehicle weight rating ranging from 8501 to 10,000 lb (3856 to 4536 kg); considered by many as a light-duty vehicle.

Class 3 commercial vehicle A vehicle with a gross vehicle weight rating ranging from 10,001 to 14,000 lb (4536 to 6350 kg).

Class 4 commercial vehicle A vehicle with a gross vehicle weight rating ranging from 14,001 to 16,000 lb (6351 to 7257 kg).

Class 5 commercial vehicle A vehicle with a gross vehicle weight rating ranging from 16,001 to 19,500 lb (7258 to 8845 kg).

Class 6 commercial vehicle A vehicle with a gross vehicle weight rating ranging from 19,501 to 26,000 lb (8846 to 11,793 kg).

Class 7 commercial vehicle A vehicle with a gross vehicle weight rating ranging from 26,001 to 33,000 lb (11,794 to 14,969 kg).

Class 8 commercial vehicle A vehicle with a gross vehicle weight rating of more than 33,000 lb (14,969 kg).

Class A foam Class A foam is for use on fires in Class A fuels, materials such as vegetation, wood, cloth, paper, and some plastics where combustion can occur at or below the surface of the material.

Class B foam Foam used to extinguish flammable and combustible liquid (Class B) fires.

Cognitive reactions Negative reactions that may present as attention deficit disorder, nightmares, confusion, lack of concentration, decreased ability to problem solve, or constant reliving of the event through flashbacks.

Cold zone The control zone of an incident that contains the command post and other support functions deemed necessary to control the incident. (NFPA 1500)

Come along A ratchet lever winching tool that can provide up to several thousand pounds of pulling force, with the standard model for extrication being 2000 to 4000 lb (907 to 1814 kg) of pulling force.

Commercial motor vehicle (CMV) Defined by the DOT as a motor vehicle or combination of motor vehicles used in commerce to transport passengers or property if the motor vehicle has a gross vehicle weight rating (GVWR) of 26,001 lb (11,794 kg) or more inclusive of a towed unit(s) with a GVWR of more than 10,000 lb (4536 kg); or has a GVWR of 26,001 lb

(11,794 kg) or more; or is designed to transport 16 or more passengers, including the driver; or is of any size and is used in the transportation of hazardous materials.

Common passenger vehicle Light or medium duty passenger and commercial vehicles commonly encountered in the jurisdiction and presenting no unusual construction, occupancy, or operational characteristics to rescuers during an extrication event. (NFPA 1006)

Compressed natural gas (CNG) A natural lighter-than-air gas compressed for use as a fuel that consists principally of methane in gaseous form plus naturally occurring mixtures of hydrocarbon gases. (NFPA 302)

Contact point When sections of cribbing are set on top of one another, the weight-bearing section of cribbing that crosses over the other. When using a 4-in. × 4-in. (10-cm × 10-cm) piece of timber, each contact point has an estimated weight-bearing capacity of 6000 lb (3 short tons).

Conventional cab Design in which the driver's seat is positioned behind the engine and front axle. The front end of the vehicle extends approximately 6 to 8 ft (1.8 to 2.4 m) from the front windshield.

Conventional-type vehicles Vehicles that use an internal combustion engine (ICE) for power.

Core support A key component of the front end of the vehicle, designed to secure the radiator to the engine assembly frame and tie the upper and lower rails together. It also houses the lights, horn, and other components while maintaining alignment of the hood with the hood latch.

Cowl section Upper area of the front passenger compartment directly in front of the windshield.

C-post A vertical support member located behind the rear doors of a vehicle.

Crash rail A rail designed to protect students from impact intrusions into the passenger compartment of a school bus; normally composed of 14-gauge steel and extending the entire length of the school bus just above the floor area between the floor and the seat rub rail.

Crew A group of personnel working without apparatus and led by a leader or boss.

Crew resource management (CRM) A program focused on improved situational awareness, sound critical decision-making, effective communication, proper task allocation, and successful teamwork and leadership. (NFPA 1500)

Cribbing Short lengths of timber/composite materials, usually 4 in. × 4 in. (101.60 mm × 101.60 mm) and 18 to 24 in. (457.20 to 609.60 mm) long, that are used in various configurations to stabilize loads in place or while load is moving. (NFPA 1670)

Critical incident stress management (CISM) A type of behavioral health mechanism for crisis intervention specifically designed to help emergency personnel who have been exposed to a traumatic event process their response to the incident in a way that validates the normal stress reactions and stabilizes the potential negative results of the individual's response.

Cross-ramming technique The use of a hydraulic ram to push off of the opposite door post, B-post, floor transmission hump, or inside rocker panel to move the interior of the vehicle away from the entrapped occupant.

Crumple zones Engineered collapsible zones that are incorporated into the frame of a vehicle to absorb energy during a collision.

Cutting torches A tool that produces an extremely high-temperature flame capable of heating steel until it melts, burns, and oxidizes, thus cutting through the object. This tool is sometimes used for rescue situations such as cutting through heavy steel objects.

D

Dash lift technique A technique used to lift and release a section of the dash from the front end of the vehicle using a powered tool, such as the hydraulic spreader, or a combination of hand tools and powered tools. It is performed by making precise relief cuts in the hood's upper rail and between the hinges of the firewall area, separating the dash section from the front end of the vehicle.

Dash reinforcement bar A metal beam or bar that runs the entire width of the dash.

Dash roll technique The standard technique for many years for displacing the dashboard using a powered tool, such as the hydraulic ram, or a combination of hand tools and powered tools. The process involves the force of pushing or rolling the entire front end of the vehicle upward and forward, including the dashboard and steering wheel assembly, off of the entrapped occupant.

Dead axle An axle used for load support more commonly set in the front section of a semi-truck; also functions for steering and is therefore also known as a steer axle.

Dead-man control A control feature designed to return the control of the hydraulic tool to the neutral position automatically in the event the control is released.

Defensive apparatus placement The positioning of apparatus to block and protect the scene from the flow of traffic.

Department of Transportation's (DOT's) Emergency Response Guidebook (ERG) A reference book, written in plain language, to guide emergency responders in their initial actions at the incident scene. (NFPA 475)

Disentanglement The spreading, cutting, or removal of a vehicle away from trapped or injured victims.

Distress Stress that generally produces a negative response, such as that experienced through the exposure to a critical incident.

Division A supervisory level established to divide an incident into geographic areas of operations. (NFPA 1561)

Door hinge A mechanism that provides the opening and closing movements for a door. Door hinges commonly range from 8- to 15-gauge metal and can be a full-body or layered-leaf system.

Door limiting device A hardened section of steel or composite material that is designed to assist the door in opening and closing. It can be located between the top and bottom hinge.

Drive train (power train) A system that transfers rotational power from the engine to the wheels, which makes the vehicle move.

Dromedary (drom) A separate box, deck, or plate mounted behind the cab and in front of the fifth wheel on the frame of a semi-truck.

Dry bulk cargo tanks A tank designed to carry dry bulk goods such as powders, pellets, fertilizers, or grain. Such tanks are generally V-shaped with rounded sides that funnel toward the bottom of the tank.

E

Electric vehicle (EV) A vehicle that is 100 percent electric, emits no air pollutants, and is propelled by one or more electric motors, which are powered by rechargeable battery packs.

Electric-powered tools Tools that utilize a general current or generator to operate.

Electrical generators Generators that utilize a general current or generator to operate. Primarily used to power scene lighting and to run power tools and equipment; may be portable or fixed.

Electronic control unit (ECU) Also known as the air bag control unit (ACU), this is the brains of an air bag system, consisting of a small processing unit generally located in the center of the vehicle.

Electropositive Electrically positive.

Emergency air line (supply line) One of two air lines of an air brake system connecting a tractor to a trailer; the emergency air line is red.

Emergency brake A brake that utilizes a combination of both the service and parking brakes to engage when a brake failure or air line break occurs.

Emergency escape plan A plan for immediate, unexpected hazards that affect the rescuers and/or victim.

Emergency response guide A booklet prepared by vehicle manufacturers to educate and assist emergency response personnel in responding to emergencies dealing with specific types and models of vehicles, such as hybrid/electric, hydrogen fuel-cell, and alternative-fuel systems.

Emotional reactions Negative reactions that may present as depression, guilt, anger, fear, anxiety, feeling of doom, grief, or perceived loss of control.

Energy A fundamental entity of nature that is transferred between parts of a system in the production of physical change within the system and is usually regarded as the capacity for doing work.

Engine cradle Attached to the frame rails and houses the engine and, in some vehicles, the bolt heads, which lock the engine in place; they are designed to shear off on impact to drop the engine under the vehicle instead of into the passenger compartment.

Ethanol A fuel composed of an alcohol base that is normally processed from crops, such as corn, sugar, trees, or grasses.

Eustress Stress that produces a positive response in the mind, body, and spirit, such as that experienced through physical exercise or a team sport. Eustress actually builds resistance to the negative aspects of stress.

Exhaust after-treatment device A device that replaced the standard muffler assembly. It captures and converts soot to carbon dioxide and water through the combination of a diesel particulate filter (DPF) and a diesel oxidation catalyst (DOC).

Expose and cut The process of creating a wide enough opening with the hydraulic spreader to expose the locking/latching mechanism or hinges and to insert a hydraulic cutter to cut.

Extended range electric vehicle (EREV) A vehicle that uses a series-type propulsion system that allows the vehicle to run on all-battery or all-electric power until it is near depletion, which occurs in the range of 40 mi (64 km) or more depending on the manufacturer.

Extrication The process of removing a trapped victim from a vehicle.

F

Federal Motor Vehicle Safety Standards (FMVSS) Safety standards enacted to protect the public from unreasonable risk of crashes, injury, or death resulting from the design, construction, or performance of a motor vehicle.

Ferrous metals Metals that contain iron, cast iron, low- and medium-alloyed steels, and specialty steels, such as tool steels and stainless steels.

Fifth wheel A turntable hitch mounted at the rear of the towing truck or semi-truck.

Finance/administration section Section responsible for all costs and financial actions of the incident or planned event, including the time unit, procurement unit, compensation/claims unit, and the cost unit. (NFPA 1026)

Firewall Also known as the bulkhead; this makes up the front section of the passenger compartment, separating the engine compartment from the passenger compartment.

Flat-form air-lift bags Pneumatic-filled bladders designed to retain their flat profile in the center as they are inflated to lift an object or spread one or more objects away from each other to assist in freeing a victim.

Flexible fuel vehicle (FFV) A vehicle capable of running on gasoline alone or utilizing the E85 blend of up to 85 percent ethanol and 15 percent gasoline.

Footprint A generic term used to describe an object's balance in relation to its center of mass as determined by how much of the object's base touches the surface and how much of the object spans the surface.

Formal incident action plans An IAP that is a formally written document and designed within an ICS for operational periods that generally run 12 or 24 hours and last from several days to weeks.

Fuel cell An electrochemical device that uses a catalyst-facilitated chemical reaction of hydrogen and oxygen to create electricity, which is then used to power an electric motor or generator, with the by-products of this process being water and heat.

Fuel-cell vehicle A hybrid vehicle system in which two separate sources of power are used individually or combined as a propulsion mechanism for the vehicle.

Full hybrid vehicle A vehicle that uses its electric motor or its internal combustion engine or a combination of both to propel itself.

G

Gas-generation system An inflation system that completely fills the air bag to the appropriate inflation ratio to protect the occupant.

Gel cell A type of battery that uses a silica base additive that firms up the electrolyte in a gel state.

Glad hands Couplers that are used to supply air to the braking system of the trailer.

Glass management The process of controlling the voluntary or involuntary fragmentation of glass by applying proper removal techniques and/or securing glass in place.

Golden Period The time during which treatment of shock and traumatic injuries is most critical and the potential for survival is best accomplished through rapid medical intervention.

Grab hook A device designed to take up the slack needed to make a chain the appropriate size for the task at hand; it is utilized by inserting a link of the chain into the slot of the hook. The grab hook may also be referred to as a chain shortener.

Graphene Strongest molecular compound known on the planet; flexible as rubber.

Gravitational acceleration sensor (G-sensor) A sensor that detects a vehicle's weightlessness, such as that experienced in a free fall, when the vehicle starts to roll and come down.

Gross combined weight rating (GCWR) A rating set by the vehicle manufacturer that determines the vehicle's cargo capacity limitations.

Gross vehicle weight rating (GVWR) A rating set by the manufacturer; it shall not be less than the sum of the unloaded vehicle weight, rated cargo load, and 150 lb times the vehicle's designated seating capacity (49 CFR 567.4[g] [3]).

Gross weight The weight of the single item package plus its contents.

Group A supervisory level established to divide the incident into functional areas of operation. (NFPA 1561)

H

Hand tool Any tool or equipment operating from human power.

Hazard analysis A documented assessment performed by personnel knowledgeable of the specific hazards of the material and that is acceptable to the AHJ.

Hazard control zones Delineates the operational boundaries, which are divided into three areas: hot, warm, and cold.

Hazardous material A substance or material including an explosive; radioactive material; infectious substance; flammable or combustible liquid, solid, or gas; toxic, oxidizing, or corrosive material; and compressed gas that the Secretary of Transportation has determined is capable of posing an unreasonable risk to health, safety, and property when transported in commerce and has been designated as hazardous under Section 5103.

Heavy vehicle Heavy duty highway, off-road, construction, or mass transit vehicles constructed of materials presenting resistance to common extrication procedures, tactics, and resources and posing multiple concurrent hazards to rescuers from occupancy, cargo, size, construction, weight, or position. (NFPA 1006)

High-pressure air-lift bags The most commonly used bags among rescue agencies, these bags utilize a working air pressure of approximately 100 to 145 psi (689 to 1000 kPa) to lift an object or spread one or more objects away from each other to assist in freeing a victim. The high-pressure kits come with hoses, a regulator, a master control module, and various other attachments.

High-strength steel (HSS) Steel with an ultimate tensile strength between 39 and 102 ksi (269 and 703 MPa).

Horizontal movement One of five directional movements; the vehicle moves forward or rearward on its longitudinal axis or moves horizontally along its lateral axis.

Hot zone The control zone immediately surrounding a hazardous area, which extends far enough to prevent adverse effects to personnel outside the zone. (NFPA 1500)

Hybrid electric commercial motor vehicle (HECMV) A CMV that utilizes either the internal combustion engine or an electric motor for propulsion.

Hybrid electric vehicle (HEV) A vehicle that combines two or more power sources for propulsion, one of which is electric power.

Hybrid-type inflator Common to side-impact air bags, this device is composed of two chambers. The first-stage chamber uses a small amount of a pyrotechnic gas-producing propellant, and the second-stage chamber is filled with a compressed inert gas or another type of gas. In combination, each chamber produces and/or releases the correct amount of gas to inflate an air bag.

Hybrid vehicle A vehicle that combines two or more power sources for propulsion, generally consisting of generated electricity through a high-voltage electrical system and a petroleum-based fuel or alternative-fuel system through the process of an internal combustion engine.

Hydraulic combination tool A powered rescue tool capable of both spreading and cutting.

Hydraulic cutter A powered rescue tool consisting of at least one movable blade used to cut, shear, or sever material.

Hydraulic ram A powered rescue tool with a piston or other type of extender that generates extending forces or both extending and retracting forces.

Hydraulic rescue tools Tools that operate by transferring energy or force from one area to another by using a hydraulic fluid such as high-density oil.

Hydraulic spreader A powered rescue tool consisting of at least one movable arm that opens to move or spread apart material or to crush or lift material.

Hydrogen An odorless, colorless, flammable, nontoxic gas that combines easily with other elements.

I

Immediate danger to life and health (IDLH) Any condition that would do one or more of the following: pose an immediate or delayed threat to life, cause irreversible adverse health effects, or interfere with an individual's ability to escape unaided from a hazardous environment.

Impact beam A steel section located within a door frame designed to absorb the impact energy of another vehicle or object and lessen the intrusion into the passenger compartment.

Incident action plan (IAP) (1) A verbal or written plan containing incident objectives reflecting the overall strategy and specific control actions where appropriate for managing an incident or planned event. (NFPA 1026) (2) The objectives reflecting the overall incident strategy, tactics, risk management, and member safety that are developed by the incident commander. Incident action plans are updated throughout the incident. (NFPA 1500)

Incident clock A procedure where dispatch will automatically notify the IC at 10-minute intervals until the incident becomes static.

Incident command system (ICS) A management structure that provides a standard approach and structure to managing operations, ensuring that operations are coordinated, safe, and effective, especially when multiple agencies are working together.

Incident commander (IC) The individual responsible for all incident activities, including the development of strategies and tactics and the ordering and release of resources. (NFPA 1026)

Inclinometer sensor A tilt sensor that detects vehicle inclination or tilt with lateral acceleration (detects how fast the vehicle's tilt is changing).

Inflators One of the most critical design features for an air bag, which provides the ability to fill up the bag instantaneously in milliseconds from the onset of the collision. There are two basic inflation systems—a stored compressed-gas system and a gas-generation system.

Informal incident action plans An IAP that is not a formally written document and is designed for small incidents that are mitigated before an operational period is designated.

Initiator A device, such as a squib (a pyrotechnic device), that activates the air bag through an electrical current, which becomes instantly hot and ignites the combustible material inside the containment housing or through ignition of a burst disk, which releases compressed gas.

Inner survey A four-point inspection of the vehicle's front, driver's side, rear, and passenger's side, including the roof and undercarriage on all sides of the vehicle. This survey is conducted approximately 3 to 5 ft (0.9 to 1.5 m) from the vehicle and is performed by the first-arriving company officer or experienced personnel.

Integrated motor assist (IMA) mild hybrid system A hybrid system used by Honda that is designed to start and stop the hybrid electric vehicle's internal combustion engine; in addition, it will assist the internal combustion engine when acceleration is needed.

Intercity bus A company providing for-hire, long-distance passenger transportation between cities over fixed routes with regular schedules.

Internal combustion engine (ICE) Any engine in which the working medium consists of the products of combustion of the air and fuel supplied. (NFPA 20)

J

Jacking the trunk (cracking the undercarriage and lifting the rear end of a vehicle) An extreme technique to be used when something such as a fuel tank or battery pack stored in the trunk blocks any attempt to enter the vehicle through tunneling.

K

Kinetic energy The energy of motion, which is based on vehicle mass (weight) and the speed of travel (velocity).

Kingpin A large locking pin that connects the cargo trailer of a semi-tractor trailer or semi-trailer to the semi-truck or tractor.

L

Ladder cribbing Several 2-in. × 4-in. (5-cm × 10-cm) sections of wood attached together by a strip of webbing running along the sides.

Ladder frame Body-over-frame construction whose cross members and beams resemble a ladder.

Laminated safety glass (LSG) Glass that contains a layer of clear plastic film between two layers of glass.

Landing gear A stabilizing device that can be lowered to support a trailer when not attached to the tractor. This device is usually operated manually by a hand crank.

Law of conservation of energy A law of physics stating that energy can be neither created nor destroyed; it can only change from one form to another.

Law of motion A law of physics describing momentum, acceleration, and action/reaction.

Liaison officer (LO) A member of the command staff, the point of contact for assisting or coordinating agencies. (NFPA 1026)

Lift axle An axle that can be raised or lowered by an air suspension system to increase the weight-carrying capacity of the vehicle or to distribute the cargo weight more evenly across all the axles.

Liquefied natural gas (LNG) A colorless, odorless, nontoxic natural gas that floats on water and is lighter than air when released as a vapor.

Liquefied petroleum gas (LPG) Also known as propane, a fossil fuel produced from the processing of natural gas and also produced as part of the refining process of crude oil. Propane is the third most widely used fuel source behind gasoline and diesel; it is commonly used with forklifts and other similar work units.

Live axle An axle that transmits propulsion or causes the wheels to turn.

Load limiting device A safety design feature that reduces the force applied by the seat belt when it locks in place from the sudden force applied to it. It can be incorporated in the webbing material of the belt or in a torsion bar attached to the retractor gear.

Lockout/tagout systems Methods of ensuring that systems and equipment have been shut down and that switches and valves are locked and cannot be turned on at the incident scene.

Logistics section Section responsible for providing facilities, services, and materials for the incident or planned event, including the communications unit, medical unit, and food unit within the service branch and the supply unit, facilities unit, and ground support unit within the support branch. (NFPA 1026)

Low-pressure air-lift bags Air bags with a very high lift with a maximum working air pressure of approximately 7 psi (48 kPa); they are used to lift an object or spread one or more objects away from each other to assist in freeing a victim.

M

Magnesium alloy A metal that is gaining popularity because of its unique properties and highly sought-after high strength-to-weight characteristics the auto industry requires.

Manual regeneration The last of three stages of regeneration that occurs only when the parking brake is set and the engine is running. It is normally completed when the active regeneration fails to clear the system sufficiently.

Marrying The process of joining vehicles together to eliminate any independent movement.

Mass casualty incident (MCI) An emergency situation that involves more than one victim that places great demand on equipment or personnel, stretching the system to its limit or beyond.

MC-306/DOT 406 flammable liquid tanker A tanker that typically carries between 6000 and 10,000 gal (22,712 and 37,854 L) of a product such as gasoline or other flammable and combustible materials. The tank is nonpressurized.

MC-307/DOT 407 chemical hauler A tanker with a rounded or horseshoe-shaped tank capable of holding 6000 to 7000 gal (22,712 to 37,854 L) of flammable liquid, mild corrosives, and poisons. The tank has a high internal working pressure.

MC-312/DOT 412 corrosives tanker A tanker that often carries aggressive (highly reactive) acids such as concentrated sulfuric and nitric acid. It is characterized by several heavy-duty reinforcing rings around the tank and holds approximately 6000 gal (22,712 L) of product.

MC-331 pressure cargo tanker A tanker that carries materials such as ammonia, propane, Freon, and butane. This type of tank is commonly constructed of steel and has rounded ends and a single open compartment inside. The liquid volume inside the tank varies from the 1000-gal (3785-L) delivery truck to the full-size 11,000-gal (41,640-L) cargo tank.

MC-338 cryogenic tanker A low-pressure tanker designed to maintain the low temperature required by the cryogens it carries. A boxlike structure containing the tank control valves is typically attached to the rear of the tanker.

Mechanism of injury (MOI) The way in which traumatic injuries occur; it describes the forces (or energy transmission) acting on the body that cause injury.

Medium-pressure air-lift bags Air bags that have a rugged design and utilize a working air pressure of approximately 15 psi (103 kPa) used to lift an object or spread one or more objects away from each other to assist in freeing a victim. These bags are not as common as the low- and high-pressure rescue air-lift bags.

Metal A classification or group of elements that possess positive ions, such as iron, gold, silver, and copper; can be ferrous or nonferrous.

Methanol An alcohol-based fuel similar to ethanol. It is also known as a wood alcohol because it is processed from natural wood sources, such as trees and yard clippings. It may be used as a flex fuel in a ratio of 85 percent methanol to 15 percent gasoline, better known as M85.

Mild hybrid vehicle A vehicle that uses electric power in conjunction with an internal combustion engine for vehicle propulsion.

Multi-cell high-pressure air-lift bags Air bags that offer a distinct height advantage over traditional flat bags and utilize a unique lifting system. The more current design is two-cell bags that are joined together and pre-connected. Another version still in use is a round-shaped bag that can be locked together with a threaded connector, creating one bag with multiple cells.

Multistage inflators Also known as hybrid inflators; cylinders that can comprise two separate chambers of compressed gas—one with a large amount of product and the other with a smaller amount of product.

N

Nader pin/bolt A door striker latch pin or bolt composed of heavy-gauge metal that is round in shape with a cap at the end of it. It is a section of the latching mechanism; named after consumer rights advocate Ralph Nader.

Natural gas A fossil fuel primarily composed of methane that can be used as a compressed natural gas (CNG) or liquefied natural gas (LNG).

Neighborhood electric vehicle (NEV) A vehicle that is classified as a battery-operated low-speed vehicle with a top speed of 25 mi/h (40 km/h) and that is approved for street use on public roadways with speeds posted of no greater than 35 mi/h (56 km/h).

NFPA 1006 The standard that establishes the minimum job performance requirements/qualifications necessary for fire service and other emergency response personnel who perform technical rescue. This standard outlines three qualification levels: awareness, operations, and technician.

NFPA 1670 The standard that identifies and qualifies levels of functional capabilities for safely and effectively conducting operations at technical rescue incidents. This standard outlines three operational capability levels: awareness, operations, and technician.

No-entry zone Those areas at an incident scene that no person(s) are allowed to enter, regardless of what personal protective equipment (PPE) they are wearing due to dangerous conditions or crime scene investigation. (NFPA 1500)

Nonferrous metals Metals or alloys free of iron, such as aluminum, copper, nickel, lead, zinc, and tin.

O

O-ring An attachment designed to join chains together or join a chain to a come along utilizing a hook.

Oblong ring See *O-ring*.

Occupant classification system A system consisting of three types of sensors: the seat position sensor, which detects the proximity of the occupant to the air bag; the seat belt sensor, which detects whether the occupant's seat belt is engaged and locked in the housing unit; and the occupant weight sensor, which measures the weight of the occupant, determining whether the occupant has met a preset weight threshold limit.

Operations level (1) This level represents the capability of individuals to respond to technical search and rescue incidents and to identify hazards, use equipment, and apply limited techniques specified in this standard to support and participate in technical search and rescue incidents. (NFPA 1006) (2) This level represents the capability of organizations to respond to technical search and rescue incidents and to identify hazards, use equipment, and apply limited techniques specified in this standard to support and participate in technical search and rescue incidents. (NFPA 1670)

Operations section Section responsible for all tactical operations at the incident or planned event, including up to 5 branches, 25 divisions/groups, and 125 single resources, task forces, or strike teams. (NFPA 1026)

Organizational analysis A process to determine if it is possible for an organization to establish and maintain a given capability.

Outer survey A survey conducted simultaneously with the inner survey; the rescuer performing the outer survey moves in the same or opposite direction as the rescuer performing the inner survey. Distance from the vehicle will vary with each incident, but it is generally a distance of 25 to 50 ft (7.6 to 15.2 m) starting from the perimeter of the inner survey position outward.

P

Parallel drive system A system that can use either the vehicle's internal combustion engine or the electric motor to power the vehicle's transmission and provide propulsion.

Passenger vehicle All sedans, coupes, and station wagons manufactured primarily for the purpose of carrying passengers, including those passenger cars pulling recreational or other light trailers.

Passive regeneration The first of three stages of regeneration that occurs automatically when the particulate matter (soot) that is caught in the DPF is burned off naturally by the elevated temperatures of the exhaust system.

Passive restraint device A device that the occupant does not have to activate for it to function; the system is automatically activated when power is applied to the vehicle.

Peer support groups A group to help alleviate the stress and trauma from the experiences encountered on the job. The group employs trusted members of the organization who have had similar experiences to provide emotional support through nonclinical conversation and guidance.

Physical reactions Negative reactions that may present as headaches, muscle twitching/tremors, dry mouth, elevated blood pressure and/or heart rate, nausea, hyperpnea, profuse sweating, or chest pains.

Pitch movement One of five directional movements; the vehicle moves up and down about its lateral axis, causing the vehicle's front and rear portions to move left or right in relation to their original position.

Planning section Section responsible for the collection, evaluation, dissemination, and use of information related to the incident situation, resource status, and incident forecast. (NFPA 1026)

Plug-in hybrid electric vehicle (PHEV) A hybrid vehicle that can recharge its battery system using a plug-in cord that can run off general house current in the range of 120 volts, also known as a Level 1 charging system.

Pneumatic chisels Pneumatic tools used to cut through various types and sizes of metal.

Pneumatic cut-off tool A pneumatic tool utilizing a small carbide disk, normally 3 in. (8 mm) in diameter, which rotates at high revolutions per minute to cut through most metals.

Pneumatic tools Tools that use air under pressure to operate.

Polycarbonate A clear thermoplastic material that is very strong and can endure impacts without breaking.

Polymer exchange membrane (PEM) Also known as a proton exchange membrane, a thin membrane used in a fuel-cell system that is placed between the anode and cathode and through which positive electrons are passed.

Post-traumatic stress disorder (PTSD) A delayed stress reaction to a prior incident. This delayed reaction is often the result of one or more unresolved issues concerning the incident.

Potential energy Stored energy or the energy of position.

Pounds per square inch (psi) A unit of measure used to describe pressure; it is the amount of force that is exerted on an area equaling 1 in.^{2}

Pressure release device (PRD) A safety feature built into high-pressure storage cylinders that is designed to rapidly release gas contents when exposed to high temperatures, such as during a fire.

Pretensioner seat belt system A seat belt system designed to pull back and tighten when activated by a collision. The most common pretensioner seat belt system uses a pyrotechnic propulsion device to engage a gear that pulls back on the belt.

Primary access (Plan A) The existing openings of doors and/or windows that provide a pathway to the trapped and/or injured victim(s). (NFPA 1670)

Protective ensemble Multiple elements of compliant protective clothing and equipment that when worn together provide protection from some risks, but not all risks, of emergency incident operations. (NFPA 1500)

Public information officer (PIO) A member of the command staff responsible for interfacing with the public and media or with other agencies with incident-related information requirements. (NFPA 1026)

Purchase point The location at which access can best be gained.

Q

Qualification Having satisfactorily completed the requirements of the objectives. (NFPA 1006)

R

Ratchet strap A mechanical tensioning device with a manual gear-ratcheting drum to put tension on an object, utilizing a webbing material.

Rear deck/shelf Also known as package tray; a panel behind the rear seat and in front of the rear window.

Reciprocating saw A power-driven saw in which the cutting action occurs through a back-and-forth motion (reciprocating) of the blade.

Response planning (preincident planning) The process of compiling, documenting, and dispersing information that will assist the organization should an incident occur at a particular location.

Risk assessment An assessment of the likelihood, vulnerability, and magnitude of incidents that could result from exposure to hazards. (NFPA 1670)

Risk–benefit analysis An assessment of the risk to the rescuers versus the benefits that can be derived from their intended actions.

Rocker panel A hollow section of metal running along the outer sections of the floorboard on the driver and passenger sides.

Roll movement One of five directional movements; the vehicle rocks side to side while rotating about on its longitudinal axis and remaining horizontal in orientation.

Rollover protection system (ROPS) A system designed to protect occupants in vehicle rollover incidents by means of a deployable roll bar.

Roof posts/pillars Posts/pillars that are designed to add vertical support to the roof structure of the vehicle. These are generally labeled with an alphanumeric type description (A, B, and C), starting with the post closest to the front windshield, which is known as the A-post.

Rotary saws Fuel-powered saws capable of cutting wood, concrete, and metal; two types of blades are used on rotary saws: a round metal blade with teeth and an abrasive disk. The application of rotary saws in vehicle extrication is limited.

Rub rails Visible exterior steel attachments that consist of 16-gauge corrugated metal. These steel members are 4 in. (102 mm) or more in width and are attached to the bow trusses. They run the entire length of the school bus, wrapping around to the rear of the vehicle.

S

Safety officer (SO) An individual appointed by the AHJ as qualified to maintain a safe working environment. (NFPA 1670)

Safing sensor A type of air bag sensor that has a deceleration setting lower than the crash-type sensor. This sensor prevents false deployments.

Scene safety zones or operational zones Zones that are divided into hot, warm, and cold zones. These zones are strictly enforced by a designated incident safety officer.

Scene size-up A mental process of evaluating the influencing factors at an incident prior to committing resources to a course of action. (NFPA 1006)

School bus Any public or private school or district or contracted carrier operating on behalf of the entity, providing transportation for kindergarteners through grade 12 pupils.

Seat belt pretensioning system A system designed to automatically tighten, or take up slack, in a seat belt when a crash is detected.

Secondary access (Plan B) Openings created by rescuers that provide a pathway to trapped and/or injured victims. (NFPA 1670)

Glossary

Self-contained breathing apparatus (SCBA) An atmosphere-supplying respirator that supplies a respirable air atmosphere to the user from a breathing air source that is independent of the ambient environment and designed to be carried by the user. (NFPA 1981)

Semi-tractor trailer (semi-trailer) A semi-truck, or semi-tractor, combined with a trailer; normally designed with three axles, one in the front for steering purposes and two tandem axles in the rear.

Semi-truck A commercial truck capable of towing a separate trailer, which has wheels at only one end (semi-trailer); may also be referred to as a tractor.

Series drive system A system that uses the internal combustion engine alone to run an onboard generator, which in turn can either run the electric motor that turns the vehicle's transmission (providing propulsion) or be used to charge the batteries or store power in a capacitor. The internal combustion engine does not provide direct propulsion to the vehicle.

Series-operated propulsion system A system that utilizes the electric motor by itself to propel a school bus, and the internal combustion engine is used only to regenerate the battery pack. These systems may be found on type A school buses.

Service air line One of two air lines of an air brake system connecting a tractor to a trailer; the emergency air line is blue.

Service brake The usual driving brake that is applied by the driver to slow and/or stop the vehicle during normal driving operations.

Shims Objects that are smaller than wedges used to snug loose cribbing under a load or to fill void spaces.

Shoring A stabilization technique used where the vertical distances are too great to use cribbing or the load must be supported horizontally, such as in a trench, or diagonally, such as in a wall shore.

Side-impact air bags Air bags designed to activate immediately upon impact to protect the following areas of the occupant: the head, the chest/upper torso, and a combination of the head and the chest/upper torso. There are three types, and all three types can be found in the door, seat backs, roof posts, or roof rails. These air bags may be labeled HPS (head protection system), IC (inflatable curtain), SIPS (side-impact protection system), or ROI (rollover inflator air bag).

Side-out technique A technique used to gain access to a four-door vehicle involved in a side-impact collision.

Single resource An individual, a piece of equipment and its personnel, or a crew or team of individuals with an identified supervisor that can be used on an incident or planned event. (NFPA 1026)

Sleeper A compartment attached to the cab of a truck that allows the driver to rest while making stops during a long transport.

Slide cribbing Two sections of 4-in. × 4-in. (10-cm × 10-cm) cribbing positioned parallel to each other with a third section of cribbing on top traversing the two bottom sections.

Slide hook A hook that allows chain links to pass freely through the throat of the hook to tighten around an object.

Smart air bag system An air bag system that automatically adjusts the pressure in the air bag by using multistage inflators and basing the deployment force on a number of calculated factors, such as crash severity, occupant's weight, proximity to the air bag, seat belt usage, and seat position.

Smart key A device that uses a computerized chip that communicates through radio frequencies to unlock or lock a vehicle as well as start a vehicle remotely without the requirement of traditional keys.

Space frame A frame made up of multiple lengths and angles of tubing welded into a rigid, but light, web or truss-like structure; the vehicle's outer panels are attached independently to the frame after its completion.

Spiral wound A type of battery that uses lead plates that are tightly wound in a spiral formation within each cell.

Spring-loaded center punch A glass removal tool used on tempered glass that, when engaged, uses a spring-loaded plunger to fire off a steel rod with a sharpened point directly into a pinpoint area of glass, causing the glass to shatter.

Squib A pyrotechnic device used to ignite the propellant that produces the gas filling an air bag.

Staging area manager ICS position responsible for ensuring that all resources in the staging area are available and ready for assignment.

Standard An NFPA Standard, the main text of which contains only mandatory provisions using the word "shall" to indicate requirements and that is in a form generally suitable for mandatory reference by another standard or code or for adoption into law. Nonmandatory provisions are not to be considered a part of the requirements of a standard and shall be located in an appendix, annex, footnote, informational note, or other means as permitted in the NFPA Manuals of Style. When used in a generic sense, such as in the phrase "standards development process" or "standards development activities," the term "standards" includes all NFPA Standards, including Codes, Standards, Recommended Practices, and Guides. (NFPA 1006)

Standard operating procedure (SOP) A written organizational directive that establishes or prescribes specific operational or administrative methods to be followed routinely for the performance of designated operations or actions. (NFPA 1521)

Standard seat belt harness A seat belt system that helps distribute the energy of a collision over larger areas of the body, such as the chest, pelvis, and shoulders. The three-point belt mechanism uses a retractor gear that locks in place when activated. Also known as a three-point harness system.

Start/stop mild hybrid system A vehicle that is not a true hybrid system by definition. The motor/generator is not used to propel the vehicle; it is designed to turn off the vehicle's internal combustion engine when the vehicle is idle and turn it back on when the accelerator is activated.

Static risk–benefit analysis An analysis conducted in an office setting prior to any incident. This type of analysis is an evaluation and justification of whether to acquire/support the required level of service needed to manage a technician-level technical rescue incident that has the potential to occur or has occurred in the past within the jurisdiction.

Step chocks Specialized cribbing assemblies made out of wood or plastic blocks in a step configuration. They are typically used to stabilize vehicles.

Stored compressed-gas system An inflation system comprising a single-stage or multistage inflation process. The igniter, or squib, sets off a burst, or rupture, disk that acts as a seal, holding back the compressed gas. When activated, the disk breaks open, releasing the gas from the chamber, which expands and instantly fills the air bag.

Stress Any type of change, whether pleasant or unpleasant, that manifests itself in cognitive, physical, emotional, or behavioral signs.

Strike team Specified combinations of the same kind and type of resources, with common communications and a leader. (NFPA 1026)

Stringers Steel longitudinal structural members that give the bow frame truss members structural support at the roof level; they run continuously from the front to the rear of a school bus.

Strut tower A structural component of the suspension system that normally has both a coil spring and shock absorber. Its main function is to resist compression.

Struts A compression element used in the support of structures, excavation openings, or other loads. (NFPA 1006)

Supplemental restraint system (SRS) A system that uses supplemental restraint devices, such as air bags, to enhance safety in conjunction with properly applied seat belts. Seat belt pretensioning systems are also considered part of an SRS.

Supplied air respirator/breathing apparatus (SAR/SABA) A respirator in which breathing air is supplied by an air line from either a compressor or stored air (bottle) system located outside the work area.

Suppression system A device that shuts down the air bag if an occupant classification system detects a child in the air bag deployment zone or if one of the sensors detects a high-risk potential by acquiring the occupant's weight, height, proximity to the air bag, seat belt usage, and seat position; the system sends this information to the electronic control unit, which will then shut off the air bag if a high risk to the occupant is determined.

SWOT analysis A self-examination model that can be adjusted, adapted, and applied to any situation, incident, or project, large or small, that an organization is currently or will be involved in.

T

Task force A group of resources with common communications and a leader that can be pre-established and sent to an incident or planned event or formed at an incident or planned event. (NFPA 1026)

Technical rescue The application of special knowledge, skills, and equipment to safely resolve unique and/or complex rescue situations. (NFPA 1670)

Technical rescuer A person who is trained to perform or direct the technical rescue. (NFPA 1006)

Technical search and rescue incidents Complex search and/or rescue incidents requiring specialized training of personnel and special equipment to complete the mission. (NFPA 1006)

Technical specialists A person with specialized skills, training, and/or certification who can be used anywhere within the incident management system organization where his or her skills might be required. (NFPA 1561)

Technician level (1) This level represents the capability of individuals to respond to technical search and rescue incidents and to identify hazards, use equipment, and apply advanced techniques specified in this standard necessary to coordinate, perform, and supervise technical search and rescue incidents. (NFPA 1006) (2) This level represents the capability of organizations to respond to technical search and rescue incidents and to identify hazards, use equipment, and apply advanced techniques specified in this standard necessary to coordinate, perform, and supervise technical search and rescue incidents. (NFPA 1670)

Temperature relief device (TRD) A device that rapidly releases product through a small metal tube attachment when detecting excessive amounts of heat at a preset temperature.

Tempered safety glass (TSG) A type of glass that has been heated and then quickly cooled; this process gives the glass its strength and resistance to impact.

Tension buttress stabilization A strut stabilization system that uses a strap in a ratchet or jacking device to add tension to the object being stabilized, locking the vehicle in place by using a diagonal force that lowers the vehicle's center of mass by increasing the vehicle's entire footprint.

Tepee, or tenting, effect A peak or tent shape that can result when using an ineffective dash roll technique; the floorboard and rocker panel area push up where the relief cuts are made when the dash area is locked down by an object or vehicle.

TPI rating A rating that indicates how many teeth per inch a blade has.

Traffic incident management A management tool that establishes roadway safety procedures and traffic control measures for emergency operations at a motor vehicle accident.

Transit bus An entity providing passenger transportation over fixed, scheduled routes, within primarily urban geographic areas.

Triage The sorting of casualties at an emergency according to the nature and severity of their injuries. (NFPA 1006)

Tube trailers A high-volume transportation device made up of several individual compressed gas cylinders banded together and affixed to a trailer. Tube trailers carry compressed gases such as hydrogen, oxygen, helium, and methane. One trailer may carry several different gases in individual tubes.

Tunneling The process of gaining entry through the rear trunk area of a vehicle, a process more commonly used for a post-crash vehicle resting on its roof.

Type A school bus A conversion-type bus constructed utilizing a cutaway front section vehicle with a left-side driver's door. This definition includes two subclassifications: type A-1, with a GVWR of 14,500 lb (6577 kg) or less, and type A-2, with a GVWR greater than 14,500 lb (6577 kg) and less than or equal to 21,500 lb (9752 kg).

Type B school bus A school bus that is constructed utilizing a stripped chassis. The entrance door is behind the front wheels. This definition includes two subclassifications: type B-1, with a GVWR of 10,000 lb (4536 kg) or less, and type B-2, with a GVWR greater than 10,000 lb (4536 kg).

Type C school bus (also known as a conventional school bus) A school bus that is constructed utilizing a chassis with a hood and front fender assembly. The entrance door is behind the front wheels. This type of school bus has a GVWR greater than 21,500 lb (9752 kg). Eighty-five to 90 percent of all school buses are type C or D.

Type D school bus (also known as a transit-style rear or front engine school bus) A school bus that is constructed utilizing a stripped chassis where the outer body of the bus is mounted to the bare chassis. The entrance door is ahead of the front wheels, and the face, or front section, of the bus is flat. Type D buses have a passenger capacity of 80 to 90 people.

U

Ultimate tensile strength (UTS) A measurement of the amount of force required to tear a section of steel apart.

Unibody construction A vehicle with a frame and body that are constructed as a single assembly that does not have a separate frame on which the body is mounted. (NFPA 58)

Unified command A team effort that allows all agencies with jurisdictional responsibility for an incident or planned event, either geographic or functional, to manage the incident or planned event by establishing a common set of incident objectives and strategies. (NFPA 1026)

Upper rails Two side beams located in the front of the vehicle that hold the hood in place and attach the front wheel strut system to the chassis.

U-shaped striker plate latch pin A latch mechanism generally made of smaller-gauge steel, which makes it easier to cut through and/or release from the latch mechanism of the door.

V

Vehicle identification badge A type of label that vehicle manufacturers use to identify the type of vehicle or the fuel that is used in the vehicle.

Vertical movement One of five directional movements; the vehicle moves up and down in relation to the ground while moving along its vertical axis.

Vertical spread A door access procedure utilizing a hydraulic spreader; the tool is placed vertically in the window frame of the door and pushes off of the roof rail and window frame to create an access point to the door's latching mechanism.

W

Warm zone The control zone outside the hot zone where personnel and equipment decontamination and hot zone support take place. (NFPA 1500)

Wedges Objects used to snug loose cribbing under a load or to fill a void between the crib and the object as it is raised.

Wet cell (flooded cell) The standard 12-volt battery that contains active electrolyte solution; must be mounted in an upright position.

Wheel well crush technique A technique utilized to gain access to door hinges from the outside.

Winches Chains or cables used for a variety of lifting, pulling, and holding operations.

Window spidering An effect caused when an object breaks laminated glass and causes spiraling rings at the area of impact resembling a spider's web.

Work A mechanism for the transfer of energy.

Working load limit (WLL) The maximum force that may be applied before failure occurs to an assembly or a component of a device or rope/line/cable in straight tension.

Y

Yaw movement One of five directional movements; the vehicle twists or turns about its vertical axis, causing the vehicle's front and rear portions to move left or right in relation to their original position.

Yield strength The amount of force or stress that a section of steel can withstand before permanent deformation occurs.

Index

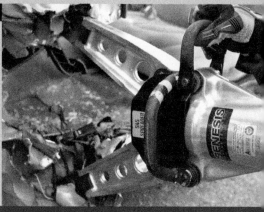

Note: Page numbers followed by "*f*" denote figures; those followed by "*t*" denote tables.

A

A-posts/pillars, 136, 136*f*
  air bag cylinder in, 251, 252*f*
AAR. *See* after-action report
absorbed glass mat (AGM), 127
AC power locator, 92, 92*f*
accelerometer, 152, 157
access, 223*f*
  air-lift bag operation, school buses, 388–389
  backboard slide technique, 226–227
  ballistic-rated glass, 235
  commercial trucks, 348–349, 348–349*f*
  dash section relocation
    dash lift technique, 260–266
    dash roll technique, 255–260
  doors, 222–224, 224*f*
    front, in school buses, 379, 382, 382*f*, 383–384
    from hinge side, 239, 243*f*
    from latch side, 237–239, 238–239*f*, 239–244
    rear, in school buses, 376, 378–379
    using hydraulic rescue tools, 235, 237, 237*f*
  lifting operations, school buses, 382, 385–387, 390–392
  points
    doors as, 222–224
    primary, 223
    secondary, 223
  roof
    removal, for upright vehicle, 252–254
    removal of, 247, 249–252
    in school buses, 373, 376–377
    using hydraulic rescue tools, 235, 237, 237*f*
  seat removal, in school buses, 370, 372–373
  side
    removal, side-out technique, 245–249, 247–249
    in school buses, 373–375
  steering wheel assembly relocation, 266–270, 390
    in school buses, 390
    utilizing 2/4-ton–rated come along, 267–269
    utilizing First Responder Jack, 269–270
  windows, 224–226, 224–225*f*
    backboard slide technique, 226–227
    breaking with center punch, 58, 59*f*
    front, in school buses, 369–371
    polycarbonate, 235
    using glass handsaw for glass removal, 60, 60*f*
  windshield
    removal from partially ejected victim, 235
    using glass handsaw, 230

  using reciprocating saw, 230, 234
accomplishments, in status report, 28
accountability, 32, 34*f*
  equipment inventory and, 34, 34*f*
action zone. *See* hot zone
active hearing protectors, 54–55, 55*f*
active regeneration, 360
active restraint device, 150
active risk–benefit analysis, 24
ACU. *See* air bag control unit
adapters, 75
additional personnel resources, 42, 42*f*
advanced high-strength steel (AHSS), 129
advanced life support (ALS), 41
AFFF. *See* Aqueous Film-Forming Foam
after-action report (AAR), 324–325
aggregate weight, 346
AGM. *See* absorbed glass mat
AHJ. *See* authority having jurisdiction
AHSS. *See* advanced high-strength steel
air ambulances, 115, 115*f*
air bag control unit (ACU), 154–155, 154*f*
air bag cylinder, location of, 234, 234*f*
air bags, 150–152, 151*f*. *See also specific types*
  components of
    air bag control unit, 154–155, 154*f*
    air bags, 152–154, 153*f*
    inflator/propellant, 155–157, 156*f*
    initiator, 154, 154*f*
    sensors, 157–158, 157*f*
  deployment process, 152
  disconnecting power, 161
  emergency procedures, 161
  first-generation, 151
  as passive restraint device, 150–151
  recognizing and identifying, 162–163
    distancing from deployment zone, 163
    extrication precautions, 163–164, 163*f*
    labeling system using acronyms, 162–163, 162*f*
  second-generation, 151
  size of, 151
  standard acronyms, 162, 162*f*
  third-generation, 151
air brake (parking brake), 341–342, 342*f*
air chisels. *See* pneumatic chisels
air compressors, 66, 67*f*
air cushions. *See* low-pressure air-lift bags
air-filtering face piece respirators, 56

air impact wrench, 70, 70f
air-lift bags, 71–72, 71f
    flat-form bags, 71, 71f
    general rules, 72
    high-pressure, 73, 73f
    high-pressure flat-form, 73
    low-pressure, 72, 73f
    medium-pressure, 72–73, 73f
    multi-cell high-pressure, 73, 73f
    removing victim from under school buses, 388–389
air medical operations, 115f
    landing zone
        establishing, 115–116, 116f
        safety, 116–117, 117f
air ride system, 336–337, 337f
air shores, 70, 70f
airway, opening, methods for, 272, 272f
Alcohol Resistant Aqueous Film-Forming Foam (AR-AFFF), 90
alloyed, 127
alloyed steels, 129
ALS. *See* advanced life support
alternative extrication techniques, 169–170, 172
    door removal on hinge side, 308–310
    impingement, 291–295, 291f, 295f
    jacking the trunk, 284–287, 294f
    pedal displacement and removal, 310, 311–312, 312–313, 312f
    penetrating objects, 298–300
    roof
        lift, 295, 298, 298f
        removal, 300–307, 301f
    seat removal
        front seat-back relocation, 290
        front seat-back removal, 287, 289
    side removal, 310
    tunneling, 283–284, 283–284f
    victim removal under vehicle, 313–314
alternative-fuel vehicles
    biodiesel, 179–180, 180f
    electricity. *See* electric vehicles; hybrid electric vehicles
    ethanol, 172–173
    hydrogen. *See* hydrogen
    liquefied petroleum gas, 177–179, 178f
    methanol, 173
    natural gas, 173–177, 174–176f
    ongoing education, 194–195
    safety, 170, 172f
    school buses, 393–394, 393f
        emergency procedures for hybrid bus, 394–395
    standard procedures, 171
    vehicle identification badge, 172, 172f
Alternative-Fuel Vehicles Safety Training Program Emergency Field Guide, 12, 13f
aluminum alloyed metal, 128
American Society for Testing and Materials (ASTM) International, 202
ammonium nitrate, 156
animals/livestock at crash scene, 115, 115f
Aqueous Film-Forming Foam (AFFF), 91
authority having jurisdiction (AHJ), 5
automatic seat belt system, 138
awareness level, 5–6, 8
    requirements of, 9–10
axles, 339–340, 340f

B

B-post, 138, 138–139f
    hydraulic tool to push, 245, 246f
    initial impact on vehicle causing, 291, 291f
    relocation
        with First Responder Jack, 294
        with hydraulic ram, 291–292
backboard slide technique, 226–227
ballistic glass, 142
bar-code systems, 34
barrier crash test, 151, 151f
basic life support (BLS), 9, 41
basket stretchers, 93
battery compartment, for school bus, 359–360, 360f
battery electric vehicle (BEV). *See* electric vehicles
battery-powered drill set, 74, 75f
battery-powered hydraulic rescue tools, 84–85, 85f
battery/batteries
    12-volt lead acid battery system, 127
    disconnecting, 161
    in hydrogen fuel cell vehicles, 183
    location of, 217, 217f
    powered tools. *See specific tools*
    systems
        for commercial motor vehicle, 342, 342f
        for electric vehicle, 193–194
        for hybrid electric vehicles, 188, 189f
    types of, 76
behavioral reactions, 323
bench seats, for school bus, 359
beneficial systems, 161
biodiesel, 179–180, 180f
    emergency procedures, 180
    identification badge, 180, 180f
blades
    for hydraulic cutter, 83
    for pneumatic chisels, 69
    for reciprocating saw, 75
BLEVE. *See* boiling liquid/expanding vapor explosion
BLS. *See* basic life support
body-over-frame construction, 130, 130f
body protection, 51–52, 52f
boiling liquid/expanding vapor explosion (BLEVE), 113, 179
bolt cutters, 58f, 63, 67
boom's cable system, 348, 349f
boots, protective, 54, 54f
boron-alloyed steel, 129–130, 129f
bow frame trusses, 357–358, 358f
bow saw, 62
bow trusses, 357
braking systems, for commercial motor vehicle, 341–342, 342f
branches, 31
breathing air compressors, 66
breathing, checking for, 273, 273t
bulkhead. *See* firewall
bullet-resistant glass. *See* ballistic glass
bumper system, 132
buses. *See specific types*
buttress stabilization, 209, 210, 210f

C

C-post, 138–139
cab beside engine (CBE), 335, 335f
cab of semi-truck, 333

cab over engine (COE), 333, 335*f*
cable cutters, 63
cables, color coding, 185, 189–190, 190*f*, 192*f*, 194
cabs, 344
    cab beside engine, 335, 335*f*
    cab over engine, 333, 335*f*
    conventional cab, 335, 335*f*
    height of, 336, 336*f*
carbon, 127
carbon fiber reinforced polymer (CFRP), 127, 128*f*
carbon steel, 127, 129
cargo area, of commercial motor vehicle, 338–339, 338–339*f*
cargo tank, 344, 346*f*
CBE. *See* cab beside engine
center air bag, 153
Center for Public Safety Excellence (CPSE), 103
center of mass, 85, 201, 209
center punch
    spring-loaded, 59, 227, 228, 228*f*
    as striking tools, 58, 59*f*
CFRP. *See* carbon fiber reinforced polymer
chain package, for come along, 64–66, 64–65*f*
chain saws, 79, 89
chain shortener. *See* grab hook
challenge events, as extrication resource, 13–14, 13*f*
charge-depleting hybrid system, 394
charge-sustaining hybrid system, 394
charter/tour bus, 355, 355*f*
chassis, 130
    for commercial motor vehicle, 336–338, 337–338*f*
    frame of school bus, 357
Chevrolet Volt, 189
chisels
    air. *See* pneumatic chisels
    hand-operated, 63
    metal, 63
"Cielo" roof, 142
circular saw, 75
    electric, 76–77
    metal-cutting, 76, 76*f*
circulation, checking for, 274, 274*f*
CISD. *See* critical incident stress debriefing
CISM. *See* critical incident stress management
class 1 commercial vehicle, 332, 332*t*
class 2a commercial vehicle, 332*t*, 333
class 2b commercial vehicle, 332*t*, 333
class 3 commercial vehicle, 332*t*, 333
class 4 commercial vehicle, 332*t*, 333
class 5 commercial vehicle, 332*t*, 333
class 6 commercial vehicle, 332*t*, 333
class 7 commercial vehicle, 332*t*, 333
class 8 commercial vehicle, 332*t*, 333
Class A foam, 91
Class B foam, 91
cleaning, of hand tools, 62*t*
clothesline effect, 154
cluster hook, 66, 66*f*
CMVs. *See* commercial motor vehicles
CNG. *See* compressed natural gas
COE. *See* cab over engine
cognitive reactions, 323
cold chisels. *See* metal chisels
cold zone, 45, 110
collisions. *See specific collisions*

come along
    chain package for, 64–66, 64–65*f*
    for steering wheel assembly relocation, 266–267
command staff
    liaison officer, 30
    public information officer, 29
    safety officer, 29–30, 30*f*
commercial motor vehicles (CMVs), 331, 331*f*
    commercial trucks, 331–332, 332*f*
        anatomy, 333–343, 333*f*, 333–343*f*
        classifications, 332–333, 332*t*
        hazardous materials, 343–347, 344–346*f*
        site operations, 347–348
        victim access, 348–349, 348–349*f*
common passenger vehicle, 6
communication
    integrated, 27
    during site operations, 103
communications unit, in logistics section, 31–32
compartment syndrome, 275
compensation/claims unit, finance/administration section, 32
composite, 127–130, 128–129*f*
    for cribbing, 86
compressed natural gas (CNG), 174, 174*f*
contact point, 202
conventional cab, 333, 335, 335*f*
conventional school bus. *See* Type C school bus
conventional vehicles, 144
core support, 132
cost unit, finance/administration section, 32
cowl section, 132
CPSE. *See* Center for Public Safety Excellence
crash rail, 358
crash sensors, 157
crew, 32
crew resource management (CRM), 37
cribbing, 86–87, 86*f*
    contact points, 202, 203*f*
    designs, 202
    height, 204
    ladder, 267
    placement
        goal of, 204, 205*f*
        with normal upright position of vehicle, 203, 205*f*
        for vehicle resting on its side, 210, 210*f*
        vehicle suspension system, 204
        for vehicle upside down or resting on roof, 212
    strength of, 202
    wood box, 202–203, 203*f*
    wood characteristics, 202
crime scenes, law enforcement management of, 318
critical incident stress, 321–323
critical incident stress debriefing (CISD), 323, 323*f*
critical incident stress management (CISM), 323, 323*f*
CRM. *See* crew resource management
cross-ramming technique, 291, 293, 295*f*
    using hydraulic ram, 297
crosstie cribbing configuration, 202–203, 203*f*
crowd control, 40, 40*f*
crumple zones, 131, 131*f*
cut-off tool, pneumatic, 58*f*, 62–63, 62–63*f*, 67, 67*f*
cutting tools
    electric
        circular saw, 76–77, 76*f*

reciprocating saw, 76, 76f
fuel-powered. *See* fuel-powered cutting tools
pneumatic
  chisels, 67, 69–70, 69f
  cut-off tool, 67, 67f
cutting torches, 79–80

D

dash lift technique, 260–266
  hydraulic, 261–263
  non-hydraulic, 264–265
dash reinforcement bar, 132, 133f
dash roll technique, 255–260
  hydraulic, 257–258
  non-hydraulic, 258–259
dead axle, 339
dead-man control, 82
defensive apparatus placement, 38
Department of Energy (DOE), 142, 356
Department of Transportation (DOT)
  classification of vehicle, 142
  Emergency Response Guidebook, 169, 174, 176f
  hazardous materials, defined, 114
die grinders. *See* cut-off tool, pneumatic
disability, 274
disentanglement, 4
dispatch information, 36–37
distress, 321
divisions, 31
documentation
  during site operations, 103
  termination of incident, 324–325
DOE. *See* Department of Energy
dogs/pets at crash scenes, 114–115
door hinges, 103, 134f
  for commercial motor vehicle, 340–341, 340f
  designs, 133, 134f
doors
  access
    from hinge side, 239, 243f
    from latch side, 237–239, 238–239f, 239–244
    points, 222–224, 224f
    using hydraulic rescue tools, 235, 237, 237f
  for commercial motor vehicle, 340–341, 340f
  frame relocation
    with First Responder Jack, 294
    with hydraulic ram, 291–292
  front access, 379, 382, 382f, 383–384
  impact beam, 135, 135f
  latching mechanisms, 135, 135f
  limiting device, 134, 134f
  outer skin/panel of, 136
  rear access
    school bus in normal position, 378–379
    school bus resting on side, 378–379, 380–381
    removal on hinge side, 308–310
DOT. *See* Department of Transportation
drive systems, hybrid electric vehicles, 190, 190–191f
drive train (power train), 333
driver air bag, 153
driver-side air bag, 156, 163
driver's seat, for school bus, 359
dromedary (drom), 339, 339f

dry bulk cargo tanks, 346, 346f
dual-stage/multistage inflation process, 151

E

E10, 173
E85 flex fuel, 173
earmuffs, 55, 55f
earplugs, 55, 55f
ECU. *See* Electronic Control Unit
electric-powered tools, 74
electric-powered vehicles, 144
electric tools, 74–75, 74–75f
  cutting tools
    circular saw, 76–77, 76f
    reciprocating saw, 76, 76f
  lifting and pulling tools, 77–78, 77f
  lighting, 78–79, 78f
electric vehicles (EVs), 193–194, 193f. *See also* electric-powered vehicles
  emergency procedures, 193–194
  neighborhood electric vehicle, 193, 193f
  Nissan LEAF, 193–194, 193f
  summary of
electric winches, 77–78, 77f
electrical generators, 74, 74f
electrical hazards, 112–113, 112–113f
  mitigating at motor vehicle collision, 218, 218f
electrical system, isolating/eliminating, 216–218, 218f
electrical transformers, position of, 112
electricity, 126–127
electronic control unit (ECU), 154–155, 154f. *See also* air bag control unit
electronic satellite sensor, 157
electropositive, 127
emergency air line (supply line), 341–342, 342f
emergency brake, 341
emergency dispatch centers, 36
emergency escape plan, 107
emergency exits, for school bus
  rear doors, 358, 359
  roof, 359, 359f
  side window, 359
emergency field guide, as extrication resource, 12–13, 13f
emergency medical services (EMS)
  airway maintaining, 271, 271f
  personnel, 41–42, 42f, 121
  relationship with fire department, 41
  single-tiered system, 41
  three-tiered system, 41
  trauma scissors, 63
  two-tiered system, 41
emergency procedures
  air bags, 161
  biodiesel, 180
  electric vehicles, 193–194
  ethanol and methanol, 173
  for hybrid bus, 394–395
  hybrid electric vehicles, 191–193, 192f
  hydrogen, 182–183
  hydrogen fuel-cell, 186–188
  liquefied petroleum gas, 178–179
  natural gas, 175–177
Emergency Response Guidebook, 169, 174, 176f
emergency roof hatches, for school bus, 359, 359f

emotional reactions, 323
EMS. *See* emergency medical services
energy
    kinetic, 121, 122*f*
    law of conservation of energy, 121
    potential, 121, 122*f*
    transfer of. *See* work
Energy Independence and Security Act of 2007, 127
Energy Policy Act of 1992, 172
Energy Policy and Conservation Act, 127
engine cradle, 132
entrance door, for school bus, 358
entrapment, classifications, 105, 105*t*
Environmental Protection Agency (EPA), 55, 360
EPA. *See* Environmental Protection Agency
equipment. *See also specific equipment*
    accountability and maintenance of, 319–321, 319*f*
    foam, 90–91, 91*f*
    inventory, and tracking systems, 34, 34*f*
    organization of, 90, 90*f*
    power detection, 92, 92*f*
    resources, 102–103, 102*f*
    securing, upon termination of incident, 319–321, 319*f*
    signaling devices, 91–92, 92*f*
    victim packaging and removal, 93, 93*f*
EREV. *See* extended range electric vehicle
ethanol, 172–173, 173*f*
ethyl mercaptan, 175, 177
Euro-style helmet, 50, 51*f*
eustress, 321
EVs. *See* electric vehicles
exhaust after-treatment device, 360
exothermic torch, 80
expose and cut, 163, 237, 237*f*, 274–275
extended range electric vehicle (EREV), 189, 190*f*
extrication, 4. *See also* vehicle rescue and extrication
    alternative techniques. *See* alternative extrication techniques
    jumpsuit, 51, 52*f*
    precautions, air bags, 163–164, 163*f*
eye and face protection, 52–53, 53*f*

F

face shield, 52–53, 53*f*
facilities unit, in logistics section, 32
Federal Hazardous Materials Transportation Law, 343
Federal Motor Carrier Safety Administration, 354
Federal Motor Vehicle Safety Standard (FMVSS), 150, 255, 356
    air bags, 151
    bumper system, 132
    and regulations, 140
    roof crush resistance, 212
    roof strength requirement, 212
ferrous metals, 76
FFVs. *See* flexible fuel vehicles
fifth wheel, 338, 338–339*f*
finance/administration section, 32
fire department
    relationship with EMS, 41
    single-tiered system, 41
    three-tiered system, 41
    two-tiered system, 41
fire hazards, 111–112, 111*f*
fire helmet, 50, 51*f*
firewall, 132

First Responder Jack (FRJ), 63, 88, 88*f*
    B-post/door frame relocation with, 294
    force applied to, 238, 238*f*
    raising roof using, 298*f*
    removing victim from under school buses, 385–387
    steering wheel assembly relocation, 269–270
fixed-wing aircraft, 115, 115*f*
flat blade, 69
flat-form air-lift bags, 71, 71*f*, 73
flat-head axe, 62, 62*f*
flex fuel identification badge, 173, 173*f*
flexible fuel vehicles (FFVs), 173
floor deck, for school bus, 357
FMVSS. *See* Federal Motor Vehicle Safety Standard
foam eductor, 91
foam equipment, 91, 91*f*
food unit, in logistics section, 32
foot protection, 54, 54*f*
footprint, 209
formal incident action plans, 6
formal postincident analysis, 324
frame systems, vehicles
    body-over-frame construction, 130, 130*f*
    space frame construction, 131, 131*f*
    unibody construction, 130–131, 130–131*f*
FRJ. *See* First Responder Jack
front impact collisions, 124–125
front-passenger air bags, 153
front seat-back
    relocation, 290
    removal, 287, 289
front wheel well crush, 239, 243*f*
fuel cell, 183
fuel-powered cutting tools
    chain saws, 79
    cutting torches, 79–80
    rotary saws, 79
fuels
    biodiesel, 179–180, 180*f*
    for commercial motor vehicle, 342–343, 343*f*
    ethanol, 172–173
    ignition sources, 113–114
    liquefied petroleum gas, 177–179, 178*f*
    methanol, 173
    natural gas, 173–177, 174–176*f*
    runoff, 113
    sources, 113
    types, for commercial motor vehicles, 342–343, 343*f*
full hybrid vehicle, 188

G

G-sensor. *See* gravitational acceleration sensor
gas-generation system, 155–156
gasohol. *See* E10
GCS. *See* Glasgow Coma Scale
GCWR. *See* gross combined weight rating
gel cell, 127
Genesis battery-operated hydraulic tools, 85*f*
glad hands, 342, 343*f*
Glasgow Coma Scale (GCS), 274
glass
    ballistic-rated, 142, 235
    Gorilla® glass, 141
    laminated safety. *See* laminated safety glass

management, 140, 224–226, 225*f*
    self-adhesive film for, 60, 61*f*
polycarbonate, 141–142
shearing tool, 230, 231*f*
tempered safety. *See* tempered safety glass
windshield, for commercial motor vehicles, 336
glass handsaw
    breaking tempered glass using, 60, 60*f*
    removal
        laminated safety glass, 230–231
        tempered safety glass, 230
glazing, 140–142
gloves, 53, 53*f*
goggles, 52, 53*f*
Golden Period, 35
Gorilla® glass, 141
grab hook, 66, 66*f*, 89
grain alcohol. *See* ethanol
graphene, 127
gravitational acceleration sensor (G-sensor), 158
grip hoist, 64, 65*f*
gross combined weight rating (GCWR), 338
gross vehicle weight rating (GVWR), 331
gross weight, 346
ground support unit, in logistics section, 32
groups, 31
GVWR. *See* gross vehicle weight rating

H

hacksaws, 62, 62*f*
Halligan bar, 58*f*, 60, 61
    for clean out tempered glass fragments, 228, 234
    to create artificial push point, 255
    separation of ball joints from housing, 140
    for tire deflation, 206, 209*f*
hammer-type punch, 59, 60*f*
hand protection, 53–54, 53*f*
hand tools, 57–58
    cleaning and inspecting, 62*t*
    cutting tools, 62–63, 62–63*f*
    leverage tools, 60–62, 61*f*
    lifting/pushing/pulling tools, 63–64, 64*f*
        come along and chain package, 64–66, 64–65*f*
        grip hoist, 64, 65*f*
    striking tools, 58–60, 58–60*f*
hazard analysis, 21–22
hazard control zones, 109, 170
hazardous materials, 114, 114*f*, 343–347
    classifications, 344
    personnel, 42, 348
    placards, 346–347, 347*f*
    shipping papers, 347
    transport vehicles for, 345–346, 345–346*f*
    United Nations/North American Hazardous Materials Code, 347
Hazardous Materials Regulations, 343–344
hazardous/potentially hazardous conditions, in status report, 28
hazards
    dogs/pets at crash scenes, 114–115
    electrical, 112–113, 112–113*f*
    fire, 111–112, 111*f*
    fuel runoff, 113
    fuel sources, 113
    hazardous materials, 114, 114*f*
    ignition sources, 113–114
    livestock/horses at crash, 115, 115*f*
    others, 114–115, 115*f*
head protection, 50–51, 51*f*
headphones, noise-reducing/canceling, 55, 55*f*
hearing protection, 54–56, 55–56*f*
heavier-gauge steel backer, 238, 239*f*
heavy vehicle, 8
HECMV. *See* hybrid-electric commercial motor vehicle
helicopter, 115–117, 115–117*f*
helmets, 50–51, 51*f*
hemorrhage, exsanguinating, 272, 272*f*
HEVs. *See* hybrid electric vehicles
high-pressure air-lift bags, 73, 73*f*
high-pressure flat-form air-lift bags, 73
high-strength steel (HSS), 129
Hindenburg airship tragedy of 1937, 180, 180*f*
hoist, 64, 64*f*
horizontal movement, 203
hot stick, 92
hot zone, 44, 110
HSS. *See* high-strength steel
hybrid-electric commercial motor vehicle (HECMV), 343
hybrid electric vehicles (HEVs), 188–193, 188*f*. *See also* hybrid vehicle
    drive systems, 190, 190*f*
    emergency procedures, 191–193, 192*f*
    extended range electric vehicle, 189, 190*f*
    full and mild designs, 188–189, 189*f*
    plug-in hybrid electric vehicle, 189
    voltage color coding, 189–190
hybrid inflators. *See* multistage inflators
hybrid-type inflator, 157
hybrid vehicle, 144
hydraulic combination tool, 81*f*, 84, 84*f*
hydraulic cutter, 81*f*, 83–84
hydraulic jacks, hand-operated, 88
hydraulic pumps, 80, 81*f*
hydraulic ram, 81*f*, 84, 84*f*
    B-post or door frame relocation with, 291–292
    cross-ramming operation, 297
hydraulic rescue tools, 80, 81–82*f*
    battery-powered, 84–85, 85*f*
    hydraulic combination tool, 84, 84*f*
    hydraulic cutter, 81*f*, 83–84
    hydraulic ram, 84, 84*f*
    hydraulic spreader, 81*f*, 82–83
hydraulic spreader, 81*f*, 82–83, 82*f*
    for making purchase point, 237, 237*f*
    raising roof using, 298*f*
hydraulic telescoping ram, 294, 295*f*
    raising roof using, 298*f*
hydrogen, 180–181, 180*f*
    emergency procedures, 182–183
    fuel-cell vehicles, 144, 183, 183*f*, 183*t*
        electrical design, 185
        emergency procedures, 186–188
        hydrogen storage system for, 185–186, 185*f*
        vehicle identification badge for, 186*f*, 187
    Hindenburg airship tragedy of 1937, 180, 180*f*
    identification label for, 182, 182*f*
    properties of, 180
    pump, 181, 182*f*
    storage tanks, 181–183

hydrogen storage system
    fuel-cell vehicle for, 185–186, 185f
        reinforced framing material, 185, 185f

I

IAP. *See* incident action plan
IC. *See* incident commander
ICE. *See* internal combustion engine
ICS. *See* incident command system
IDLH. *See* immediate dangerous to life and health
ignition sources, as hazards, 113–114
immediate danger to life and health (IDLH), 36
    stabilization of vehicle and, 216
immobilization devices, 93, 93f
impact beam, 135, 135f
impact sensors, 157
impaled objects. *See* penetrating objects
impingement, 291–295, 295f
incident action plan (IAP), 3, 9, 20, 26
    components of, 109t
    consolidated, 27
    formal, 7
    informal, 7
    information required to develop, 12
    sample, 109f
    scene size-up, 108–109
incident clock, 36
incident command system (ICS), 7, 20
    common terminology, 27
    consolidated IAPs, 27
    designated incident facilities, 27–28
    emergency and nonemergency events, 26, 26f
    integrated communications, 27
    jurisdictional authority, 26, 26f
    modular organization, 27
    organization, 28–32, 29f
        command staff, 29–30, 30f
        incident commander, 28–29
        sections, 30–32
        terminology, 32
    resource management, 28, 28f
    span of control, 27
    unity of command, 27
    victim reconnaissance, 28
incident commander (IC), 27, 28–29
incident response planning, 25–26
    jurisdictional authority, 26
    operational procedures, 26
    problem identification, 25
    resource identification and allocation, 25–26, 26f
incidents, 10
inclinometer sensor, 158
independent suspension system, 336–337, 337f
inflation system
    gas-generation system, 155–156, 156f
    hybrid-type inflator, 157
    stored compressed gas system, 155, 156f
inflator, 151, 152f, 155–157, 156f
informal incident action plans, 7
informal postincident analysis, 324, 324f
initiator, in air bag system, 152f, 154, 154f
inner survey, 105–108, 106f
inspection
    of eye protection, 53
    of hand tools, 62t
    of nondisposable hearing protection, 55–56
    of respiratory protection, 57
insulated wire cutters, 63
Insurance Institute for Highway Safety, 136
integrated motor assist (IMA) mild hybrid system, 188
intercity bus, 354, 355f
internal combustion engine (ICE), 144
Internet
    as research tools, 93
    for vehicle extrication, 12, 13f

J

J-hooks, 66
jacking the trunk, 284–287, 287f
jacks. *See specific jacks*
jaw thrust maneuver, 272, 272f
JumpSTART triage system, 276

K

KED. *See* Kendrick Extrication Device
Kendrick Extrication Device (KED), 93, 93f, 276–277, 277f
kinetic energy, 121, 122f
kingpin, 338
knee air bag, 153, 153f
knee bolster bag. *See* knee air bag
knives, 63, 63f

L

L-bracket, 255
labeling system, for supplemental restraint system, 162–163, 162f
ladder cribbing, 267
ladder frame, 130, 130f
laminated safety glass (LSG), 140–141, 141f
    markings for safety, 224, 225f
    removal, 231
        using glass handsaw, 231–232
        using reciprocating saw, 230, 234
landing gear, 339, 339f
landing zone
    establishing, 115–116, 116f
    safety, 116–117, 117f
large-tooth saws, 62
lateral (side-impact) collisions, 125, 125f
law enforcement personnel, 40–41, 41f
    crime scenes, 318
law of conservation of energy, 121
law of motion, 122
LEDs. *See* light-emitting diodes
Level 1 charging system, 189
Level 2 charging system, 189
Level 3 charging system, 189
leverage tools, 60–62, 61f
Lexan™, 141
Li-ion batteries, 74, 75f
liaison officer (LO), 30
lift axle, 339, 340f
lifting, 61f, 63–64, 64f
    come along and chain package, 64–66, 64–65f
    grip hoist, 64, 65f
    winches, 64, 64f
lifting tools
    electric, 77–78, 77f
    pneumatic

air-lift bags, 71–73, 71–74f
air shores, 70, 70f
light-emitting diodes (LEDs), 79
light towers, 78, 78f
lighting, electric, 78–79, 78f
liquefied natural gas (LNG), 173
liquefied petroleum gas (LPG), 177
   emergency procedures, 178–179
   identification label for, 178, 178f
   properties, 177–178
litters, 93
live axles, 339
live wires, 92, 92f
livestock at crash scene, 114–115, 115f
LNG. *See* liquefied natural gas
LO. *See* liaison officer
load limiting device, 159
load rating grades, 65f, 66
lockout/tagout systems, 110, 111f
logistics section, 31–32
long-term operations, 34–35
lorry, 331
low-pressure air-lift bags, 72, 73f
LPG. *See* liquefied petroleum gas
lye, 156

M

M85, 173
magnesium alloy, 128
magnetic bias sensor, 157
Makrolon®, 141
Manual on Uniform Traffic Control Devices (MUTCD), 38
manual regeneration, 360
marrying of vehicles, 89, 214–215, 216f
mask/face piece fit testing, 57
mass casualty incident (MCI), 28, 28f
master link, 66, 66f
MC-306/DOT 406 flammable liquid tanker, 344–345, 344–345f
MC-307/DOT 407 chemical hauler, 344–345, 345f
MC-312/DOT 412 corrosives tanker, 345, 345f
MC-331 pressure cargo tanker, 345, 345f
MC-338 cryogenic tanker, 345–346, 346f
MCI. *See* mass casualty incident
mechanical energy. *See* energy
mechanical jacks, 88, 88f
mechanism of injury (MOI), 122, 124
medevac. *See* medical evacuation
medical care, initial, 271–276, 271–272f
   airway, 272, 272f
   breathing, 273, 273t
   circulation, 274, 274f
   compartment syndrome, 275
   disability, 274
   expose, 274–275
   exsanguinating hemorrhage, 272, 272f
   triage, 275–276, 275t, 276f
medical evacuation, 115
medical gloves, 54
medical unit, in logistics section, 32
medium-pressure air-lift bags, 72–73, 73f
metal, 127
metal chisels, 63
metal collapsible step chocks, 87
metal-cutting circular saw, 75, 75f

methanol, 173
Mil-spec AFFF, 91
mild hybrid vehicle, 188
mineral base oil, 82, 82f
MOI. *See* mechanism of injury
motor vehicle collisions
   classifications
      front impact collisions, 124–125
      lateral (side-impact) collisions, 125, 125f
      rear-end collisions, 125, 125f
      rollovers, 125–126, 126f
      rotational collisions, 126
   events in, 122–123
      occupant impact with vehicle, 123–124, 123f
      occupant organs impact solid structures of body, 124, 124f
      vehicle impact with object, 123, 123f
   number of, 3, 3f
MS steel, 130
multi-cell high-pressure air-lift bags, 73, 73f
multi-gas meters, 170, 172f
multiple gas cylinders, 155, 156f
multistage inflators, 155

N

Nader pin/bolt, 4, 135, 135f
National Fire Protection Association (NFPA) standards
   1001, for fire fighter professional qualifications, 4
   1006, for technical rescue personnel professional qualifications, 5–7, 14–15
   and NFPA 1670, compliance with, 10, 12
   1500, fire department occupational safety, health, and wellness program, 50
   1670, operations and training for technical search and rescue incidents, 7–10, 14–15
      compliance with NFPA 1006 and, 10, 12
      evaluation, 8–9
      operational levels, 8
      requirements, 9–10
      safety procedures, 9
      training requirements, 8–9
   1951, protective ensembles for technical rescue incidents, 50
   Alternative-Fuel Vehicles Safety Training Program Emergency Field Guide, 12, 13f
   Manual on Uniform Traffic Control Devices, 38
National Highway Traffic Safety Administration (NHTSA), 3, 150, 355–356
National Incident Management System (NIMS), 7, 26, 36
National Institute of Safety and Health (NIOSH) Sound Level Meter app, 56, 56f
natural gas, 173
   compressed, 174, 174f, 181
   emergency procedures, 175–177, 181
   identification label for, 175, 175f
   liquefied, 177–179, 178f
   storage pressure, 174, 174f
NAVRA. *See* North American Vehicle Rescue Association
neighborhood electric vehicle (NEV), 193, 193f
NEV. *See* neighborhood electric vehicle
NHTSA. *See* National Highway Traffic Safety Administration
Nimitz Freeway, 42, 42f
NIMS. *See* National Incident Management System
Nissan LEAF, 193–194, 193f

no-entry zone, 45, 110
Noise Reduction Rating (NRR), 55
nonferrous metals, 76
North American Vehicle Rescue Association (NAVRA), 13
NRR. *See* Noise Reduction Rating

O

O-ring, 66, 66*f*
oblong ring. *See* O-ring
occupant
    classification system, 158
    ejection from vehicle, 125, 126*f*
    impact with vehicle, 123–124, 123*f*
    organs impact solid structures of body, 124, 124*f*
    weight sensor, 158
Occupational Safety and Health Administration (OSHA)
    hearing protection, 55
    respiratory protection devices, 56
online resources, for vehicle extrication, 12, 13*f*
operational procedures, in incident response planning, 26
operational zones. *See* scene safety zones
operations effectiveness assessment, in status report, 28–29
operations level, 7–8
    requirements of, 10
operations section, 30–31
operations section chief, 30
organizational analysis, 22–23, 23*f*
OSHA. *See* Occupational Safety and Health Administration
outer survey, 105, 108
outside pedestrian protection system, 154
override collision, 124
oxyacetylene torch, 80
oxygen/propane torch, 80

P

package tray. *See* rear deck/shelf
Packexe SMASH®, 60, 61*f*, 225*f*
parallel drive system, 190
passenger-side air bag, 156, 163
passenger vehicle, 142
passive hearing protectors, 55
passive regeneration, 360
passive restraint device, 150–151
pedal displacement and removal, 310, 311–312, 312*f*
peer support groups, 323–324
PEM. *See* polymer exchange membrane
penetrating objects, 298–300
personal protective equipment (PPE), 36
    body protection, 51–52, 52*f*
    decontamination, 7, 57, 319–321
    eye and face protection, 52–53, 53*f*
    foot protection, 54, 54*f*
    hand protection, 53–54, 53*f*
    head protection, 50–51, 51*f*
    hearing protection, 54–56, 55–56*f*
    maintenance of, 57
    requirements, 50
    respiratory protection
        air-filtering face piece respirators, 56
        fit testing, 57
        self-contained breathing apparatus, 57, 57*f*
        supplied air respirator, 57
personnel
    accountability system, 32, 34*f*

law enforcement personnel, 40–41, 41*f*
rehabilitation, 102
resources, 40
    additional personnel resources, 42, 42*f*
    EMS personnel, 41–42, 42*f*
    hazardous materials personnel, 42
    law enforcement personnel, 40–41, 41*f*
securing, upon termination of incident
    critical incident stress, 321, 323
    critical incident stress management, 323, 323*f*
    documentation and record management, 324–325
    peer support groups, 323–324
    postincident analysis, 324, 324*f*
    stress, 321
personnel resources, 40
    EMS personnel, 41–42, 42*f*
    hazardous materials personnel, 42
    law enforcement personnel, 40–41, 41*f*
Petrogen torches, 80
PHEVs. *See* plug-in hybrid electric vehicles
phosphate ester, 82
physical reactions, 323
PIA. *See* postincident analysis
piano-type hinge, 340, 340*f*
pick-head axe, 62, 62*f*
PIO. *See* public information officer
piston struts, 139–140, 140*f*
    hydraulic/gas-filled, 261, 261*f*
    in lifting vehicle's hood, 260, 261*f*
pitch movement, 203
placards, 346–347, 347*f*
planning section, 31
plasma cutter, 80
plastic molding, removing, 266, 266*f*
plug-in hybrid electric vehicles (PHEVs), 188, 189
plunger center punch, 59, 60*f*
pneumatic chisels, 67, 69, 69*f*
    types of, 69
    usage
        for door removal on hinge side, 308–310
        for roof removal, 301, 301*f*, 302–303
pneumatic cut-off tool, 67, 67*f*
pneumatic tools, 66–73, 67*f*
    cutting
        pneumatic chisels, 67, 69–70, 69*f*
        pneumatic cut-off tool, 67, 67*f*
    lifting
        air-lift bags, 71–73, 71–74*f*
        air shores, 70, 70*f*
    rotating, 70, 70*f*
polycarbonate, 141–142
    windows, 235
polymer exchange membrane (PEM), 183
portable lights, 78, 78*f*
portable propane cylinder, hidden dangers, 216, 216*f*
post-traumatic stress disorder (PTSD), 321
postincident analysis (PIA), 324, 324*f*
potential energy, 121, 122*f*
pounds per square inch (psi), 144
power detection equipment, 92, 92*f*
Power Hawk rescue tool system, 85, 85*f*
PPE. *See* personal protective equipment
PRD. *See* pressure release device
preincident assignments, 37–38, 37*f*

pressure release device (PRD), 170
pretensioning seat belt system, 138, 159, 159f, 161
primary access (Plan A), 107, 223
problem identification, in incident response planning, 25
procurement unit, finance/administration section, 32
PRO/pak system, 91, 91f
propane, 177–178. *See also* liquefied petroleum gas
propane tanks, 393, 393f
propellant, 155–157, 156f
propulsion systems, vehicles, 144
protective ensemble, 50
public information officer (PIO), 29
pulling tools, 58f, 63–64, 64f
    come along and chain package, 64–66, 64–65f
    electric, 77–78, 77f
    grip hoist, 64, 65f
    winches, 64, 64f
purchase point, 142
    hydraulic spreader for making, 237, 237f
pushing tools, 58f, 63–64, 64f
    come along and chain package, 64–66, 64–65f
    grip hoist, 64, 65f
    winches, 64, 64f

Q
qualification, 5

R
R-hook, 66
radio frequency identification (RFID), 34
ratchet lever jacks, 88, 88f
    hand-operated, 64, 64f
ratchet straps, 89, 89f
    for vehicle stabilization, 209, 214, 215f
rear deck/shelf, 139
rear-end collisions, 125, 125f
rear posts, 139, 139f
rear seat deployment air bag system, 154
reciprocating saw
    blades, 75
    electric, 75, 75f
    laminated safety glass removal, 230, 235, 235f
    roof removal using, 301, 304, 304f, 305–306
record management, termination of incident, 324–325
recovery operations, 274
reinforcement plates, 238, 239f
Rescue 42 TeleCrib® Junior, 87f
rescue operations, 274
    elements of, 103, 103t
research tools, 93
resource
    challenge events, 13–14, 13f
    current status, in status report, 29
    emergency field guide, 12–13, 13f
    equipment, 102–103, 102f
    identification and allocation, in incident response planning, 25–26, 26f
    incident command system management, 28, 28f
    online resources, 12, 13f
    personnel, 40
        additional personnel resources, 42, 42f
        EMS personnel, 41–42, 42f
        hazardous materials personnel, 42
        law enforcement personnel, 40–41, 41f

scenario-based training, 14–15, 14f
specialists, 12
respiratory protection
    air-filtering face piece respirators, 56
    fit testing, 57
    self-contained breathing apparatus, 56, 57f
    supplied air respirator, 57
response analysis, level of, 24
response planning (preincident planning), 25
RFID. *See* radio frequency identification
risk assessment, 21
risk–benefit analysis, 23–24, 23f
rocker panel, 133, 133f
Rolamite sensor, 157
roll movement, 203
rollover protection system (ROPS), 158, 158f, 161–162
rollovers, 125–126, 126f
roof
    access
        school bus, 373, 376–377
        using hydraulic rescue tools, 235, 237, 237f
    hatches, emergency, 359, 359f
    lift, 295, 298, 298f
    removal, 247, 249–252, 252f, 307–308
        for upright vehicle, 252–254
        using air chisel, 301, 301f, 302–303
        using reciprocating saw, 301, 304f, 305–306
        vehicle on its side, 304, 306–307
    strength requirements, 212
roof posts/pillars, 136
    A-posts/pillars, 136, 136f
    B-posts, 138, 138–139f
    C-post, 138–139, 139f
    piston struts, 139–140, 140f
ROPS. *See* rollover protection system
rotary saws, 79
rotary wing aircraft, 115, 115f
rotating tools, pneumatic, 70, 70f
rotational collisions, 126
rub rails, 358

S
saddle tanks, 342, 343f
safety
    alternative-fuel vehicles, 170, 172f
    dealing with electricity, 112, 112f
    landing zone, 116–117, 117f
    programs and guidelines for, 35
    site operations, 101–102, 101f
        communication and documentation, 103
        equipment resources, 102–103, 102f
        personnel rehabilitation, 102
safety belts. *See* seat belt
"safety cage", 127
safety glasses, 53
safety officer (SO), 29–30, 30f
safing sensor, 157
SAR/SABA. *See* supplied air respirator/breathing apparatus
SCBA. *See* self-contained breathing apparatus
scenario-based training, as extrication resource, 14–15, 14f
scene of incident
    communication and documentation, 103
    securing, upon termination of incident, 318–319, 319f

scene safety zones, 44–45, 109–110, 110–111f
scene size-up, 42–43, 103
    incident action plan, 108–109, 109f, 109t
    inner survey, 105–108, 106f
    outer survey, 105, 108
    report, 44, 105, 105t
    school bus, stabilization, 361
school buses, 354, 354f, 355–357
    access, 367, 369
        air-lift bag operation, 388–389
        front door, 379, 382, 382f, 383–384
        front window, 369–371
        lifting operations, 382, 385–387, 390–392
        rear door, 376, 378–379
        roof, 373, 376–377
        seat removal, 370, 372–373
        sidewall, 373–375
        steering wheel assembly, 390
    alternative-fuel, 393–394, 393f
        emergency procedures for hybrid bus, 394–395
    anatomy, 357–360, 358–360f
    classifications, 356–357
    lifting off of underride, 390–392
    site operations
        planning, 362
        priorities and objectives, 360–361
        stabilization, 361–369
scissor/screw jack, 88, 89f
scoop stretcher, 93
seat belt, 158–159
    as active restraint device, 150
    air bag, 153–154
    automatic system, 138
    cutters, 63
    heavy-gauge steel slide tracks for, 139f
    nonretractable, 159
    pretensioner system, 138
    pretensioning system, 153, 159, 159f, 161
    retractable, 159
    sensor, 158
    standard harness, 138
    types of, 159
seat cushion air bag, 154
seat position sensor, 158
seat removal
    front seat-back relocation, 290
    front seat-back removal, 287, 289
    in school buses, 370, 372–373
secondary access (Plan B), 107, 223
self-adhesive film, for glass management, 60, 61f
self-contained breathing apparatus (SCBA), 36, 56, 57f
semi-tractor. See semi-truck
semi-truck, 333, 333f
semi-tractor trailer (semi-trailer), 333, 333f
sensors, in air bag system, 157–158, 157f. See also specific types
series drive system, 190
series-operated propulsion system, 394
service air line, 341, 341f
service brake, 341
Shark-X, 89f
sheet metal snips, 63
shims, 86, 86f
shoring, 70, 70f
side-impact air bag, 153, 153f, 157

side-impact collisions
    body structure of vehicle after, 245, 245f
    vehicle on left suffered, 283–284, 284f
side-out technique, 245–249, 245–246f, 247–249
side removal, with vehicle upside down or resting on roof, 310
side window exits, for school bus, 359
sidewall access, in school buses, 373–375
sidewinder jack, 88, 89f
signaling devices, 91, 92f
single resource, 32
single-tiered system, 41
site operations, 101f
    air medical operations, 115f
        landing zone, establishing, 115–116, 116f
        landing zone safety, 116–117, 117f
    commercial trucks, 347–348
    entrapment classifications, 105, 105t
    hazards
        electrical, 112–113, 112–113f
        fire, 111–112, 111f
        fuel runoff, 113
        fuel sources, 113
        hazardous materials, 114, 114f
        ignition sources, 113–114
        others, 114–115, 115f
    planning, 362
    priorities and objectives, 360–361
    rescue operation, elements of, 103, 103t
    safety, 101–102
        communication and documentation, 103
        equipment resources, 102–103, 102f
        personnel rehabilitation, 102
    scene safety zones, 109–110, 110–111f
    scene size-up, 103
        incident action plan, 108–109, 109f, 109t
        inner survey, 105–108, 106f
        outer survey, 105, 108
        report, 105, 105t
    stabilization, 361–369
sleeper, 336
slide cribbing, 268
slide hook, 66, 66f
smart air bag systems, 151
smart key, 171
SO. See safety officer
sodium azide, 156
SOGs. See standard operating guidelines
SOPs. See standard operating procedures
space frame construction, 131, 131f
specialists
    as extrication resource, 12
    technical, 31
spiral wound, 127
spring-back–type punch, 59, 60f
spring-loaded center punch, 59, 227, 228, 228f
squib, 154, 154f
SRS. See supplemental restraint system
stabilization, 200–201, 200–201f
    electrical system, isolating/eliminating, 216–218, 218f
    mitigating electrical hazards, 218, 218f
stabilization of vehicle
    cribbing
        wood box, 202–203, 203f
        wood characteristics, 202

hidden dangers and energy sources, 216–218, 216–217f
school buses, 361–369
    in normal position, 363–364
    resting on roof, 366–367
    resting on side, 365
    on top of another vehicle, 368–369
vehicle positioning. *See* vehicle positioning for stabilization
stabilization tools, 85
    cribbing, 86–87, 86f
    jacks, 88–89, 88–89f
    ratchet strap, 89, 89f
    struts, 87–88, 87–88f
staging area manager, 31
standard, 4
standard operating procedures (SOPs), 6, 7, 10, 24–25, 25f
standard seat belt harness, 138
START triage, 276
start/stop mild hybrid system, 188
static risk–benefit analysis, 23
stationary punch, 59
steam methane reforming, 181
steel
    brackets, 132, 133f
    strength measurements, 129
    types of. *See specific types*
    in vehicle designs, 128–130
steer axle. *See* dead axle
steering wheel assembly relocation, 65, 266–270, 390
    utilizing 2/4-ton–rated come along, 267–269
    utilizing First Responder Jack, 269–270
step chock, 86, 86f, 204, 205f
storage tanks, hydrogen, 181–183
stored compressed gas system, 155, 155f
strengths, weaknesses, opportunities, and threats (SWOT) analysis, 362
stress. *See also specific stresses*
    immediate recognition and treatment of, 321, 321f
stretchers, 93
strike team, 32
striking tools, 58–60, 58–60f
stringers, 358
strut tower, 132
struts, 70, 87
Super-X Strut®, 88f, 150
supplemental restraint system (SRS), 87–88, 87–88f
    air bags. *See* air bags
    rollover protection system, 158, 158f, 161–162
    seat belt. *See* seat belt
supplied air respirator/breathing apparatus (SAR/SABA), 57
supply unit, in logistics section, 32
suppression system, 151–152
suspension, for commercial motor vehicle, 336–338, 337–338f
suspension system, 204
"swing bar", 134
SWOT analysis. *See* strengths, weaknesses, opportunities, and threats (SWOT) analysis

T
T-blade, 69
T-bone collisions. *See* lateral (side-impact) collisions
T-hook, 66
tactical priorities, in status report, 28
task force, 32
technical rescue, 4

technical rescuer, 4
    large commercial vehicle collision, 332, 332f
    positioning, for stabilizing vehicle resting on its side, 210, 210f
    safety rules, 227, 228f
    wearing personal protective equipment, 232, 232f
technical search and rescue incidents, 7
technical specialists, 31
technician level, 7, 8
    requirements of, 10
telescoping ram, 251f
    hydraulic, 294, 295f
temperature relief device (TRD), 185
tempered safety glass (TSG), 141
    breaking
        using glass handsaw, 60, 60f, 230
        using spring-loaded center punch, 59, 60f, 228–229
    markings for safety, 224, 225f
    with tinting/safety film, 228, 228f
tension buttress stabilization, 88, 88f
tepee, or tenting, effect, 238f, 260
TERC. *See* Transportation Emergency Response Committee
termination of incident, 318–321
    securing equipment, 319–321, 319f
    securing personnel, 321, 321f
        critical incident stress, 321, 323
        critical incident stress management, 323, 323f
        documentation and record management, 324–325
        peer support groups, 323–324
        postincident analysis, 324, 324f
        stress, 321
    securing the scene, 318–319, 319f
    steps in, 325–326
Tesla Semi, 343
thermal imaging camera (TIC), 92, 92f, 183
three-point harness system. *See* standard seat belt harness
three-tiered system, 41
TIC. *See* thermal imaging camera
tilt cab. *See* cab over engine (COE)
time management, 35–36
time unit, finance/administration section, 32
tire deflation, 206, 206f, 208, 208f
TIRFOR. *See* grip hoist
tools. *See also specific tools*
    categories, 50
    research, 93
    slippage, 295
    staging of, 90, 90f
torches, 80
tower ladder fire apparatus, 331f
Towing and Recovery Association of America (TRAA), 349
TPI rating, 76, 76f
TRAA. *See* Towing and Recovery Association of America
traffic, 38–40
traffic cones, 38, 39f, 112
traffic incident management, 38
training, requirements, 8–9
transit bus, 354, 355f
"transit-style" rear/front engine school bus. *See* Type D school bus
Transportation Emergency Response Committee (TERC), 13
traumatic injury, 122
TRD. *See* temperature relief device
triage, 108
    categories, 275–276, 275t, 276f
    tags, 276f

triangle crosstie cribbing configuration, 203, 203f
trucks
  chassis, 336, 337f
  commercial. *See* commercial motor vehicles
TSG. *See* tempered safety glass
tube trailers, 346, 346f
tunneling, 212, 213, 283–284, 283f, 284f
  hybrid electric vehicles, 192
  through the trunk, 284–286
turnout gear, 51
two-piece full/solid hinges, 340, 340f
two-tiered system, 41
Type A school bus, 356, 356f
Type B school bus, 356, 356f
Type C school bus, 356, 356f, 390
  disabling hybrid system on, 395
Type D school bus, 356–357, 357f
  collision with pickup truck, 366, 367f
  disabling hybrid system on, 395

U

U-shaped striker plate latch pin, 135, 135f
ultimate tensile strength (UTS), 129
underride collision, 124
unibody construction, 130–131, 130–131f
unified command, 26
United Nations/North American Hazardous Materials Code, 347
upper rails, 132, 132f
USAR helmet, 50, 51f
UTS. *See* ultimate tensile strength

V

vehicle identification badge, 172, 172f
  biodiesel, 180, 180f
  flex fuel, 173, 173f
  hybrid electric vehicles, 191, 192f
  hydrogen fuel-cell vehicle, 186f, 187
vehicle identification number (VIN), 142–144
vehicle positioning for stabilization, 3–4f, 4, 203
  in normal position, 203, 204f
    balanced platform, creating, 204
    cribbing placement for, 204, 205f
    tire deflation, 206, 206f, 208, 208f
  with one vehicle on another, 214–216, 214f, 216f
    marrying method, 214–215, 216f
    prevention of sliding, 216, 216f
  resting on its side, 209, 209f, 212
    buttress stabilization struts for, 209, 210f
    center of mass for, 209
    creating A-frame configuration for, 210
    cribbing placement for, 210, 210f
    technical rescuer position in, 210, 210f
  upside down or resting on its roof, 212–213, 212f
    A-frame configuration for, 212
    cribbing placement for, 212
vehicle rescue and extrication
  continuous improvement, 16
  resources
    challenge events, 13–14, 13f
    emergency field guide, 12–13, 13f
    online resources, 12, 13f
    scenario-based training, 14–15, 14f
    specialists, 12
  stabilization of scene. *See* site operations
  stabilization of vehicle. *See* stabilization of vehicle
  stabilization of victim. *See* access
  standards and qualifications. *See also* National Fire Protection Association (NFPA) standards
vehicle rescue incident awareness, 20–21
  incident command system. *See* incident command system
  incident response planning
    operational procedures, 26
    problem identification, 25
    resource identification and allocation, 25–26, 26f
  inner and outer surveys, 44
  level of service
    hazard analysis, 21–22
    level of response analysis, 24
    organizational analysis, 22–23, 23f
    risk assessment, 21
    risk–benefit analysis, 23–24, 23f
  long-term operations, 34–35
  responding to scene
    crowd control, 40, 40f
    dispatch information, 36–37
    personal protective equipment, 36
    personnel resources, 40–42
    preincident assignments, 37–38, 37f
    traffic, 38–40
  safety, 35
  scene safety zones, 44–45
  scene size-up, 42–43
    report, 44
  standard operating procedures, 24–25, 25f
  time management, 35–36
  tracking systems
    equipment inventory and, 34, 34f
    personnel accountability, 32, 34f
vehicle stabilization. *See* stabilization of vehicle
vehicles. *See also specific types*
  anatomy and composition
    electricity, 126–127
    metal, carbon, and composites, 127–130, 128–129f
  classifications, 142–144, 143t
  federal safety standards and regulations, 140
  frame systems
    body-over-frame construction, 130, 130f
    space frame construction, 131, 131f
    unibody construction, 130–131, 130–131f
  glass and glazing
    ballistic glass, 142
    Gorilla® glass, 141
    laminated safety glass, 140–141, 141f
    polycarbonate, 141–142
    tempered safety glass, 141
  impact with object, 123, 123f
  occupant impact with, 123–124, 123f
  propulsion systems, 144
    conventional vehicles, 144
    electric-powered vehicles, 144
    hybrid electric vehicles, 144
    hydrogen fuel cell vehicles, 144
  structural components, 132–133, 132–133f
    doors, 133–136, 134–136f
    rocker panel, 133, 133f
    roof posts, 136–140, 136f, 136–140f
vertical movement, 203
vertical spread, 237–239, 238–239f, 239–244

victim(s)
　　access, 367, 369–390
　　equipment, packaging and removal, 93, 93f
　　extricating from passenger car, 277–278
　　gaining access to. *See* access
　　packaging and removal, 276–278, 277f
　　reconnaissance, 28
　　removal under vehicle, 313–314
　　removing vehicle from, 249–254
　　stabilization, 361
　　transport, 277
VIN. *See* vehicle identification number
visual devices, 92
void space filling, for stabilization, with normally positioned vehicle, 204, 205f
voltage color coding, 189–190

W

warm zone, 44, 110
wedge insertion, into cribbing, 204, 205f, 206
wedges, 86, 86f
wet cell, 127
wheel well crush technique, 244
white wave, 110
whizzer saws. *See* cut-off tool, pneumatic
winches, 64, 64f
　　electric, 77–78, 77f
windows. *See also* glass
　　access through, 224–225, 224–225f
　　backboard slide technique, 226–227
　　breaking with center punch, 59, 60f
　　front access on school buses, 369–371
　　polycarbonate, removal of, 235
　　spidering, 140–141
　　using glass handsaw for glass removal, 60, 60f
windshield
　　entering through, 224
　　fractured, 156, 156f
　　glass, for commercial motor vehicles, 336
　　removal
　　　　from partially ejected victim, 235
　　　　using glass handsaw, 230–231
　　　　using reciprocating saw, 232, 235, 235f
WLL. *See* working load limit
wood
　　for cribbing, 203
　　cribbing, 87
　　struts, 86
wood alcohol. *See* methanol
wood box configuration, for cribbing, 203, 203f
work, 121
　　negative, 122
working environment, safe, 14, 14f
working load limit (WLL), 65, 65f
World Rescue Challenge, 14
World Rescue Organization (WRO), 14
WRO. *See* World Rescue Organization

Y

yaw movement, 203
yield strength, 129